THE
T CELL
RECEPTOR
FactsBook

Other books in the FactsBook Series:

Robin Callard and Andy Gearing
The Cytokine FactsBook

Steve Watson and Steve Arkinstall
The G-Protein Linked Receptor FactsBook

Shirley Ayad, Ray Boot-Handford, Martin J. Humphries, Karl E. Kadler
and C. Adrian Shuttleworth
The Extracellular Matrix FactsBook, 2nd edn

Grahame Hardie and Steven Hanks
The Protein Kinase FactsBook
The Protein Kinase FactsBook CD-Rom

Edward C. Conley
The Ion Channel FactsBook
I: Extracellular Ligand-Gated Channels

Edward C. Conley
The Ion Channel FactsBook
II: Intracellular Ligand-Gated Channels

Edward C. Conley and William J. Brammar
The Ion Channel FactsBook
IV: Voltage-Gated Channels

Kris Vaddi, Margaret Keller and Robert Newton
The Chemokine FactsBook

Marion E. Reid and Christine Lomas-Francis
The Blood Group Antigen FactsBook

A. Neil Barclay, Marion H. Brown, S.K. Alex Law, Andrew J. McKnight,
Michael G. Tomlinson and P. Anton van der Merwe
The Leucocyte Antigen FactsBook, 2nd edn

Robin Hesketh
The Oncogene and Tumour Suppressor Gene FactsBook, 2nd edn

Jeffrey K. Griffith and Clare E. Sansom
The Transporter FactsBook

Tak W. Mak, Josef Penninger, John Rader, Janet Rossant
and Mary Saunders
The Gene Knockout FactsBook

Bernard J. Morley and Mark J. Walport
The Complement FactsBook

Steven G.E. Marsh, Peter Parham and Linda Barber
The HLA FactsBook

Hans G. Drexler
The Leukemia-Lymphoma Cell Line FactsBook

Clare M. Isacke and Michael A. Horton
The Adhesion Molecule FactsBook, 2nd edn

Marie-Paule Lefranc and Gérard Lefranc
The Immunoglobulin FactsBook

THE T CELL RECEPTOR
FactsBook

Marie-Paule Lefranc
Gérard Lefranc

IMGT, the international ImMunoGeneTics database
Laboratoire d'ImmunoGénétique Moléculaire
Université Montpellier II,
Institut de Génétique Humaine CNRS,
Montpellier, France

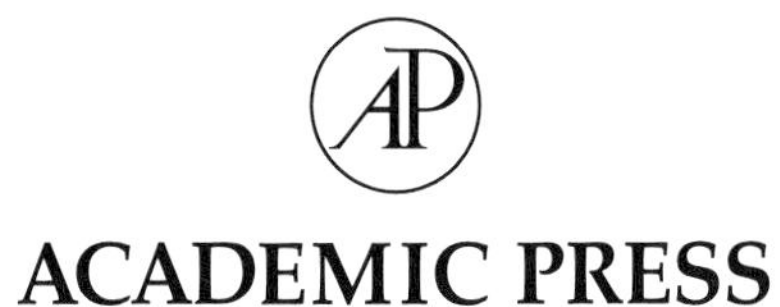

ACADEMIC PRESS

A Harcourt Science and Technology Company

San Diego San Francisco New York Boston
London Sydney Tokyo

Academic Press
A Harcourt Science and Technology Company
Harcourt Place, 32 Jamestown Road, London NW1 7BY, UK
http://www.academicpress.com

Academic Press
A Harcourt Science and Technology Company
525 B Street, Suite 1900, San Diego, California 92101-4495, USA
http://www.academicpress.com

ISBN 0-12-441352-8

Library of Congress Catalog Number: 2001 091534

A catalogue record for this book is available from the British Library

Typeset by Mackreth Media Services, Hemel Hempstead, UK
Printed in Great Britain by St Edmundsbury Press Limited,
Bury St Edmunds, Suffolk

01 02 03 04 05 SE 9 8 7 6 5 4 3 2 1

Contents

Section III THE HUMAN T CELL RECEPTOR TRB GENES

Section IV THE HUMAN T CELL RECEPTOR TRG GENES

Section V THE HUMAN T CELL RECEPTOR TRD GENES

Preface

The authors wish to acknowledge the IMGT team that contributed to the completion of this book. In particular, we would like to thank Nathalie Bosc, Valérie Contet, Géraldine Folch, Christèle Jean, and Dominique Scaviner, the motivated and enthusiastic IMGT annotators for their invaluable contribution and expertise. Sandrine Béranger, Chantal Ginestoux, Chrystel Godiris, and Manuel Ruiz helped with figures for the introductory chapters. We are very grateful to Gérard Mennessier for the IMGT/Collier de Perles tool development, and to Véronique Giudicelli and Denys Chaume for the bioinformatics and computer management of IMGT, the international ImMunoGeneTics database (http://imgt.cines.fr:).

The authors wish to acknowledge the funding by the Ministère de l'Education Nationale, the Ministère de la Recherche, the Université Montpellier II, the CNRS, the European Community, and the Région Languedoc-Roussillon.

The authors hope that there are a minimum of omissions and inaccuracies and that these can be rectified in later editions. We would appreciate if such points were forwarded to the Editor, The T Cell Receptor FactsBook, Academic Press Ltd, Harcourt Place, 32 Jamestown Road, London NW1 7BY, UK.

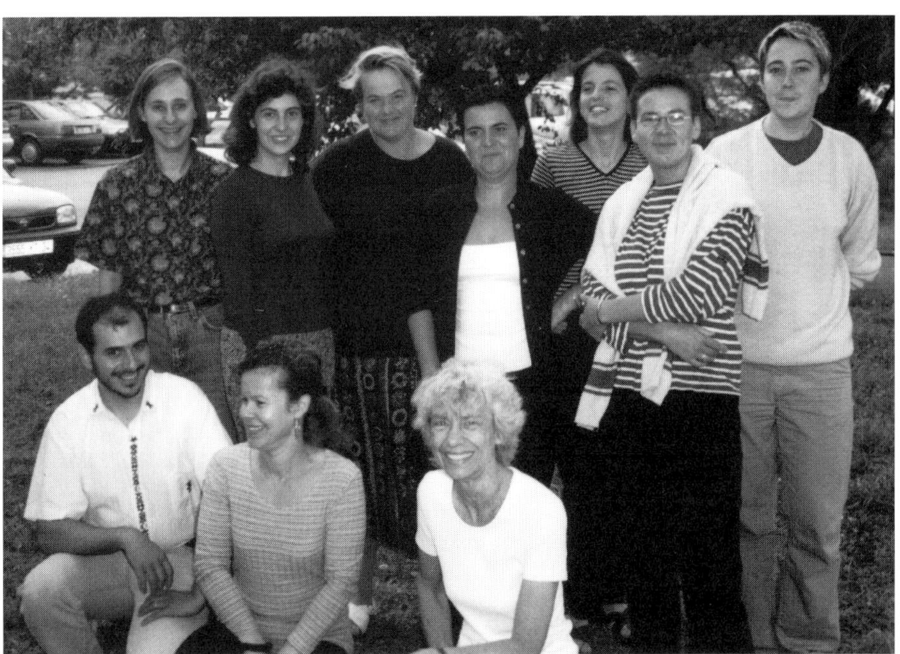

Back row from left: *Sandrine Béranger, Christèle Jean, Valérie Contet, Géraldine Folch, Chantal Ginestoux, Dominique Scaviner, Nathalie Bosc*
Front row from left: *Manuel Ruiz, Chrystel Godiris,* **Marie-Paule Lefranc.**

Abbreviations

a or A	Adenine (purine base of DNA and RNA)
c or C	Cytosine (pyrimidine base of DNA and RNA)
C	Constant
CDR	Complementarity Determining Region
CH	Immunoglobulin heavy constant exon or domain
CNRS	Centre National de la Recherche Scientifique
D	Diversity
DDBJ	DNA DataBank of Japan
E	Enhancer
EMBL	European Molecular Biology Laboratory Nucleotide Sequence Database
ER	Endoplasmic reticulum
FR	Framework
g or G	Guanine (purine base of DNA and RNA)
GDB	Genome Database
GenBank	US Nucleotide Sequence Database
HUGO	HUman Genome Organization
Ig	Immunoglobulin
IG	Immunoglobulin gene
IMGT	The international ImMunoGeneTics database
J	Joining
kb	Kilobase
kDa	Kilodalton
LIGM-DB	Laboratoire d'ImmunoGénétique Moléculaire DataBase (Immunoglobulin and T cell receptor database), part of IMGT
MHC	Major Histocompatibility Complex
nt	Nucleotide
OMIM	Online Mendelian Inheritance in Man (MIM)
ORF	Open Reading Frame
pMHC	peptide-MHC complex
RS	Recombination signal
SRS	Sequence Retrieval System, a database query system developed by EMBL
t or T	Thymine (pyrimidine base of DNA)
TcR	T cell Receptor
TR	T cell Receptor gene
V	Variable

Links to database or molecular biology server web sites quoted in this book are available from IMGT Bloc-notes, http://imgt.cines.fr

Label name	Definition
1st–CYS	codon (3 nucleotides) for cysteine in conserved position in FR1-IMGT
2nd–CYS	codon (3 nucleotides) for cysteine in conserved position in FR3-IMGT
3'D-HEPTAMER	7-nucleotide recombination site like CACAGTG, part of a 3'D-RS
3'D-NONAMER	9-nucleotide recombination site like ACAAAAACC, part of a 3'D-RS
3'D-RS	recombination signal including the 3'D-HEPTAMER, 3'D-SPACER, and 3'D-NONAMER in 3' of the D-REGION of a D-GENE
3'UTR	3' untranslated sequence, EMBL feature Key signification
5'D-HEPTAMER	7-nucleotide recombination site like CACTGTG, part of a 5'D-RS
5'D-NONAMER	9-nucleotide recombination site like GGTTTTTGT, part of a 5'D-RS
5'D-RS	recombination signal including the 5'D-NONAMER, 5'D-SPACER and 5'D-HEPTAMER in 5' of the D-REGION of a D-GENE or in 5' of the D-REGION of D-J-GENE
5'UTR	5' untranslated sequence, EMBL feature Key signification
ACCEPTOR-SPLICE	splicing site in 5' of coding region (nagnn), with splicing occurring after g
C-GENE	genomic DNA including C-REGION (and INTRONs if present) with 5'UTR and 3'UTR
C-REGION	coding region of C-GENE or corresponding region in cDNA
CDR1-IMGT	first complementarity determining region according to the IMGT unique numbering
CDR2-IMGT	second complementarity determining region according to the IMGT unique numbering
CDR3-IMGT	third complementarity determining region according to the IMGT unique numbering
CONSERVED-TRP	codon (3 nucleotides) for tryptophan in conserved position in FR2-IMGT
D-J-C-CLUSTER	genomic DNA in germline configuration including at least one D-GENE, one J-GENE and one C-GENE
D-REGION	coding region of D-SEGMENT (plus 1 or 2 nucleotide(s) after the 5'D-HEPTAMER and/or before the 3'D-HEPTAMER, if present), or corresponding region in cDNA
D-GENE	germline genomic DNA including D-REGION with 5'UTR and 3'UTR
DELETION	point out a deletion compared to other sequences
DONOR-SPLICE	splicing site in 3' of coding region (ngt), with splicing occurring before g

Label name	Definition
EX1	first exon of TR C-GENE, or corresponding region in cDNA
EX2	second exon of TR C-GENE, or corresponding region in cDNA
EX2R	duplicated exon 2 of human TRG C-GENE, or corresponding region in cDNA
EX2T	triplicated exon 2 of human TRG C-GENE, or corresponding region in cDNA
EX3	third exon of TR C-GENE, or corresponding region in cDNA
EX4	fourth exon of TR C-GENE, or corresponding region in cDNA
FR1-IMGT	first framework according to the IMGT unique numbering
FR2-IMGT	second framework according to the IMGT unique numbering
FR3-IMGT	third framework according to the IMGT unique numbering
INSERTION	point out an insertion of one or more nucleotide compared with old release of the sequence or with a similar sequence
INT–DONOR–SPLICE	alternative donor splice site located in a coding region
J-C-CLUSTER	genomic DNA in germline configuration including at least one J-GENE and one C-GENE
J-HEPTAMER	7-nucleotide recombination site, like CACAGTG, part of a J-RS
J-NONAMER	9-nucleotide recombination site, like GGTTTTTGT, part of a J-RS
J-REGION	coding region of J-GENE (plus 1 or 2 nucleotide(s) after J-HEPTAMER, if present) or corresponding region in cDNA
J-RS	recombination signal including J-HEPTAMER, J-SPACER and J-NONAMER in 5' of J-REGION of a J-GENE or J-SEQUENCE
J-GENE	germline genomic DNA including J-REGION with 5'UTR and 3'UTR
JUNCTION	coding region encompassing the V-J or V-D-J junction from 2nd-CYS to the J-PHE or J-TRP of the J-REGION
L-INTRON-L	sequence including L-PART1, V-INTRON and L-PART2 in genomic DNA or corresponding sequence in unspliced cDNA
L-PART1	exon encoding the first part of the leader peptide of a V-, V-D-, V-D-J-, or V-J-GENE or corresponding region in unspliced cDNA
L-PART2	5' region of V-EXON encoding the second part of leader peptide of a V-, V-D-, V-D-J- or V-J-GENE or corresponding region in unspliced cDNA
N-AND-D-REGION	coding region encompassing the N diversity sequence and coding region of D-GENE(s) when limits between N- and D-REGIONS are unknown or corresponding region in cDNA
N-REGION	coding region encompassing the N diversity sequence
OCTAMER	8-nucleotide regulation site or octanucleotide, in the 5'UTR of a V-, V-D-, V-D-J- or V-J-GENE
STOP-CODON	codon that stops gene translation
TATA_BOX	TATA signal in eukaryotic promoters
V-CLUSTER	genomic DNA in germline configuration including more than one V-GENE
V-D-J-EXON	rearranged genomic DNA including L-PART2, V-, any D- and N-REGION, and J-REGION

Label name	Definition
V-D-J-GENE	rearranged genomic DNA including L-PART1, V-INTRON, and V-D-J-EXON, with the 5'UTR and 3'UTR
V-D-J-REGION	coding region including V-, any D- and N-REGION, and J-REGION, in rearranged genomic DNA, or corresponding region in cDNA
V-EXON	germline genomic DNA including L-PART2 and V-REGION
V-HEPTAMER	7-nucleotide recombination site, like CACAGTG, part of V-RS
V-INTRON	non-coding sequence between L-PART1 and V-EXON in genomic DNA or corresponding sequence in unspliced cDNA
V-J-EXON	rearranged genomic DNA including L-PART2, V- and J- REGION
V-J-GENE	rearranged genomic DNA including L-PART1, V-INTRON and V-J-EXON, with the 5'UTR and 3'UTR
V-J-REGION	coding region including V- and J-REGION, in rearranged genomic DNA or corresponding region in cDNA
V-NONAMER	9-nucleotide recombination site, like ACAAAAACC, part of V-RS
V-REGION	coding region of V-GENE without the leader peptide (plus 1 or 2 nucleotide(s) before the V-HEPTAMER, if present) or corresponding region in cDNA
V-RS	recombination signal including V-HEPTAMER, V-SPACER and V-NONAMER in 3' of V-REGION of a V-GENE or V-SEQUENCE
V-SPACER	12- or 23-nucleotide spacer between the V-HEPTAMER and the V-NONAMER of a V-RS

Aide-Mémoire

Useful restriction sites

*Bam*HI	G⬇GATCC
*Eco*RI	G⬇AATTC
*Hin*dIII	A⬇AGCTT
*Kpn*I	GGTAC⬇C
*Pst*I	CTGCA⬇G
*Pvu*II	CAG⬇CTG
*Sac*I (*Sst*I)	GAGCT⬇C
*Taq*I	T⬇CGA
*Xba*I	T⬇CTAGA
*Xho*I	C⬇TCGAG

Amino Acid Abbreviations

Amino acid	Abbreviations	
Alanine	Ala	A
Arginine	Arg	R
Asparagine	Asn	N
Aspartic acid	Asp	D
Asparagine or Aspartic acid	Asx	B
Cysteine	Cys	C
Glutamine	Gln	Q
Glutamic acid	Glu	E
Glutamine or Glutamic acid	Glx	Z
Glycine	Gly	G
Histidine	His	H
Isoleucine	Ile	I
Leucine	Leu	L
Lysine	Lys	K
Methionine	Met	M
Phenylalanine	Phe	F
Proline	Pro	P
Serine	Ser	S
Threonine	Thr	T
Tryptophan	Trp	W
Tyrosine	Tyr	Y
Valine	Val	V

Genetic code

first	Nucleotide position in codon				third
	second				
	U	C	A	G	
U	UUU Phe	UCU Ser	UAU Tyr	UGU Cys	U
	UUC Phe	UCC Ser	UAC Tyr	UGC Cys	C
	UUA Leu	UCA Ser	UAA Stop	UGA Stop	A
	UUG Leu	UCG Ser	UAG Stop	UGG Trp	G
C	CUU Leu	CCU Pro	CAU His	CGU Arg	U
	CUC Leu	CCC Pro	CAC His	CGC Arg	C
	CUA Leu	CCA Pro	CAA Gln	CGA Arg	A
	CUG Leu	CCG Pro	CAG Gln	CGG Arg	G
A	AUU Ile	ACU Thr	AAU Asn	AGU Ser	U
	AUC Ile	ACC Thr	AAC Asn	AGC Ser	C
	AUA Ile	ACA Thr	AAA Lys	AGA Arg	A
	AUG Met	ACG Thr	AAG Lys	AGG Arg	G
G	GUU Val	GCU Ala	GAU Asp	GGU Gly	U
	GUC Val	GCC Ala	GÁC Asp	GGC Gly	C
	GUA Val	GCA Ala	GAA Glu	GGA Gly	A
	GUG Val	GCG Ala	GAG Glu	GGG Gly	G

THE INTRODUCTORY CHAPTERS

1 Introduction

SCOPE OF THE BOOK

The primary aim of this book is to provide a compendium of the human germline T cell Receptor genes which are used to create the human T cell receptor repertoire. The book includes entries for 168 genes and for 271 alleles, with a total of 393 sequences displayed (Section II). Prior to the entries there are four introductory chapters (Section I). The first introductory chapter defines the data content and data selection criteria based on the International ImMunoGeneTics database (IMGT) Scientific chart[1] and IMGT-ONTOLOGY concepts[2]. Chapter 2 is a short overview on the structural and biological properties of the human T cell receptors. Chapter 3 provides a summary of the molecular mechanisms of the synthesis of the human T cell receptor chains. Chapter 4 represents a major IMGT contribution by providing, in a unique document, the first complete description of the T cell receptor germline repertoire in the human.

SELECTION OF THE DATA

The individual entries comprise all the human T cell receptor constant genes, and germline variable, diversity, and joining genes which have at least one functional or ORF (Open Reading Frame) allele, and which are localized in the four major loci. Selected data are from IMGT, the international ImMunoGeneTics database[1,3–5] (http://imgt.cines.fr), created in Montpellier in 1989 by M.-P. Lefranc (Université Montpellier II, CNRS), and more particularly from the IMGT/LIGM-DB database, and from the IMGT Repertoire[6]. The selection criteria of the individual entries are defined in the IMGT Scientific chart[1] (http://imgt.cines.fr) and in the IMGT-ONTOLOGY 'IDENTIFICATION' and 'CLASSIFICATION' concepts[2], some of which are briefly summarized in the following paragraphs.

The 'IDENTIFICATION' concept

The 'IDENTIFICATION' concept allows scientists to identify T cell receptor sequences according to fundamental biological and immunogenetic characteristics[2]. These are as follows.

'molecule type':
Three instances are considered: genomic DNA), cDNA, and protein.

'gene type':
Four types of genes are involved in T cell receptor synthesis, the variable (V), diversity (D) and joining (J) genes which encode the antigen binding sites, and the constant (C) genes which encode the part of the polypeptide chains that has effector properties.

'configuration':
The configuration defines the status of the genes: 'germline' or 'rearranged' for the V, D, and J genes. This concept is particularly important because it is unique to the immunoglobulin and T cell receptor V, D, and J genes. Note that the C genes do not rearrange directly and therefore their configuration is not defined.

'chain type':
The chain type identifies the nature of the polypeptide chain potentially encoded by the T cell receptor genes. There are four main instances which are defined by the C gene sequence characteristics: TcR-Alpha, TcR-Beta, TcR-Gamma, and TcR-Delta.

'functionality':
The definition of functionality is based on the sequence analysis. As examples, the instances functional (for germline V, D, J, and for C genes), and productive (for rearranged V-J-C and V-D-J-C sequences) mean that the coding regions have an open reading frame without a stop codon, and that there is no described defect in the splicing sites, and/or recombination signals and/or regulatory elements. According to the gravity of the identified defects, the functionality can be defined as ORF, pseudogene, or vestigial (for germline V, D, J, and for C genes)[7]. Complete definitions are available in the IMGT Scientific chart at http://imgt.cines.fr.

The 'CLASSIFICATION' concept

The 'CLASSIFICATION' concept (Fig. 1) organizes the immunogenetic knowledge useful to name and classify the T cell receptor (TR) genes[2].

'locus':
A locus is a group of T cell receptor genes that are ordered and are localized in the same chromosomal location in a given species. The human genome includes four main T cell receptor loci: TRA (14q11.2), TRB (7q34), TRG (7p14), and TRD (14q11.2), this last one being nestled within the TRA locus. T cell receptor genes have also been identified in other chromosomal locations outside the main loci which represent new instances of the concept locus. However, the genes they contain, designated as orphons, are not functional.

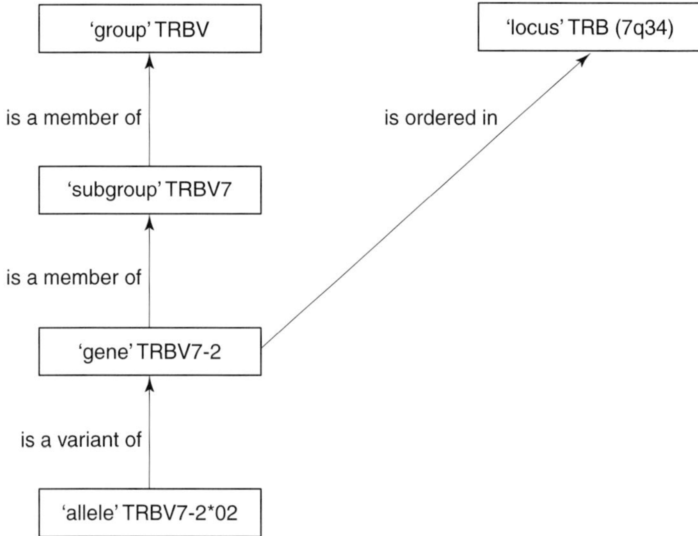

Figure 1. *The 'CLASSIFICATION' concept in the IMGT-ONTOLOGY.*

'group':
A group is a set of genes that share the same 'gene type' (V, D, J or C) and participate potentially in the synthesis of a polypeptide of the same 'chain type'. By extension, a group includes the related pseudogenes and orphons.

'subgroup':
A subgroup is a set of genes that belong to the same group, in a given species, and that share at least 75% identity at the nucleotide level (in the germline configuration for V, D, and J).

'gene':
A gene is defined as a DNA sequence that can be potentially transcribed and/or translated (this definition includes the regulatory elements in 5' and 3', and the introns, if present). Instances of the 'gene' concept are gene names. By extension, orphons and pseudogenes are also instances of the 'gene' concept. For each gene, IMGT has defined a reference sequence[1]. For the V, D, and J genes, the reference sequence corresponds to a germline entity. The rules for the choice of the reference sequences are described in the IMGT Scientific chart.

'allele':
An allele is a polymorphic variant of a gene. Alleles are described, exhaustively and in a standardized way, for the four 'core' coding regions, that is for the germline V-REGIONs, D-REGIONs, and J-REGIONs, and for the C-REGIONs, from T cell receptor genes. These alleles refer to sequence polymorphisms, with mutations described at the sequence level[4,7]. Their sequences are compared to the reference sequence designated as *01 (see IMGT Scientific chart at for IMGT description of mutations, and IMGT allele nomenclature for sequence polymorphisms).

Due to the usual absence of somatic hypermutations in V-REGIONs from T cell receptors, rearranged genomic DNA or cDNA can be found included in the alignments of alleles (Section II), when the corresponding germline gene has not yet been isolated. Note that nucleotide mutations and amino acid changes in the CDR3-IMGT of these TR V-REGIONs are not taken into account for the description of allele polymorphisms.

DESCRIPTION OF THE DATA

The description of the individual gene entries is based on the 'DESCRIPTION' concept of the IMGT-ONTOLOGY[2], and, for the V-REGIONs, on the setting up of the IMGT unique numbering[7-9].

The 'DESCRIPTION' concept

The 'DESCRIPTION' concept provides a standardized description of the organization and of the components of the T cell receptor sequences, and a characterization of their specific and conserved motifs. A list of the IMGT labels used in this book is provided. Prototypes have been set up to graphically represent the description and configuration of a T cell receptor gene[3] (Fig. 2). For example, the prototype V-GENE represents a genomic V gene in the germline configuration, whereas V-J-GENE represents genomic V and J genes in the rearranged configuration for an alpha or a gamma chain, and V-D-J-GENE represents genomic V, D, and J genes in the rearranged configuration for a beta or a delta chain (Fig. 2).

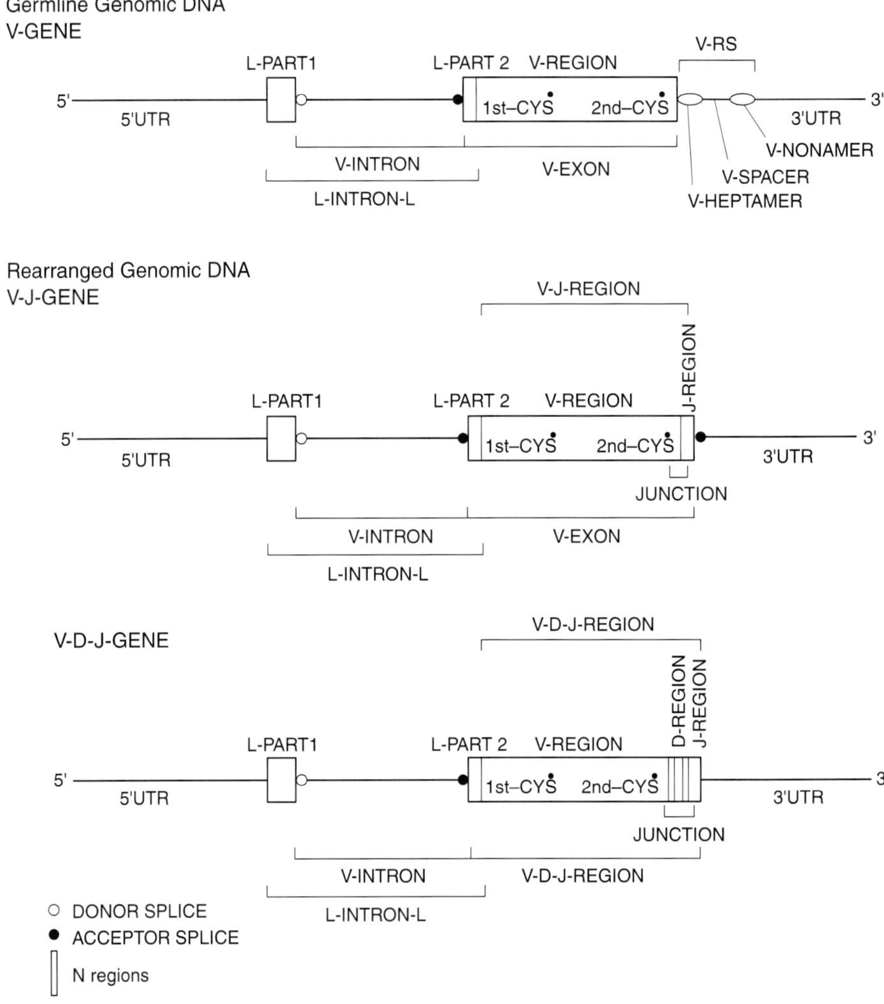

Figure 2. *Prototypes of a variable gene in the germline (V-GENE) or rearranged (V-J-GENE for a T cell receptor alpha or gamma chain, V-D-J-GENE for a T cell receptor beta or delta chain) configuration. Labels (in capital letters) are those used for the sequence description in IMGT (http://imgt.cines.fr).*

THE IMGT UNIQUE NUMBERING FOR THE V-REGIONS

The IMGT unique numbering[7-9] relies on the high conservation of the structure of the variable region. This numbering, set up after aligning more than 5000 sequences, takes into account and combines the definition of the framework (FR) and complementarity determining regions (CDR)[10], structural data from X-ray diffraction studies[11], and the characterization of the hypervariable loops[12]. The delimitations of the FR-IMGT and CDR-IMGT regions have been defined, and correspondence between the IMGT numbering and the other numberings has been established[9].

The IMGT unique numbering has many advantages:

- It allows an easy comparison between sequences coding the variable regions, whatever the antigen receptor (immunoglobulins or T cell receptors), the chain type (alpha, beta, gamma, or delta chains for T cell receptors), or the species.

- In the IMGT unique numbering, the conserved amino acids always have the same position, for instance Cysteine 23, Tryptophan 41, Leucine 89, Cysteine 104. The hydrophobic amino acids of the framework regions are also found in conserved positions.

- This unique numbering has allowed the redefinition of the limits of the FR and CDR. The FR-IMGT and CDR-IMGT lengths themselves become crucial information characterizing the variable regions belonging to a group, a subgroup and/or a gene.

- Framework amino acids (and codons) located at the same position in different sequences can be compared without requiring sequence alignments. This also holds for amino acids belonging to CDR-IMGT of the same length.

- The IMGT unique numbering has allowed a standardized IMGT description of mutations for the IMGT description of allele polymorphisms of the T cell receptor variable regions[4,7].

- The unique numbering is used as the output of the IMGT/V-QUEST alignment tool (http://imgt.cines.fr) which analyses your T cell receptor variable (germline or rearranged) sequences according to IMGT criteria[1]. In IMGT/V-QUEST, a variable rearranged sequence is compared to the appropriate sets of V-REGION, D-REGION, and J-REGION alleles from the IMGT reference directory. The results show, aligned with the input sequence, the sequences of the most homologous V-REGION alleles and, if appropriate, D-REGION (for beta and delta chains) and J-REGION alleles. The aligned V-REGION sequences are displayed according to the IMGT unique numbering and with the FR-IMGT and CDR-IMGT delimitations.

By facilitating comparisons between the sequences and the descriptions of alleles and mutations, the IMGT unique numbering represents a big step forward in the analysis of the T cell receptor sequences of all species. Moreover, it gives insight to the structural configuration of the variable domain and opens interesting views on the evolution of the sequences of the V-set, since this numbering has been applied with success to all the sequences belonging to the V-set of the immunoglobulin superfamily, including nonrearranging sequences in vertebrates (CD4, *Xenopus* CTX,...) and in invertebrates (*Drosophila* Amalgam, *Drosophila* Fasciclin II, etc.)[7-9].

Correspondence between numberings

Table 1 gives the correspondence between the IMGT unique Lefranc numbering[7–9] and the different Kabat numberings [13] for the T cell receptor variable regions.

Table 1. *Correspondence between the V-REGION numberings.*

| | TRBV | | | | TRAV | | | | TRDV | | | | TRGV | | |
	Human TRBV6-5				Human TRAV8-6				Human TRDV2				Human TRGV3		
1	1	aat	ASN	N	1	0	agc	ALA	A	1	00	gcc	ALA	A	1	01	tct	SER	S
2	2	gct	ALA	A	2	1	cag	GLN	Q	2	1	att	ILE	I	2	00	tcc	SER	S
3	3	ggt	GLY	G	3	2	tct	SER	S	3	2	gag	GLU	E	3	1	aac	ASN	N
4	4	gtc	VAL	V	4	3	gtg	VAL	V	4	3	ttg	LEU	L	4	2	ttg	LEU	L
5	5	act	THR	T	5	4	acc	THR	T	5	4	gtg	VAL	V	5	3	gaa	GLU	E
6	6	cag	GLN	Q	6	5	cag	GLN	Q	6	5	cct	PRO	P	6	4	ggg	GLY	G
7	7	acc	THR	T	7	6	ctt	LEU	L	7	6	gaa	GLU	E	7	5	aga	ARG	R
8	8	cca	PRO	P	8	7	gac	ASP	D	8	7	cac	HIS	H	8	6	acg	THR	T
9	9	aaa	LYS	K	9	8	agc	SER	S	9	8	caa	GLN	Q	9	7	aag	LYS	K
10	10	ttc	PHE	F	10	9	caa	GLN	Q	10	9	aca	THR	T	10	8	tca	SER	S
11	11	cag	GLN	Q	11	10	gtc	VAL	V	11	10	gtg	VAL	V	11	9	gtc	VAL	V
12	12	gtc	VAL	V	12	11	cct	PRO	P	12	11	cct	PRO	P	12	10	acc	THR	T
13	13	ctg	LEU	L	13	12	gtc	VAL	V	13	12	gtg	VAL	V	13	11	agg	ARG	R
14	14	aag	LYS	K	14	13	ttt	PHE	F	14	13	tca	SER	S	14	12	cag	GLN	Q
15	15	aca	THR	T	15	14	gaa	GLU	E	15	14	ata	ILE	I	15	13	act	THR	T
16	16	gga	GLY	G	16	15	gaa	GLU	E	16	15	ggg	GLY	G	16	14	ggg	GLY	G
17	17	cag	GLN	Q	17	16	gcc	ALA	A	17	16	gtc	VAL	V	17	15	tca	SER	S
18	18	agc	SER	S	18	17	cct	PRO	P	18	17	cct	PRO	P	18	16	tct	SER	S
19	19	atg	MET	M	19	18	gtg	VAL	V	19	18	gcc	ALA	A	19	17	gct	ALA	A
20	20	aca	THR	T	20	19	gag	GLU	E	20	19	acc	THR	T	20	18	gaa	GLU	E
21	21	ctg	LEU	L	21	20	ctg	LEU	L	21	20	ctc	LEU	L	21	19	atc	ILE	I
22	22	cag	GLN	Q	22	21	agg	ARG	R	22	21	agg	ARG	R	22	20	act	THR	T
23	23	tgt	**CYS**	**C**	23	22	tgc	**CYS**	**C**	23	22	tgc	**CYS**	**C**	23	21	tgc	**CYS**	**C**
24	24	gcc	ALA	A	24	23	aac	ASN	N	24	23	tcc	SER	S	24	22	gat	ASP	D
25	25	cag	GLN	Q	25	24	tac	TYR	Y	25	24	atg	MET	M	25	23	ctt	LEU	L
26	26	gat	ASP	D	26	25	tca	SER	S	26	25	aaa	LYS	K	26	24	act	THR	T
27	27	atg	MET	M	27	26	tcg	SER	S	27	26	gga	GLY	G	27	25	gta	VAL	V
28	28	aac	ASN	N	28	27	tct	SER	S	28	27	gaa	GLU	E	28	26	aca	THR	T
29	29	cat	HIS	H	29	28	gtt	VAL	V	29	28	gcg	ALA	A	29	27	aat	ASN	N
30	30	gaa	GLU	E	30	29	tca	SER	S	30	29	atc	ILE	I	30	28	acc	THR	T
31	*31	tac	TYR	Y	31	30	gtg	VAL	V	31	30	ggt	GLY	G	31	29	ttc	PHE	F
32	*	--- ---		–	32	*31	tat	TYR	Y	32	31	aac	ASN	N	32	30	tac	TYR	Y
33		--- ---		–	33	*	--- ---		–	33	32	tac	TYR	Y	33	31	--- ---		–
34		--- ---		–	34	*	--- ---		–	34	33	tat	TYR	Y	34	32	--- ---		–
35		--- ---		–	35		--- ---		–	35		--- ---		–	35		--- ---		–
36		--- ---		–	36		--- ---		–	36		--- ---		–	36		--- ---		–
37		--- ---		–	37		--- ---		–	37		--- ---		–	37		--- ---		–
38		--- ---		–	38		--- ---		–	38		--- ---		–	38		--- ---		–

Left margin labels: rows 1–26 are marked **FR1-IMGT**; rows 27–38 are marked **CDR1-IMGT**.

Table 1. *Continued.*

		TRBV					TRAV					TRDV					TRGV			
		Human TRBV6-5					Human TRAV8-6					Human TRDV2					Human TRGV3			
FR2-IMGT	**39**	32	atg	MET	M	**39**	32	ctc	LEU	L	**39**	34	atc	ILE	I	**39**	33	atc	ILE	I
	40	33	tcc	SER	S	**40**	33	ttc	PHE	F	**40**	34A	aac	ASN	N	**40**	34	cac	HIS	H
	41	34	tgg	**TRP**	**W**	**41**	34	tgg	**TRP**	**W**	**41**	35	tgg	**TRP**	**W**	**41**	35	tgg	**TRP**	**W**
	42	35	tat	TYR	Y	**42**	35	tat	TYR	Y	**42**	36	tac	TYR	Y	**42**	36	tac	TYR	Y
	43	36	cga	ARG	R	**43**	36	gtg	VAL	V	**43**	37	agg	ARG	R	**43**	37	cta	LEU	L
	44	37	caa	GLN	Q	**44**	37	caa	GLN	Q	**44**	38	aag	LYS	K	**44**	38	cac	HIS	H
	45	38	gac	ASP	D	**45**	38	tac	TYR	Y	**45**	39	acc	THR	T	**45**	39	cag	GLN	Q
	46	39	cca	PRO	P	**46**	39	ccc	PRO	P	**46**	40	caa	GLN	Q	**46**	40	gag	GLU	E
	47	40	ggc	GLY	G	**47**	40	aac	ASN	N	**47**	41	ggt	GLY	G	**47**	41	ggg	GLY	G
	48	41	atg	MET	M	**48**	41	caa	GLN	Q	**48**	42	aac	ASN	N	**48**	42	aag	LYS	K
	49	42	ggg	GLY	G	**49**	42	gga	GLY	G	**49**	43	aca	THR	T	**49**	43	gcc	ALA	A
	50	43	ctg	LEU	L	**50**	43	ctc	LEU	L	**50**	44	atc	ILE	I	**50**	44	cca	PRO	P
	51	44	agg	ARG	R	**51**	44	cag	GLN	Q	**51**	45	act	THR	T	**51**	45	cag	GLN	Q
	52	45	ctg	LEU	L	**52**	45	ctt	LEU	L	**52**	46	ttc	PHE	F	**52**	46	cgt	ARG	R
	53	46	att	ILE	I	**53**	46	ctc	LEU	L	**53**	47	ata	ILE	I	**53**	47	ctt	LEU	L
	54	47	cat	HIS	H	**54**	47	ctg	LEU	L	**54**	48	tac	TYR	Y	**54**	48	ctg	LEU	L
	55	48	tac	TYR	Y	**55**	48	aag	LYS	K	**55**	49	cga	ARG	R	**55**	49	tac	TYR	Y
CDR2-IMGT	**56**	49	tca	SER	S	**56**	*49	tat	TYR	Y	**56**	50	gaa	GLU	E	**56**	50	tat	TYR	Y
	57	50	gtt	VAL	V	**57**	*50	tta	LEU	L	**57**	51	aag	LYS	K	**57**	51	gac	ASP	D
	58	51	ggt	GLY	G	**58**	*51	tca	SER	S	**58**	52	gac	ASP	D	**58**	52	gtc	VAL	V
	59	52	gct	ALA	A	**59**	*52	gga	GLY	G	**59**	*	---	---	-	**59**	53	tcc	SER	S
	60	53	ggt	GLY	G	**60**		---	---	-	**60**		---	---	-	**60**	54	acc	THR	T
	61	54	atc	ILE	I	**61**		---	---	-	**61**		---	---	-	**61**	55	gca	ALA	A
	62		---	---	-	**62**		---	---	-	**62**		---	---	-	**62**	56	agg	ARG	R
	63		---	---	-	**63**		---	---	-	**63**		---	---	-	**63**	*57	gat	ASP	D
	64		---	---	-	**64**		---	---	-	**64**		---	---	-	**64**		---	---	-
	65		---	---	-	**65**		---	---	-	**65**		---	---	-	**65**		---	---	-
FR3-IMGT	**66**	55	act	THR	T	**66**	*53	tcc	SER	S	**66**	*53	atc	ILE	I	**66**	*58	gtg	VAL	V
	67	56	gac	ASP	D	**67**	*54	acc	THR	T	**67**	*54	tat	TYR	Y	**67**	*59	ttg	LEU	L
	68	57	caa	GLN	Q	**68**	*55	ctg	LEU	L	**68**	*55	ggc	GLY	G	**68**	*60	gaa	GLU	E
	69	58	gga	GLY	G	**69**	*56	gtt	VAL	V	**69**	*56	cct	PRO	P	**69**	*61	tca	SER	S
	70	59	gaa	GLU	E	**70**	*57	gaa	GLU	E	**70**	*57	ggt	GLY	G	**70**	*62	gga	GLY	G
	71	60	gtc	VAL	V	**71**	*58	agc	SER	S	**71**	*57A	ttc	PHE	F	**71**	*63	ctc	LEU	L
	72	61	ccc	PRO	P	**72**	*59	atc	ILE	I	**72**	*57B	aaa	LYS	K	**72**	*64	agt	SER	S
	73	*62	---	---	-	**73**	*	---	---	-	**73**	*57C	---	---	-	**73**	*64A	cca	PRO	P
	74	*63	aat	ASN	N	**74**	*60	aac	ASN	N	**74**	58	gac	ASP	D	**74**	*65	gga	GLY	G
	75	*64	ggc	GLY	G	**75**	61	ggt	GLY	G	**75**	59	aat	ASN	N	**75**	*66	aag	LYS	K
	76	65	tac	TYR	Y	**76**	62	ttt	PHE	F	**76**	60	ttc	PHE	F	**76**	*67	tat	TYR	Y
	77	66	aat	ASN	N	**77**	63	gag	GLU	E	**77**	61	caa	GLN	Q	**77**	*68	tat	TYR	Y
	78	67	gtc	VAL	V	**78**	64	gct	ALA	A	**78**	62	ggt	GLY	G	**78**	*69	act	THR	T
	79	68	tcc	SER	S	**79**	65	gaa	GLU	E	**79**	63	gac	ASP	D	**79**	*70	cat	HIS	H
	80	69	aga	ARG	R	**80**	66	ttt	PHE	F	**80**	64	att	ILE	I	**80**	*71	aca	THR	T
	81	70	tca	SER	S	**81**	67	aac	ASN	N	**81**	65	gat	ASP	D	**81**	*72	ccc	PRO	P
	82		---	---	-	**82**	68	aag	LYS	K	**82**	66	att	ILE	I	**82**	*	---	---	-

Table 1. *Continued.*

	TRBV				TRAV				TRDV				TRGV			
	Human TRBV6-5				Human TRAV8-6				Human TRDV2				Human TRGV3			
83	71	acc	THR	T	**83**	69	agt	SER	S	**83**	67	gca	ALA	A	**83**	73	agg	ARG	R
84	72	aca	THR	T	**84**	70	caa	GLN	Q	**84**	68	aag	LYS	K	**84**	74	agg	ARG	R
85	73	gag	GLU	E	**85**	71	act	THR	T	**85**	69	aac	ASN	N	**85**	75	tgg	TRP	W
86	74	gat	ASP	D	**86**	72	tcc	SER	S	**86**	70	ctg	LEU	L	**86**	76	agc	SER	S
87	75	ttc	PHE	F	**87**	73	ttc	PHE	F	**87**	71	gct	ALA	A	**87**	77	tgg	TRP	W
88	76	ccg	PRO	P	**88**	74	cac	HIS	H	**88**	72	gta	VAL	V	**88**	78	ata	ILE	I
89	77	ctc	LEU	L	**89**	75	ttg	LEU	L	**89**	73	ctt	LEU	L	**89**	79	ttg	LEU	L
90	78	agg	ARG	R	**90**	76	agg	ARG	R	**90**	74	aag	LYS	K	**90**	80	aga	ARG	R
91	79	ctg	LEU	L	**91**	77	aaa	LYS	K	**91**	75	ata	ILE	I	**91**	81	ctg	LEU	L
92	80	ctg	LEU	L	**92**	78	ccc	PRO	P	**92**	76	ctt	LEU	L	**92**	82	caa	GLN	Q
93	81	tcg	SER	S	**93**	79	tca	SER	S	**93**	77	gca	ALA	A	**93**	83	aat	ASN	N
94	82	gct	ALA	A	**94**	80	gtc	VAL	V	**94**	78	cca	PRO	P	**94**	84	cta	LEU	L
95	83	gct	ALA	A	**95**	81	cat	HIS	H	**95**	79	tca	SER	S	**95**	85	att	ILE	I
96	84	ccc	PRO	P	**96**	82	ata	ILE	I	**96**	80	gag	GLU	E	**96**	86	gaa	GLU	E
97	85	tcc	SER	S	**97**	83	agc	SER	S	**97**	81	aga	ARG	R	**97**	87	aat	ASN	N
98	86	cag	GLN	Q	**98**	84	gac	ASP	D	**98**	82	gat	ASP	D	**98**	88	gat	ASP	D
99	87	aca	THR	T	**99**	85	acg	THR	T	**99**	83	gaa	GLU	E	**99**	89	tct	SER	S
100	88	tct	SER	S	**100**	86	gct	ALA	A	**100**	84	ggg	GLY	G	**100**	90	ggg	GLY	G
101	89	gtg	VAL	V	**101**	87	gag	GLU	E	**101**	85	tct	SER	S	**101**	91	gtc	VAL	V
102	90	tac	TYR	Y	**102**	88	tac	TYR	Y	**102**	86	tac	TYR	Y	**102**	92	tat	TYR	Y
103	91	ttc	PHE	F	**103**	89	ttc	PHE	F	**103**	87	tac	TYR	Y	**103**	93	tac	TYR	Y
104	92	tgt	**CYS**	**C**	**104**	90	tgt	**CYS**	**C**	**104**	88	tgt	**CYS**	**C**	**104**	94	tgt	**CYS**	**C**
105	93	gcc	ALA	A	**105**	91	gct	ALA	A	**105**	89	gcc	ALA	A	**105**	95	gcc	ALA	A
106	94	agc	SER	S	**106**	92	gtg	VAL	V	**106**	90	tgt	CYS	C	**106**	96	acc	THR	T
107	95	agt	SER	S	**107**	93	agt	SER	S	**107**	91	gac	ASP	D	**107**	97	tgg	TRP	W
108	96	tat	TYR	Y						**108**	92	acc	THR	T	**108**	98	gac	ASP	D
109	97	---	---	-											**109**	99	agg	ARG	R

The left margin of the TRBV column is labelled vertically *FR3-IMGT – continued* for rows 83–103 and **CDR3-IMGT** for rows 104–109.

For each V-REGION group, one germline sequence is shown with, on the left hand side of each column, the IMGT unique Lefranc numbering (in bold)[7–9] and the corresponding Kabat numbering[13].

Positions of missing amino acids (shown with dashes) are reported to the 3' end of the CDR-IMGT. Asterisks (*) indicate positions for which it is not possible to make changes from one numbering to the other, automatically.

1st–CYS 23, CONSERVED–TRP 41, and 2nd–CYS 104 are in bold.

ORGANIZATION OF THE DATA

Nomenclature

The IMGT gene name (gene symbol) and the IMGT full name are given. The concepts of classification (Fig. 1) have been used to set up a unique nomenclature of the T cell receptor genes[14–23]. A four-letter root designates the 'group': TRAV,

TRAJ, and TRAC for the T cell receptor alpha genes; TRBV, TRBD, TRBJ, and TRBC for the T cell receptor beta genes; TRGV, TRGJ, and TRGC for the T cell receptor gamma genes; and TRDV, TRDD, TRDJ, and TRDC for the T cell receptor delta genes.

Gene names are derived from the four-letter root, by adding, if necessary, number(s) and/or letter(s) to allow unambiguous identification of the gene, a single number or letter being used whenever it is possible. IMGT nomenclature was approved by the HUGO (HUman Genome Organization) Nomenclature Committee (http://www.gene.ucl.ac.uk/nomenclature) in 1999.

Definition and functionality

The definition includes information on the functionality of a gene, and if necessary, that of its alleles. It also comprises eventual structural or biological particularities.

Gene location

The chromosomal location of the gene is given.

Nucleotide and amino acid sequences

Alignments of all known germline sequences assigned to the different alleles, by comparison to the allele*01, are displayed. The translation of the allele*01, and the nucleotide mutations and corresponding amino acid changes of the other alleles, are shown.

Dashes indicate identical nucleotides. Dots indicate gaps according to the IMGT numbering.

Allele names of the V-REGIONs, D-REGIONs, J-REGIONs, and C-REGIONs comprise the IMGT gene name followed by an asterisk and a two-figure number. The V-REGIONs, D-REGIONs, J-REGIONs and C-REGIONs selected as references for the allele polymorphism description have the number *01; other alleles are designated by increasing numbers (*02, *03, ...) based, if possible, on chronological order of their publication, and/or confirmation of data by different authors.

Note that the number *01 does not mean necessarily that other alleles are already known; it signifies that any new polymorphic sequence will be described by comparison to that allele, *01.

IMGT accession numbers are indicated for each allele. Although the IMGT accession numbers are the same as those from the EMBL/GenBank/DDBJ generalist databases, the content of the IMGT/LIGM-DB flat files differs by the expertised annotations added by IMGT. IMGT data are available from the IMGT/LIGM-DB sequence database, from the IMGT Repertoire, and via SRS sites (available from the IMGT Home page, http://imgt.cines.fr). References indicated by a number between brackets are listed at the end of the group entries.

Framework and complementarity determining regions

For the V-GENE entries, the length (in number of amino acids) of the framework (FR) and Complementarity Determining Regions (CDR) are indicated. The limits of the FR and CDR are based on the IMGT unique numbering[7-9].

Colliers de Perles

The IMGT Colliers de Perles[1,4,5,9] are 2D graphical representations of the T cell receptor variable regions, with FR-IMGT and CDR-IMGT delimitations. Colliers de Perles 2D representation provides information on the amino acid positions in the beta-strands and loops of the variable domain and allows quick visualization of amino acids which are important for the structural configuration of the V-REGION.

Amino acids are shown in the one letter abbreviation. Hydrophobic amino acids (hydropathy index with positive value) and Tryptophan (W) found at a given position in more than 50% of analysed T cell receptor sequences are shown in dark grey. All Proline (P) are shown in pale grey. The CDR-IMGT are limited by amino acids shown in squares, which belong to the neighbouring FR-IMGT. Hatched circles or squares correspond to missing positions according to the IMGT unique numbering.

Arrows indicate the direction of the beta-strands and their different designations in 3D structure. This information has to be used carefully if not supported by experimental data.

For a given germline V-GENE, the lengths of the three CDR-IMGT are shown in brackets after the gene name, and separated by full points. For example, TRGV9 [8.7.5] means that in the germline TRGV9 gene, the CDR1-IMGT, CDR2-IMGT, and CDR3-IMGT regions are 8, 7, and 5 amino acids long, respectively.

Genome database accession numbers

All IMGT human T cell receptor genes[14-23] have been entered into GDB, Genome Database, Toronto, Canada (http://www.gdb.org), and into LocusLink at NCBI (National Center for Biotechnology Information), Bethesda, USA (http.//www.ncbi.nlm.nih.gov/LocusLink), and accession numbers are provided. Links to the individual IMGT, GDB and LocusLink gene entries are available from http.//imgt.cines.fr from IMGT Repertoire>List of human Ig and TcR genes>T cell receptors. Links to OMIM (Online Mendelian Inheritance in Man, MIM) (http.//www.ncbi.nlm.nih.gov/Omim) are cited when there are existing entries in OMIM.

References

1 Lefranc, M.-P. et al. (1999) Nucleic Acids Res. 27, 209–212.
2 Giudicelli, V., et al. (1999) Bioinformatics 15, 1047–1054.
3 Giudicelli, V., et al. (1997) Nucleic Acids Res. 25, 206–211.
4 Lefranc, M.-P. et al. (1998) Nucleic Acids Res. 26, 297–303.
5 Ruiz, M. et al. (2000) Nucleic Acids Res. 28, 219–221.
6 Lefranc, M.-P. (2000) BIOforum International 4, 98–100.
7 Lefranc, M.-P. (1998) Exp. Clin. Immunogenet. 15, 1–7.
8 Lefranc, M.-P. (1997) Immunol. Today 18, 509.
9 Lefranc, M.-P. (1999) The Immunologist. 7, 132–136.
10 Kabat, E.A. et al. (1987) In 'Sequences of Proteins of Immunological Interest'. Public Health Service, NIH, Washington DC.
11 Satow, Y. et al. (1986) J. Mol. Biol. 190, 593–604.
12 Chothia, C. and Lesk, A.M. (1987) J. Mol. Biol. 196, 901–917.

[13] Kabat, E.A. et al. (1991) In 'Sequences of Proteins of Immunological Interest'. NIH Publication 91–3242 Washington DC.

[14] Lefranc, M.-P. et al. (1989) Eur. J. Immunol. 19, 989–994.

[15] Lefranc, M.-P. and Rabbitts, T.H. (1990) Res. Immunol. 141, 615–618.

[16] Lefranc, M.-P. (1990) Res. Immunol. 141, 692–695.

[17] Lefranc, M.-P. (2000) In Curr. Protocols Immunol. A.1O.1–A.1O.23, John Wiley and Sons, New York, USA.

[18] Folch, G. and Lefranc, M.-P. (2000) Exp. Clin. Immunogenet. 17, 42–54.

[19] Folch, G. and Lefranc, M.-P. (2000) Exp. Clin. Immunogenet. 17, 107–114.

[20] Scaviner, D. and Lefranc, M.-P. (2000) Exp. Clin. Immunogenet. 17, 83–96.

[21] Scaviner, D. and Lefranc, M.-P. (2000) Exp. Clin. Immunogenet. 17, 97–106.

[22] Folch, G. et al. (2000) Exp. Clin. Immunogenet. 17, 205–215.

[23] Lefranc, M.-P. The Immunologist 8, 72–79.

2 T cell receptor structural and biological properties

INTRODUCTION

The T cell receptors (TcR), like the immunoglobulins (Ig) or antibodies, are clonotypic antigen-specific receptors which are essential to the immune response. T cell receptors which are present on the cell surface of T lymphocytes (T cells) differ in several ways from the immunoglobulins: (1) immunoglobulins are tetramers, made up of four polypeptide chains (two heavy chains and two light chains) and possess two antigen-recognition sites, T cell receptors are dimers and possess only one antigen-recognition site (Fig. 1) (2) immunoglobulins are found either as membrane bound surface receptors on B lymphocytes or in a secreted form, T cell receptors exist only as membrane-bound surface receptors (3) immunoglobulins recognize soluble and native antigens (Ag), T cell receptors recognize protein antigens once they have been processed and converted into small surface peptides and bound to the major histocompatibility complex (MHC) molecules at the surface of antigen-presenting cells (APC) (e.g., macrophages, monocytes, B cells, and dendritic cells). This phenomenon is known as MHC-restricted recognition, or MHC restriction.

The 'education' of T cells to recognize the MHC molecules of their own body (i.e., self-MHC) takes place in the thymus. The conventional T cell receptor, or $\alpha\beta$ TcR, is expressed on most T lymphocytes and consists of two glycosylated polymorphic disulfide-linked chains α and β (Fig. 2), noncovalently associated with the nonpolymorphic membrane-bound CD3 proteins to form the functional TcR-CD3 at the cell surface. The $\alpha\beta$ TcR must discriminate among different peptides embedded in the surfaces of the MHC molecules whose dimensions and shape are relatively constant. The α and β chains participate in the interaction with the pMHC (peptide–MHC) complex, whereas the CD3 proteins participate in signal transduction. Recombinant DNA technology has led to the identification of another locus γ, in the mouse[1] and in humans[2]. Two years thereafter, the γ chain was demonstrated to be part of another type of T cell receptor, or $\gamma\delta$ TcR, which comprises two chains, γ and δ, also associated with the CD3 proteins, at the cell surface of a subset of T cells[3-6] (Fig. 2). The $\gamma\delta$ TcR recognize carbohydrate-, nucleotide-, or phospho-carrying antigens for which the mode of presentation is still poorly characterized. T cells express either the $\alpha\beta$ TcR or the $\gamma\delta$ TcR[7,8].

The $\alpha\beta$ and $\gamma\delta$ T cell receptors are associated with the CD3 complex (Fig. 2), which comprises the CD3γ, CD3δ, CD3ϵ, CD3ζ (dzêta), and CD3η (êta) proteins organized in CD3$\gamma\epsilon$, $\delta\epsilon$, and $\zeta\zeta$ or $\zeta\eta$ dimers[9-10]; CD4 and CD8, which act as coreceptors for MHC class II or class I molecules, respectively, with their attendant T cell specific tyrosine kinase p56lck[11]; and the transmembrane protein tyrosine phosphatase CD45.

After specific recognition of foreign antigen by the T cell receptor, T cells are activated. They acquire activation antigens such as CD69, and express cytokine receptors including CD25 (IL-2 receptor α chain), and start to proliferate. Both $\alpha\beta$ and $\gamma\delta$ T cells display two types of effector functions: cytokine production and cytotoxic activity against microorganisms and tumor cells[12-14]. The effector cytotoxic activity of $\alpha\beta$ and $\gamma\delta$ T cells comprises two pathways: cytotoxicity mediated via the granzyme/perforin pathway and apoptosis via the Fas/Fas-ligand interaction.

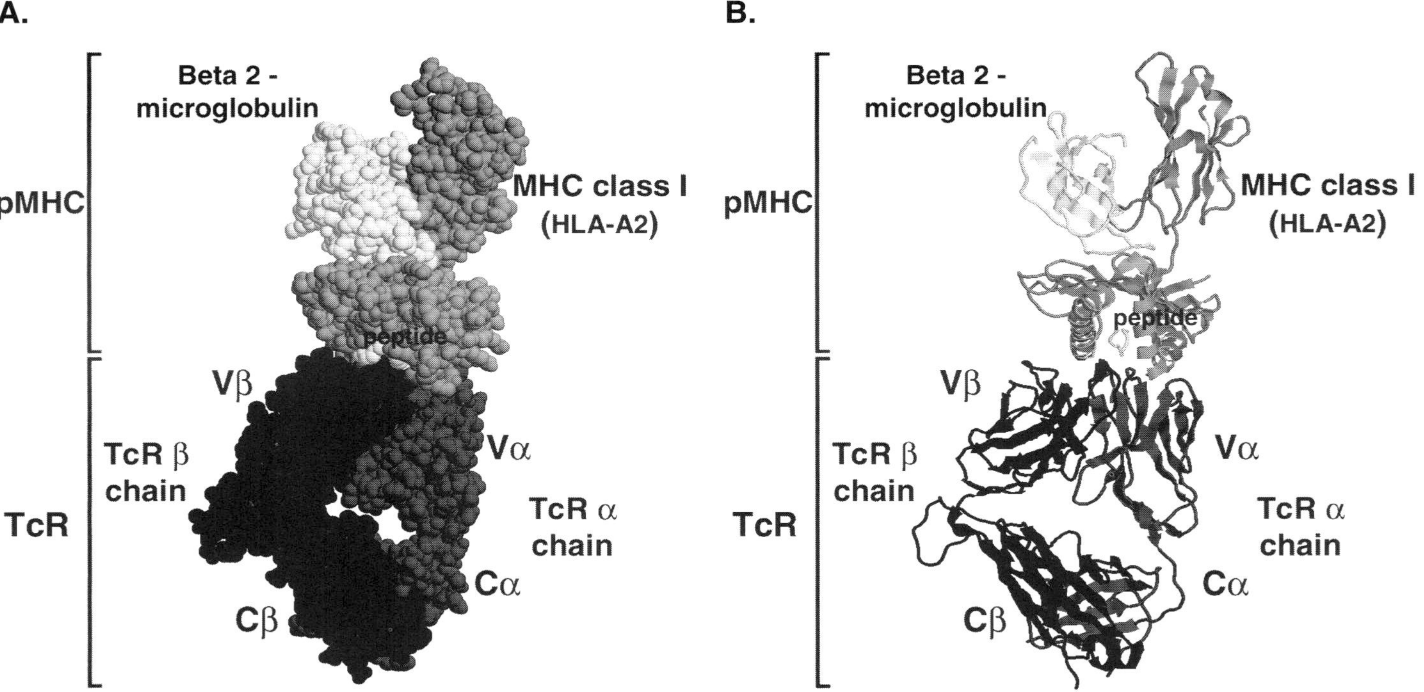

Figure 1. *3D representations of a human αβ T cell receptor recognizing a viral peptide presented by the human Major Histocompatibility Complex (MHC) class I molecule HLA-A2.* ***(A)*** *Spacefill model.* ***(B)*** *Cartoon model. The corresponding PDB file is 1BD2. Carbohydrates are not shown. Only the extracellular domains of the TcR and of the MHC are displayed. In vivo, the TcR and the pMHC (peptide-MHC) are membrane-bound on the surface of a T cell, and of an antigen presenting cell (APC), respectively. V = variable domain, C = constant domain.*

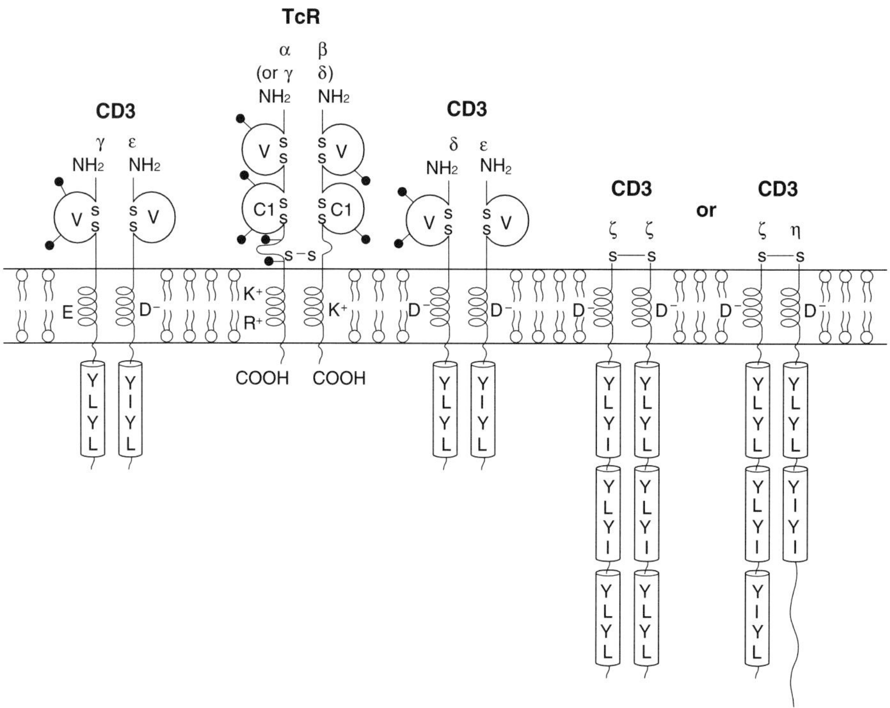

Figure 2. *Representation of an αβ (or γδ) TcR-CD3 complex. Positively and negatively charged amino acids of the transmembrane region as well as intracytoplasmic CD3 ITAMs are indicated. ITAMs, shown as grey cylinders, are not to scale. The TcR N-glycosylation sites are from an αβ TcR. The γδ TcR N-glycosylation sites are shown in Fig. 4.*

αβ AND γδ T CELLS

αβ T cells

The αβ T cell receptors are expressed at the surface of T cells that also express the CD antigens CD3 and either CD4 or CD8, these CD3⁺CD4⁺CD8⁻ and CD3⁺CD4⁻CD8⁺ αβ T cells represent 90–99 % of the mature peripheral T cells in humans. The CD3⁺CD4⁺ αβ T cells (about 60% of the αβ T cells) recognize peptides (generally derived from exogenous antigens such as microorganisms) bound to MHC class II molecules and are, for the most part, helper T cells. The CD3⁺CD8⁺ αβ T cells (about 30% of the αβ T cells) recognize peptides (generated by endogenous processing) bound to MHC class I molecules and are mostly cytotoxic T cells, responsible for finding infected or cancerous cells[15,16]. CD4 and CD8 are molecules that interact with a nonpolymorphic region of class II and class I molecules, respectively. There is a small subset of αβ T cells that lack CD4 and

CD8 ('double negative'). These cells, as well as some CD8$^+$ αβ T cells, recognize microbial lipid antigens in a CD1-restricted fashion[17].

The ability of αβ T cells to recognize a potentially infinite array of antigen–MHC combinations resides in the variable N-terminal portions of the TcR α and β chains. A single pMHC on an APC cell surface can sequentially engage and trigger as many as 200 αβ TcR[18], consistent with the low affinities and rapid dissociation rates that have been measured for TcR binding to pMHC[19,20]. A major issue is to explain how a TcR can recognize specific pMHC which are as few as 100 among the 100 000 irrelevant pMHC found on the surface of an APC[21–23].

TcR α and β chains are subject to allelic exclusion so that a unique αβ receptor type is usually expressed at the surface of a given T cell clone. However, αβ T cells expressing two different alpha chains, and therefore two different αβ receptors, have been identified on the membrane surface of up to one-third of mature T cells[24]. A small proportion (approximately 1%) of human peripheral T cells has also been shown to express two different V beta[25,26].

γδ T cells

The γδ T cells represent 1–10% of peripheral T cells (mean 3%) and 0.2–0.9% of the thymocytes in humans. The γδ T cell receptors are mainly expressed at the surface of T cells that express CD3, but lack CD4 or CD8. Thus the CD4$^-$CD8$^-$ γδ T cells (about 60% of the γδ T cells) recognize antigens independently of the classic MHC class I or class II molecules. A subset of CD4$^-$CD8$^+$ γδ T cells exist (about 30% of the γδ T cells), along with some very rare CD4$^+$CD8$^-$ γδ T cells. The CD4$^-$CD8$^+$ γδ T cells usually express CD8αα, not the CD8αβ heterodimer expressed by conventional αβ T cells.

The γδ T cells can recognize a heterogeneous array of ligands, for example in mouse, stress-induced heat-shock proteins from either bacteria or autologous cells[27,28], and in human, stress-induced MHC molecules (MICA and MICB), and non-peptidic carbohydrate-, nucleotide- and mycobacterial phospho-carrying antigens[12–14]. The function of these γδ cells could be to eliminate body cells that are under stress, for example as a result of infection or transformation to malignancy. The function of the γδ T cell receptors, the nature of their cognate antigens, and the context in which these antigens are recognized are still poorly characterized and are the object of extensive studies.

Like the α and β chains, the γ and δ chains have clonally unique structures and are subject to allelic exclusion. However, γδ T cells expressing two different gamma chains[29,30] and, at a lower frequency, two different delta chains[31], have been identified.

THE T CELL RECEPTOR CHAINS

Structure of the T cell receptor chains

The α and β chains of the αβ TcR, and the γ and δ chains of the γδ TcR possess an N-terminal extracellular region which comprises a variable domain of 104–125 amino acids and a constant domain of 91–129 amino acids, a connecting peptide of 21–62 amino acids, a transmembrane region of 17–26 amino acids, and a small cytoplasmic tail of 0–7 amino acids[7,8] (Table 1). Each variable and constant domain

Table 1. *Human T cell Receptor and CD3 chain characteristics.*

Chain Types												
	T cell Receptor							CD3				
	alpha	beta		gamma			delta	gamma	delta	epsilon	zeta	eta
Chain characteristics	α	$\beta1$	$\beta2$	$\gamma1$	$\gamma2$ (2x)	$\gamma2$ (3x)	δ	γ	δ	ϵ	ζ	η
Molecular weight (kDa) (1)	43–49 (32)		38–44 (34)	40 (30)	40,44 (32)	55 (34)	40–45 (37)	25 (16)	20 (16)	20 (20)	16 (16)	21 (21)
Number of Ig-like domains (2)	2	2	2	2	2	2	2	1	1	1	0	0
Total length (3)	~241	~277	~279	~273	~289	~305	~254	160	150	185	142	184
Constant domain (for TcR) (4) or Ig-like domain (for CD3)	91	129	129	110	110	110	93	80	67	91	–	–
Connecting peptide (4)	30	21	21	30	46	62	36	9	12	13	9	9
Transmembrane region	17	22	22	26	26	26	25	27	27	26	21	21
Intracytoplasmic region	3	5	7	7	7	7	0	44	44	55	112	154
N-glycosylation sites (5)	4	1	1	3	4 or 5	5	2	2	2	0	0	0
Charges in transmembrane region (6)	2+ (K, R)	1+ (K)	1+ (K)	3+ (K, R, R)	2 or 3+ (K, R*, R)	2+ (K,R)	3+ (R, K, K)	1– (E)	1– (D)	1– (D)	1– (D)	1– (D)
ITAMs	–	–	–	–	–	–	–	1	1	1	3	2

Note — the leftmost rows "Total length (3)" through "Intracytoplasmic region" are bracketed in the source by the rotated label "Length in number of amino acids".

(1) The relative masses are given in kilodalton (kDa), with those of the backbone proteins in parentheses.
(2) The Ig-like domains of the TcR chain comprises one variable (V) domain and one constant (C) domain of type C1. The Ig-like domain of the CD3γ, CD3δ, and CD3ϵ chains is of type C2[32].
(3) The total length for the TcR chains has been calculated by including a V domain with an arbitrary length of 100 amino acids, to facilitate data comparison of the length of the C domain, connecting peptide, and transmembrane and intracytoplasmic regions which, thus, is equal to the total length minus 100.
(4) The TcR chain constant domain is encoded by EX1 whereas the connecting peptide is encoded by EX2 and the 5′ part of EX3 (see Chapter 3).
(5) For the TcR chains, N-glycosylation sites of the variable domains (zero or one N-glycosylation site) are not taken into account (see Section II).
(6) Number of negatively (−) or positively (+) charged amino acids are indicated with, between parentheses, involved amino acids. An asterisk indicates an Arginine which can be either present or absent depending on the allelic polymorphism.

has a structure similar to that of the immunoglobulin domain[32] and is characterized by a series of multistranded antiparallel β-sheet bilayers and an intradisulfide loop of 51–66 amino acids (Fig. 3). The strands weave back and forth, forming a pleated sheet which folds into a sandwich-like structure. X-ray crystallographic structures of αβ TcR components have been reported[34–42], including murine β chain [34,35], Vα homodimer[36], and intact αβ TcR[37]; complex between a human TcR, a viral peptide, and a human class I MHC molecule[38,39]; complex between a murine TcR, a peptide, and MHC class II[40]; human Vδ domain[41]; and murine TcR in complex with an anti-

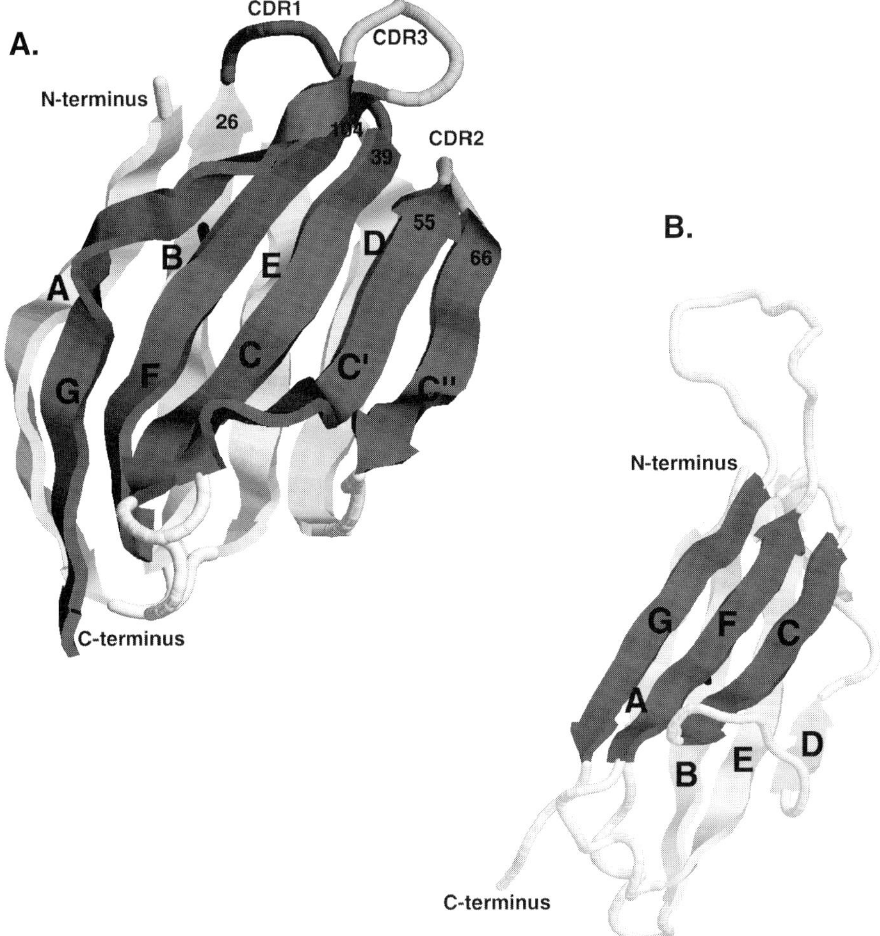

Figure 3. *3D representation (cartoon model) of the variable domain **(A)** and of the constant domain **(B)** of a TcR beta chain. These figures show the spreading of the strands labeled A to G, in the two antiparallel sheets (the beta sheet in contact with the domain of the other chain is in dark grey, and the external beta sheet is in light grey). The disulfide bridges of the domains are shown as black cylinders. The FR-IMGT amino acids positions which limit the CDR-IMGT of the variable domain (A) are indicated[33] (see Section II, Colliers de Perles).*

TcR Fab[42]. Each chain contains a Cysteine proximal to the transmembrane region which is involved in the formation of an α–β and γ–δ interchain disulfide bond, respectively. The human TcR γ2 chain, encoded by the constant gene TRGC2, is an exception in that it has no Cysteine in that region and is non-disulfide-linked to the δ chain (Fig. 4)[7,8]. The γ2 chain is 16 or 32 amino acids longer than γ1. This results from an allelic polymorphism of the TRGC2 gene which displays a duplication [TRGC2(2x)] or a triplication [TRGC2 (3x)] of exon 2[43–45]. All the clonotypic α, β, γ, and δ chains and the associated CD3 proteins possess a hydrophobic and probably helicoidal membrane-spanning region that has the unusual feature of containing charged amino acids: one or two positive charges for the TcR α, β, γ and δ chains, and one negative charge for the CD3 proteins, which probably interact to stabilize the TcR-CD3 complex (Fig. 2).

Glycosylation of the T cell receptor chains

The T cell receptor chains are glycoproteins. The human TcR α chain (43–49 kDa) contains four to five N-linked oligosaccharides of the complex type, attached to a polypeptide backbone of 32 kDa (Table 1). The human TcR β chain (38–44 kDa) contains one or two (one high-mannose and one complex) N-linked glycan side chains attached to a polypeptide backbone of 34 kDa [7,8].

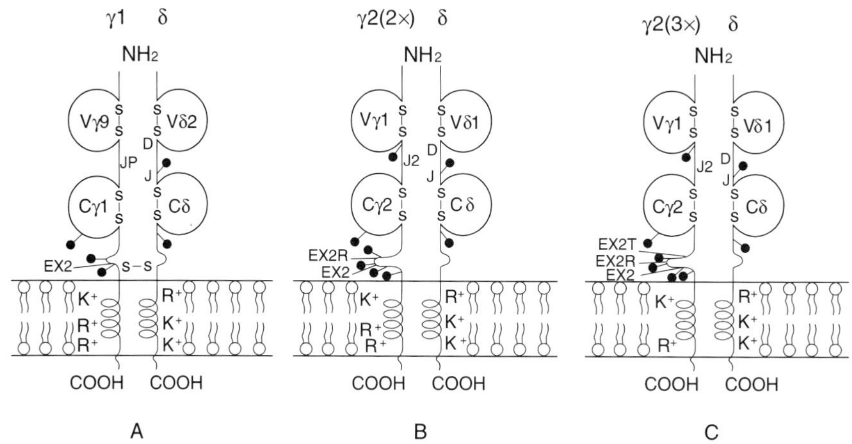

Figure 4. *Schematic representation of the three types of human γδ T cell receptor. There are three types of human γδ TcR, distinguished by their γ chains[7,8]: **(A)** the γ1δ TcR, in which the 40 kDa γ1 chain is disulfide-linked to the δ chain; **(B)** the γ2(2x)δ TcR; and **(C)** the γ2(3x)δ TcR, in which the 40 or 44 kDa γ2(2x) chain and the 55 kDa γ2(3x) chain are characterized by a duplication or triplication of exon 2, respectively, and are non-disulfide-linked to the δ chain. The γ2(2x) 'exon 2 region' may comprise EX2R (with one N-glycosylation site) or EX2T (no N-glycosylation site). The γ2(3x) 'exon 2 region' comprises EX2, EX2R and EX2T [7,8]. The Vγ9, Cγ1, Cγ2, Vδ1, Vδ2, and Cδ domains are encoded by the TRGV9, TRGC1, TRGC2, TRDV1, TRDV2, and TRDC genes, respectively. The VγI domain can be encoded by any of the 3–5 functional TRGV1 subgroup genes (see Section II).*

There are three types of human γ chains depending on the constant domain[7,8] (Fig. 4): the γ1 chain (40 kDa), whose constant region encoded by the TRGC1 gene is disulfide-linked to the δ chain and has three N-glycosylation sites; the γ2(2x) chains (40 and 44 kDa, which represent two different degrees of glycosylation), encoded by the allelic TRGC2 gene, with duplication of exon 2 (and therefore 16 amino acids longer than γ1); and the γ2(3x) chains (55 kDa) encoded by the allelic TRGC2 gene, with triplication of exon 2 (and therefore 32 amino acids longer than γ1). The γ2(2x) and γ2(3x) chains are non-disulfide-linked to the δ chain and have four or five N-glycosylation sites (Table 1). These variations in the number of exons and differences in the degree of glycosylation explain the difference in relative molecular mass of the γ1 (40 kDa) and γ2 (40 or 44 kDa, 55 kDa) chains. Depending on the γ chain, there are, therefore, three types of T cell receptor γδ dimers: the disulfide-linked γ1δ receptor, and the nondisulfide-linked γ2(2x)δ and γ2(3x)δ receptors (Fig. 4).

THE T CELL RECEPTOR-CD3 COMPLEX

Organization of the T cell receptor-CD3 complex

In addition to the αβ or γδ heterodimers which are structurally unique for each clone of T cells, the T cell receptor-CD3 complex comprises the additional nonpolymorphic CD3γ, CD3δ, CD3ε, CD3ζ, and CD3η proteins, which are identical in all T cells[9,10]. The CD3 proteins are responsible for coupling TcR occupancy to intracellular signal transduction pathways that result in the events comprising T cell activation. The CD3γ, CD3δ, and CD3ε chains contain an N-terminal Ig-like extracellular domain of type C2[32], a connecting peptide, a transmembrane region, and a cytoplasmic region (Fig. 2) (Table 1). The CD3ζ and CD3η lack the Ig-like domain. The transmembrane regions of the CD3 proteins have a predicted α-helix configuration and contain a negatively charged amino acid (aspartic acid for the CD3δ, CD3ε, CD3ζ, and CD3η chains, glutamic acid for the CD3γ chain) (Table 1). The cytoplasmic regions of the CD3 chains are considerably longer than those of the TcR α, β, γ, and δ chains and have an important role in the interaction with cytoplasmic components that are directly involved in the transduction of the antigen-binding signal. Indeed, the cytoplasmic region of the CD3 proteins possesses a characteristic motif $Yxx(L/I)x_{6-8}Yxx(L/I)$, designated as ITAM (Immunoreceptor Tyrosine-based Activation Motif). CD3γ, CD3δ, and CD3ε have one ITAM, whereas CD3ζ and CD3η have three and two ITAMs, respectively (Fig. 2) (Table 1). The phosphorylation of the CD3ζ ITAMs leads to the recruitment of SH2 (src homology 2) carrying proteins such as ZAP-70 (Zeta Associated Protein of 70 kDa).

The CD3γ, CD3δ, and CD3ε chains

The human CD3γ (25 kDa) and CD3δ (20 kDa) are glycoproteins bearing two N-linked oligosaccharide side chains and whose protein size is 16 kDa. CD3ε (20 kDa) is not glycosylated. These chains contain one Ig-like domain with an intrachain disulfide bond. The CD3G, CD3D, and CD3E genes encoding the γ, δ, and ε chains, respectively, are found within 60 kb on human chromosome 11q23 and probably arose by gene duplication. The highly homologous CD3G and CD3D genes lie within 1.5 kb of each other. Activation of T cells results in phosphorylation of CD3γ and CD3δ.

The CD3ζ and CD3η chains

The human CD3ζ chain is a 16 kDa nonglycosylated protein with no sequence or structural homology to the other CD3 or TcR chains. In contrast to the other chains, ζ has a very short extracellular region of 9 amino acids, with the vast majority of the ζ protein (112 amino acids out of 142) existing as the cytoplasmic region. As for the other CD3 chains, the transmembrane region has a negatively charged amino acid. The ζ chain is encoded by the CD3Z gene found on chromosome 1 at 1q22-q23.

In the majority of receptors, ζ exists as a disulfide-linked 32 kDa (ζζ) homodimer. Five to twenty percent of ζ is disulfide-linked to CD3η (CD3 eta), a 21 kDa splice variant of ζ, in a 37 kDa (ζη) heterodimer. Note that the ζ chain is related to the γ chain of the FcεRI, FcγRI (CD64) and FcγRIII (CD16) and can associate with CD16. Cells possess both ζζ homodimers and ζη heterodimers, with a ratio of homodimers to heterodimers ranging from 5:1 to 10:1. Activation of T cells results in tyrosine phosphorylation of CD3ζ and CD3η.

Biosynthesis and assembly of the T cell receptor-CD3 complex

A T cell cannot recognize antigen unless the TcR-CD3 complex is correctly asssembled and efficiently transported and expressed at the cell surface[9,10,46]. The genes encoding the TcR-CD3 proteins are expressed sequentially during the stages of T cell maturation. CD3γ, CD3δ, and CD3ε are synthesized by the earliest recognizable thymocytes, but the proteins remain inside the cell. Assembly of the TcR components takes place within the endoplasmic reticulum (ER) and begins soon after biosynthesis. Within the endoplasmic reticulum there is a transient, noncovalent association with a 26 kDa nonglycosylated protein, the CD3ω (omega) or TRAP (T cell Receptor Associated Protein). Upon further maturation, T cells begin to express the pre-T cell receptor, a heterodimer of pTα (pre-T cell receptor alpha chain 'substitute') and TcR β chains, on the cell surface of the pre-T cells. After synthesis of the TcR α chain, there is assembly of the full TcR receptor within the ER, and glycosylation processing of the N-linked side chains of the TcR and CD3 chains in the Golgi apparatus. The TcR-CD3 complex is then transported to the plasma membrane. Incomplete TcRs are directed from the Golgi to the lysosomes, where they are rapidly degraded, or are retained for a long period within the ER.

Activation of the T cell receptor-CD3 complex

The TcR-CD3 complex initiates signaling by engaging proximal src-related protein tyrosine kinases (PTKs), such as p56lck and p59fyn. Binding of p56lck to the CD4 and CD8 coreceptors brings the kinases into proximity with the TcR-CD3 complex. A CXCP motif in the cytoplasmic domain of CD4 and CD8 mediates binding to p56lck. This non-covalent interaction requires two cysteines in the N-terminal portion of lck. The activity of p56lck is under the control of CD45, which initially dephosphorylates the inhibitory site of p56lck. Following the antigen recognition by the αβ or γδ T cell receptors[47,48], phosphorylation of the ITAM Tyrosines of the CD3γ, CD3δ, CD3ε and CD3ζ chains by p56lck and p59fyn represents one of the earliest events on the signaling cascade. Phosphorylation of both Tyrosines within an ITAM (diphosphorylation) is essential for signaling, as this is required for efficient recruitment of the tandem SH2 domain of ZAP-70. Subsequent phosphorylation of ZAP-70 by p56lck leads to ZAP-70 activation and results in the recruitment and ZAP-70-mediated phosphorylation of effector molecules such as the adaptor proteins LAT (Linker for Activation of T cells) and SLP-76 (SH2 domain-containing Leukocyte Protein of 76 kDa), which couple immune receptors to downstream signaling pathways[49]. Thus these adaptor proteins link the T cell receptors to PLC-γ1, Grb-2/Sos, and PI3K, resulting in the activation of the calcium and MAP (Mitogen-Activated Protein) kinase pathways[48–50].

T cell activation leads to membrane reorganization and to the formation of a SMAC (SupraMolecular Activation Cluster) or mature immunological synapse with the APC. This contact shows a TcR receptor segregation together with their signaling protein complexes and is associated to coalescing lipid rafts[51]. These rafts, also referred to as GEMs, membrane glycosphingolipid-enriched microdomains, contain GPI (Glycosylphosphatidylinositol)-linked proteins, src-like tyrosine kinases and other proteins targeted to rafts through saturated acyl chains[52–55]. The central area of a SMAC contains the TcR-CD3 complex, CD4 or CD8 coreceptors, CD28 costimulatory molecule, CD2 adhesion molecule, p56lck and p59fyn kinases, and the Ca^{2+} independent Protein Kinase C (PKC) θ (thêta), while the peripheral regions are enriched in LFA-1 (Lymphocyte Function-Associated-1) adhesion molecule and the cytoskeletal protein talin[56]. TcR induced cytoskeletal changes involve signaling through SLP76-Vav-Nck to activate effectors of the Rho-family of GTPases[50]. CD45 is excluded from the vicinity of the ligated TcR[57]. The segregation of TcR and signaling molecules appears critical for lymphocyte activation[56].

References

[1] Saito, H. et al. (1984) Nature 309, 757–762.
[2] Lefranc, M.-P. and Rabbitts T. H. (1985) Nature 316, 464–466.
[3] Brenner, M.B. et al. (1986) Nature 322, 145–149.
[4] Bank, I. et al. (1986) Nature 322, 179–181.
[5] Weiss, A. et al. (1986) Proc. Natl Acad. Sci. USA 83, 6998–7002.
[6] Moingeon, P. et al. (1986) Nature 323, 638–640.
[7] Lefranc, M.-P. (1990) Eur. Cytokine Network 1, 121–130.
[8] Lefranc, M.-P. (1994) *In*: Immunochemistry, van Oss C. J. and van Regenmortel M.H.V. eds. Marcel Dekker Inc., New York, pp 129–157.
[9] Clevers, H. et al. (1988) Annu. Rev. Immunol. 6, 629–662.
[10] Ashwell, J.D. and Klausner, R. D. (1990) Annu. Rev. Immunol. 8, 139–167.
[11] Bierer, B.E. et al. (1989) Annu. Rev. Immunol. 7, 579–599.
[12] Kabelitz, D. et al. (1999) Microbes and Infection 1, 255–261.
[13] Kabelitz, D. et al. (1999) Springer Semin. Immunopathol. 21, 55–75.
[14] Kabelitz, D. et al. (2000) Int. Arch. Allergy Immunol. 122, 1–7.
[15] Kronenberg, M. et al. (1986) Annu. Rev. Immunol. 4, 529–591.
[16] Harty, J.T. et al. (2000) Annu. Rev. Immunol. 18, 275–308.

17 Rosat, J.P. et al. (1999) J. Immunol. 162, 366–371.
18 Valittuti, S. et al. (1995) Nature 375, 148–151.
19 Matsui, K. et al. (1994) Proc. Natl Acad. Sci. USA 91, 862–866.
20 Corr, M. et al. (1994) Science 265, 946–948.
21 Demotz, S. et al. (1990) Science 249, 1028–1031.
22 Harding, C.V. and Unanue, E.R. (1990) Nature 346, 574–576.
23 Christinck, E.R. et al. (1990) Nature 352, 67–70.
24 Padovan, E. et al. (1993) Science 262, 422–424.
25 Padovan, E. et al. (1995) J. Exp. Med. 181, 1587–1591.
26 Davodeau, F. et al. (1995) J. Exp. Med. 181, 1391–1398.
27 Haas, W. et al. (1993) Annu. Rev. Immunol. 11, 637–685.
28 Hayday, A.C. (2000) Annu. Rev. Immunol. 18, 975–1026.
29 Davodeau, F. et al. (1993) Science 260, 1800–1802.
30 Hinz, T. et al. (1996) Br. J. Hematol. 94, 62–64.
31 Peyrat, M.A. et al. (1995) J. Immunol. 155, 3060–3067.
32 Williams, A. F. and Barclay, A. N. (1988) Annu. Rev. Immunol. 6, 381–405.
33 Lefranc, M.-P. (1999) The Immunologist 7, 132–136.
34 Bentley, G.A. et al. (1995) Science 267, 1984–1987.
35 Fields, B.A. et al. (1996) Science 270, 1821–1824.
36 Fields, B.A. et al. (1995) Nature 384, 188–192.
37 Garcia, K.C. et al. (1996) Science 274, 209–219.
38 Garboczi, D.N. et al. (1996) Nature 384, 134–141.
39 Ding, Y.H. et al. (1998) Immunity 8, 409–411.
40 Reinherz, E.L. et al. (1999) Science 286, 1913–1921.
41 Li, H. et al. (1998) Nature 391, 502–506.
42 Wang, J. et al. (1998) EMBO J. 17, 10–26.
43 Lefranc, M.-P. et al. (1986) Proc. Natl Acad. Sci. USA 83, 9596–9600.
44 Lefranc, M.-P. and Rabbitts, T. H. (1989) TIBS 14, 214–218.
45 Buresi, C. et al. (1989) Immunogenetics 29, 161–172.
46 Klausner, R. D. et al. (1990) Annu. Rev. Cell. Biol. 6, 403–431.
47 Janeway, C.A., Jr. (1992) Annu. Rev. Immunol. 10, 645–674.
48 Love, P.E. and Shores E. W. (2000) Immunity 12, 591–597.
49 Rudd, C.E. (1999) Cell 96, 5–8.
50 Van Leeuwen, J.E. and Samelson, L. E. (1999) Curr. Opin. Immunol. 11, 242–248.
51 Xavier, R. et al. (1998) Immunity 8, 723–732.
52 Montixi, C. et al. (1998) EMBO J. 17, 5334–5348.
53 Simons, K. and Ikonen, E. (1997) Nature 387, 569–572.
54 Harder, T. et al. (1998) J. Cell. Biol. 141, 929–942.
55 Acuto, O. and Cantrell, D. (2000) Annu. Rev. Immunol. 18, 165–184.
56 Penninger, J.M. and Crabtree, G.R. (1999) Cell 96, 9–12.
57 Sykulev, Y. (2000) The Immunologist 8, 51–57.

3 Synthesis of the T cell receptor chains

Synthesis of the T cell receptor chains occurs during T cell differentiation in the thymus. The normal human thymus develops early on in fetal development, and is colonized by stem cells at 7 to 8 weeks of gestational age. Recent data on human postnatal thymus function support the notion that the human thymus is functional well into adult life (into the sixth decade)[1]. The thymus is essential for the initial establishment of the peripheral T cell pool expressing the αβ and γδ TcR. Children born without a thymus (complete DiGeorge syndrome) lack functional peripheral T cells.

As for immunoglobulins[2], the constant region (C-REGION) of the TcR chains is encoded by a constant gene, whereas the variable domain (V-J-REGION of an α or γ chain, V-D-J-REGION of a β or δ chain) is encoded by the joining together of noncontiguous DNA genes: a variable (V) gene and a joining (J) gene for the α and γ chains, a V gene, a diversity (D) gene, and a J gene for the β and δ chains (Fig. 1). As with immunoglobulins, three hypervariable regions or CDR (Complementarity Determining Regions) determine the recognition and binding to the antigen, in the three-dimensional structure. Both CDR1 and CDR2 are encoded within the V genes, whereas the CDR3 occur at the V-J junction in the α and γ chains, and at the V-D-J junction in the β and δ chains. The somatic V-J and V-D-J rearrangements occur during lymphocyte development in the thymus (Fig. 2). There is a chronological order of the rearrangements, with the TRD locus rearranging first, then TRG, TRB, and, at the last, TRA[3].

SYNTHESIS OF THE T CELL RECEPTOR CHAINS

Somatic V-J rearrangements in the TRA and TRG loci

For the synthesis of a TcR α chain or a TcR γ chain (Fig. 3), there is first a joining of a V gene to one of the J genes, with deletion of the DNA located between these genes (V-J rearrangement). The rearranged V-J gene, the intermediary DNA between the J gene that has been used and the C gene, and the C gene itself, are transcribed. The primary transcript is then spliced (RNA maturation). The messenger RNA is translated into a polypeptide chain by the ribosomes. The signal peptide is cleaved off following the entry of the polypeptide chain into the endoplasmic reticulum (ER) and a mature TcR α or γ chain is produced.

Somatic V-D-J rearrangements in the TRB and TRD loci

For the synthesis of a TcR β chain (Fig. 4) or a TcR δ chain, two successive rearrangements are required: first, one of the D and one of the J genes are joined together, then one of the V genes is joined to the partially rearranged D-J genes. The rearranged V-D-J gene is transcribed with the downstream C gene into a V-D-J-C premessenger RNA. The primary transcript is then spliced into mature RNA. The messenger RNA is translated into a polypeptide chain by the ribosomes. The signal peptide is cleaved off following the entry of the polypeptide chain into the ER and a mature TcR β or δ chain is produced.

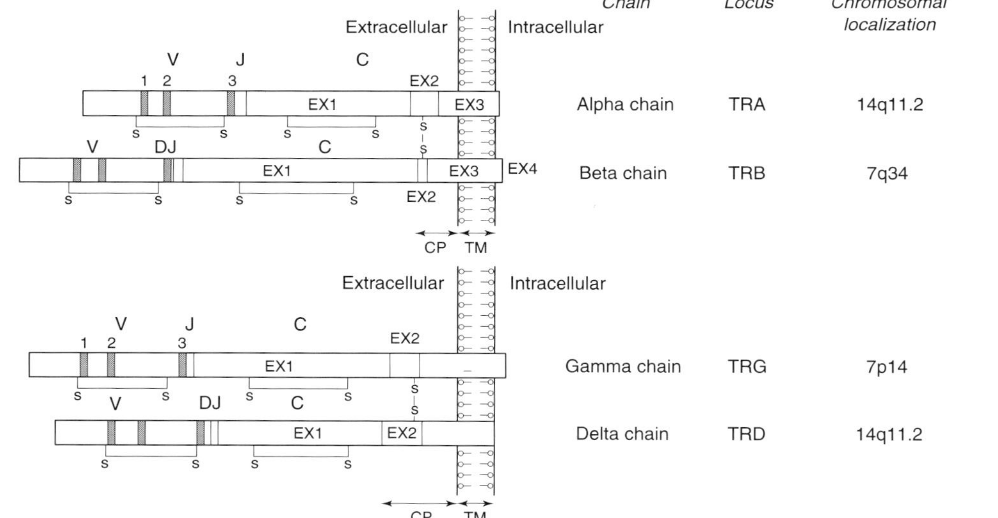

Figure 1. *Schematic representation of αβ and γδ T cell receptors. The variable domain of an alpha or gamma chain, or V-J-REGION, is encoded by two rearranged genes (one TRAV rearranged to one TRAJ for an alpha chain, one TRGV rearranged to one TRGJ for a gamma chain). The variable domain of a beta or delta chain, or V-D-J-REGION, is encoded by three rearranged genes (TRBV, TRBD, and TRBJ for a beta chain; TRDV, TRDD, and TRDJ for a delta chain). The three hypervariable regions or CDR (Complementarity Determining Regions) 1, 2, and 3 (hatched in the figure) determine the recognition and binding site to the antigen, in the three-dimensional structure. The C-REGION of the alpha, beta, gamma, and delta chains, is encoded by the TRAC, TRBC, TRGC, and TRDC genes, respectively, and comprises a constant (C) domain, a connecting peptide (CP), a transmembrane region (TM), and a very short (absent for the delta chain) intracytoplasmic region. A γ1 chain as represented in the figure, has a single exon 2 and is disulfide-linked to the δ chain. In contrast the two types of γ2 chain, γ2(2x) and γ2(3x), have a duplicated and triplicated exon 2 coding region, respectively, without cysteine in the connecting peptide and, therefore, there is no γ2-δ interchain disulfide bridge. V = V-REGION, J = J-REGION, D = D-REGION (or more exactly N-AND-D-REGION to take into account the N-diversity), C = C-REGION.*

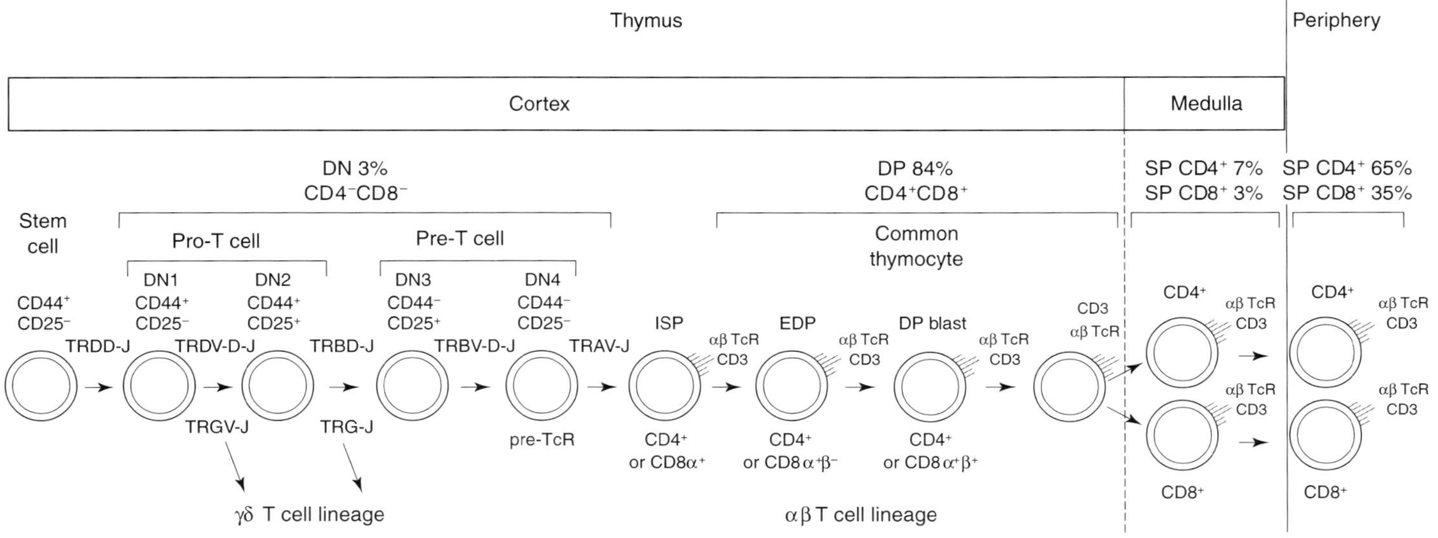

Figure 2. *T cell differentiation from the hematopoietic stem cell to the mature αβ T cells. See also paragraph 'Chronological order of the T cell receptor gene rearrangements' in this chapter. CD44 and CD25 are surface markers, extensively used to characterize the mouse early T cell differentiation populations. The ISP and EDP cells have been characterized in the human thymus[3]. The pre-TcR plays a crucial role at the checkpoint between DN and DP stages. The γδ T cell lineage diverges from the αβ T cell lineage prior to the expression of the pre-TcR. DN = double negative (CD4⁻CD8⁻), DP = double positive (CD4⁺CD8⁺ α⁺β⁺), SP = single positive (CD4⁺ or CD8⁺), ISP = immature single positive (CD4⁺ or CD8⁺), EDP = early double positive (CD4⁺ CD8α⁺β⁻), lo = low, hi = high.*

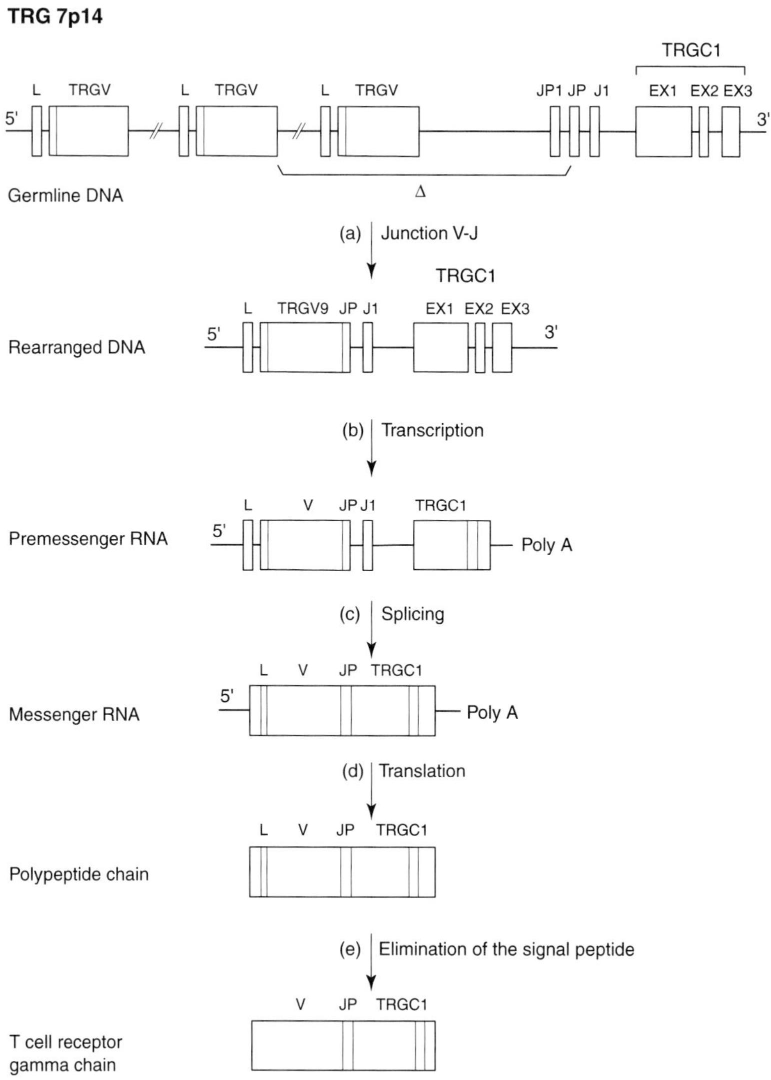

Figure 3. *Synthesis of a TcR gamma chain. (a) At the DNA level, one of the TRGV genes is joined to one of the TRGJ genes, with deletion of the intermediary DNA, to create a rearranged TRGV-J gene. (b) The rearranged TRGV-J gene is transcribed with the downstream TRGC gene into a TRGV-J-C premessenger RNA. (c) The RNA sequences corresponding to the introns and to non-used TRGJ genes are excised by splicing, and a mature messenger which comprises the spliced coding regions, and the 5' and 3' untranslated sequences, is obtained. (d) The messenger RNA is translated into a polypeptide chain by the ribosomes. (e) The signal peptide is cleaved off by a peptidase following the entry of the polypeptide chain into the endoplasmic reticulum, and a mature TcR gamma chain is produced. L = L-PART1 (L for Leader).*

ORIGIN OF THE VARIABLE DOMAIN DIVERSITY OF THE T CELL RECEPTORS

The diversity of the T cell receptor chains depends on two mechanisms: combinatorial diversity, which is a consequence of the number of V, D, and J genes (Chapter 4), and the N-region diversity, which creates an extensive and clonal somatic diversity at the V-J and V-D-J junctions.

Combinatorial diversity

Recombination signals

The junction of T cell receptor genes results, as for the immunoglobulin genes, from the activity of the recombinase enzyme which recognizes the recombination signals, or heptamer-nonamer, present 3′ (downstream) from the V genes, 5′ (upstream) from the J genes, and on both sides of the D genes (Fig. 5). The heptamer-nonamer sequences are separated by 12 ± 1 or 23 ± 1 nucleotides. Effective recombination takes place between signals separated by a 12 ± 1 base pair (bp) spacer and a 23 ± 1 bp spacer (12/23 rule), as first observed in immunoglobulin rearrangements[4]. Therefore, rearrangements between two V genes or two J genes do not usually occur. In contrast, the TRBD and TRDD genes possess a 12 bp spacer in 5′ and a 23 bp spacer in 3′, which allow V-D-D-J rearrangements (rare for the TRB locus, but quite common for the TRD locus, where V-D1-D2-D3-J joinings have even been described). These types of rearrangements are not possible in the immunoglobulin heavy chain locus.

Rearrangements by deletion or inversion

In most cases, rearrangements in the T cell receptor loci result from deletional joining. This is in agreement with the V genes being localized upstream from the J (or D and J) and C genes, and in the same orientation of transcription. In such deletional rearrangements, the V and J (or D-J) genes form a contiguous coding sequence, or coding joint, whereas the reciprocal fusion of the recombination signals, or signal joint, leads to the excision of a circular DNA molecule[5-7](Fig. 6A). When the V and J (or D-J) genes to be joined are in opposite orientation of transcription on the chromosome, rearrangements occur by inversional joinings.

As a result, the DNA sequences initially located between the V and J (or D-J) genes which rearrange, as well as the signal joints, remain on the chromosome (Fig. 6B). This is exemplified by the rearrangements of the murine TRBV31[8] and human TRBV30[9] located downstream from the TRBC2 gene, the murine TRDV5[10] and human TRDV3[11-13] located downstream from the TRDC gene. According to the recombination model proposed by Alt and Baltimore[14] and by Alt and Yancopoulos[15], whether or not joining leads to deletion or inversion is simply based on the relative orientation of the participating genes in the chromosome.

Recombinase

Two genes, RAG1[16] (Recombination Activating Gene 1) and RAG2[17], were characterized in 1989 and 1990, respectively. These two genes are transcribed in

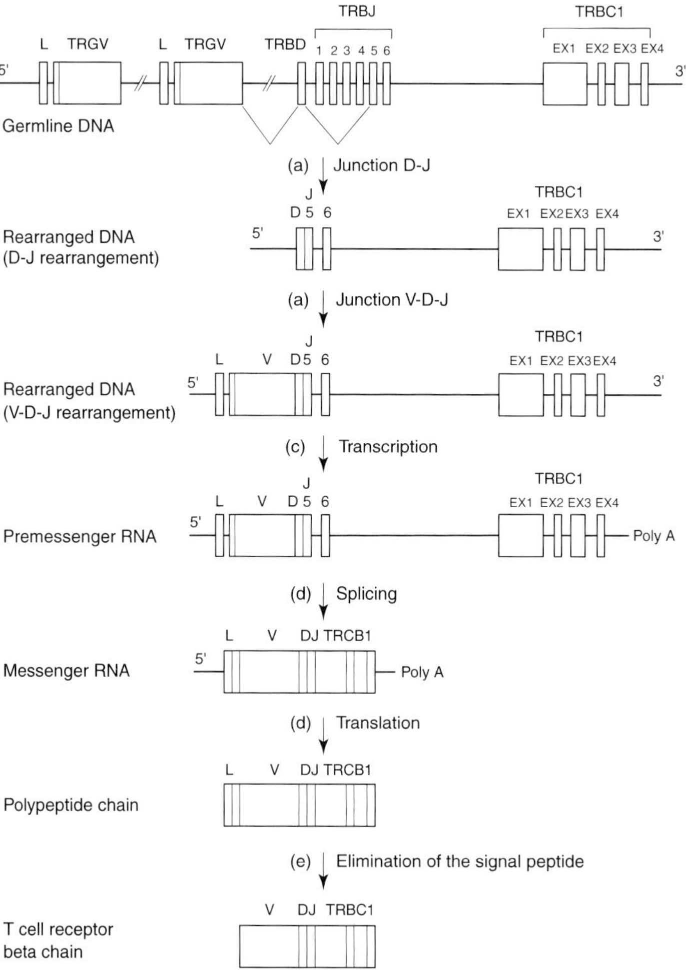

Figure 4. *Synthesis of a TcR beta chain. (a) At the DNA level, in a first step, one of the TRBD genes is joined to one of the TRBJ genes, with deletion of the intermediary DNA, to create a partially rearranged D-J gene. In a second step, one of the TRBV gene is joined to D-J, with deletion of the intermediary DNA, to generate a completely rearranged TRBV-D-J gene. (b) The rearranged TRBV-D-J gene is transcribed with the downstream TRBC gene into a TRBV-D-J-C premessenger RNA. (c) The RNA sequences corresponding to the introns and to the non-used TRBJ genes are excised by splicing, and a mature messenger which comprises the spliced coding regions, and the 5' and 3' untranslated sequences, is obtained. (d) The messenger RNA is translated into a polypeptide chain by the ribosomes. (e) The signal peptide is cleaved off by a peptidase following the entry of the polypeptide chain into the endoplasmic reticulum, and a mature TcR beta chain is produced. L = L-PART1 (L for Leader).*

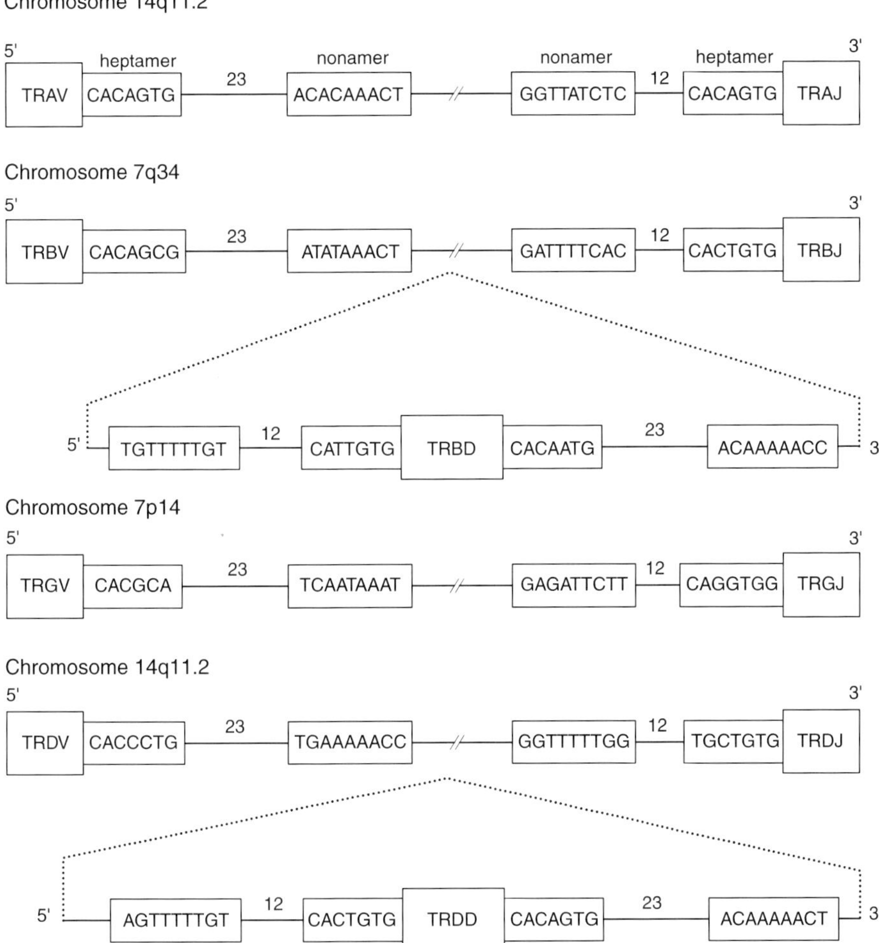

Figure 5. *Examples of human T cell receptor V, D, and J gene recombination signals. Although the heptamer and the nonamer sequences are well conserved, there are sequence differences between individual genes as shown in the recombination signal tables in Section II. Spacer lengths are 12 ± 1 or 23 ± 1 bp. This is known as the 12/23 rule.*

lymphocytes that have a recombinase activity (that is, the B and T lymphocytes at an early stage of their development). In-vitro nonlymphoid cells are able to recombine transfected V-D-J recombination substrates following introduction of expressed RAG1 and RAG2[17]. These two genes are unrelated in amino acid sequence, but are located only 8 kb apart on the same chromosome (11p13). Although the 5' untranslated regions of the cDNAs of both genes contain spliced exons, the RAG1 and RAG2 coding sequences are contained within a single exon. The two genes and their organization have been highly conserved in vertebrate evolution. By homologous recombination, Mombaerts et al.[18] and Shinkai et al.[19]

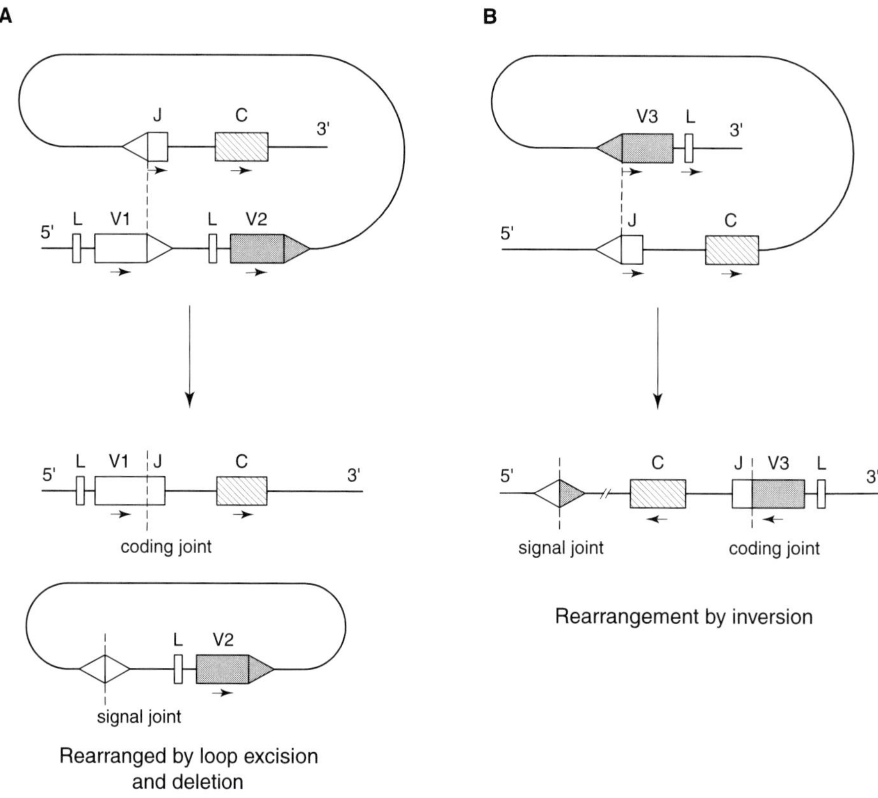

Figure 6. *Rearrangements by loop excision and deletion (**A**), and by inversion (**B**).*
L = L-PART1 (L for Leader).

have disrupted RAG1 and RAG2, respectively, in the mouse genome. The RAG1 or RAG2 deficient mice have identical phenotypes (i.e., their lymphoid organs are devoid of mature B and T cells). The arrest of B and T cell development occurs at a very early stage, preventing a significant accumulation of immature lymphoid cells. Apart from the complete deficiency of B and T cells, the knock-out RAG1 or RAG2 mice have no other developmental defects and are fertile. The RAG1 and RAG2 proteins are responsible for sequence-specific recognition and DNA cleavage, and they appear to perform multiple post-cleavage roles in the reaction as well[20].

Junctional diversity

The N-diversity results from the deletion of nucleotides at the extremities of the coding V, D and J genes by action of an exonuclease and the addition, at random, of nucleotides by the terminal deoxynucleotidyl transferase (TdT)[14]. This enzyme preferentially adds G and C nucleotides at the junctions and is specifically transcribed during lymphocytic maturation. In contrast with the immunoglobulin

N-regions, T cell receptor N-regions are less rich in G and C and occasionally display short nucleotide sequences, identical with those found at the extremities of the coding region of the germline V and J genes. These sequences from the V and J ends could be used, in some cases, as templates by the enzyme[21].

The rearranged TcR genes have a junctional diversity that is more important than that of the immunoglobulins. Indeed, (1) the N-diversity affects all the TcR loci, whereas it affects only the immunoglobulin heavy chain genes; (2) the possibility to join two or even three D genes in the TRD locus still increases the diversity in originating three (or four) N-sequences at the V-D-D-(D-)J junctions; (3) the TRBD and TRDD genes can be read in the three reading frames (which is not generally the case for the IGHD genes).

Nucleotides that are palindromic to the last nucleotides of the germline V genes, to the first nucleotides of the germline J genes, and to the ends of the germline D genes, are designated as 'P' nucleotides and are found at the V-J or V-D-J junctions in cells in which the TcR genes seem not to have been submitted to the exonuclease activity. Indeed, these P nucleotides are only identified when the ends of the respective V, D, and J coding regions are intact[22].

In the T cell receptor loci, there are no somatic mutations. This has been demonstrated by the complete identity of several rearranged genes with their germline counterparts and represents an important difference from the immunoglobulin genes [23]. As a consequence, oligonucleotides that correspond to V and J sequences can be used as specific primers for in-vitro DNA amplification by the polymerase chain reaction (PCR)[24-27], and the sequencing of the N-region of the rearranged genes. This method can be applied to the identification of the N-region of malignant clones. Specific oligonucleotides can then be used to detect the residual malignant cells during the treatment of leukemia or in bone marrow samples before an autograft. Anchored-PCR, which uses only one specific primer, has been extensively used for the analysis of TcR V, D, and J gene usage, and for the detection of TcR expression[27,28].

THE T CELL RECEPTOR CONSTANT REGIONS AND GENES

The constant regions of the TcR chains are encoded by the constant genes. Figure 7 shows the characteristics of the TRAC, TRBC1 and TRBC2, TRGC1 and TRGC2, and TRDC genes which encode the constant region of the TcR alpha, beta 1 and beta 2, gamma 1 and gamma 2, and delta chains, respectively. TRBC1 and TRBC2, and TRGC1 and TRGC2, represent duplicated genes. TRGC2(2x) and TRGC2(3x) are allelic forms of the TRGC2 gene with duplication (2x) or triplication (3x) of exon 2. These constant genes encode the constant domain, the connecting peptide, the transmembrane region and the intracytoplasmic region as described in Table 1 of Chapter 2. At the genomic level, each constant gene consists of several exons, EX1 to EX4 (Table 1). EX1 encodes the constant domain (91 to 129 amino acids). The EX2, EX2T and/or EX2R, and the 5' part of EX3 encode the connecting peptide, whereas the 3' part of EX3 encodes the transmembrane region. The TRBC1 and TRBC2 EX4 exon encodes the short intracytoplasmic region (the TRAC and TRDC EX4 are not translated).

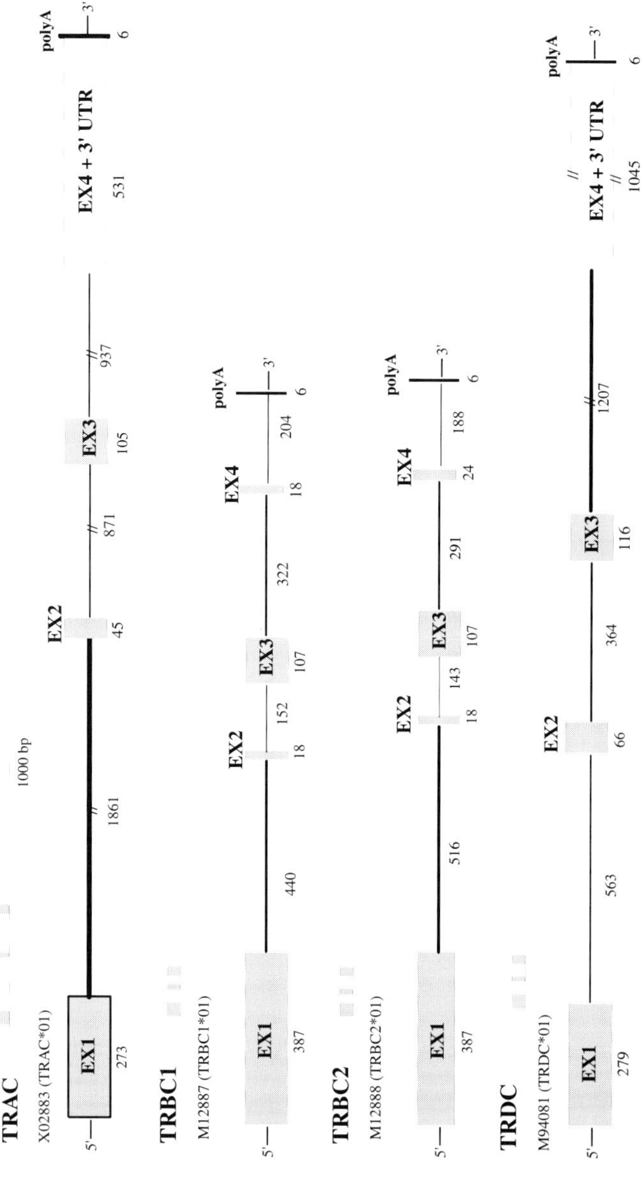
1000 bp
TRAC
X02883 (TRAC*01)
5'
EX1
273
1861
EX2
45
871
EX3
105
937
EX4 + 3' UTR
531
polyA
3'
6
TRBC1
M12887 (TRBC1*01)
5'
EX1
387
440
EX2
18
152
EX3
107
322
EX4
18
204
polyA
3'
6
TRBC2
M12888 (TRBC2*01)
5'
EX1
387
516
EX2
18
143
EX3
107
291
EX4
24
188
polyA
3'
6
TRDC
M94081 (TRDC*01)
5'
EX1
279
563
EX2
66
364
EX3
116
1207
EX4 + 3' UTR
1045
polyA
3'
6

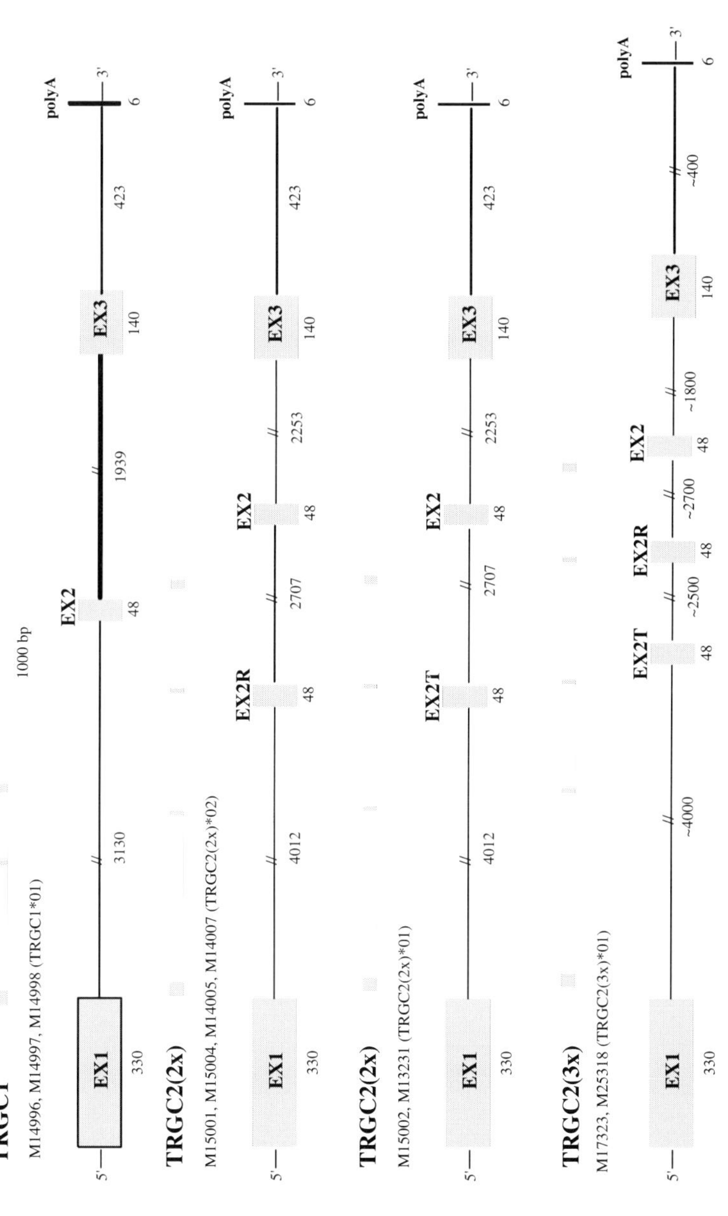

Figure 7. *Structure of the human T cell receptor constant genes. Sequences and references for the individual genes and alleles are given in Section II. Size of the exons and introns are in base pairs (bp). Schematic gene representations (scale indicated on the first line) are also shown besides each gene name. The TRAC and TRDC "EX4 + 3' UTR" are untranslated. The genomic organization of TRGC1 and TRGC2(2x)*02 is from reference 29. Size of the introns is from AF159056. The genomic organization of the TRGC2(2x)*03 and TRGC2(3x) is from reference 30.*

Table 1. *Characteristics of the human T cell receptor constant regions*

C genes Characteristics		TRAC	TRBC1	TRBC2	TRGC1	TRGC2 (2x)	TRGC2 (3x)	TRDC
EX1	Length in number of amino acids	91	129	129	110	110	110	93
	1st–CYS (1)	23	31	31	32	32	32	21
	2nd–CYS (1)	73	96	96	88	88	88	72
	N-glycosylation sites (1)	33 67 78	70	70	66	66	66	15 78
EX2T	Length in number of amino acids	–	–	–	–	16*	16	–
	N-glycosylation sites (1)	–	–	–	–	0	0	–
EX2R	Length in number of amino acids	–	–	–	–	16*	16	–
	N-glycosylation sites (1)	–	–	–	–	10	10	–
EX2	Length in number of amino acids	15	6	6	16	16	16	22
	N-glycosylation sites (1)	–	–	–	10, 16	10,16	10,16	–
EX3	Length in number of amino acids	35	36	36	47	47	47	39
	N-glycosylation sites (1)	8	–	–	–	9	9	–
	Cysteine (1) (2)	4	2	2	11	–	–	18
EX4	Length in number of amino acids	n.t.	6	8	0	0	0	n.t.
C–REGION Length in number of amino acids		141	177	179	173	189	205	154

* polymorphism of the TRGC2(2x) duplicated exon 2 which can be from the EX2T or EX2R type.
n.t. not translated.
(1) Amino acid position. Numbering starts from the first codon of each individual exon.
(2) Cysteine involved in the interdisulfide bridge, and localized in the TcR chain connecting peptide.

REPERTOIRE OF THE $\alpha\beta$ AND $\gamma\delta$ T CELLS

The diversity of the T cell receptors that results from both the combinatorial association of α and β chains, or γ and δ chains, and the junctional N-diversity affect the specificity of the T cell receptors and, therefore, play a major role in the development of the T cell repertoire.

Repertoire of the $\alpha\beta$ T cells

The functional $\alpha\beta$ TcR repertoire in an individual is selected from a population of cells containing randomly rearranged TRAV and TRBV genes, by a combination of positive and negative selective events that occur during intrathymic maturation. Both helper and cytotoxic $\alpha\beta$ T cells draw upon the same pool of germline TRAV and TRBV genes in the production of their antigen receptors (Chapter 4). Both Vα and Vβ domains contribute to the antigen-binding site. There is no simple and general correlation between use of any TRAV or TRBV genes and phenotype, function, specificity, or MHC restriction. However, in some systems, receptors encoded by particular TRAV and TRBV genes may be selected by particular antigen-MHC configurations.

Repertoire of the $\gamma\delta$ T cells

The potential combinatorial diversity of the γ and δ chains is more limited than that of the α and β chains (Chapter 4). Moreover, it is restricted by the preferential usage of some V, D and J genes. In humans, most of the peripheral $\gamma\delta$ T cells express a preferential TRGV and TRDV rearrangement[31–33]. Indeed, TRGV9-JP and TRDV2 are preferentially expressed in human peripheral $\gamma\delta$ T cells (80–95 % of the $\gamma\delta$ T cells) and the corresponding TRGV9-JP-C1 chains are frequently associated with TRDV2-D3-J-C chains[31–33]. These $\gamma\delta$ T cells respond to microbial phosphoantigens.

Antibodies that recognize specifically epitopes of the human Cδ (TCRδ-1[34], TCR $\gamma\delta$-1[35]), Vδ1-Jδ1 (δTCS-1[36]), Vδ2 (BB3[37]), Vδ3 (p11.10b[38]), Vγ1 subgroup, and Vγ9 regions[39–41] are precious tools in the characterization of the human $\gamma\delta$ T cells.

In the human, epithelial tissues contain $\gamma\delta$ T cells in significantly lower numbers than in the mouse. Representation of the $\gamma\delta$ T cells in adult human skin is not significantly different from that in peripheral blood, whereas, in intestinal intraepithelium, most of the $\gamma\delta$ T cells express TRGV1 subgroup genes and the TRDV1 gene. The $\gamma\delta$:$\alpha\beta$ ratio among intestinal intraepithelial lymphocytes (IELs) is about 1:5, compared with about 1:50 in the lymph node.

Polymorphism of the TRGV1 subgroup genes by insertion/deletion[42,43] and differences in the structural characteristics of the TRGC2 alleles[30,43] create a polymorphic repertoire in the different populations (Fig. 8).

CHRONOLOGICAL ORDER OF THE T CELL RECEPTOR GENE REARRANGEMENTS

The human T cell receptor genes are rearranged and expressed in a specific order, TRD, TRG, TRB, and TRA[3], during thymic development, and the $\gamma\delta$ T cells appear before the $\alpha\beta$ T cells during thymic ontogeny[44]. In humans, a distinct wave has been described in the early fetal thymus, and a chronology of the TRG rearrangements has

A

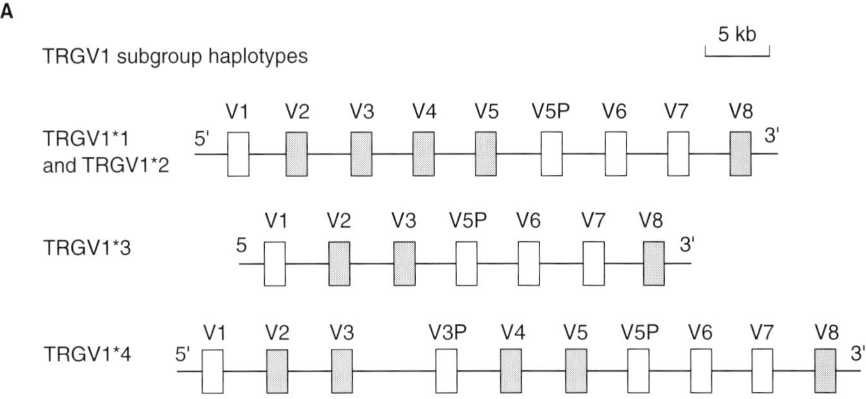

B

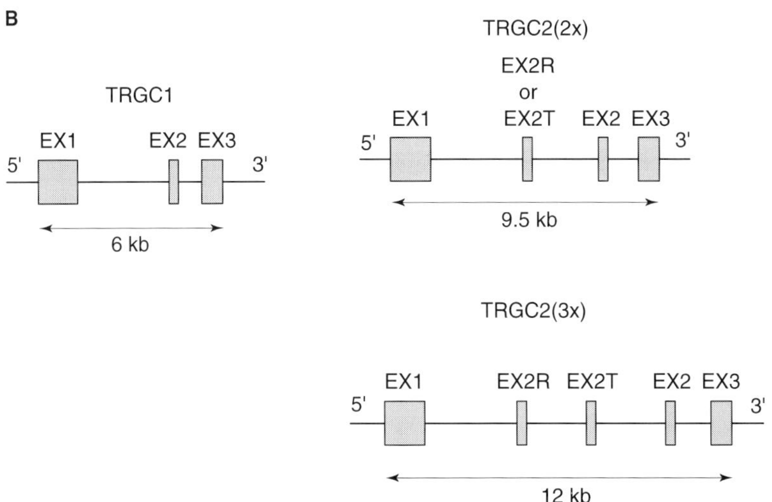

Figure 8. *Allelic polymorphism of the human TRG genes. (A) Schematic representation of the TRGV1 subgroup haplotypes[42,43]. Functional variable genes are shown as grey boxes, and pseudogenes or ORF as white boxes. The TRGV1*1 and TRGV1*2 subgroup haplotypes result from the presence or absence, respectively, of polymorphic restriction sites. The TRGV1*3 subgroup haplotype corresponds to a deletion of the V4 and V5 genes and the TRGV1*4 subgroup haplotype to an insertion of 6 kb corresponding to an additional gene, V3P. (B) Schematic representation of the TRGC genes[30,43]. Exons are shown as boxes. The allelic TRGC2 genes with duplication or triplication of exon 2 are designated as TRGC2(2x) and TRGC2(3x), respectively.*

been proposed[45,46]. Indeed, most of the γδ T cells from the peripheral blood express TRGV9-JP[31], with frequently a nonproductive TRGV10-JP1 subgroup rearrangement on the other chromosome [32]. The other γδ T cells express a TRGVI gene joined to J1 or J2. These rearrangements, which use genes that are located upstream of TRGV9 and downstream from JP on the chromosome, most probably occur after the TRGV9-JP rearrangements. This has been suggested by two observations: (1) all αβ T cells (which appear after the γδ T cells) display TRGV1 subgroup genes rearranged to J1 or J2, and this on both chromosomes[47]; (2) two successive rearrangements, first TRGV9-JP, and second involving TRGV3 and TRGJ1, have been described on the same chromosome in the SP-F7 cell line[45]. Such a situation was observed because the second rearrangement occurred by inversion and, therefore, maintained the intermediary DNA and the first TRGV9-JP rearrangement on the chromosome (Fig. 9). Thus, the order of the rearrangements and the developmentally regulated V gene expression seem to depend, in part, on the location of V and J genes in the TRG and TRD loci, the first waves using the most proximal V and J genes, and the last waves using the most distal V and J genes[46] (Fig. 10). However, other factors may also be involved, such as transcriptional regulation of V genes, structural constraint for the pairing of some γ and δ chains, and intrathymic selection by determinants with a programmed expression during thymic development.

The TRD and TRG loci are the first loci to rearrange during thymic ontogeny (Fig. 1). If both loci show a functional (in-frame) rearrangement, and if both the γ and δ chains are synthesized, the T cells express a γδ TcR at the cell surface. Partial TRBD-J rearrangements may be observed in the γδ T cells, and some of them express immature TRBC transcripts or even sterile TRAC transcripts. However, the expression of a functional γδ TcR at the surface stops further rearrangements of the TRB and TRA loci. If the γδ TcR cannot be expressed at the cell surface, either as a consequence of nonfunctional (out-of-frame) or nonproductive (absence of γ or δ membrane protein) rearrangements, or as a consequence of the activity of a silencer downregulating the TRG locus in *cis*, the TRB locus continue to rearrange. Partial TRBD-J rearrangements are followed by complete TRBV-D-J rearrangements. The pre-TcR, a heterodimer which consists of a rearranged TcR β chain disulfide-linked to the invariant surrogate α chain, pTα, is expressed at the cell surface of immature thymocytes. The expression of the pre-TcR associated with the CD3 proteins signals cessation of TRBV-D-J rearrangements, and thymocyte developmental progression in the αβ T cell lineage. Indeed, signals delivered through the pre-TcR are crucial for cell survival and for proper transition from the DN (CD4$^-$CD8$^-$) to DP (CD4$^+$CD8$^+$) stage of the immature αβ lineage thymocytes. TRAV-J rearrangements start to occur. Functional rearrangements of one TRA locus and one TRB locus, if productive, allow the expression of a αβ TcR at the surface of a T cell.

As a consequence of the chronological order of rearrangements, all γδ and αβ T cells display rearranged TRG genes, which are, therefore, excellent markers of clonality for the cells of both phenotypes: γδ and αβ[21,23,48–51]. The localization of the TRD locus, nestled in the TRA locus, results in its deletion on rearrangement of TRAV and TRAJ genes and, therefore, at least one of the two TRD loci is deleted in αβ T cells. That deletion could occur in two steps: a deletion of the TRD locus, involving specific sequences located upstream from TRDD1 (sequence δ REC) and downstream from the TRDC gene (sequence φJα)[52,53], would take place before the TRAV-J rearrangements.

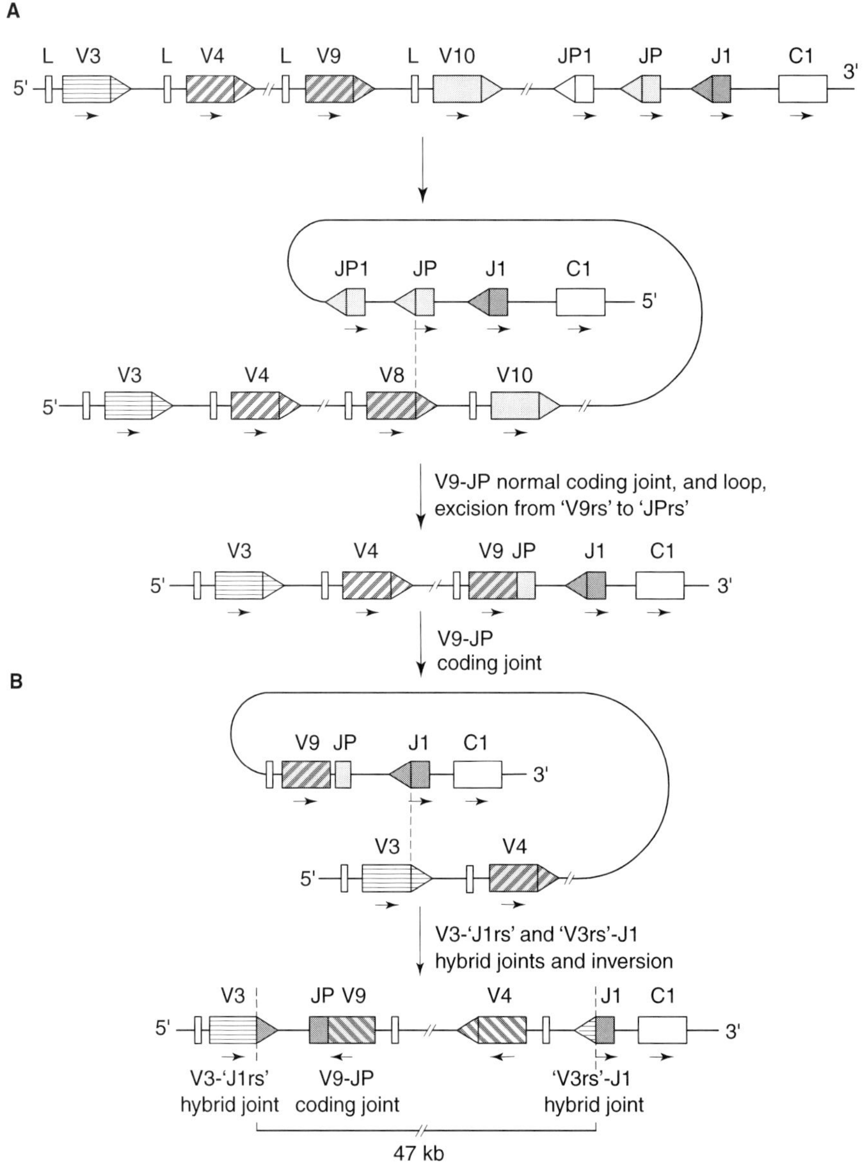

Figure 9. *Schematic representation of two successive TRGV-J rearrangements on the same chromosome[45]. (A) A standard rearrangement by loop excision and deletion led to a V9-JP joining. (B) A second rearrangement between V3 and J1 resulted in the formation of reciprocal hybrid joints, and in a 47 kb inversion and, therefore, the maintenance on the chromosome of the previous V9-JP rearrangement. Horizontal arrows indicate orientation of the transcription. Recombination signals are shown by triangles, and coding regions by rectangles. L = L-PART1 (L for leader).*

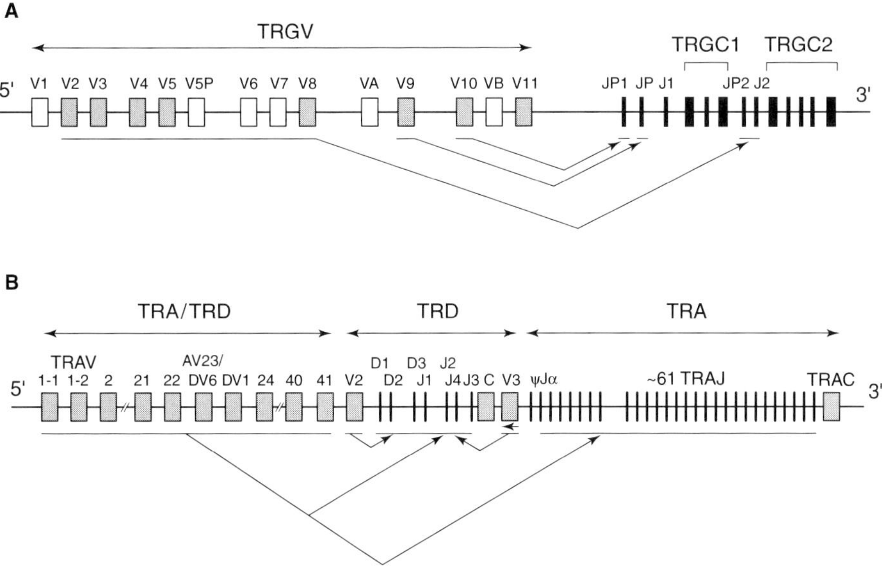

Figure 10. *Chronological order of the human TRG **(A)** and TRD/TRA **(B)** rearrangements (modified from reference 46). Exons of the TRAC and TRDC genes are not shown. The non-productive TRGV10-JP1 rearrangements (TRGV10 is not functional) precede the frequent TRGV9-JP rearrangements which characterize most of the circulating γδ T cells. Later productive rearrangements involve functional TRGV1 subgroup genes (V2, V3, V4, V5, V8) and more downstream TRGJ genes (J1, JP2, J2). The TRDV and TRAV/DV (for example, AV23/DV6) rearrangements to TRDD and TRDJ genes precede the TRA rearrangements in the TRA/TRD locus. In the αβ T cell lineage the TRAV and TRAV/DV genes rearrange to the TRAJ genes, therefore deleting the intermediate TRA genes and the TRD locus.*

ANALYSIS OF THE T CELL RECEPTOR GENE REARRANGEMENTS IN HUMANS

The TRG and TRB rearrangements are the most commonly analyzed[54]. Indeed, (1) the TRA rearrangements are difficult to study. Given the extent of the TRAJ region, a high number of Jα probes are necessary to cover all the region. Moreover, nonfunctional J-J rearrangements can be observed upstream of the functional TRAV-J rearrangement, making the Southern blot interpretation difficult[55]; (2) TRD rearrangements can be studied in immature T cells or in γδ T cells. However, in most of the αβ T cells, the TRD locus is deleted on at least one chromosome as a consequence of the TRAV-J rearrangement.

Practically, the TRG and TRB rearrangements are studied with the TRGJ1 probe pH60[48,56] and the Cβ probe, respectively, which detect the rearranged restriction fragments in Southern blot analysis[54] (Fig. 11). A TRBV-D-J rearrangement leads to a decrease, by half, in the intensity of the 24 kb germline *Bam*HI band and to the appearance of a new rearranged *Bam*HI band. The analysis of the *Eco*RI and *Hin*dIII restriction fragments allow assignment of the TRGV rearrangements to the TRBJ1 or TRBJ2 genes, respectively[54]. Since the TRGJ1 and TRGJ2 genes are highly homologous[48], it is possible by using the pH60 probe to first detect the V rearrangements with respect to J1 and J2 and, second, to identify the rearranged TRGV genes by the sizes of the rearranged *Bam*HI, *Eco*RI, and *Hin*dIII restriction fragments[49] (Table 2). Moreover, rearrangements to the additional TRGJ genes JP, JP1, and JP2, can be identified by hybridization of the *Kpn*I digests to the TRGJ1 pH60 probe[50] (Table 2, Fig. 11). Therefore, this unique probe can detect all the TRG rearrangements, whatever the TRGJ gene involved in the rearrangements[49,50]. Thus, it is a very useful tool to establish the clonality of αβ T cell clones[48], leukemic cells[57,58], and T lymphocytes expressing γδ receptor[31,32,59]. The TRDJ1 and TRDJ2 probes allow the characterization of the TRD rearrangements in the γδ T cells[59,60].

TRANSCRIPTIONAL REGULATION OF T CELL RECEPTOR GENE EXPRESSION: ENHANCERS AND SILENCERS

Rearrangements and expression of the TcR genes are coordinate- and lineage-specific. Extensive studies are currently underway to characterize the regulatory elements (promoters, enhancers, or silencers) and to identity the nuclear proteins that bind to these elements involved in the transcriptional regulation of the TcR genes. Promoters of some TcR genes, such as the TRGV9 and TRDV2 genes, do not display a TATA box[61]. A TRA enhancer has been identified at 4.5 kb 3' from the TRAC gene[62], and several nuclear transcription factors have been characterized[63–66]. A TRA enhancer has been described between the most 3' TRAJ and the TRAC gene in humans[67] but it has not been confirmed in the mouse[68] and its existence in humans is controversial. A TRB enhancer has been mapped to 5.5 kb 3' from the human TRBC2 gene[69]. A TRD enhancer has been located between TRDJ3 and TRDC in the human TRD locus[70,71]. Negative regulatory elements or silencers seem to play an important role in restricting the lineage specificity of certain TcR genes.

Three *cis*-acting sequences in 3' of the human TRG locus, and upstream of an enhancer located 6.5 kb downstream of the TRGC2 gene have been characterized[72]. The association of the enhancer with either silencer was shown to restrict transcription to the γδ T cell lines[72]. Some regulatory elements seem to function as both a silencer and an enhancer, depending on the particular set of nuclear proteins expressed by a given cell type or the precise DNA context in which they are located[65].

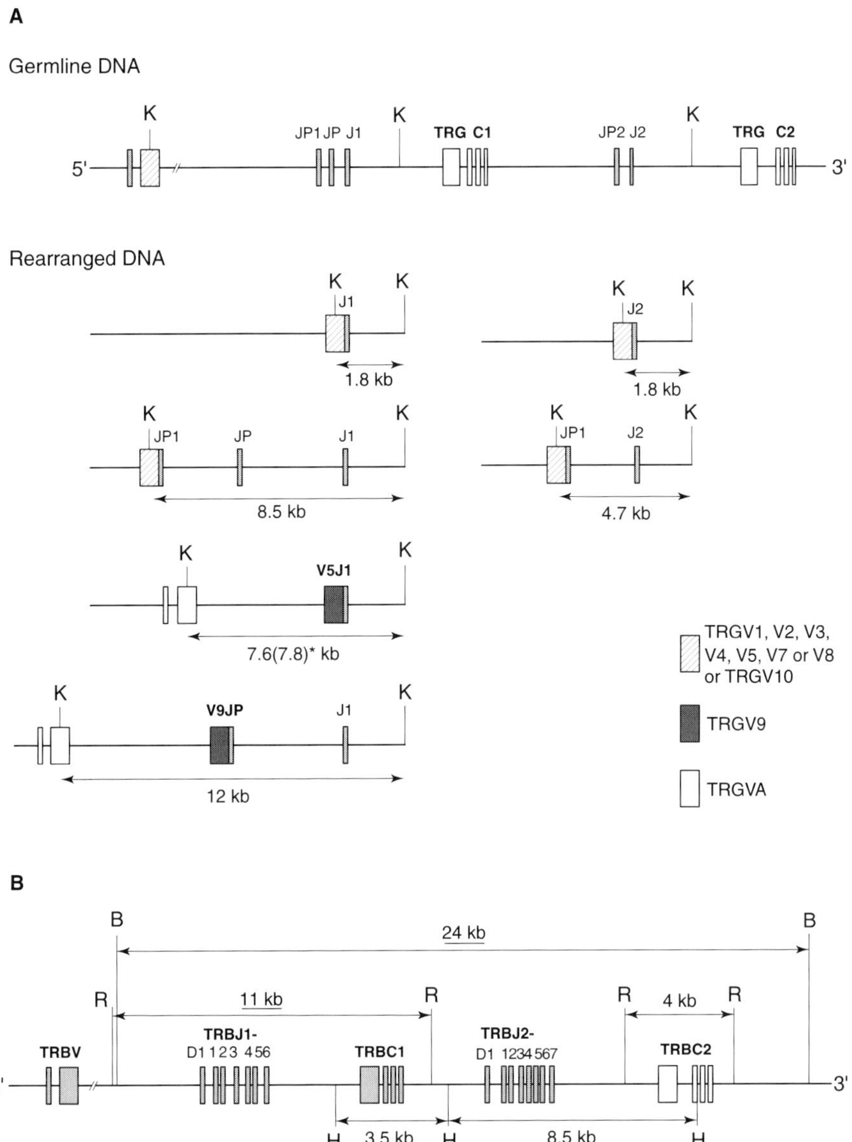

Figure 11. *Restriction fragments for the analysis of the human TRGV-J (A) and TRBV-D-J (B) rearrangements. KpnI restriction fragments hybridized to the pH60 probe[48,56] allow the assignment of the TRGV-J rearrangements to given TRGJ-genes[50] (see Table 2 for a complete description of the TRGV-J rearrangement restriction fragments). The asterisk indicates a rearranged fragment related to a RFLP (Restriction Fragment Length Polymorphism). Lengths of the BamHI, EcoRI, and HindIII restriction fragments that are informative for the detection of the TRBV-D-J rearrangements[54] are underlined. B = BamHI, H = HindIII, K = KpnI, R = EcoRI.*

Table 2. *Assignments of the human TRGV-J rearranged restriction fragments to given TRGV and TRGJ genes by hybridization to the pH60 probe*[49,50]. *Note that V7 is a pseudogene, and V10 and V11 are ORF.*

A. Assignments of the TRGV-J rearrangements to given TRGV genes (joined to J1 or J2) by hybridization to *Bam*HI, *Hin*dIII, and *Eco*RI restriction fragments to the pH60 probe[49].

Assignment to TRGV genes		Restriction fragments		
TRGV subgroup	TRGV gene	*Bam*HI	*Hin*dIII	*Eco*RI
TRGV1	V2	11.7	4.3	0.9
	V3	16	3.7	5.4 (+V2)
	V4	21	4.3	0.9
	V5	25	3.6	2.2
	V7	35	2.9	3.1
	V8	40	2.9	4.2
TRGV2	V9	15.5	4.0	2.4
TRGV3	V10	19	5.1	0.65
TRGV4	V11	12	5.6	9.5

B. Assignments of the human TRGV-J rearrangements to given TRGJ genes by hybridization of *Kpn*I restriction fragments to the pH60 probe[50]. TRGV genes that have been found rearranged are shown in parentheses.

TRGV subgroup TRGJ	TRGV1 (V2,V3,V4, V5,V7,V8)	TRGV2 (V9)	TRGV3 (V10)	TRGV4 (V11)
J1 or 2	**1.8**	7.5 (7.8)*	**1.8**	6.0
JP1	**8.5**	14.5	**8.5**	12.7
JP	5.9	**12**	5.9	10
JP2	**4.7**	10.7	**4.7**	9.0

Sizes of the *Kpn*I rearranged restriction fragments are indicated in kilobases (kb). The asterisk indicates a rearranged fragment related to an RFLP (Restriction Fragment Length Polymorphism). The rearrangements illustrated in Fig. 11 are shown in bold.

References

1 Haynes, B.H. et al. (2000) Annu. Rev. Immunol. 18, 529–560.
2 Tonegawa, S. (1983) Nature 302, 575–581.
3 Blom, B. et al. (1999) Blood 93, 3033–3043.

[4] Early, P. et al. (1980) Cell 19, 981–992.

[5] Fujimoto, S. and Yamagishi, H. (1987) Nature 327, 242–243.

[6] Okazaki, K. et al. (1987) Cell 49, 477–485.

[7] Toda, M. et al. (1988) J. Mol. Biol. 202, 219–231.

[8] Malissen, M. et al. (1986) Nature 319, 28–33.

[9] Rowen, L. et al. (1996) Science 272, 1755–1762.

[10] Iwashima, M. et al. (1988) Proc. Natl Acad. Sci. USA 85, 8161–8165.

[11] Hata, S. et al. (1989) J. Exp. Med. 169, 41–57.

[12] Loh, E.Y. et al. (1988) Proc. Natl Acad. Sci. USA 85, 9714–9718.

[13] Takihara, Y. et al. (1989) Eur. J. Immunol. 19, 571–574.

[14] Alt, F. and Baltimore, D. (1982) Proc. Natl Acad. Sci. USA 79, 4118–4122.

[15] Alt, F. and Yancopoulos, G. D. (1987) Nature 327, 189–190.

[16] Schatz, D.G. et al. (1989) Cell 59, 1035–1048.

[17] Oettinger, M.A. et al. (1990) Science 248, 1517–1522.

[18] Mombaerts, P. et al. (1992) Cell 68, 869–877.

[19] Shinkai, Y. et al. (1992) Cell 68, 855–867.

[20] Fugmann, S.D. et al. (2000) Annu. Rev. Immunol. 18, 495–527.

[21] Lefranc, M.-P. et al. (1986) Cell 45, 237–246.

[22] Lafaille, J.L. et al. (1989) Cell 59, 857–870.

[23] Huck, S. et al. (1988) EMBO J. 7, 719–726.

[24] Saiki, R. et al. (1985) Science 230, 1350–1354.

[25] Saiki, R.K. et al. (1988) Science 239, 487–491.

[26] Erlich, H.A. et al. (1991) Science 252, 1643–1651.

[27] Panzara, M.A. et al. (1992) Curr. Opin. Immunol. 4, 205–210.

[28] Loh, E.Y. et al. (1989) Science 243, 217–220.

[29] Lefranc, M.-P. et al. (1989) Proc. Natl Acad. Sci. USA 83, 9596–9600.

[30] Buresi, C. et al. (1989) Immunogenetics 29, 161–172.

[31] Triebel, F. et al. (1988) J. Exp. Med. 167, 694–699.

[32] Triebel, F. et al. (1988)) Eur. J. Immunol. 18, 789–794.

[33] Triebel, F. and Hercend, T. (1989) Immunol. Today 10, 186–188.

[34] Band, H. et al. (1987) Science 238, 682–684.

[35] Borst, J. et al. (1988) J. Exp. Med. 167, 1625–1644.

[36] Ciccone, E. et al. (1988) J. Exp. Med. 168, 1–11.

[37] Wu, Y.J. et al. (1988) J. Immunol. 141, 1476–1479.

[38] Peyrat, M.A. et al. (1995) J. Immunol. 155, 3060–3067.

[39] Kabelitz, D. et al. (1994) J. Immunol. 152, 3128–3136.

[40] Hinz, T. et al. (1997) Int. Immunol. 9, 1065–1072.

[41] Kabelitz, D. (1999) Microbes and Infection 1, 255–261.

[42] Ghanem, N. et al. (1989) Immunogenetics 30, 350–360.

[43] Ghanem, N. et al. (1991) Hum. Genet. 6, 450–456.

[44] Ikuta, K. et al. (1992) Annu. Rev. Immunol. 10, 759–783.

[45] Alexandre, D. et al. (1991) Int. Immunol. 3, 973–982.

[46] Alexandre, D. and Lefranc, M-P. (1992) Mol. Immunol. 29, 447–451.

[47] Moisan, J.P. et al. (1989) Hum. Immunol. 24, 95–110.

[48] Lefranc, M.-P. et al. (1986) Nature 319, 420–422.

[49] Forster, A. et al. (1987) EMBO J. 6, 1945–1950.

[50] Huck, S. and Lefranc, M-P. (1987) FEBS Lett. 224, 291–296.

[51] Lefranc, M.-P. (1990) Eur. Cytokine Network 1, 121–130.

[52] De Villartray, J.P. et al. (1988) Nature 335, 170–174.

53 Begley, C.G. et al. (1989) J. Exp. Med. 170, 339–342.

54 Soua, Z., et al. (1995) Exp. Clin. Immunogenet. 12, 16–30.

55 Baer, R. et al. (1988) EMBO J. 7, 1661–1668.

56 Lefranc, M.-P. and Rabbitts T.H. (1985) Nature 316, 464–466.

57 Chen, Z. et al. (1988) Blood 72, 776–783.

58 Migone, N. et al. (1988) Eur. J. Immunol. 18, 173–178.

59 Sturm, E. et al. (1989) Eur. J. Immunol. 19, 1261–1265.

60 Kanavaros, P. et al. (1991) J. Clin. Invest. 87, 666–672.

61 Dariavach, P. and Lefranc, M.-P. (1988) FEBS Lett. 256, 185–191.

62 Ho, I.C. et al. (1989) Proc. Natl Acad. Sci. USA 86, 6714–6718.

63 Ho, I.C. et al. (1990) Science 250, 814–818.

64 Ho, I.C. and Leiden, J.M. (1990) Mol. Cell. Biol. 10, 4720–4727.

65 Ho, I.C. and Leiden, J.M. (1990) J. Exp. Med. 172, 1443–1449.

66 Leiden, J.M. (1992) Immunol. Today 13, 22–30.

67 Luria, S. et al. (1987) EMBO J. 6, 3307–3312.

68 Winoto, A. and Baltimore, D. (1989) EMBO J. 8, 729–733.

69 Gottschalk, L.R. and Leiden, J.M. (1990) Mol. Cell. Biol. 10, 5486–5495.

70 Bories, J.C. et al. (1990) J. Exp. Med. 171, 75–83.

71 Redondo, J.M. et al. (1990) Science 247, 1225–1229.

72 Lefranc, M.-P. and Alexandre, D. (1995) Eur. J. Immunol. 25, 617–622.

THE HUMAN TRA LOCUS

Chromosomal localization of the human TRA locus

The human TRA locus is located on chromosome 14[1-3], on the long arm at band 14q11.2 (Fig. 1). The TRD locus is nestled within the TRA locus. The orientation of the TRA and TRD loci has been determined by the analysis of translocations involving these loci, in leukemia and lymphoma.

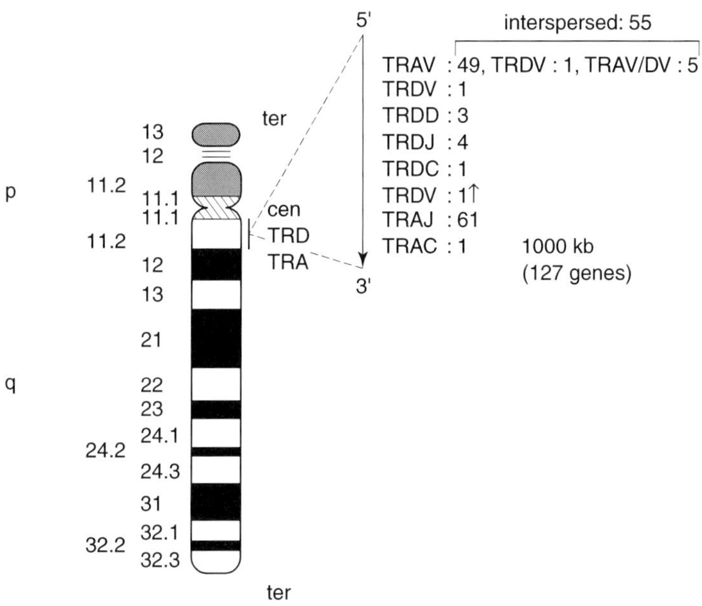

Figure 1. *Chromosomal localization of the human TRA locus at 14q11.2. A vertical line indicates the localization of the TRA and TRD loci at 14q11.2. The arrow indicates the orientation 5' -> 3' of the loci, and the gene group order in the loci. The length of the arrow is proportional to the total size of the loci, indicated in kilobases (kb). The total number of genes in the TRA and TRD loci is shown between parentheses. The number of functional genes defines the potential TRA repertoire which comprises 95–97 genes (40–41 TRAV, 4–5 TRAV/DV, 50 TRAJ, and 1 TRAC) per haploid genome. The five genes, designated as TRAV/DV, have been found rearranged to J genes of the TRA locus, and to D and J genes of the TRD locus, and can therefore be used in the synthesis of alpha or delta chains[4].*

Organization of the human TRA locus

The human TRA locus at 14q11.2 spans 1000 kilobases (kb) (Fig. 2). It consists of 54 TRAV genes belonging to 41 subgroups[4-8], 61 TRAJ genes localized on 71 kb[9-10], and a unique TRAC gene[11-12]. The most 5' TRAV genes occupy the most centromeric position, whereas the TRAC gene, 3' of the locus, is the most telomeric gene in the TRA locus. The organization of the TRAJ genes on a large area is quite unusual and has not been observed in the other immunoglobulin or T cell receptor loci[12]. Moreover, the TRD locus is nestled in the TRA locus between the TRAV and TRAJ genes. V-J rearrangements in the TRA locus therefore result in deletion of the TRD genes localized on the same chromosome[13]. That deletion occurs in two steps, that is a deletion of the TRD genes, involving specific sequences located upstream from TRDC (sequence ϕJα)[14,15], would take place before the TRAV-J rearrangement.

The potential genomic TRA repertoire comprises 44–46 functional TRAV genes belonging to 32–34 subgroups, 50 functional TRAJ genes, and the unique TRAC gene[4,10]. Among the variable genes are included five genes designated as TRAV/DV which belong to five different subgroups and which have been found rearranged either to TRAJ or to TRDD genes and can therefore be used in the synthesis of alpha or delta chains[4].

The total number of human TRA genes per haploid genome (including the 5 TRAV/DV genes) is 116, of which 95 to 97 genes are functional (see Tables 9 and 10). Enhancer sequences have been characterized 4.5kb 3' from TRAC [16].

List of the TRA genes on chromosome 14 at 14q11.2, and correspondence between nomenclatures

TRAJ gene nomenclature
TRAJ genes are designated by a number for the localization from 3' to 5' in the locus[10].

TRAV gene nomenclature
TRAV genes are designated by a number for the subgroup, followed whenever there are several genes belonging to the same subgroup, by a hyphen and a number for their relative localization in the locus[4]. Numbers increase from 5' to 3' in the locus. Functionality is shown in parentheses when the germline TRAV genes have not yet been isolated. The TRAV14/DV4, TRAV23/DV6, TRAV29/DV5, TRAV36/DV7, and TRAV38-2/DV8 genes have been found rearranged to J genes of the TRA locus, and to D and J genes of the TRD locus.

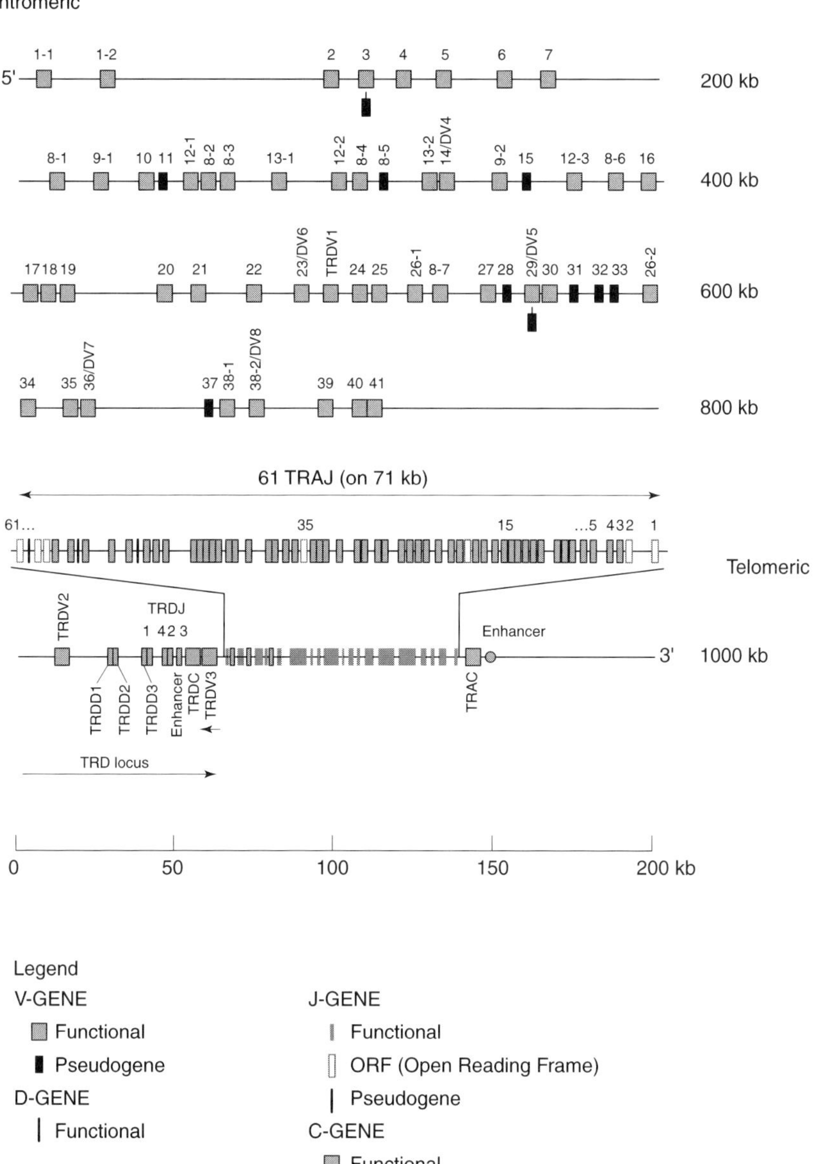

Figure 2. *Representation of the human TRA locus at 14q11.2. The boxes representing the genes are not to scale. Exons are not shown. The TRAV genes are designated by a number for the subgroup, followed, whenever there are several genes belonging to the same subgroup, by a hyphen and a number for their relative localization in the locus. Numbers increase from 5′ to 3′ in the locus. The TRD genes which are nestled in the TRA locus are also represented.*

Table 1. *List of functional or ORF human TRA genes. Only the genes with at least one functional or ORF allele are shown. For a complete listing of the human TRA genes including the pseudogenes, see references 4 and 10 and IMGT gene data: http://imgt.cines.fr/cgi-bin/IMGTlect.jv?query=203.*
For information on individual TRA genes:
http://imgt.cines.fr/cgi-bin/IMGTlect.jv?query=202 +genename.
Example: IMGT Repertoire for TRAV6:
http://imgt.cines.fr/cgi-bin/IMGTlect.jv?query=202+TRAV6.

IMGT gene groups	IMGT gene names	IMGT functionality	IMGT number of alleles	Other nomenclatures TRAV (1)	Ref. 7
TRAC	TRAC	F	1		
TRAJ	TRAJ1	ORF	1		
	TRAJ2	ORF	1		
	TRAJ3	F	1		
	TRAJ4	F	1		
	TRAJ5	F	1		
	TRAJ6	F	1		
	TRAJ7	F	1		
	TRAJ8	F	1		
	TRAJ9	F	1		
	TRAJ10	F	1		
	TRAJ11	F	1		
	TRAJ12	F	1		
	TRAJ13	F	1		
	TRAJ14	F	1		
	TRAJ15	F	2		
	TRAJ16	F	1		
	TRAJ17	F	1		
	TRAJ18	F	1		
	TRAJ19	ORF	1		
	TRAJ20	F	1		
	TRAJ21	F	1		
	TRAJ22	F	1		
	TRAJ23	F	1		
	TRAJ24	F	2		
	TRAJ25	ORF	1		
	TRAJ26	F	1		
	TRAJ27	F	1		
	TRAJ28	F	1		
	TRAJ29	F	1		
	TRAJ30	F	1		

Continued

Table 1. *Continued.*

IMGT gene groups	IMGT gene names	IMGT functionality	IMGT number of alleles	Other nomenclatures TRAV (1)	Ref. 7
	TRAJ31	F	1		
	TRAJ32	F	1		
	TRAJ33	F	1		
	TRAJ34	F	1		
	TRAJ35	ORF	1		
	TRAJ36	F	1		
	TRAJ37	F	1		
	TRAJ38	F	1		
	TRAJ39	F	1		
	TRAJ40	F	1		
	TRAJ41	F	1		
	TRAJ42	F	1		
	TRAJ43	F	1		
	TRAJ44	F	1		
	TRAJ45	F	1		
	TRAJ46	F	1		
	TRAJ47	F	1		
	TRAJ48	F	1		
	TRAJ49	F	1		
	TRAJ50	F	1		
	TRAJ52	F	1		
	TRAJ53	F	1		
	TRAJ54	F	1		
	TRAJ56	F	1		
	TRAJ57	F	1		
	TRAJ58	ORF	1		
	TRAJ59	ORF	1		
	TRAJ61	ORF	1		
TRAV	TRAV1-1	F	2	1S1	7S1
	TRAV1-2	F	2	1S2	7S2
	TRAV2	F	2	2S1	11S1
	TRAV3	F, (P)	2	3S1	16S1
	TRAV4	F	1	4S1	20S1
	TRAV5	F	1	5S1	15S1
	TRAV6	F	6	6S1	5S1
	TRAV7	F	1	7S1	
	TRAV8-1	F	2	8S1	1S1
	TRAV8-2	F	2	8S2	1S5

Continued

Table 1. *Continued.*

IMGT gene groups	IMGT gene names	IMGT functionality	IMGT number of alleles	Other nomenclatures TRAV (1)	Ref. 7
	TRAV8-3	F	3	8S3	1S4
	TRAV8-4	F	7	8S4	1S2
	TRAV8-6	F	2	8S6	1S3
	TRAV8-7	F	1	8S7	
	TRAV9-1	F	1	9S1	
	TRAV9-2	F	4	9S2	22S1
	TRAV10	F	1	10S1	24S1
	TRAV12-1	F	2	12S1	2S3
	TRAV12-2	F	3	12S2	2S1
	TRAV12-3	F	2	12S3	2S2
	TRAV13-1	F	3	13S1	8S1
	TRAV13-2	F	2	13S2	8S2
	TRAV14/DV4	F	4	hADV14S1	6S1-ADV6S1
	TRAV16	F	1	16S1	9S1
	TRAV17	F	1	17S1	3S1
	TRAV18	F	1	18S1	
	TRAV19	F	1	19S1	12S1
	TRAV20	F	4	20S1	30S1
	TRAV21	F	2	21S1	23S1
	TRAV22	F	1	22S1	13S1
	TRAV23/DV6	F	4	hADV23S1	17S1-ADV17S1
	TRAV24	F	2	24S1	18S1
	TRAV25	F	1	25S1	32S1
	TRAV26-1	F	3	26S1	4S2
	TRAV26-2	F	2	26S2	4S1
	TRAV27	F	3	27S1	10S1
	TRAV29/DV5	F, (P)	3	hADV29S1	21S1-ADV21S1
	TRAV30	F	4	30S1	29S1
	TRAV34	F	1	34S1	26S1
	TRAV35	F	2	35S1	25S1
	TRAV36/DV7	F	4	hADV36S1	28S1-DV28S1
	TRAV38-1	F	4	38S1	14S2
	TRAV38-2/DV8	F	1	hADV38S2	14S1-ADV14S1
	TRAV39	F	1	39S1	27S1
	TRAV40	F	1	40S1	31S1
	TRAV41	F	1	41S1	19S1

(1) Boysen, C. et al. (AE000658-AE000661) unpublished

Number of the human TRAV germline variable genes at 14q11.2 and potential repertoire

Overview

54 TRAV and TRAV/DV genes belonging to 41 subgroups, on 700 kilobases:
    44 FUNCTIONAL
    8 PSEUDOGENE
    2 FUNCTIONAL or PSEUDOGENE (TRAV3, TRAV29/DV5)

Potential repertoire

40–41 FUNCTIONAL TRAV genes belonging to 28 to 29 subgroups, and 4–5 FUNCTIONAL TRAV/DV genes belonging to 4 to 5 subgroups. One subgroup (TRAV38) has one 'TRAV' gene and one 'TRAV/DV' gene. There is therefore a total of 44–46 FUNCTIONAL TRAV and TRAV/DV genes belonging to 32 to 34 subgroups.

Table 2. *Repertoire of the human TRAV germline variable genes at 14q11.2.*

Subgroup	Functional	ORF	Pseudogene	Total
TRAV1	2	–	–	2
TRAV2	1	–	–	1
TRAV3	(1)*	–	(1)*	1
TRAV4	1	–	–	1
TRAV5	1	–	–	1
TRAV6	1	–	–	1
TRAV7	1	–	–	1
TRAV8	6	–	1	7
TRAV9	2	–	–	2
TRAV10	1	–	–	1
TRAV11	–	–	1	1
TRAV12	3	–	–	3
TRAV13	2	–	–	2
TRAV14/DV4	1	–	–	1
TRAV15	–	–	1	1
TRAV16	1	–	–	1
TRAV17	1	–	–	1
TRAV18	1	–	–	1
TRAV19	1	–	–	1
TRAV20	1	–	–	1
TRAV21	1	–	–	1
TRAV22	1	–	–	1
TRAV23/DV6	1	–	–	1
TRAV24	1	–	–	1
TRAV25	1	–	–	1

Continued

Table 2. *Continued.*

Subgroup	Functional	ORF	Pseudogene	Total
TRAV26	2	–	–	2
TRAV27	1	–	–	1
TRAV28	–	–	1	1
TRAV29/DV5	(1)*	–	(1)*	1
TRAV30	1	–	–	1
TRAV31	–	–	1	1
TRAV32	–	–	1	1
TRAV33	–	–	1	1
TRAV34	1	–	–	1
TRAV35	1	–	–	1
TRAV36/DV7	1	–	–	1
TRAV37	–	–	1	1
TRAV38/DV8[a]	2	–	–	2
TRAV39	1	–	–	1
TRAV40	1	–	–	1
TRAV41	1	–	–	1
Total	44(+2)*	0	8(+2)*	54

* Indicates that the following genes have alleles with different functionality: FUNCTIONAL or PSEUDOGENE (TRAV3, TRAV29/DV5)
[a] Only the TRAV38-2 gene has so far been found rearranged to TRDD genes.

THE HUMAN TRB LOCUS

Chromosomal localization of the human TRB locus

The human TRB locus is located on chromosome 7[17-19], on the long arm, at band 7q34[19] (Fig. 3). The orientation of the locus has been determined by the analysis of translocations, involving the TRB locus, in leukemia and lymphoma.

Organization of the human TRB locus

The human TRB locus at 7q34 spans 620 kb (Fig. 4). It consists of 64–67 TRBV genes belonging to 32 subgroups[7,8,20-26]. Except for TRBV30, localized downstream of the TRBC2 gene, in inverted orientation of transcription[25], all the other TRBV genes are located upstream of a duplicated D-J-C-cluster, which comprises, for the first part one TRBD, six TRBJ, and the TRBC1 gene, and for the second part, one TRBD, eight TRBJ, and the TRBC2 gene[13,27-29]. The two constant genes, TRBC1 and TRBC2, encode proteins which differ by six amino acids. TRBV30 rearranges by an inversion mechanism as this has been described for the murine TRBV31 gene, similarly located in the mouse TRB locus, downstream of the TRBC2 gene, and in inverted orientation of transcription[30]. Twenty-three of the 32 TRBV subgroups are

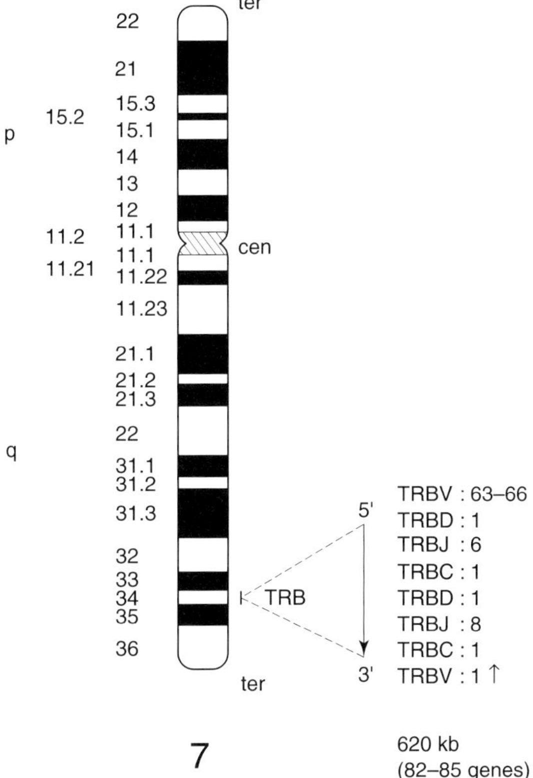

Figure 3. *Chromosomal localization of the human TRB locus at 7q34. A vertical line indicates the localization of the TRB locus at 7q34. The arrow indicates the orientation 5' -> 3' of the locus, and the gene group order in the locus. The TRBV gene localized at the 3' end of the TRB locus is in inverted orientation of transcription (shown by a small arrow). The length of the arrow is proportional to the size of the locus, indicated in kilobases (kb). The total number of genes in the locus is shown between parentheses. The number of functional genes defines the potential TRB repertoire, which comprises 56–65 genes (40–48 TRBV, 2 TRBD, 12–13 TRBJ, and 2 TRBC) per haploid genome.*

found to consist of a single member each. The most 5' TRBV genes occupy the most centromeric position, whereas the TRBV30 gene, 3' of the locus, is the most telomeric gene in the TRB locus. The potential repertoire consists of 40–48 functional TRBV genes belonging to 21–23 subgroups, the two TRBD, twelve to thirteen TRBJ (6 from the first cluster and 6–7 from the second cluster), and the two TRBC genes. Six TRBV orphons have been localized on chromosome 9 at 9p21[31-32]. Enhancer sequences have been characterized 5.5 kb 3' from TRBC2 [33].

The total number of human TRB genes per haploid genome is 82 to 85 (88 to 91 genes, if the orphons are included) of which 56 to 65 are functional (see Tables 9 and 10).

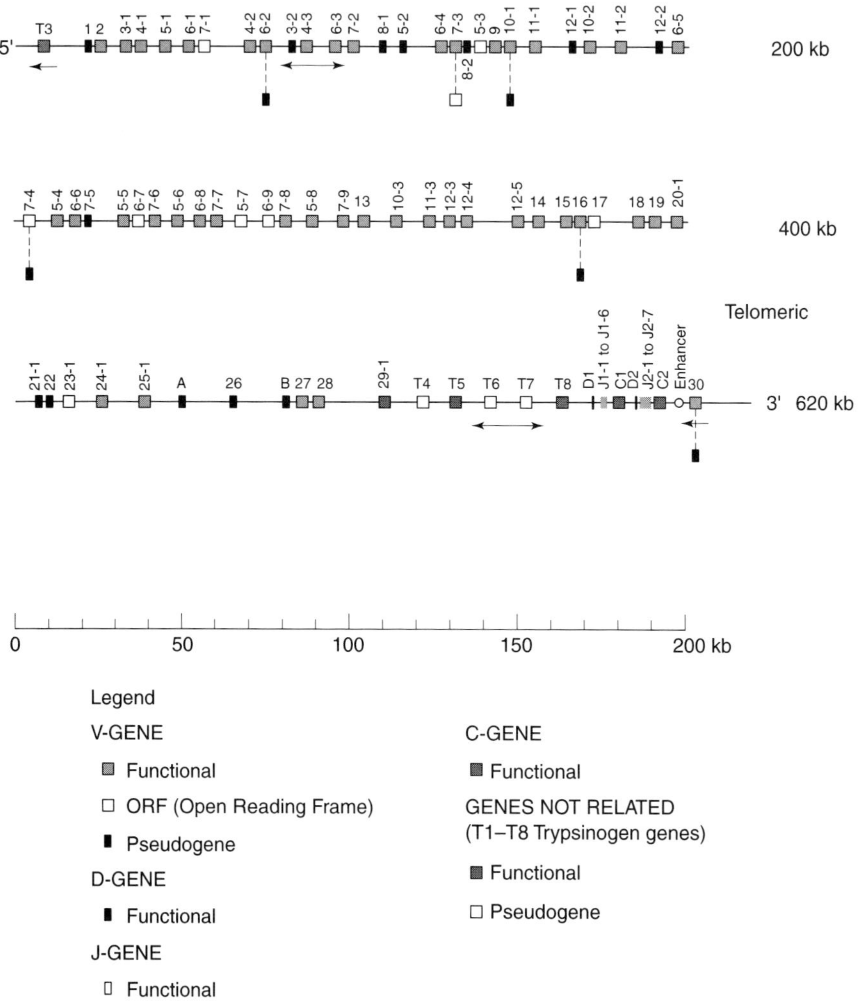

Figure 4. *Representation of the human TRB locus at 7q34. The boxes representing the genes are not to scale. Exons are not shown. The TRBV genes are designated by a number for the subgroup followed, whenever there are several genes belonging to the same subgroup, by a hyphen and a number for their relative localization in the locus. Numbers increase from 5′ to 3′ in the locus. Single arrows show genes whose polarity is opposite to that of the D-J-C-CLUSTER. Double arrows indicate insertion/deletion polymorphisms.*

List of the TRB genes on chromosome 7 at 7q34, and correspondence between nomenclatures

TRBV gene nomenclature

TRBV genes are designated by a number for the subgroup followed, whenever there are several genes belonging to the same subgroup, by a hyphen and a number for their relative localization in the locus. Numbers increase from 5' to 3' in the locus[26].

Functionality is shown in:

- parentheses when the accession number refers to a rearranged sequence and the corresponding germline gene has not yet been isolated;
- brackets when the accession number refers to a DNA genomic sequence, but not known as being germline or rearranged.

Since orphons have been described for each of the following TRBV subgroups: 20, 21, 23, 24, 25, and 29, the single member gene in the main locus is designated by the subgroup number followed by a hyphen and the number 1. To date, no orphon has been reported that belongs to subgroup 22, therefore the IMGT designation of the single member gene is TRBV22.

Table 3. *List of functional or ORF human TRB genes. Only the genes with at least one functional or ORF allele are shown. For a complete listing of the human TRBV genes including the pseudogenes, see references 26 and 29, and IMGT gene data: http://imgt.cines.fr/cgi-bin/IMGTlect.jv?query=203.*
For information on individual TRA genes:
http://imgt.cines.fr/cgi-bin/IMGTlect.jv?query=202+genename.
Example: IMGT Repertoire for TRBV3-1:
http://imgt.cines.fr/cgi-bin/IMGTlect.jv?query=202+TRBV3-1.

IMGT gene groups	IMGT gene names	IMGT functionality	IMGT number of alleles	Other nomenclatures Ref. 23	Ref. 7	Ref. 25
TRBC	TRBC1	F	2			
	TRBC2	F	2			
TRBD	TRBD1	F	1			
	TRBD2	F	2			
TRBJ	TRBJ1-1	F	1			
	TRBJ1-2	F	1			
	TRBJ1-3	F	1			
	TRBJ1-4	F	1			
	TRBJ1-5	F	1			
	TRBJ1-6	F	1			

Continued

Table 3. *Continued.*

IMGT gene groups	IMGT gene names	IMGT functionality	IMGT number of alleles	Other nomenclatures		
				Ref. 23	Ref. 7	Ref. 25
	TRBJ2-1	F	1			
	TRBJ2-2	F	1			
	TRBJ2-2P	ORF	1			
	TRBJ2-3	F	1			
	TRBJ2-4	F	1			
	TRBJ2-5	F	1			
	TRBJ2-6	F	1			
	TRBJ2-7	F, ORF	2			
TRBV	TRBV2	F	3	22S1	22S1	2
	TRBV3-1	F	2	9S1	9S1	3-1
	TRBV4-1	F	2	7S1	7S1	4-1
	TRBV4-2	F	2	7S3	7S3	4-2
	TRBV4-3	F	4	7S2	7S2	4-3
	TRBV5-1	F	2	5S1	5S1	5-1
	TRBV5-3	ORF	2	5S5	5S5	5-3
	TRBV5-4	F	4	5S6	5S6	5-4
	TRBV5-5	F	3	5S3	5S3	5-5
	TRBV5-6	F	1	5S2	5S2	5-6
	TRBV5-7	ORF	1	5S7	5S7	5-7
	TRBV5-8	F	2	5S8	5S4	5-8
	TRBV6-1	F	1	13S3	13S3	6-1
	TRBV6-2	F, (P)	3	13S2a	13S2a	6-2
	TRBV6-3	F	1	13S2b	13S2b	6-3
	TRBV6-4	F	2	13S5	13S5	6-4
	TRBV6-5	F	1	13S1	13S1	6-5
	TRBV6-6	F	5	13S6	13S6	6-6
	TRBV6-7	ORF	1	13S8	13S8	6-7
	TRBV6-8	F	1	13S7	13S7	6-8
	TRBV6-9	F	1	13S4	13S4	6-9
	TRBV7-1	ORF	1	6S10	6S7	7-1
	TRBV7-2	F	4	6S7	6S5	7-2
	TRBV7-3	F, ORF	5	6S1	6S1	7-3
	TRBV7-4	F, (P)	3	6S11	6S8	7-4
	TRBV7-6	F	2	6S4	6S3	7-6
	TRBV7-7	F	2	6S14	6S6	7-7
	TRBV7-8	F	3	6S3	6S2	7-8
	TRBV7-9	F	7	6S5	6S4	7-9
	TRBV9	F	3	1S1	1S1	9

Continued

Table 3. *Continued.*

IMGT gene groups	IMGT gene names	IMGT functionality	IMGT number of alleles	Other nomenclatures Ref. 23	Ref. 7	Ref. 25
	TRBV10-1	F, [P]	3	12S4	12S2	10-1
	TRBV10-2	F	2	12S3	12S3	10-2
	TRBV10-3	F	4	12S2	12S1	10-3
	TRBV11-1	F	1	21S1	21S1	11-1
	TRBV11-2	F	3	21S3	21S3	11-2
	TRBV11-3	F	4	21S4	21S2	11-3
	TRBV12-3	F	1	8S1	8S1	12-3
	TRBV12-4	F	2	8S2	8S2	12-4
	TRBV12-5	F	1	8S3	8S3	12-5
	TRBV13	F	2	23S1	23S1	13
	TRBV14	F	2	16S1	16S1	14
	TRBV15	F	3	24S1	24S1	15
	TRBV16	F, P	3	25S1	25S1	16
	TRBV17	ORF	1	26S1[1]	26S1	17
	TRBV18	F	1	18S1	18S1	18
	TRBV19	F	3	17S1	17S1	19
	TRBV20-1	F	7	2S1	2S1	20-1
	TRBV23-1	ORF	1	19S1	19S1	23-1
	TRBV24-1	F	1	15S1	15S1	24-1
	TRBV25-1	F	1	11S1	11S1	25-1
	TRBV27	F	1	14S1	14S1	27
	TRBV28	F	1	3S1	3S1	28
	TRBV29-1	F	3	4S1	4S1	29-1
	TRBV30	F, P	5	20S1	20S1	30

[1] 26S1 was defined in Slightom et al. (1994).

Number of the human TRBV germline variable genes at 7q34 and potential repertoire

Overview

64–67 TRBV genes belonging to 30 subgroups, on 620 kilobases:
    40–42 FUNCTIONAL
    6 ORF (Open Reading Frame)
    12–13 PSEUDOGENE
    5 FUNCTIONAL or PSEUDOGENE
    1 FUNCTIONAL or ORF

Potential repertoire

40–48 FUNCTIONAL TRBV genes belonging to 21–23 subgroups

Table 4. *Repertoire of the human TRBV germline variable genes at 7q34.*

Subgroup	Functional	ORF	Pseudogene	Total
TRBV1	–	–	1	1
TRBV2	1	–	–	1
TRBV3	1	–	0–1**	1–2**
TRBV4	2–3**	–	–	2–3**
TRBV5	5	2	1	8
TRBV6	6–7** (+1)*	1	(1)*	8–9**
TRBV7	5(+2)*	1(+1)*	1(+1)*	9
TRBV8	–	–	2	2
TRBV9	1	–	–	1
TRBV10	2(+1)*	–	(1)*	3
TRBV11	3	–	–	3
TRBV12	3	–	2	5
TRBV13	1	–	–	1
TRBV14	1	–	–	1
TRBV15	1	–	–	1
TRBV16	(1)*	–	(1)*	1
TRBV17	–	1	–	1
TRBV18	1	–	–	1
TRBV19	1	–	–	1
TRBV20	1	–	–	1
TRBV21	–	–	1	1
TRBV22	–	–	1	1
TRBV23	–	1	–	1
TRBV24	1	–	–	1
TRBV25	1	–	–	1
TRBV26	–	–	1	1
TRBV27	1	–	–	1
TRBV28	1	–	–	1
TRBV29	1	–	–	1
TRBV30	(1)*	–	(1)*	1
TRBVA	–	–	1	1
TRBVB	–	–	1	1
Total	40–42(+6)*	6(+1)*	12–13(+5)*	64–67

*Indicates that the following genes have alleles with different functionality:
FUNCTIONAL or PSEUDOGENE (TRBV6-2, TRBV7-4, TRBV10-1, TRBV16, TRBV30)
FUNCTIONAL or ORF (TRBV7-3)
** Indicate allelic polymorphisms by insertion/deletion which concern TRBV3-2, TRBV4-3, TRBV6-3.

THE HUMAN TRG LOCUS

Chromosomal localization of the human TRG locus

The human TRG locus[34–48] is located on chromosome 7[49], at band 7p14[50,51]. The orientation of the locus has been determined by the analysis of chromosome 7 inversions inv(7)(p14-q34), involving the TRG and TRB loci in ataxia telangiectasia patients, and in leukemia.

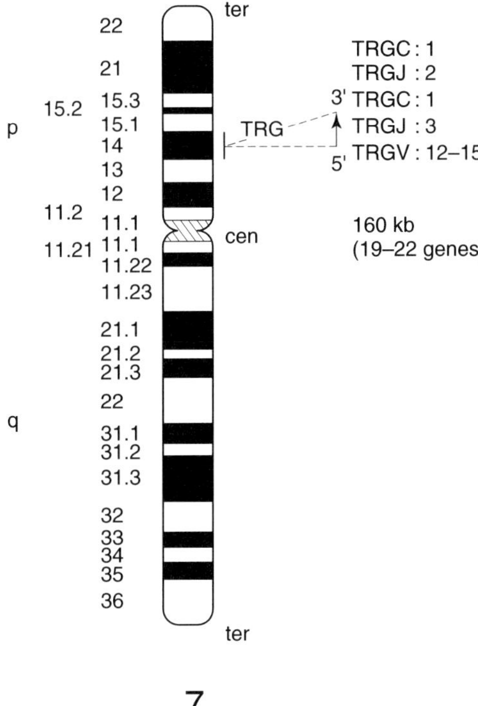

Figure 5. *Chromosomal localization of the human TRG locus at 7p14. A vertical line indicates the localization of the TRG locus at 7p14. The arrow indicates the orientation 5' -> 3' of the locus, and the gene group order in the locus. The length of the arrow is proportional to the size of the locus, indicated in kilobases (kb). The total number of genes in the locus is shown in parentheses.*

Organization of the human TRG locus

The human TRG locus[34–48] at 7p14 spans 160 kb[41]. It consists of 12–15 TRGV genes belonging to 6 subgroups[34–36,38,40,47–48], upstream of a duplicated J-C cluster, which comprises, for the first part, three TRGJ and the TRGC1 gene, and for the second part, two TRGJ and the TRGC2 gene [35,37,39,43]. The most 5' TRGV genes occupy the most centromeric position, whereas the TRGC2 gene, 3' of the locus, is the most telomeric in the TRG locus[41]. There is no cross-hybridization between the TRGV genes belonging to the six different subgroups, which are only 30% homologous at the protein level[36,40]. TRGV9, expressed in 80–95% of the human peripheral γδ T cells, is the unique member of subgroup 2. TRGV10 and TRGV11, single members of subgroups 3 and 4, respectively, have been found rearranged[40] and transcribed, but they are ORF that cannot be expressed in a gamma chain, due to a splicing defect of the premessenger[47,48]. The potential repertoire consists of 4–6 functional TRGV genes belonging to two subgroups, the five TRGJ and the two TRGC genes[34–41,47,48].

Polymorphisms in the number of TRGV genes and in the exon number of the TRGC2 gene have been described in different populations[43,44,46]. A variation of the number of the TRGV subgroup genes (from seven to ten) has been observed[44,46]. These allelic polymorphisms, which result from the deletion of V4 and V5, or from the insertion of an additional V gene, V3P, between V3 and V4, can be detected by restriction fragment length polymorphism (RFLP)[44,46] (see Chapter 3). The two TRGC genes, which are 16 kb apart, result, with their associated TRGJ genes, from a recent duplication in the locus. However, there are several structural differences[42]. TRGJP1, TRGJ1, and TRGC1 cross-hybridize to TRGJP2, TRGJ2, and TRGC2, respectively[34,37,39], whereas the TRGJP has no equivalent in the duplicated TRGJP2-J2-C2 cluster[36]. The TRGC1 gene has three exons[37], whereas the TRGC2 gene has four or five exons, owing to the duplication or triplication of a region that includes exon 2[43]. The allelic polymorphism of the TRGC2 gene with duplication (C2(2x)) or triplication (C2(3x)) of exon 2 can be identified by RFLP[43] (see Chapter 3). The exon 2 of the TRGC1 gene has a cysteine[37] involved in the interchain disulfide bridge, whereas this cysteine in not conserved in the exon 2 of the human TRGC2 gene. Enhancer and silencer sequences have been characterized 6.5 kb downstream of the TRGC2 gene[52].

The total number of TRG genes per haploid genome is 19 to 22 of which 11 to 13 are functional (Tables 9 and 10).

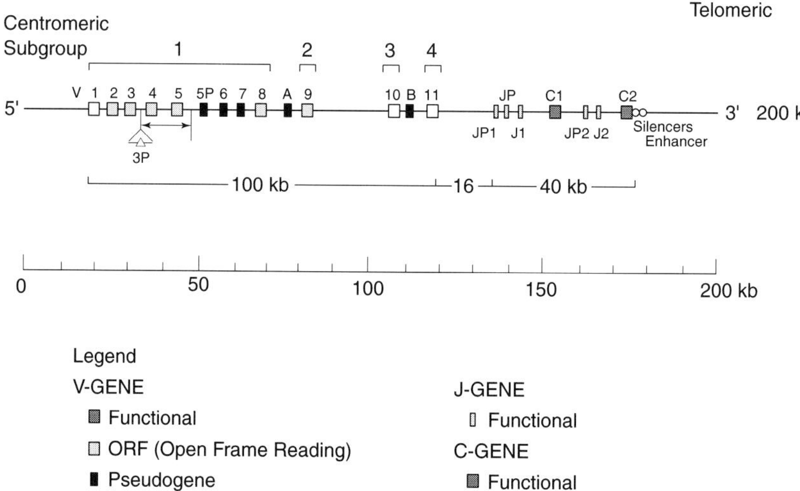

Figure 6. *Representation of the human TRG locus at 7p14. The boxes representing the genes are not to scale. Exons are not shown. A double arrow indicates an insertion/deletion polymorphism. The TRGV3P gene, a polymorphic gene by insertion, has been identified by Southern hybridization in a rare haplotype but has not been sequenced[46].*

List of the TRG genes on chromosome 7 at 7p14, and correspondence between nomenclatures

TRGV gene nomenclature

TRGV genes are designated by a number for the localization from 5′ to 3′ in the locus[36,41]. Two pseudogenes, single members of their subgroup, are designated by a letter[40,41].

Table 5. *List of functional or ORF human TRGV genes. Only the genes with at least one functional or ORF allele are shown. For a complete listing of the human TRGV genes including the pseudogenes, see reference 41 and IMGT gene data: http://imgt.cines.fr/cgi-bin/IMGTlect.jv?query=203.*
For information on individual TRG genes:
http://imgt.cines.fr/cgi-bin/IMGTlect.jv?query=202+genename.
Example: IMGT Repertoire for TRGV4:
http://imgt.cines.fr/cgi-bin/IMGTlect.jv?query=202+TRGV4.

IMGT gene groups	IMGT gene names	IMGT functionality	IMGT number of alleles
TRGC	TRGC1	F	2
	TRGC2(2x)	F	4
	TRGC2(3x)	F	1
TRGJ	TRGJ1	F	2
	TRGJ2	F	1
	TRGJP	F	1
	TRGJP1	F	1
	TRGJP2	F	1
TRGV	TRGV1	ORF	1
	TRGV2	F	2
	TRGV3	F	2
	TRGV4	F	2
	TRGV5	F	1
	TRGV8	F	1
	TRGV9	F	2
	TRGV10	ORF	2
	TRGV11	ORF	2

Number of the human TRGV germline variable genes at 7p14 and potential repertoire

Overview

12–15 TRGV genes belonging to 6 subgroups, on 120 kilobases:
    4–6 FUNCTIONAL
    3 ORF (Open Reading Frame)
    5 PSEUDOGENE

Potential repertoire

4–6 FUNCTIONAL TRGV genes belonging to 2 subgroups.

Table 6. *Repertoire of the human TRGV germline variable genes at 7p14.*

Subgroup	Gene name	Functional	ORF	Pseudogene	Total
1	TRGV1	–	1	–	1
	TRGV2	1	–	–	1
	TRGV3	1	–	–	1
	TRGV3P				0–1*
	TRGV4	0–1*	–	–	0–1*
	TRGV5	0–1*	–	–	0–1*
	TRGV5P	–	–	1	1
	TRGV6	–	–	1	1
	TRGV7	–	–	1	1
	TRGV8	1	–	–	1
2	TRGV9	1	–	–	1
3	TRGV10	–	1	–	1
4	TRGV11	–	1	–	1
A	TRGVA	–	–	1	1
B	TRGVB	–	–	1	1
	Total	4–6	3	5	12–15

* Indicates allelic polymorphism by insertion/deletion.
The TRGV3P gene, a polymorphic gene by insertion, has been identified by Southern hybridization in a rare haplotype but has not been sequenced[46].
The most frequent haplotype comprises 14 TRGV genes (6 FUNCTIONAL + 3 ORF + 5 PSEUDOGENES) with V4 and V5 present, and V3P absent[41,46].

THE HUMAN TRD LOCUS

Chromosomal localization of the human TRD locus

The human TRD locus is located on chromosome 14, on the long arm at band 14q11.2 (Fig. 7). The TRD locus is embedded in the TRA locus, between the TRAV and TRAJ genes[53-55]. The orientation of the locus has been determined by the analysis of translocations involving the TRD locus, in leukemia and lymphoma.

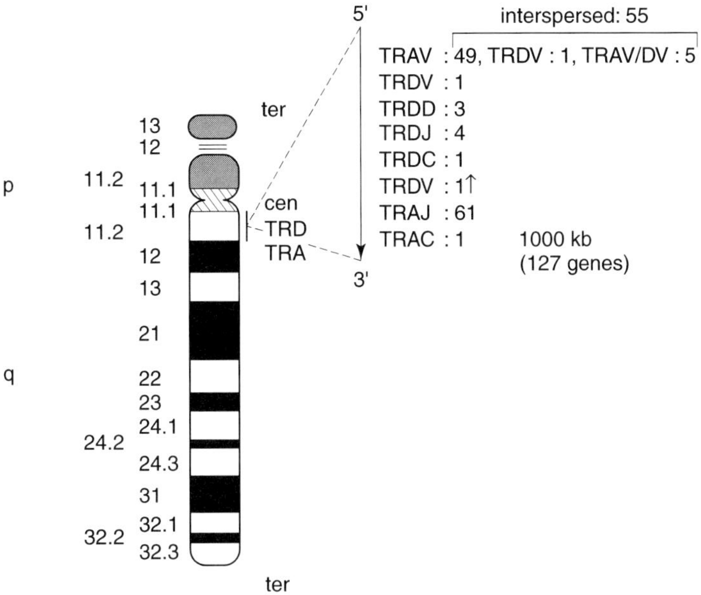

Figure 7. *Chromosomal localization of the human TRD locus embedded in the TRA locus at 14q11.2. A vertical line indicates the localization of the TRA and TRD loci at 14q11.2. The arrow indicates the orientation 5' -> 3' of the loci, and the gene group order in the loci. The length of the arrow is proportional to the total size of the loci, indicated in kilobases (kb). The total number of genes in the TRA and TRD loci is shown in parentheses. The five genes, designated TRAV/DV, have been found rearranged to J genes of the TRA locus, and to D and J genes of the TRD locus and can therefore be used in the synthesis of alpha or delta chains[4].*

Organization of the human TRD locus

The human TRD locus at 14q11.2 comprises a cluster of one TRDV gene (TRDV2)[56–58], three TRDD genes[59,60], and four TRDJ genes[54,60–63], upstream of the unique TRDC gene[59]; another TRDV gene (TRDV3) is localized downstream of the TRDC gene, in inverted orientation of transcription[56,60,64]. This cluster spans 60 kb and is localized inside the TRA locus, between the TRAV genes and the TRAJ genes[13]. One TRDV gene (TRDV1)[65,66] is localized at 360 kb upstream of the TRDC gene, among the TRAV genes[67]. Five variable genes have been found rearranged to both (D)J genes of the TRD locus and TRAJ genes, and can therefore be used for the synthesis of both delta and alpha chains[4,68,69]. These genes are described as TRAV/DV[4]. The TRDV genes are unique members of different subgroups. All the TRD genes are functional, with the exception of one TRAV/DV, which has been found either functional or as a pseudogene[4]. Enhancer sequences have been described between the TRDJ3 and the TRDC gene[70,71].

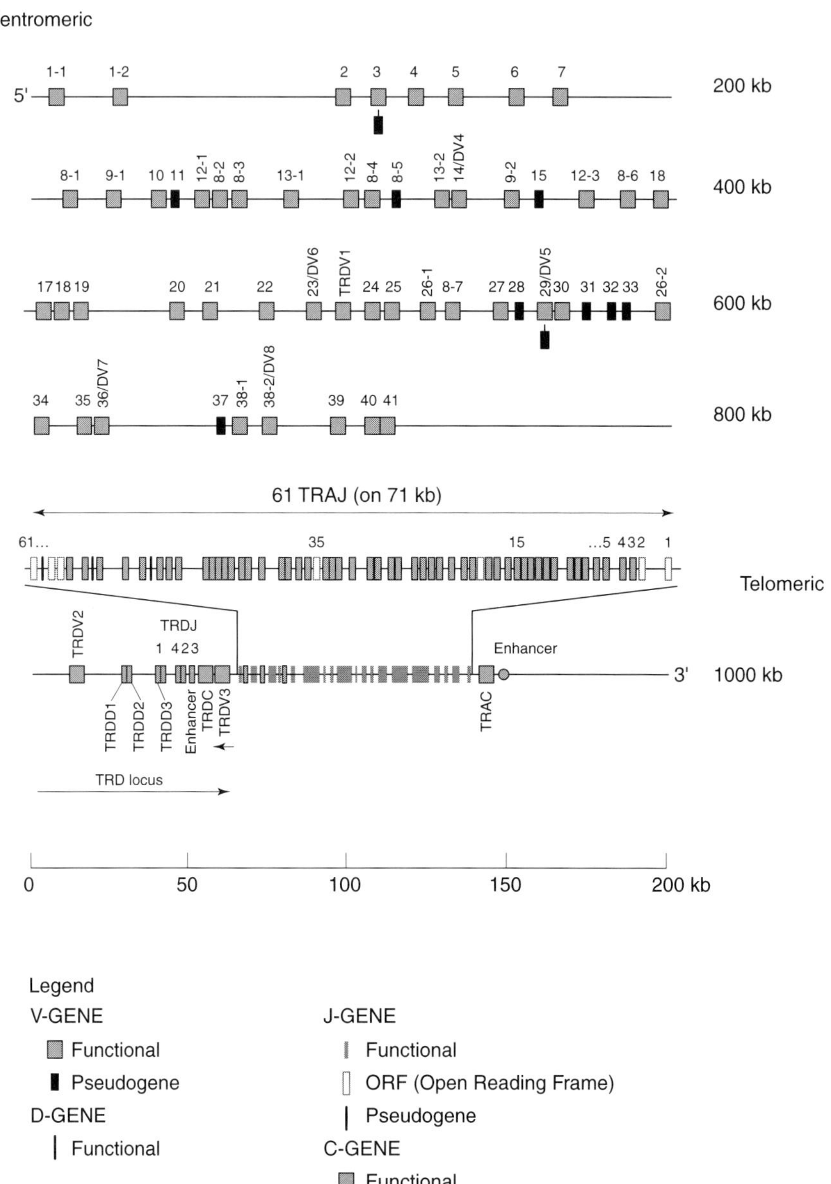

Figure 8. *Representation of the human TRD locus nestled in the TRA locus at 14q11.2. The boxes representing the genes are not to scale. Exons are not shown. The three TRDV genes are designated by a number for the subgroup which corresponds to the position from 5' to 3' in the locus. The five TRAV/DV genes can be used for the synthesis of both delta and alpha chains.*

List of the TRD genes on chromosome 14 at 14q11.2, and correspondence between nomenclatures

TRDV and TRAV/DV gene nomenclature

TRDV genes (genes only found rearranged to TRDD genes) are designated by a number for the subgroup which corresponds to the position from 5′ to 3′ in the locus.

TRAV/DV genes (genes found rearranged to TRDD genes nd to TRAJ genes) are designated according to the TRAV nomenclature. To indicate that these genes can be involved in TRD rearrangements, a slash is added, followed by the letters DV and a number. These genes have been reported in the TRAV table.

Table 7. *List of functional or ORF human TRD genes. Only the genes with at least one functional or ORF allele are shown. The TRAV14/DV4, TRAV23/DV6, TRAV29/DV5, TRAV36/DV7, and TRAV38-2/DV8 genes which have been found rearranged to J genes of the TRA locus, and to D and J genes of the TRD locus are displayed in the human TRAV table. For a complete listing of the human TRD genes including the pseudogenes, see references 4 and 10 and IMGT gene data: http://imgt.cines.fr/cgi-bin/IMGTlect.jv?query=203.*
For information on individual TRD genes:
http://imgt.cines.fr/cgi-bin/IMGTlect.jv?query=202+genename.
Example: IMGT Repertoire for TRDV2
http://imgt.cines.fr/cgi-bin/IMGTlect.jv?query=202+TRDV2.

IMGT gene groups	IMGT gene names	IMGT functionality	IMGT number of alleles
TRDC	TRDC	F	1
TRDD	TRDD1	F	1
	TRDD2	F	1
	TRDD3	F	1
TRDJ	TRDJ1	F	1
	TRDJ2	F	1
	TRDJ3	F	1
	TRDJ4	F	1
TRDV	TRDV1	F	1
	TRDV2	F	3
	TRDV3	F	2

Number of the human TRDV germline variable genes at 14q11.2 and potential repertoire

Overview

3 TRDV genes belonging to 3 subgroups
 TRDV1 at 360 kb upstream of TRDC, among the TRAV genes
 TRDV2 at 44 kb upstream of TRDC
 TRDV3 at 3 kb downstream of TRDC and in an inverted orientation of transcription.

5 TRAV/DV genes belonging to 5 subgroups
 The TRAV/DV genes have been found rearranged either to TRAJ genes or to D and J genes of the TRD locus, and can therefore be used in the synthesis of alpha or delta chains.

Potential repertoire

3 FUNCTIONAL TRDV genes belonging to 3 subgroups, and 4–5 FUNCTIONAL TRAV/DV genes belonging to 4 to 5 subgroups.

Table 8. *Repertoire of the human TRDV and TRAV/DV germline variable genes at 14q11.2.*

Subgroup	Functional	ORF	Pseudogene	Total
TRDV1	1	–	–	1
TRDV2	1	–	–	1
TRDV3	1	–	–	1
Total	3	0	0	3
TRAV14/DV4	1	–	–	1
TRAV23/DV6	1	–	–	1
TRAV29/DV5	(1)*	–	(1)*	1
TRAV36/DV7	1	–	–	1
TRAV38-2/DV8 [a]	1	–	–	1
Total	4(+1)*	0	(1)*	5

*Indicates that the following gene has alleles with different functionality: FUNCTIONAL or PSEUDOGENE (TRAV29/DV5)
[a] The TRAV38/DV8 subgroup comprises two genes; only the TRAV38-2/DV8 gene has so far been found rearranged to TRDD genes.

Table 9. *Total number of human T cell receptor genes per haploid genome.*

Locus	Major loci						Number of orphons	Total number of genes (including orphons)
	Chromosomal localization	V	D	J	C	Total number of genes in the major locus		
TRA	14q11.2	54[a]	0	61	1	116[a]	–	116[a]
TRB	7q34	64–67	2	14	2	82–85	6	88–91
TRG	7p14	12–15	0	5	2	19–22	–	19–22
TRD	14q11.2	3				11		
		8[a]	3	4	1		–	11
						16[a]		

[a] including the 5 TRAV/DV genes.
Major loci refer to the TRA locus at 14q11.2, TRB locus at 7q34, TRG locus at 7p14, and TRD locus at 14q11.2, genes of which are involved in T cell receptor chain synthesis.
Orphons are genes located outside of the main loci, which cannot contribute to the TcR chain synthesis. Six TRBV orphons have been identified on chromosome 9 at 9p21.

Table 10. *Number of functional human T cell receptor genes per haploid genome.*

Locus	Chromosomal localization	Locus size in kb (kilobases)	V	D	J	C	Number of functional genes	Combinatorial diversity (range per locus)
TRA	14q11.2	1000	44–46[a]	0	50	1	95–97[b]	$44 \times 50 = 2200$ (m) $46 \times 50 = 2300$ (M)
TRB	7q34	620	40–48	2	12–13	2	56–65	$40 \times 2 \times 12 = 960$ (m) $48 \times 2 \times 13 = 1248$ (M)
TRG	7p14	160	4–6	0	5	2	11-13	$4 \times 5 = 20$ (m) $6 \times 5 = 30$ (M)
TRD	14q11.2	60[b] 530[c]	3 8[a]	3	4	1	11 16[a]	$3 \times 3 \times 4 = 36$ (m) $8 \times 3 \times 4 = 96^{a}\ 8 \times 7 \times 4 = 224^{d}$ (M)

[a] including the 5 TRAV/DV genes,
[b] size of the cluster from TRDV2 to TRDV3,
[c] distance between the most 5′ TRAV/DV gene (TRAV14/DV4) and the most 3′ gene of the TRD locus (TRDV3).
[d] taking into account the rearrangement with 2 or 3 TRDD (4 possible combinations: D1,D2; D1,D3; D2,D3; D1,D2,D3)

The range of the theoretical combinatorial diversity is indicated taking into account the minimum (m) and the maximum (M) number of functional V, D, and J genes in each of the major TRA, TRB, TRG, and TRD loci.

References

1 Collins, M.K.L. et al. (1984) EMBO J. 3, 2347–2349.
2 Croce, C. et al. (1984) Science 227, 1044–1047.
3 Rabbitts, T.H. et al. (1985) EMBO J. 4, 1461–1465.
4 Scaviner, D. and Lefranc, M.-P. (2000) Exp. Clin. Immunogenet. 17, 83–96.
5 Wilson, R.K. et al. (1988) Immunol. Rev. 101, 149–172.
6 Roman-Roman, S. et al. (1991) Eur. J. Immunol. 21, 927–933.
7 Arden, B. et al. (1995) Immunogenetics 42, 455–500.
8 Folch, G. et al. (2000) Exp. Clin. Immunogenet. *in press.*
9 Koop, B.F. et al. (1994) Genomics 19, 478–493.
10 Scaviner, D. and Lefranc, M.-P. (2000) Exp. Clin. Immunogenet. 17, 97–106.
11 Baer, R. et al. (1986) Mol. Biol. Med. 3, 265–277.
12 Yoshikai, Y. et al. (1985) Nature 316, 837–740.
13 Lefranc, M.-P. (1990) Eur. Cytokine Net. 1, 121–130.
14 De Villartray, J.P. et al. (1988) Nature 335, 170–174.
15 Begley, C.G. et al. (1989) J. Exp. Med. 170, 339–342.
16 Ho, I.C. et al. (1989) Proc. Natl Acad. Sci USA. 86, 6714–6718.
17 Barker, P.E. et al. (1984) Science 226, 348–349.
18 Caccia, N. et al. (1984) Cell. 37, 1091–1099.
19 Isobe, M. et al. (1985) Science 228, 580–582.
20 Wilson, R.K. et al. (1988) Immunol. Rev. 101, 149–172.
21 Lai, E. et al. (1988) Nature 333, 543–588.
22 Ferradini, L. et al. (1991) Eur. J. Immunol. 21, 935–942.
23 Wei, S. et al. (1994) Immunogenetics 40, 27–36.
24 Posnett, D.N. et al. (1996) The Immunologist 4, 5–8.
25 Rowen, L. et al. (1996) Science 272, 1755–1762.
26 Folch, G. and Lefranc, M.-P. (2000) Exp. Clin. Immunogenet. 17, 42–54.
27 Toyonaga, B. et al. (1985) Proc. Natl Acad. Sci. USA 82, 8624–8628.
28 Tunnacliffe, A. et al. (1985) Proc. Natl Acad. Sci. USA 82, 5068–5072.
29 Folch, G. and Lefranc, M.-P. (2000) Exp. Clin. Immunogenet. 17, 107–114.
30 Malissen, M. et al. (1986) Nature 319, 28–33.
31 Robinson, M.A. et al. (1993) Proc. Natl Acad. Sci. USA 90, 2433–2437.
32 Charmley, P. et al. (1995) Genomics 25, 150–156.
33 Gottschalk, L.R. and Leiden, J.M. (1990) Mol. Cell. Biol. 10, 5486–5495.
34 Lefranc, M.-P. and Rabbitts, T.H. (1985) Nature 316, 464–466.
35 Lefranc, M.-P. et al. (1986) Nature 319, 420–422.
36 Lefranc, M.-P. et al. (1986) Cell 45, 237–246.
37 Lefranc, M.-P. et al. (1986) Proc. Natl Acad. Sci. USA 83, 9596–9600.
38 Forster, A. et al. (1987) EMBO J. 6, 1945–1950.
39 Huck, S. and Lefranc, M.-P. (1987) FEBS Lett. 224, 291–296.
40 Huck, S. et al. (1988) EMBO J. 7, 719–726.
41 Lefranc, M.-P. et al. (1989) Eur. J. Immunol. 19, 989–994.
42 Lefranc, M.-P. and Rabbitts, T.H. (1989) TIBS 14, 214-218.
43 Buresi, C. et al. (1989) Immunogenetics 29, 161–172.
44 Ghanem, N. et al. (1989) Immunogenetics 30, 350–360.
45 Lefranc, M.-P. and Rabbitts, T.H. (1990) Res. Immunol. 141, 565–577 ; 615-618.
46 Ghanem, N. et al. (1991) Hum. Genet. 86, 450–456.
47 Zhang, X.M. et al. (1994) Eur. J. Immunol. 24, 571–578.

[48] Zhang, X.M. et al. (1996) Immunogenetics 43, 196–203.
[49] Rabbitts, T.H. et al. (1985) EMBO J. 4, 1461–1465.
[50] Murre, C. et al. (1985) Nature 316, 549–552.
[51] Bensmana, M. et al. (1991) Cytogenet. Cell Genet. 56, 31–32.
[52] Lefranc, M.-P. and Alexandre, D. (1995) Eur. J. Immunol. 25, 617–622.
[53] Baer, R. et al. (1988) EMBO J. 7, 1661–1668.
[54] Satyanarayana, K. et al. (1988) Proc. Natl Acad. Sci. USA 85, 8166–8170.
[55] Griesser, H. et al. (1988) Eur. J. Immunol. 18, 641–644.
[56] Hata, S. et al. (1989) J. Exp. Med. 169, 41–57.
[57] Triebel, Y. et al. (1988) Eur. J. Immunol. 18, 2021–2027.
[58] Dariavach, P. and Lefranc, M.-P. (1989) Nucleic Acids Res. 17, 4880.
[59] Takihara, Y. et al. (1988) Proc. Natl Acad. Sci. USA 85, 6097–6101.
[60] Loh, E.Y. et al. (1988) Proc. Natl Acad. Sci. USA 85, 9714–9718.
[61] Isobe, M. et al. (1988) Proc. Natl Acad. Sci. USA 85, 3933–3937.
[62] Boehm, T. et al. (1988) EMBO J. 7, 385–394.
[63] Davodeau, F. et al. (1994) J. Immunol. 153, 137–142.
[64] Takihara, Y. et al. (1989) Eur. J. Immunol. 19, 571–574.
[65] Hata, S. et al. (1987) Science 238, 678–682.
[66] Loh, E.Y. et al. (1987) Nature 330, 569–572.
[67] Boysen, C. et al. unpublished (AE000660, AE000661).
[68] Guglielmi, P. et al. (1988) Proc. Natl Acad. Sci. USA 85, 5634–5638.
[69] Casorati, G. and Migone, N. (1989) Res. Immunol. 141, 624–626.
[70] Redondo, J.M. et al. (1990) Science 247, 1225–1229.
[71] Bories, J.C. et al. (1990) J. Exp. Med. 171, 75–83.

THE HUMAN T CELL RECEPTOR TRA GENES

Part 1

TRAC

Nomenclature

TRAC: T cell receptor alpha constant.

Definition and functionality

TRAC is the functional and unique constant gene in the TRA locus.

Gene location

TRAC is in the TRA locus on chromosome 14 at 14q11.2. TRAC is the most 3′ gene in the TRA/TRD locus.

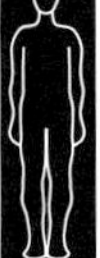

Nucleotide and amino acid sequences for human TRAC

The nucleotide between parentheses at the beginning of exons comes from a DONOR–SPLICE (n from ngt).

The Cysteines involved in the intrachain disulfide bridges are shown with their number and letter **C** in bold.

N-Glycosylation sites (NXS/T, where X is different from P) are underlined.

A DONOR–SPLICE, located just after the termination codon, uses a downstream ACCEPTOR–SPLICE, placing part of the 3′ non-coding sequence on a separate untranslated exon, designated as EX4. Since EX4 is untranslated, nucleotide differences observed in EX4 are not taken into account for the description of alleles.

		1	2	3	4	5	6	7	8	9	10	11	12	13	14	15	16	17	18	19	20
		N	I	Q	N	P	D	P	A	V	Y	Q	L	R	D	S	K	S	S	D	K
X02883 ,TRAC*01 (EX1)	[1]	(A)AT	ATC	CAG	AAC	CCT	GAC	CCT	GCC	GTG	TAC	CAG	CTG	AGA	GAC	TCT	AAA	TCC	AGT	GAC	AAG
X02592 ,TRAC*01 (cDNA)	[2]	(-)--	---	---	---	---	---	---	---	---	---	---	---	---	---	---	---	---	---	---	---
M14858 ,TRAC*01	[3]	(-)--	---	---	---	---	---	---	---	---	---	---	---	---	---	---	---	---	---	---	---
AE000662,TRAC*01	[5]	(-)--	---	---	---	---	---	---	---	---	---	---	---	---	---	---	---	---	---	---	---
M94081 ,TRAC*01	[4]	(-)--	---	---	---	---	---	---	---	---	---	---	---	---	---	---	---	---	---	---	---

	21	22	**23**	24	25	26	27	28	29	30	31	32	33	34	35	36	37	38	39	40
	S	V	**C**	L	F	T	D	F	D	S	Q	T	N	V	S	Q	S	K	D	S
X02883 ,TRAC*01	TCT	GTC	TGC	CTA	TTC	ACC	GAT	TTT	GAT	TCT	CAA	ACA	AAT	GTG	TCA	CAA	AGT	AAG	GAT	TCT
X02592 ,TRAC*01	---	---	---	---	---	---	---	---	---	---	---	---	---	---	---	---	---	---	---	---
M14858 ,TRAC*01	---	---	---	---	---	---	---	---	---	---	---	---	---	---	---	---	---	---	---	---
AE000662,TRAC*01	---	---	---	---	---	---	---	---	---	---	---	---	---	---	---	---	---	---	---	---
M94081 ,TRAC*01	---	---	---	---	---	---	---	---	---	---	---	---	---	---	---	---	---	---	---	---

	41	42	43	44	45	46	47	48	49	50	51	52	53	54	55	56	57	58	59	60
	D	V	Y	I	T	D	K	T	V	L	D	M	R	S	M	D	F	K	S	N
X02883 ,TRAC*01	GAT	GTG	TAT	ATC	ACA	GAC	AAA	ACT	GTG	CTA	GAC	ATG	AGG	TCT	ATG	GAC	TTC	AAG	AGC	AAC
X02592 ,TRAC*01	---	---	---	---	---	---	---	---	---	---	---	---	---	---	---	---	---	---	---	---
M14858 ,TRAC*01	---	---	---	---	---	---	---	---	---	---	---	---	---	---	---	---	---	---	---	---
AE000662,TRAC*01	---	---	---	---	---	---	---	---	---	---	---	---	---	---	---	---	---	---	---	---
M94081 ,TRAC*01	---	---	---	---	---	---	---	---	---	---	---	---	---	---	---	---	---	---	---	---

	61	62	63	64	65	66	67	68	69	70	71	72	**73**	74	75	76	77	78	79	80
	S	A	V	A	W	S	N	K	S	D	F	A	**C**	A	N	A	F	N	N	S
X02883 ,TRAC*01	AGT	GCT	GTG	GCC	TGG	AGC	AAC	AAA	TCT	GAC	TTT	GCA	TGT	GCA	AAC	GCC	TTC	AAC	AAC	AGC
X02592 ,TRAC*01	---	---	---	---	---	---	---	---	---	---	---	---	---	---	---	---	---	---	---	---
M14858 ,TRAC*01	---	---	---	---	---	---	---	---	---	---	---	---	---	---	---	---	---	---	---	---
AE000662,TRAC*01	---	---	---	---	---	---	---	---	---	---	---	---	---	---	---	---	---	---	---	---
M94081 ,TRAC*01	---	---	---	---	---	---	---	---	---	---	---	---	---	---	---	---	---	---	---	---

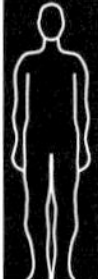

```
                    81  82  83  84  85  86  87  88  89  90  91
                    I   I   P   E   D   T   F   F   P   S   P
X02883  ,TRAC*01    ATT ATT CCA GAA GAC ACC TTC TTC CCC AGC CCA G
X02592  ,TRAC*01    --- --- --- --- --- --- --- --- --- --- --- -
M14858  ,TRAC*01    --- --- --- --- --- --- --- --- --- --- --- -
AE000662,TRAC*01    --- --- --- --- --- --- --- --- --- --- --- -
M94081  ,TRAC*01    --- --- --- --- --- --- --- --- --- --- --- -

                    1   2   3   4   5   6   7   8   9   10  11  12  13  14  15
                    E   S   S   C   D   V   K   L   V   E   K   S   F   E   T
X02883  ,TRAC*01 (EX2)   AA AGT TCC TGT GAT GTC AAG CTG GTC GAG AAA AGC TTT GAA ACA G
X02592  ,TRAC*01 (cDNA)  -- --- --- --- --- --- --- --- --- --- --- --- --- --- --- -
M14859  ,TRAC*01         -- --- --- --- --- --- --- --- --- --- --- --- --- --- --- -
AE000662,TRAC*01         -- --- --- --- --- --- --- --- --- --- --- --- --- --- --- -
M94081  ,TRAC*01         -- --- --- --- --- --- --- --- --- --- --- --- --- --- --- -

                    1   2   3   4   5   6   7   8   9   10  11  12  13  14  15  16  17  18  19  20
                    D   T   N   L   N   F   Q   N   L   S   V   I   G   F   R   I   L   L   L   K
X02883  ,TRAC*01 (EX3)   AT ACG AAC CTA AAC TTT CAA AAC CTG TCA GTG ATT GGG TTC CGA ATC CTC CTC CTG AAA
X02592  ,TRAC*01 (cDNA)  -- --- --- --- --- --- --- --- --- --- --- --- --- --- --- --- --- --- --- ---
M14860  ,TRAC*01         -- --- --- --- --- --- --- --- --- --- --- --- --- --- --- --- --- --- --- ---
AE000662,TRAC*01         -- --- --- --- --- --- --- --- --- --- --- --- --- --- --- --- --- --- --- ---
M94081  ,TRAC*01         -- --- --- --- --- --- --- --- --- --- --- --- --- --- --- --- --- --- --- ---

                    21  22  23  24  25  26  27  28  29  30  31  32  33  34  35
                    V   A   G   F   N   L   L   M   T   L   R   L   W   S   S   *
X02883  ,TRAC*01    GTG GCC GGG TTT AAT CTG CTC ATG ACG CTG CGG CTG TGG TCC AGC TGA G
X02592  ,TRAC*01    --- --- --- --- --- --- --- --- --- --- --- --- --- --- --- --- -
M14860  ,TRAC*01    --- --- --- --- --- --- --- --- --- --- --- --- --- --- --- --- -
AE000662,TRAC*01    --- --- --- --- --- --- --- --- --- --- --- --- --- --- --- --- -
M94081  ,TRAC*01    --- --- --- --- --- --- --- --- --- --- --- --- --- --- --- --- -


X02883  ,TRAC*01 (Untranslated EX4   ATCTGCAAGATTGTAAGACAGCCTGTGCTCCCTCGCTCCTTCCTCTGCATTGCCCCTCTTCTCCCTCTCCAAACAGAGG
                  and 3'UTR)
X02592  ,TRAC*01 (cDNA)               ------------------------------------------------------------------------------
X05002/M14861,TRAC*01        [3]      ------------------------------------------------------------------------------
AE000662,TRAC*01                      ------------------------------------------------------------------------------
M94081  ,TRAC*01                      ------------------------------------------------------------------------------

X02883  ,TRAC*01    GAACTCTCCCACCCCCAAGGAGGTGAAAGCTGCTACCACCTCTGTGCCCCCCCGC-AATGCCACCAACTGGATGGGATCC
                                                                    #                   #   #
X02592  ,TRAC*01    ---------T-----------------------------GT-----------------.....--
                                                                    #                   #   #
X05002/M14861,TRAC*01  ---------T-----------------------------GC-----------------.....--
                                                                    #        #          #   #
AE000662,TRAC*01    ---------T-----------------------------GC-----.-----------.....--
                                                                    #        #          #   #
M94081  ,TRAC*01    ---------T-----------------------------GC-----.-----------.....--

X02883  ,TRAC*01    TACCCGAATTTATGATTAAGATTGCTGAAGAGCTGCCAAACACTGCTGCCACCCCCTCTGTTCCCTTATTGCTGCTTGTC
X02592  ,TRAC*01    ------------------------------------------------------------------------------
X05002/M14861,TRAC*01  ---------------------------------------------------------------------------
AE000662,TRAC*01    ------------------------------------------------------------------------------
M94081  ,TRAC*01    ------------------------------------------------------------------------------

X02883  ,TRAC*01    ACTGCCTGACATTCACGGCAGAGGCAAGGCTGCTGCAGCCTCCCCTGGCTGTGCACATTCCCTCCTGCTCCCCAGAGACT
X02592  ,TRAC*01    ------------------------------------------------------------------------------
X05002/M14861,TRAC*01  ---------------------------------------------------------------------------
                                                             #
AE000662,TRAC*01    -----------------------------------------.---G--------------------------------
                                                             #
M94081  ,TRAC*01    -----------------------------------------.---G--------------------------------

X02883  ,TRAC*01    GCCTCCGCCATCCCACAGATGATGGATCTTCAGTGGGTTCTCTTGGGCTCTAGGTCCTGGAGAATGTTGTGAGGGTT-TA
                                                                                              #
X02592  ,TRAC*01    -----------------------------------------------------------------------G--
                                                                                              #
X05002/M14861,TRAC*01  --------------------------------------------------------------------G--
                                                                                              #
AE000662,TRAC*01    -------------------------------------------------------------C-----------G--
                                                                                              #
M94081  ,TRAC*01    -------------------------------------------------------------C-----------G--

X02883  ,TRAC*01    TTTTTTTTTAATAGTGTTCATAAAGAAATACATAGTATTCTTCTTCTCAAGACGTGGGGGGAAATTATCTCATTATCGAG
X02592  ,TRAC*01    ------------------------------------------------------------------------------
X05002/M14861,TRAC*01  ---------------------------------------------------------------------------
AE000662,TRAC*01    -----------------------------G------------------------------------------------
M94081  ,TRAC*01    -----------------------------G------------------------------------------------
```

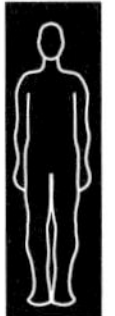

```
X02883   ,TRAC*01           GCCCTGCTATGCTGTGTGTCTGGGCGTGTTGTATGTCCTGCTGCCGATGCCTTC
X02592   ,TRAC*01           ------------------------------------------------------
X05002/M14861,TRAC*01       ------------------------------------------------------
AE000662,TRAC*01            ------------------------------------------------------
M94081   ,TRAC*01           ------------------------------------------------------

#: Nucleotide deletion or insertion
```

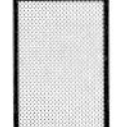

Genome database accession numbers

GDB:9953797   LocusLink: 28755

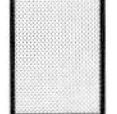

References
1 Yoshikai, Y. et al. (1985) Nature 316, 837–840.
2 Rabbitts, T.H. et al. (1985) EMBO J. 4, 1461–1465.
3 Baer, R.J. et al. (1986) Mol. Biol. Med. 3, 265–277.
4 Koop, B.F. et al. (1994) Genomics 19, 478–493.
5 Boysen, C. et al., unpublished.

Protein display

Protein display of the TRAC gene is shown on page 372.

Part 2

TRAJ

Nomenclature

T cell receptor alpha joining group.

Definition and functionality

The human TRAJ group comprises 61 mapped genes of which 52 are functional, eight are ORF (TRAJ1, TRAJ2, TRAJ19, TRAJ25, TRAJ35, TRAJ58, TRAJ59, and TRAJ61) and three are pseudogenes (TRAJ51, TRAJ55, and TRAJ60).

Gene location

The human TRAJ genes are located in the TRA/TRD locus on chromosome 14 at 14q11.2, between the TRDV3 and TRAC genes, at a distance of 71 kb.

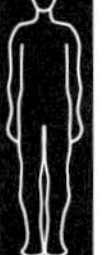

Nucleotide and amino acid sequences for the human functional or ORF TRAJ genes with nomenclature

The conserved **FGXG** motif, characteristic of the TRA J-REGION, is underlined.

```
TRAJ1
T cell receptor alpha joining 1
                              Y   E   S   I   T   S   Q   L   Q   F   G   K   G   T   R   V   S   T   S   P
   X02884  ,TRAJ1*01  [6](1)  G TAT GAA AGT ATT ACC TCC CAG TTG CAA TTT GGC AAA GGA ACC AGA GTT TCC ACT TCT CCC C

TRAJ2
T cell receptor alpha joining 2
                            N   T   G   G   T   I   D   K   L   T   F   G   K   G   T   H   V   F   I   I   S
   X02884  ,TRAJ2*01  [6](2)  TG AAT ACT GGA GGA ACA ATT GAT AAA CTC ACA TTT GGG AAA GGG ACC CAT GTA TTC ATT ATA TCT G

TRAJ3
T cell receptor alpha joining 3
                            G   Y   S   S   A   S   K   I   I   F   G   S   G   T   R   L   S   I   R   P
   X02884  ,TRAJ3*01  [6]    G GGG TAC AGC AGT GCT TCC AAG ATA ATC TTT GGA TCA GGG ACC AGA CTC AGC ATC CGG CCA A

TRAJ4
T cell receptor alpha joining 4
                            F   S   G   G   Y   N   K   L   I   F   G   A   G   T   R   L   A   V   H   P
   M94081  ,TRAJ4*01  [4]    TG TTT TCT GGT GGC TAC AAT AAG CTG ATT TTT GGA GCA GGG ACC AGG CTG GCT GTA CAC CCA T

TRAJ5
T cell receptor alpha joining 5
                            D   T   G   R   R   A   L   T   F   G   S   G   T   R   L   Q   V   Q   P
   M94081  ,TRAJ5*01  [4]    TG GAC ACG GGC AGG AGA GCA CTT ACT TTT GGG AGT GGA ACA AGA CTC CAA GTG CAA CCA A

TRAJ6
T cell receptor alpha joining 6
                            A   S   G   G   S   Y   I   P   T   F   G   R   G   T   S   L   I   V   H   P
   M16747  ,TRAJ6*01  [1]    T GCA TCA GGA GGA AGC TAC ATA CCT ACA TTT GGA AGA GGA ACC AGC CTT ATT GTT CAT CCG T

TRAJ7
T cell receptor alpha joining 7
                            D   Y   G   N   N   R   L   A   F   G   K   G   N   Q   V   V   V   I   P
   M94081  ,TRAJ7*01  [4]    T GAC TAT GGG AAC AAC AGA CTC GCT TTT GGG AAG GGG AAC CAA GTG GTG GTC ATA CCA A

TRAJ8
T cell receptor alpha joining 8
                            N   T   G   F   Q   K   L   V   F   G   T   G   T   R   L   L   V   S   P
   M94081  ,TRAJ8*01  [4]    TG AAC ACA GGC TTT CAG AAA CTT GTA TTT GGA ACT GGC ACC CGA CTT CTG GTC AGT CCA A

TRAJ9
T cell receptor alpha joining 9
                            G   N   T   G   G   F   K   T   I   F   G   A   G   T   R   L   F   V   K   A
   M94081  ,TRAJ9*01  [4]    GGA AAT ACT GGA GGC TTC AAA ACT ATC TTT GGA GCA GGA ACA AGA CTA TTT GTT AAA GCA A

TRAJ10
T cell receptor alpha joining 10
                            I   L   T   G   G   G   N   K   L   T   F   G   T   G   T   Q   L   K   V   E   L
   M94081  ,TRAJ10*01 [4]    ATA CTC ACG GGA GGA GGA AAC AAA CTC ACC TTT GGG ACA GGC ACT CAG CTA AAA GTG GAA CTC A
```

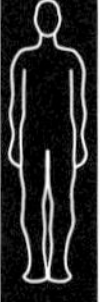

TRAJ11
T cell receptor alpha joining 11

```
                                N   S   G   Y   S   T   L   T   F   G   K   G   T   M   L   L   V   S   P
  M94081   ,TRAJ11*01 [4]      TG AAT TCA GGA TAC AGC ACC CTC ACC TTT GGG AAG GGG ACT ATG CTT CTA GTC TCT CCA G
```

TRAJ12
T cell receptor alpha joining 12

```
                                M   D   S   S   Y   K   L   I   F   G   S   G   T   R   L   L   V   R   P
  X02885   ,TRAJ12*01 [6]      GG ATG GAT AGC AGC TAT AAA TTG ATC TTC GGG AGT GGG ACC AGA CTG CTG GTC AGG CCT G
```

TRAJ13
T cell receptor alpha joining 13

```
                                N   S   G   G   Y   Q   K   V   T   F   G   I   G   T   K   L   Q   V   I   P
  M94081   ,TRAJ13*01 [4]      TG AAT TCT GGG GGT TAC CAG AAA GTT ACC TTT GGA ATT GGA ACA AAG CTC CAA GTC ATC CCA A
```

TRAJ14
T cell receptor alpha joining 14

```
                                    I   Y   S   T   F   I   F   G   S   G   T   R   L   S   V   K   P
  M94081   ,TRAJ14*01 [4]          ATT TAT AGC ACA TTC ATC TTT GGG AGT GGG ACA AGA TTA TCA GTA AAA CCT G
```

TRAJ15
T cell receptor alpha joining 15

```
                                N   Q   A   G   T   A   L   I   F   G   K   G   T   T   L   S   V   S   S
  X05775   ,TRAJ15*01 [5]      CC AAC CAG GCA GGA ACT GCT CTG ATC TTT GGG AAG GGA ACC ACC TTA TCA GTG AGT TCC A
                                                                            H
  M94081   ,TRAJ15*02 [4]      -- --- --- --- --- --- --- --- --- --- --- --- CA- C-- --- --- --- --- -
```

TRAJ16
T cell receptor alpha joining 16

```
                                F   S   D   G   Q   K   L   L   F   A   R   G   T   M   L   K   V   D   L
  M94081   ,TRAJ16*01 [4]      GG TTT TCA GAT GGC CAG AAG CTG CTC TTT GCA AGG GGA ACC ATG TTA AAG GTG GAT CTT A
```

TRAJ17
T cell receptor alpha joining 17

```
                                I   K   A   A   G   N   K   L   T   F   G   G   G   T   R   V   L   V   K   P
  X05773   ,TRAJ17*01 [5]      TG ATC AAA GCT GCA GGC AAC AAG CTA ACT TTT GGA GGA GGA ACC AGG GTG CTA GTT AAA CCA A
```

TRAJ18
T cell receptor alpha joining 18

```
                             D   R   G   S   T   L   G   R   L   Y   F   G   R   G   T   Q   L   T   V   W   P
  M94081   ,TRAJ18*01 [4]   CC GAC AGA GGC TCA ACC CTG GGG AGG CTA TAC TTT GGA AGA GGA ACT CAG TTG ACT GTC TGG CCT G
```

TRAJ19
T cell receptor alpha joining 19

```
                                Y   Q   R   F   Y   N   F   T   F   G   K   G   S   K   H   N   V   T   P
  M94081   ,TRAJ19*01 [4](3)  GC TAT CAA AGA TTT TAC AAT TTC ACC TTT GGA AAG GGA TCC AAA CAT AAT GTC ACT CCA A
```

TRAJ20
T cell receptor alpha joining 20

```
                                S   N   D   Y   K   L   S   F   G   A   G   T   T   V   T   V   R   A
  M94081   ,TRAJ20*01 [4]      GT TCT AAC GAC TAC AAG CTC AGC TTT GGA GCC GGA ACC ACA GTA ACT GTA AGA GCA A
```

TRAJ21
T cell receptor alpha joining 21

```
                                Y   N   F   N   K   F   Y   F   G   S   G   T   K   L   N   V   K   P
  M94081   ,TRAJ21*01 [4]      TAC AAC TTC AAC AAA TTT TAC TTT GGA TCT GGG ACC AAA CTC AAT GTA AAA CCA A
```

TRAJ22
T cell receptor alpha joining 22

```
                                S   S   G   S   A   R   Q   L   T   F   G   S   G   T   Q   L   T   V   L   P
  X02886   ,TRAJ22*01 [6]      TT TCT TCT GGT TCT GCA AGG CAA CTG ACC TTT GGA TCT GGG ACA CAA TTG ACT GTT TTA CCT G
```

TRAJ23
T cell receptor alpha joining 23

```
                                I   Y   N   Q   G   G   K   L   I   F   G   Q   G   T   E   L   S   V   K   P
  M94081   ,TRAJ23*01 [4]      TG ATT TAT AAC CAG GGA GGA AAG CTT ATC TTC GGA CAG GGA ACG GAG TTA TCT GTG AAA CCC A
```

TRAJ24
T cell receptor alpha joining 24

```
                                T   T   D   S   W   G   K   F   E   F   G   A   G   T   Q   V   V   V   T   P
  X02887   ,TRAJ24*01 [6]      TG ACA ACT GAC AGC TGG GGG AAA TTC GAG TTT GGA GCA GGG ACC CAG GTT GTG GTC ACC CCA G
                                                                L   Q
  M94081   ,TRAJ24*02 [4]      -- --- --- --- --- --- --- --- --G C-- --- --- --- --- --- --- --- --- --- --- -
```

TRAJ25
T cell receptor alpha joining 25

```
                                E   G   Q   G   F   S   F   I   F   G   K   G   T   R   L   L   V   K   P
  X02888   ,TRAJ25*01 [6](4)   CA GAA GGA CAA GGC TTC TCC TTT ATC TTT GGG AAG GGG ACA AGG CTG CTT GTC AAG CCA A
```

TRAJ26
T cell receptor alpha joining 26

```
                                D   N   Y   G   Q   N   F   V   F   G   P   G   T   R   L   S   V   L   P
  M94081   ,TRAJ26*01 [4]      GG GAT AAC TAT GGT CAG AAT TTT GTC TTT GGT CCC GGA ACC AGA TTG TCC GTG CTG CCC T
```

TRAJ27
T cell receptor alpha joining 27

```
                                N   T   N   A   G   K   S   T   F   G   D   G   T   T   L   T   V   K   P
  M94081   ,TRAJ27*01 [4]      T AAC ACC AAT GCA GGC AAA TCA ACC TTT GGG GAT GGG ACT ACG CTC ACT GTG AAG CCA A
```

TRAJ28
T cell receptor alpha joining 28
```
                                        Y   S   G   A   G   S   Y   Q   L   T   F   G   K   G   T   K   L   S   V   I   P
M94081  ,TRAJ28*01 [4]      CA TAC TCT GGG GCT GGG AGT TAC CAA CTC ACT TTC GGG AAG GGG ACC AAA CTC TCG GTC ATA CCA A
```

TRAJ29
T cell receptor alpha joining 29
```
                                    N   S   G   N   T   P   L   V   F   G   K   G   T   R   L   S   V   I   A
X02889  ,TRAJ29*01 [6]      GG AAT TCA GGA AAC ACA CCT CTT GTC TTT GGA AAG GGC ACA AGA CTT TCT GTG ATT GCA A
```

TRAJ30
T cell receptor alpha joining 30
```
                                    N   R   D   D   K   I   I   F   G   K   G   T   R   L   H   I   L   P
M94081  ,TRAJ30*01 [4]      TG AAC AGA GAT GAC AAG ATC ATC TTT GGA AAA GGG ACA CGA CTT CAT ATT CTC CCC A
```

TRAJ31
T cell receptor alpha joining 31
```
                                    N   N   N   A   R   L   M   F   G   D   G   T   Q   L   V   V   K   P
M14905  ,TRAJ31*01 [3]       G AAT AAC AAT GCC AGA CTC ATG TTT GGA GAT GGA ACT CAG CTG GTG GTG AAG CCC A
```

TRAJ32
T cell receptor alpha joining 32
```
                                N   Y   G   G   A   T   N   K   L   I   F   G   T   G   T   L   L   A   V   Q   P
M94081  ,TRAJ32*01 [4]      TG AAT TAT GGC GGT GCT ACA AAC AAG CTC ATC TTT GGA ACT GGC ACT CTG CTT GCT GTC CAG CCA A
```

TRAJ33
T cell receptor alpha joining 33
```
                                    D   S   N   Y   Q   L   I   W   G   A   G   T   K   L   I   I   K   P
M94081  ,TRAJ33*01 [4]      TG GAT AGC AAC TAT CAG TTA ATC TGG GGC GCT GGG ACC AAG CTA ATT ATA AAG CCA G
```

TRAJ34
T cell receptor alpha joining 34
```
                                    S   Y   N   T   D   K   L   I   F   G   T   G   T   R   L   Q   V   F   P
M35622  ,TRAJ34*01 [2]      TCT TAT AAC ACC GAC AAG CTC ATC TTT GGG ACT GGG ACC AGA TTA CAA GTC TTT CCA A
```

TRAJ35
T cell receptor alpha joining 35
```
                                    I   G   F   G   N   V   L   H   C   G   S   G   T   Q   V   I   V   L   P
M94081  ,TRAJ35*01 [4](5)    G ATA GGC TTT GGG AAT GTG CTG CAT TGC GGG TCC GGC ACT CAA GTG ATT GTT TTA CCA C
```

TRAJ36
T cell receptor alpha joining 36
```
                                Q   T   G   A   N   N   L   F   F   G   T   G   T   R   L   T   V   I   P
M94081  ,TRAJ36*01 [4]       T CAA ACT GGG GCA AAC AAC CTC TTC TTT GGG ACT GGA ACG AGA CTC ACC GTT ATT CCC T
```

TRAJ37
T cell receptor alpha joining 37
```
                                G   S   G   N   T   G   K   L   I   F   G   Q   G   T   T   L   Q   V   K   P
M94081  ,TRAJ37*01 [4]       T GGC TCT GGC AAC ACA GGC AAA CTA ATC TTT GGG CAA GGG ACA ACT TTA CAA GTA AAA CCA G
```

TRAJ38
T cell receptor alpha joining 38
```
                                N   A   G   N   N   R   K   L   I   W   G   L   G   T   S   L   A   V   N   P
M94081  ,TRAJ38*01 [4]       T AAT GCT GGC AAC AAC CGT AAG CTG ATT TGG GGA TTG GGA ACA AGC CTG GCA GTA AAT CCG A
```

TRAJ39
T cell receptor alpha joining 39
```
                                    N   N   N   A   G   N   M   L   T   F   G   G   G   T   R   L   M   V   K   P
M94081  ,TRAJ39*01 [4]      TG AAT AAT AAT GCA GGC AAC ATG CTC ACC TTT GGA GGG GGA ACA AGG TTA ATG GTC AAA CCC C
```

TRAJ40
T cell receptor alpha joining 40
```
                                T   T   S   G   T   Y   K   Y   I   F   G   T   G   T   R   L   K   V   L   A
M35620  ,TRAJ40*01 [2]      ACT ACC TCA GGA ACC TAC AAA TAC ATC TTT GGA ACA GGC ACC AGG CTG AAG GTT TTA GCA A
```

TRAJ41
T cell receptor alpha joining 41
```
                                    N   S   N   S   G   Y   A   L   N   F   G   K   G   T   S   L   L   V   T   P
M94081  ,TRAJ41*01 [4]       G AAC TCA AAT TCC GGG TAT GCA CTC AAC TTC GGC AAA GGC ACC TCG CTG TTG GTC ACA CCC C
```

TRAJ42
T cell receptor alpha joining 42
```
                                N   Y   G   G   S   Q   G   N   L   I   F   G   K   G   T   K   L   S   V   K   P
M94081  ,TRAJ42*01 [4]      TG AAT TAT GGA GGA AGC CAA GGA AAT CTC ATC TTT GGA AAA GGC ACT AAA CTC TCT GTT AAA CCA A
```

TRAJ43
T cell receptor alpha joining 43
```
                                    N   N   N   D   M   R   F   G   A   G   T   R   L   T   V   K   P
M94081  ,TRAJ43*01 [4]      AC AAT AAC AAT GAC ATG CGC TTT GGA GCA GGG ACC AGA CTG ACA GTA AAA CCA A
```

TRAJ44
T cell receptor alpha joining 44
```
                                    N   T   G   T   A   S   K   L   T   F   G   T   G   T   R   L   Q   V   T   L
M35619  ,TRAJ44*01 [2]      TA AAT ACC GGC ACT GCC AGT AAA CTC ACC TTT GGG ACT GGA ACA AGA CTT CAG GTC ACG CTC G
```

TRAJ45
T cell receptor alpha joining 45
```
                                Y   S   G   G   G   A   D   G   L   T   F   G   K   G   T   H   L   I   I   Q   P
M94081  ,TRAJ45*01 [4]      TG TAT TCA GGA GGA GGT GCT GAC GGA CTC ACC TTT GGC AAA GGG ACT CAT CTA ATC ATC CAG CCC T
```

TRAJ46
T cell receptor alpha joining 46
```
                                    K   K   S   S   G   D   K   L   T   F   G   T   G   T   R   L   A   V   R   P
M94081  ,TRAJ46*01 [4]      AG AAG AAA AGC AGC GGA GAC AAG CTG ACT TTT GGG ACC GGG ACT CGT TTA GCA GTT AGG CCC A
```

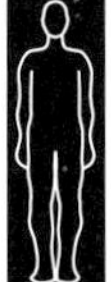

TRAJ47
T cell receptor alpha joining 47

```
                                      E   Y   G   N   K   L   V   F   G   A   G   T   I   L   R   V   K   S
  M94081  ,TRAJ47*01 [4]             TG GAA TAT GGA AAC AAA CTG GTC TTT GGC GCA GGA ACC ATT CTG AGA GTC AAG TCC T
```

TRAJ48
T cell receptor alpha joining 48

```
                                  S   N   F   G   N   E   K   L   T   F   G   T   G   T   R   L   T   I   I   P
  M94081  ,TRAJ48*01 [4]         TA TCT AAC TTT GGA AAT GAG AAA TTA ACC TTT GGG ACT GGA ACA AGA CTC ACC ATC ATA CCC A
```

TRAJ49
T cell receptor alpha joining 49

```
                                      N   T   G   N   Q   F   Y   F   G   T   G   T   S   L   T   V   I   P
  M94081  ,TRAJ49*01 [4]              G AAC ACC GGT AAC CAG TTC TAT TTT GGG ACA GGG ACA AGT TTG ACG GTC ATT CCA A
```

TRAJ50
T cell receptor alpha joining 50

```
                                    K   T   S   Y   D   K   V   I   F   G   P   G   T   S   L   S   V   I   P
  M94081  ,TRAJ50*01 [4]            TG AAA ACC TCC TAC GAC AAG GTG ATA TTT GGG CCA GGG ACA AGC TTA TCA GTC ATT CCA A
```

TRAJ52
T cell receptor alpha joining 52

```
                            N   A   G   G   T   S   Y   G   K   L   T   F   G   Q   G   T   I   L   T   V   H   P
  M94081  ,TRAJ52*01 [4]  CT AAT GCT GGT GGT ACT AGC TAT GGA AAG CTG ACA TTT GGA CAA GGG ACC ATC TTG ACT GTC CAT CCA A
```

TRAJ53
T cell receptor alpha joining 53

```
                            N   S   G   G   S   N   Y   K   L   T   F   G   K   G   T   L   L   T   V   N   P
  M94081  ,TRAJ53*01 [4]  AG AAT AGT GGA GGT AGC AAC TAT AAA CTG ACA TTT GGA AAA GGA ACT CTC TTA ACC GTG AAT CCA A
```

TRAJ54
T cell receptor alpha joining 54

```
                                  I   Q   G   A   Q   K   L   V   F   G   Q   G   T   R   L   T   I   N   P
  M94081  ,TRAJ54*01 [4]          TA ATT CAG GGA GCC CAG AAG CTG GTA TTT GGC CAA GGA ACC AGG CTG ACT ATC AAC CCA A
```

TRAJ56
T cell receptor alpha joining 56

```
                                Y   T   G   A   N   S   K   L   T   F   G   K   G   I   T   L   S   V   R   P
  M94081  ,TRAJ56*01 [4]        T TAT ACT GGA GCC AAT AGT AAG CTG ACA TTT GGA AAA GGA ATA ACT CTG AGT GTT AGA CCA G
```

TRAJ57
T cell receptor alpha joining 57

```
                              T   Q   G   G   S   E   K   L   V   F   G   K   G   T   K   L   T   V   N   P
  M94081  ,TRAJ57*01 [4]      TA ACT CAG GGC GGA TCT GAA AAG CTG GTC TTT GGA AAG GGA ACG AAA CTG ACA GTA AAC CCA T
```

TRAJ58
T cell receptor alpha joining 58

```
                              *   E   T   S   G   S   R   L   T   F   G   E   G   T   Q   L   T   V   N   P
  M94081  ,TRAJ58*01 [4](6)   TT TAA GAA ACC AGT GGC TCA TGG TTG ACC TTT GGG GAA GGA ACA CAG CTC ACA GTG AAT CCT G
```

TRAJ59
T cell receptor alpha joining 59

```
                                K   E   G   N   R   K   F   T   F   G   M   G   T   Q   V   R   V
  M94081  ,TRAJ59*01 [4](7)    GG AAG GAA GGA AAC AGG AAA TTT ACA TTT GGA ATG GGG ACG CAA GTG AGA GTG
```

TRAJ61
T cell receptor alpha joining 61

```
                                Y   R   V   N   R   K   L   T   F   G   A   N   T   R   G   I   M   K   L
  M94081  ,TRAJ61*01 [4](7)    GG TAC CGG GTT AAT AGG AAA CTG ACA TTT GGA GCC AAC ACT AGA GGA ATC ATG AAA CTC A
```

Notes:

(1) Non-canonical J-HEPTAMER: gggcatg instead of cactgtg.

(2) Non-canonical J-HEPTAMER: tacggta instead of cactgtg.

(3) 7 nucleotides instead of 12 in J-SPACER.

(4) Non-canonical J-HEPTAMER: cactatg instead of cactgtg.

(5) Non-canonical J-REGION: Cys-Gly-X-Gly instead of Phe-Gly-X-Gly.

(6) The first codon of the germline J-REGION is a STOP-CODON which may disappear during rearrangements.

(7) Defective DONOR–SPLICE.

References:

[1] Baer, R.J. et al. (1987) Cell 50, 97–105.

[2] Baer, R.J. et al. (1988) EMBO J. 7, 1661–1668.

[3] Finger, L.R. et al. (1986) Science 234, 982–985.

[5] Mengle-Gaw, L. et al. (1987) EMBO J. 6, 2273–2280.

[4] Koop, B.F. et al. (1994) Genomics 19, 478–493.

[6] Yoshikai, Y. et al. (1985) Nature 316, 837–839.

Recombination signals

Only the recombination signals of the allele *01 of each functional or ORF J-REGION are shown. Non-conserved nucleotides taken into account for the ORF functionality definition are shown in bold and italics.

J Recombination Signal (J-RS)			TRAJ gene and allele name
J-NONAMER	(bp)	J-HEPTAMER	
GGATTCTGT	12	**GGGCA**TG	TRAJ1*01 (ORF)
AGTTTGTGC	12	**TACG**GT**A**	TRAJ2*01 (ORF)
GGTTATCTC	12	CACAGTG	TRAJ3*01
AGTTCTTGT	12	GATTGTG	TRAJ4*01
GGATTTTGT	12	CAGGGTG	TRAJ5*01
GGTTTTATC	12	CACTGTG	TRAJ6*01
GGTTTTTGT	10	CACAGTG	TRAJ7*01
CCATTTTGT	12	CAGAGTG	TRAJ8*01
CCATTTTGT	12	CACTGTG	TRAJ9*01
AGTTTATGT	12	CACTGTG	TRAJ10*01
CATTTTTGT	12	TATAGTG	TRAJ11*01
TGTTTTTGA	12	CACTGTG	TRAJ12*01
TCATTTTGT	12	TACAGTG	TRAJ13*01
CATTTTTGT	12	TGCTGTG	TRAJ14*01
GGTATTTGC	12	CACTGTG	TRAJ15*01
GGTATTTGC	12	CACTGTG	TRAJ15*02
GGTTTTTGT	12	CACTGTG	TRAJ16*01
GGTATTTGC	12	CATTTGT	TRAJ17*01
GGTTCATGT	12	CATTGTG	TRAJ18*01
TGATTTTGC	7	AGATGTG	TRAJ19*01 (ORF)
GGTTTGTGT	11	CACTGTG	TRAJ20*01
ATTTTTTGT	12	CATGGTG	TRAJ21*01
GGTTTTTGT	12	CATAGTG	TRAJ22*01
TGTTTTTGA	12	CACAGTG	TRAJ23*01
CCATTTTGT	12	CACAGTG	TRAJ24*01
CCATTTTGT	12	CACAGTG	TRAJ24*02
GGTTTTTGA	12	CACT**A**TG	TRAJ25*01 (ORF)
GGTTTTTGC	12	CACTGTG	TRAJ26*01
GGTTATTGC	12	GACTGTG	TRAJ27*01
GGTTTTTGC	12	CTCTGTG	TRAJ28*01
GGTTTTTGT	12	CACTGTG	TRAJ29*01 (1)
AGTTTTTGT	12	CACAGTG	TRAJ30*01
GGTTTCAGT	12	TGCTGTG	TRAJ31*01
GGTTAGTGT	12	GACTGTG	TRAJ32*01
GGTTTTTGT	12	GTCTGTG	TRAJ33*01
GGTTTTTGT	12	CACTGTG	TRAJ34*01
GGTTTTTGT	12	CATTGTG	TRAJ35*01 (ORF)
TGTTTTTGT	12	CACTGTG	TRAJ36*01
AGTTTTTGT	12	TAGAGTG	TRAJ37*01

Recombination signals – *continued*

J Recombination Signal (J-RS)			TRAJ gene and allele name
J-NONAMER	(bp)	J-HEPTAMER	
GGTTTTGGT	12	GACTGTG	TRAJ38*01
GGTTTTTGC	12	CACTGTG	TRAJ39*01
GGTTTATGT	12	CACTGTG	TRAJ40*01
GTTTTTTGT	12	CACTGTG	TRAJ41*01
GATTATTGT	12	GACTGTG	TRAJ42*01
GGTTTTTGT	12	TACTGTG	TRAJ43*01
GGTTTCTGT	12	CACAGTG	TRAJ44*01
AGTTTATGT	12	CAGAGTG	TRAJ45*01
TGTTTCTGT	12	AGCCGTG	TRAJ46*01
TGTTTTTGT	12	CGCTGTG	TRAJ47*01
GGTTTTTGC	12	CACTGTG	TRAJ48*01
GGTTTTTGT	12	CACAGTG	TRAJ49*01
AGTTATTGT	12	GGCTGTG	TRAJ50*01
GGTTCTTGT	12	TGCAGTG	TRAJ52*01
TGTTTCTGT	12	GGCTGTG	TRAJ53*01
AGTTTCTGT	12	TGTGGTG	TRAJ54*01
AGTTTTTGT	12	CATTGTG	TRAJ56*01
AGTATTTGT	12	GGGGGTG	TRAJ57*01
GGTTTTTGC	12	CACAGTG	TRAJ58*01 (ORF)
AGTTTATGT	12	TCCTGTG	TRAJ59*01 (ORF)
GGTTTTTGT	12	TCCTGTG	TRAJ61*01 (ORF)

(1) From M94081.

Part 3

TRAV

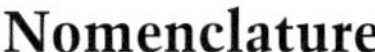

Nomenclature

TRAV1-1: T cell receptor alpha variable 1-1.

Definition and functionality

TRAV1-1 is one of the two functional genes of the TRAV1 subgroup which comprises two mapped genes.

Gene location

TRAV1-1 is in the TRA/TRD locus on chromosome 14 at 14q11.2.

Nucleotide and amino acid sequences for human TRAV1-1

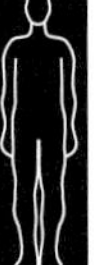

```
                        1   2   3   4   5   6   7   8   9  10  11  12  13  14  15  16  17  18  19  20
                        G   Q   S   L   E   Q       P   S   E   V   T   A   V   E   G   A   I   V   Q
AE000658,TRAV1-1*01 [6] GGA CAA AGC CTT GAG CAG ... CCC TCT GAA GTG ACA GCT GTG GAA GGA GCC ATT GTC CAG

M12070  ,TRAV1-1*01 [1] --- --- --- --- --- --- ... --- --- --- --- --- --- --- --- --- --- --- --- ---

X04939  ,TRAV1-1*02 [38]--- --- --- --- --- --- ... --- --- --- --- --- --- --- --- --- --- --- --- ---

L11161  ,TRAV1-1*02 [7] --- --- --- --- --- --- ... --- --- --- --- --- --- --- --- --- --- --- --- ---


                                                               ______________CDR1-IMGT___________________
                       21  22  23  24  25  26  27  28  29  30  31  32  33  34  35  36  37  38  39  40
                        I   N   C   T   Y   Q   T   S   G   F   Y   G                           L   S
AE000658,TRAV1-1*01    ATA AAC TGC ACG TAC CAG ACA TCT GGG TTT TAT GGG ... ... ... ... ... ... CTG TCC

M12070  ,TRAV1-1*01    --- --- --- --- --- --- --- --- --- --- --- --- ... ... ... ... ... ... --- ---

X04939  ,TRAV1-1*02    --- --- --- --- --- --- --- --- --- --- --- --- ... ... ... ... ... ... --- ---

L11161  ,TRAV1-1*02    --- --- --- --- --- --- --- --- --- --- --- --- ... ... ... ... ... ... --- ---


                                                                                       ______________CDR2-
                       41  42  43  44  45  46  47  48  49  50  51  52  53  54  55  56  57  58  59  60
                        W   Y   Q   Q   H   D   G   G   A   P   T   F   L   S   Y   N   A
AE000658,TRAV1S1*01    TGG TAC CAG CAA CAT GAT GGC GGA GCA CCC ACA TTT CTT TCT TAC AAT GCT ... ... ...

M12070  ,TRAV1-1*01    --- --- --- --- --- --- --- --- --- --- --- --- --- --- --- --- --- ... ... ...
                                                                                       G
X04939  ,TRAV1-1*02    --- --- --- --- --- --- --- --- --- --- --- --- --- --- --- -G- ... ... ...
                                                                                       G
L11161  ,TRAV1-1*02    --- --- --- --- --- --- --- --- --- --- --- --- --- --- --- -G- ... ... ...


                       IMGT_____________________
                       61  62  63  64  65  66  67  68  69  70  71  72  73  74  75  76  77  78  79  80
                                                L   D   G   L   E   E   T       G   R   F   S   S   F   L
AE000658,TRAV1-1*01    ... ... ... ... ... CTG GAT GGT TTG GAG GAG ACA ... GGT CGT TTT TCT TCA TTC CTT

M12070  ,TRAV1-1*01    ... ... ... ... ... --- --- --- --- --- --- --- ... --- --- --- --- --- --- ---

X04939  ,TRAV1-1*02    ... ... ... ... ... --- --- --- --- --- --- --- ... --- --- --- --- --- --- ---

L11161  ,TRAV1-1*02    ... ... ... ... ... --- --- --- --- --- --- --- ... --- --- --- --- --- --- ---


                       81  82  83  84  85  86  87  88  89  90  91  92  93  94  95  96  97  98  99 100
                        S   R   S   D   S   Y   G   Y   L   L   L   Q   E   L   Q   M   K   D   S   A
AE000658,TRAV1-1*01    AGT CGC TCT GAT AGT TAT GGT TAC CTC CTT CTA CAG GAG CTC CAG ATG AAA GAC TCT GCC

M12070  ,TRAV1-1*01    --- --- --- --- --- --- --- --- --- --- --- --- --- --- --- --- --- --- --- ---

X04939  ,TRAV1-1*02    --- --- --- --- --- --- --- --- --- --- --- --- --- --- --- --- --- --- --- ---

L11161  ,TRAV1-1*02    --- --- --- --- --- --- --- --- --- --- --- --- --- --- --- --- --- --- --- --


                                       _CDR3-IMGT_
                      101 102 103 104 105 106 107
                        S   Y   F   C   A   V   R
AE000658,TRAV1-1*01    TCT TAC TTC TGC GCT GTG AGA GA

M12070  ,TRAV1-1*01    --- --- --- --- --- ---          #g

X04939  ,TRAV1-1*02    --- --- --- --- --- --T          #c

L11161  ,TRAV1-1*02                                     °
```

#c: Rearranged cDNA
#g: Rearranged genomic DNA
°: Genomic DNA, but not known as being germline or rearranged

Framework and complementarity determining regions

FR1-IMGT: 25 (-1 aa: 7)
FR2-IMGT: 17
FR3-IMGT: 38 (-1 aa: 73)

CDR1-IMGT: 6
CDR2-IMGT: 2
CDR3-IMGT: 3

Collier de Perles for human TRAV1-1*01

Accession number: IMGT AE000658   EMBL/GenBank/DDBJ: AE000658

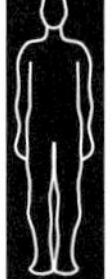

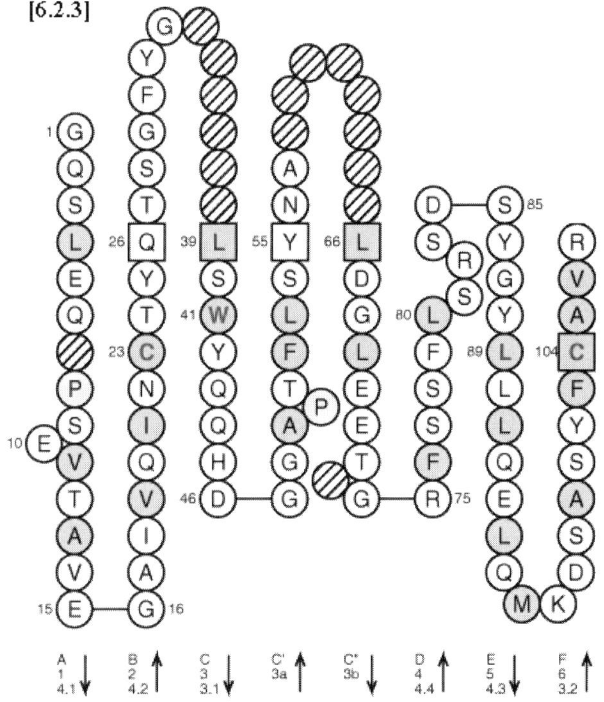

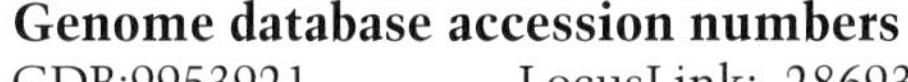

Genome database accession numbers

GDB:9953921   LocusLink: 28693

TRAV1-2

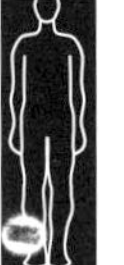

Nomenclature

TRAV1-2: T cell receptor alpha variable 1-2.

Definition and functionality

TRAV1-2 is one of the two functional genes of the TRAV1 subgroup which comprises two mapped genes.

Gene location

TRAV1-2 is in the TRA/TRD locus on chromosome 14 at 14q11.2.

Nucleotide and amino acid sequences for human TRAV1-2

```
                                  1   2   3   4   5   6   7   8   9  10  11  12  13  14  15  16  17  18  19  20
                                  G   Q   N   I   D   Q       P   T   E   M   T   A   T   E   G   A   I   V   Q
       AE000658,TRAV1-2*01   [6] GGA CAA AAC ATT GAC CAG ... CCC ACT GAG ATG ACA GCT ACG GAA GGT GCC ATT GTC CAG

       X58744  ,TRAV1-2*01  [28] --- --- --- --- --- --- ... --- --- --- --- --- --- --- --- --- --- --- --- ---

       U32544  ,TRAV1-2*02   [5] --- --- --- --- --- --- ... --- --- --- --- --- --- --- --- --- --- --- --- ---


                                                              ___________________CDR1-IMGT_____________________
                                 21  22  23  24  25  26  27  28  29  30  31  32  33  34  35  36  37  38  39  40
                                  I   N   C   T   Y   Q   T   S   G   F   N   G                           L   F
       AE000658,TRAV1-2*01       ATC AAC TGC ACG TAC CAG ACA TCT GGG TTC AAC GGG ... ... ... ... ... ... CTG TTC

       X58744  ,TRAV1-2*01       --- --- --- --- --- --- --- --- --- --- --- --- ... ... ... ... ... ... --- ---

       U32544  ,TRAV1-2*02       --- --- --- --- --- --- --- --- --- --- --- --- ... ... ... ... ... ... --- ---


                                                                                          ________________CDR2-
                                 41  42  43  44  45  46  47  48  49  50  51  52  53  54  55  56  57  58  59  60
                                  W   Y   Q   Q   H   A   G   E   A   P   T   F   L   S   Y   N   V
       AE000658,TRAV1-2*01       TGG TAC CAG CAA CAT GCT GGC GAA GCA CCC ACA TTT CTG TCT TAC AAT GTT ... ... ...

       X58744  ,TRAV1-2*01       --- --- --- --- --- --- --- --- --- --- --- --- --- --- --- --- --- ... ... ...

       U32544  ,TRAV1-2*02       --- --- --- --- --- --- --- --- --- --- --- --- --- --- --- --- --- ... ... ...


                                 IMGT_______________
                                 61  62  63  64  65  66  67  68  69  70  71  72  73  74  75  76  77  78  79  80
                                                      L   D   G   L   E   E   K       G   R   F   S   S   F   L
       AE000658,TRAV1-2*01       ... ... ... ... ... CTG GAT GGT TTG GAG GAG AAA ... GGT CGT TTT TCT TCA TTC CTT

       X58744  ,TRAV1-2*01       ... ... ... ... ... --- --- --- --- --- --- --- ... --- --- --- --- --- --- ---

       U32544  ,TRAV1-2*02       ... ... ... ... ... --- --- --- C-- --- --- --- ... --- --


                                 81  82  83  84  85  86  87  88  89  90  91  92  93  94  95  96  97  98  99 100
                                  S   R   S   K   G   Y   S   Y   L   L   L   K   E   L   Q   M   K   D   S   A
       AE000658,TRAV1-2*01       AGT CGG TCT AAA GGG TAC AGT TAC CTC CTT TTG AAG GAG CTC CAG ATG AAA GAC TCT GCC

       X58744  ,TRAV1-2*01       --- --- --- --- --- --- --- --- --- --- --- --- --- --- --- --- --- --- --- ---

       U32544  ,TRAV1-2*02


                                                 _CDR3-IMGT_
                                101 102 103 104 105 106 107
                                  S   Y   L   C   A   V   R
       AE000658,TRAV1-2*01       TCT TAC CTC TGT GCT GTG AGA GA

       X58744  ,TRAV1-2*01       --- --- --- --- ---                 #c

       U32544  ,TRAV1-2*02                                            °


#c: Rearranged cDNA
°: Genomic DNA, but not known as being germline or rearranged
```

Framework and complementarity determining regions

FR1-IMGT: 25 (-1 aa: 7)   CDR1-IMGT: 6
FR2-IMGT: 17   CDR2-IMGT: 2
FR3-IMGT: 38 (-1 aa: 73)   CDR3-IMGT: 3

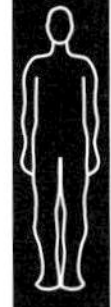

Collier de Perles for human TRAV1-2*01

Accession number: IMGT AE000658   EMBL/GenBank/DDBJ: AE000658

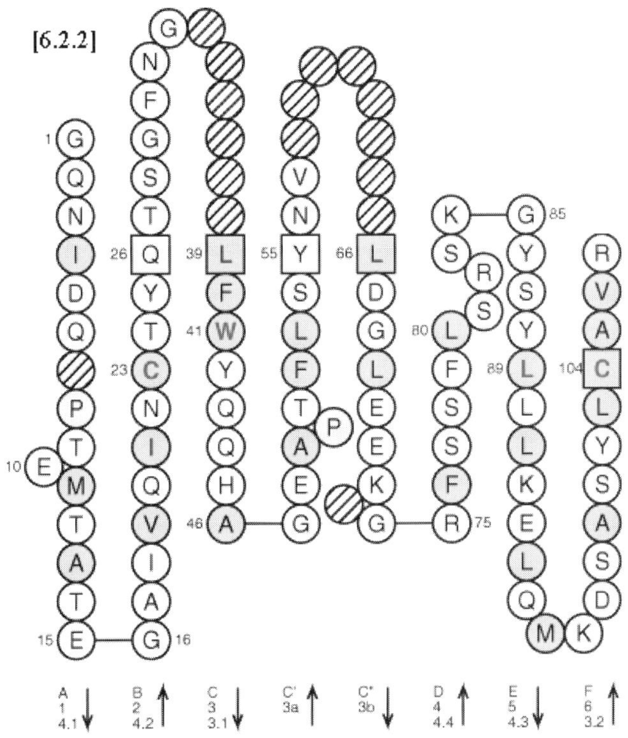

Genome database accession numbers
GDB:9953923   LocusLink: 28692

Nomenclature

TRAV2: T cell receptor alpha variable 2.

Definition and functionality

TRAV2 is the unique functional gene of the TRAV2 subgroup which only comprises this mapped gene.

Gene location

TRAV2 is in the TRA/TRD locus on chromosome 14 at 14q11.2.

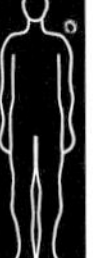

Nucleotide and amino acid sequences for human TRAV2

```
                         1   2   3   4   5   6   7   8   9  10  11  12  13  14  15  16  17  18  19  20
                         K   D   Q   V   F   Q       P   S   T   V   A   S   S   E   G   A   V   V   E
AE000658,TRAV2*01   [6]  AAG GAC CAA GTG TTT CAG ... CCT TCC ACA GTG GCA TCT TCA GAG GGA GCT GTG GTG GAA

X04936  ,TRAV2*01   [38] --- --- --- --- --- --- ... --- --- --- --- --- --- --- --- --- --- --- --- ---

U32522  ,TRAV2*01   [5]  --- --- --- --- --- --- ... --- --- --- --- --- --- --- --- --- --- --- --- ---

M17659  ,TRAV2*02   [17] --- --- --- --- --- --- ... --- --- --- --- --- --- --- --- --- --- --- --- ---

                                                                    ________________CDR1-IMGT________________
                        21  22  23  24  25  26  27  28  29  30  31  32  33  34  35  36  37  38  39  40
                         I   F   C   N   H   S   V   S   N   A   Y   N                           F   F
AE000658,TRAV2*01       ATC TTC TGT AAT CAC TCT GTG TCC AAT GCT TAC AAC ... ... ... ... ... ... TTC TTC

X04936  ,TRAV2*01       --- --- --- --- --- --- --- --- --- --- --- --- ... ... ... ... ... --- ---

U32522  ,TRAV2*01       --- --- --- --- --- --- --- --- --- --- --- --- ... ... ... ... ... --- ---

M17659  ,TRAV2*02       --- --- --- --- --- --- --- --- --- --- --- --- ... ... ... ... ... --- ---

                                                                            __________________CDR2-
                        41  42  43  44  45  46  47  48  49  50  51  52  53  54  55  56  57  58  59  60
                         W   Y   L   H   F   P   G   C   A   P   R   L   L   V   K
AE000658,TRAV2*01       TGG TAC CTT CAC TTC CCG GGA TGT GCA CCA AGA CTC CTT GTT AAA ... ... ... ... ...

X04936  ,TRAV2*01       --- --- --- --- --- --- --- --- --- --- --- --- --- --- --- ... ... ... ... ...

U32522  ,TRAV2*01       --- --- --- --- --- --- --- --- --- --- --- --- --- --- --- ... ... ... ... ...
                             H
M17659  ,TRAV2*02       --- C-- --- --- --- --- --- --- --- --- --- --- --- --- --- ... ... ... ... ...

                        IMGT________________
                        61  62  63  64  65  66  67  68  69  70  71  72  73  74  75  76  77  78  79  80
                                             G   S   K   P   S   Q   Q       G   R   Y   N   M   T   Y
AE000658,TRAV2*01       ... ... ... ... ... GGC TCA AAG CCT TCT CAG CAG ... GGA CGA TAC AAC ATG ACC TAT

X04936  ,TRAV2*01       ... ... ... ... ... --- --- --- --- --- --- --- ... --- --- --- --- --- --- ---

U32522  ,TRAV2*01       ... ... ... ... ... --- --- --- --- --- --

M17659  ,TRAV2*02       ... ... ... ... ... --- --- --- --- --- --- --- ... --- --- --- --- --- --- ---

                        81  82  83  84  85  86  87  88  89  90  91  92  93  94  95  96  97  98  99 100
                                 E   R   F   S   S   S   L   L   I   L   Q   V   R   E   A   D   A   A
AE000658,TRAV2*01       ... ... GAA CGG TTC TCT TCA TCG CTG CTC ATC CTC CAG GTG CGG GAG GCA GAT GCT GCT

X04936  ,TRAV2*01       ... ... --- --- --- --- --- --- --- --- --- --- --- --- --- --- --- --- --- ---

U32522  ,TRAV2*01

M17659  ,TRAV2*02       ... ... --- --- --- --- --- --- --- --- --- --- --- --- --- --- --- --- --- ---

                                        _CDR3-IMGT_
                       101 102 103 104 105 106 107
                         V   Y   Y   C   A   V   E
AE000658,TRAV2*01       GTT TAC TAC TGT GCT GTG GAG GA

X04936  ,TRAV2*01       --- --- --- --- --- --- ---      #c

U32522  ,TRAV2*01                                         o

M17659  ,TRAV2*02       --- --- --- --- --- --- ---      #c
```

#c: Rearranged cDNA
°: Genomic DNA, but not known as being germline or rearranged

Framework and complementarity determining regions

FR1-IMGT: 25 (-1 aa: 7)   CDR1-IMGT: 6
FR2-IMGT: 17   CDR2-IMGT: 0
FR3-IMGT: 36 (-3 aa: 73,81,82)   CDR3-IMGT: 3

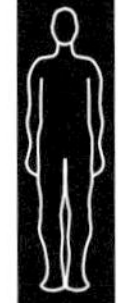

Collier de Perles for human TRAV2*01

Accession number: IMGT AE000658   EMBL/GenBank/DDBJ: AE000658

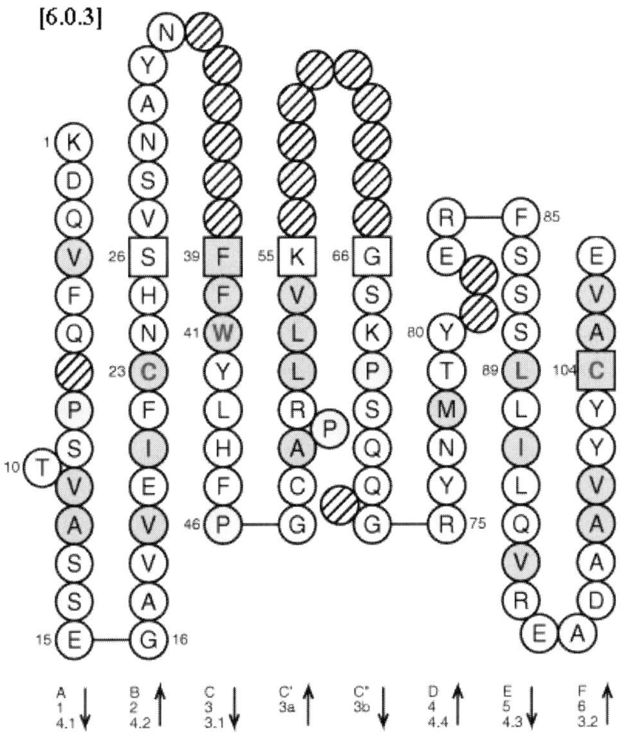

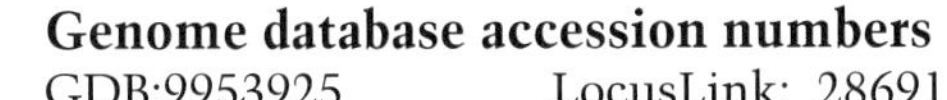

Genome database accession numbers
GDB:9953925   LocusLink: 28691

TRAV3

Nomenclature

TRAV3: T cell receptor alpha variable 3.

Definition and functionality

TRAV3 is a functional gene (allele *01) or a pseudogene (allele *02). TRAV3 belongs to the TRAV3 subgroup which only comprises this mapped gene. TRAV3*02 is a pseudogene due to a 1 nt DELETION in codon 7 leading to a frameshift in FR1-IMGT.

Gene location

TRAV3 is in the TRA/TRD locus on chromosome 14 at 14q11.2.

Nucleotide and amino acid sequences for human TRAV3

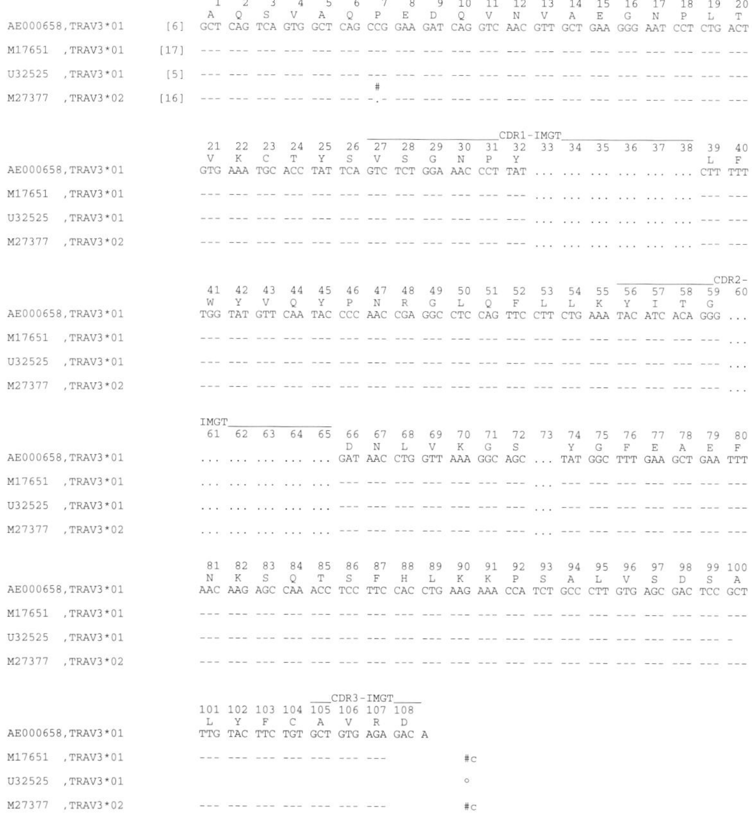

```
                  1   2   3   4   5   6   7   8   9  10  11  12  13  14  15  16  17  18  19  20
                  A   Q   S   V   A   Q   P   E   D   Q   V   N   V   A   E   G   N   P   L   T
AE000658,TRAV3*01 [6] GCT CAG TCA GTG GCT CAG CCG GAA GAT CAG GTC AAC GTT GCT GAA GGG AAT CCT CTG ACT

M17651  ,TRAV3*01 [17] --- --- --- --- --- --- --- --- --- --- --- --- --- --- --- --- --- --- --- ---

U32525  ,TRAV3*01 [5]  --- --- --- --- --- --- --- --- --- --- --- --- --- --- --- --- --- --- --- ---
                                            #
M27377  ,TRAV3*02 [16] --- --- --- --- --- --- -.- --- --- --- --- --- --- --- --- --- --- --- --- ---

                                                                        CDR1-IMGT
                 21  22  23  24  25  26  27  28  29  30  31  32  33  34  35  36  37  38  39  40
                  V   K   C   T   Y   S   V   S   G   N   P   Y                           L   F
AE000658,TRAV3*01 GTG AAA TGC ACC TAT TCA GTC TCT GGA AAC CCT TAT ... ... ... ... ... ... CTT TTT

M17651  ,TRAV3*01 --- --- --- --- --- --- --- --- --- --- --- --- ... ... ... ... ... ... --- ---

U32525  ,TRAV3*01 --- --- --- --- --- --- --- --- --- --- --- --- ... ... ... ... ... ... --- ---

M27377  ,TRAV3*02 --- --- --- --- --- --- --- --- --- --- --- --- ... ... ... ... ... ... --- ---

                                                                                        CDR2-
                 41  42  43  44  45  46  47  48  49  50  51  52  53  54  55  56  57  58  59  60
                  W   Y   V   Q   Y   P   N   R   G   L   Q   F   L   L   K   Y   I   T   G
AE000658,TRAV3*01 TGG TAT GTT CAA TAC CCC AAC CGA GGC CTC CAG TTC CTT CTG AAA TAC ATC ACA GGG ...

M17651  ,TRAV3*01 --- --- --- --- --- --- --- --- --- --- --- --- --- --- --- --- --- --- --- ...

U32525  ,TRAV3*01 --- --- --- --- --- --- --- --- --- --- --- --- --- --- --- --- --- --- --- ...

M27377  ,TRAV3*02 --- --- --- --- --- --- --- --- --- --- --- --- --- --- --- --- --- --- --- ...

                 IMGT
                 61  62  63  64  65  66  67  68  69  70  71  72  73  74  75  76  77  78  79  80
                                      D   N   L   V   K   G   S       Y   G   F   E   A   E   F
AE000658,TRAV3*01 ... ... ... ... ... GAT AAC CTG GTT AAA GGC AGC ... TAT GGC TTT GAA GCT GAA TTT

M17651  ,TRAV3*01 ... ... ... ... ... --- --- --- --- --- --- --- ... --- --- --- --- --- --- ---

U32525  ,TRAV3*01 ... ... ... ... ... --- --- --- --- --- --- --- ... --- --- --- --- --- --- ---

M27377  ,TRAV3*02 ... ... ... ... ... --- --- --- --- --- --- --- ... --- --- --- --- --- --- ---

                 81  82  83  84  85  86  87  88  89  90  91  92  93  94  95  96  97  98  99 100
                  N   K   S   Q   T   S   F   H   L   K   K   P   S   A   L   V   S   D   S   A
AE000658,TRAV3*01 AAC AAG AGC CAA ACC TCC TTC CAC CTG AAG AAA CCA TCT GCC CTT GTG AGC GAC TCC GCT

M17651  ,TRAV3*01 --- --- --- --- --- --- --- --- --- --- --- --- --- --- --- --- --- --- --- ---

U32525  ,TRAV3*01 --- --- --- --- --- --- --- --- --- --- --- --- --- --- --- --- --- --- --- -

M27377  ,TRAV3*02 --- --- --- --- --- --- --- --- --- --- --- --- --- --- --- --- --- --- --- ---

                              CDR3-IMGT
                101 102 103 104 105 106 107 108
                  L   Y   F   C   A   V   R   D
AE000658,TRAV3*01 TTG TAC TTC TGT GCT GTG AGA GAC A

M17651  ,TRAV3*01 --- --- --- --- --- --- ---         #c

U32525  ,TRAV3*01                                     o

M27377  ,TRAV3*02 --- --- --- --- --- --- ---         #c
```

\# (in the sequence): Frameshift
\#c: Rearranged cDNA
°: Genomic DNA, but not known as being germline or rearranged

Framework and complementarity determining regions

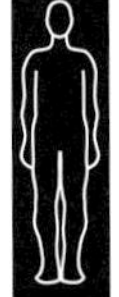

FR1-IMGT: 26
FR2-IMGT: 17
FR3-IMGT: 38 (-1 aa: 73)

CDR1-IMGT: 6
CDR2-IMGT: 4
CDR3-IMGT: 4

Collier de Perles for human TRAV3*01

Accession number: IMGT AE000658   EMBL/GenBank/DDBJ: AE000658

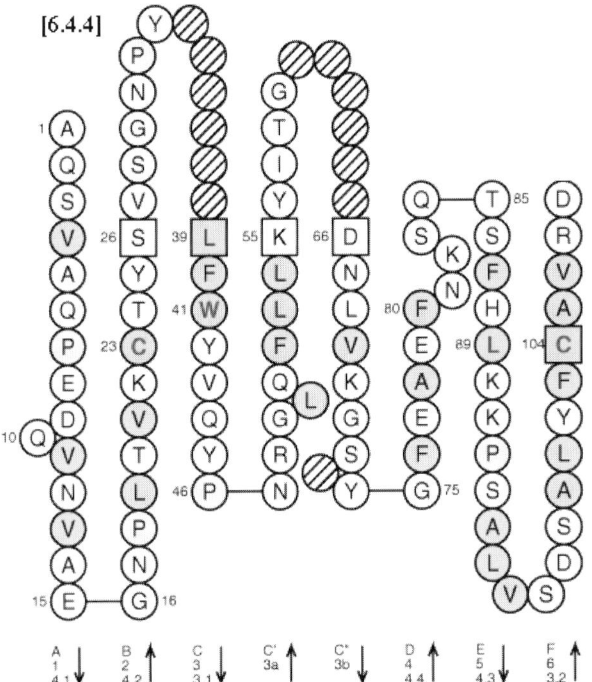

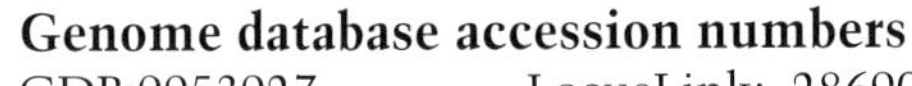

Genome database accession numbers
GDB:9953927   LocusLink: 28690

TRAV4

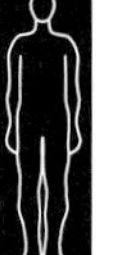

Nomenclature

TRAV4: T cell receptor alpha variable 4.

Definition and functionality

TRAV4 is the unique functional gene of the TRAV4 subgroup which only comprises this mapped gene.

Gene location

TRAV4 is in the TRA/TRD locus on chromosome 14 at 14q11.2.

Nucleotide and amino acid sequences for human TRAV4

```
                            1   2   3   4   5   6   7   8   9  10  11  12  13  14  15  16  17  18  19  20
                            L   A   K   T   T   Q       P   I   S   M   D   S   Y   E   G   Q   E   V   N
AE000658,TRAV4*01    [6]   CTT GCT AAG ACC ACC CAG ... CCC ATC TCC ATG GAC TCA TAT GAA GGA CAA GAA GTG AAC

M17663  ,TRAV4*01   [17]   --- --- --- --- --- --- ... --- --- --- --- --- --- --- --- --- --- --- --- ---

U32529  ,TRAV4*01    [5]   --- --- --- --- --- --- ... --- --- --- --- --- --- --- --- --- --- --- --- ---


                                                       _________________________CDR1-IMGT_________________________
                           21  22  23  24  25  26  27  28  29  30  31  32  33  34  35  36  37  38  39  40
                            I   T   C   S   H   N   N   I   A   T   N   D   Y                       I   T
AE000658,TRAV4*01          ATA ACC TGT AGC CAC AAC AAC ATT GCT ACA AAT GAT TAT ... ... ... ... ... ATC ACG

M17663  ,TRAV4*01          --- --- --- --- --- --- --- --- --- --- --- --- --- ... ... ... ... ... --- ---

U32529  ,TRAV4*01          --- --- --- --- --- --- --- --- --- --- --- --- --- ... ... ... ... ... --- ---


                                                                                           _________________CDR2-
                           41  42  43  44  45  46  47  48  49  50  51  52  53  54  55  56  57  58  59  60
                            W   Y   Q   Q   F   P   S   Q   G   P   R   F   I   I   Q   G
AE000658,TRAV4*01          TGG TAC CAA CAG TTT CCC AGC CAA GGA CCA CGA TTT ATT ATT CAA GGA ... ... ... ...

M17663  ,TRAV4*01          --- --- --- --- --- --- --- --- --- --- --- --- --- --- --- --- ... ... ... ...

U32529  ,TRAV4*01          --- --- --- --- --- --- --- --- --- --- --- --- --- --- --- ---


                           IMGT________________
                           61  62  63  64  65  66  67  68  69  70  71  72  73  74  75  76  77  78  79  80
                                                    Y   K   T   K   V   T   N       E   V   A   S   L   F   I
AE000658,TRAV4*01          ... ... ... ... ... TAC AAG ACA AAA GTT ACA AAC ... GAA GTG GCC TCC CTG TTT ATC

M17663  ,TRAV4*01          ... ... ... ... ... --- --- --- --- --- --- --- ... --- --- --- --- --- --- ---

U32529  ,TRAV4*01


                           81  82  83  84  85  86  87  88  89  90  91  92  93  94  95  96  97  98  99 100
                            P   A   D   R   K   S   S   T   L   S   L   P   R   V   S   L   S   D   T   A
AE000658,TRAV4*01          CCT GCC GAC AGA AAG TCC AGC ACT CTG AGC CTG CCC CGG GTT TCC CTG AGC GAC ACT GCT

M17663  ,TRAV4*01          --- --- --- --- --- --- --- --- --- --- --- --- --- --- --- --- --- --- --- ---

U32529  ,TRAV4*01


                                              ____CDR3-IMGT____
                          101 102 103 104 105 106 107 108
                            V   Y   Y   C   L   V   G   D
AE000658,TRAV4*01          GTG TAC TAC TGC CTC GTG GGT GAC A

M17663  ,TRAV4*01          --- --- --- --- ---                    #c

U32529  ,TRAV4*01                                                 o
```

#c: Rearranged cDNA
o: Genomic DNA, but not known as being germline or rearranged

Framework and complementarity determining regions

FR1-IMGT: 25 (-1 aa: 7)   CDR1-IMGT: 7
FR2-IMGT: 17   CDR2-IMGT: 1
FR3-IMGT: 38 (-1 aa: 73)   CDR3-IMGT: 4

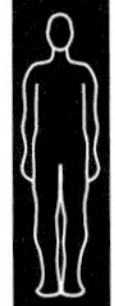

Collier de Perles for human TRAV4*01

Accession number: IMGT AE000658   EMBL/GenBank/DDBJ: AE000658

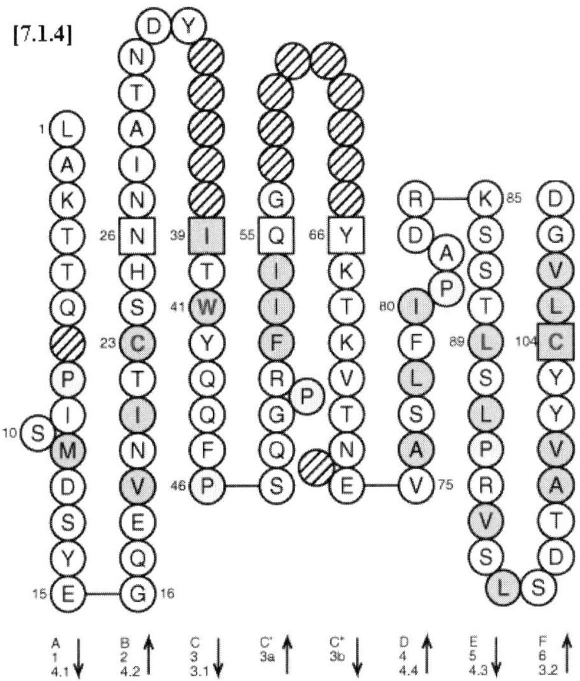

Genome database accession numbers
GDB:9953929   LocusLink: 28689

Nomenclature

TRAV5: T cell receptor alpha variable 5.

Definition and functionality

TRAV5 is the unique functional gene of the TRAV5 subgroup which only comprises this mapped gene.

Gene location

TRAV5 is in the TRA/TRD locus on chromosome 14 at 14q11.2.

Nucleotide and amino acid sequences for human TRAV5

```
                          1   2   3   4   5   6   7   8   9  10  11  12  13  14  15  16  17  18  19  20
                          G   E   D   V   E   Q   S       L   F   L   S   V   R   E   G   D   S   S   V
AE000659,TRAV5*01    [6]  GGA GAG GAT GTG GAG CAG AGT ... CTT TTC CTG AGT GTC CGA GAG GGA GAC AGC TCC GTT

M27376  ,TRAV5*01   [16]  --- --- --- --- --- --- --- ... --- --- --- --- --- --- --- --- --- --- --- ---

                                                        ______________________CDR1-IMGT____________________
                         21  22  23  24  25  26  27  28  29  30  31  32  33  34  35  36  37  38  39  40
                          I   N   C   T   Y   T   D   S   S   S   T   Y                           L   Y
AE000659,TRAV5*01        ATA AAC TGC ACT TAC ACA GAC AGC TCC TCC ACC TAC ... ... ... ... ... ... TTA TAC

M27376  ,TRAV5*01        --- --- --- --- --- --- --- --- --- --- --- --- ... ... ... ... ... ... --- ---

                                                                                    ____________CDR2-
                         41  42  43  44  45  46  47  48  49  50  51  52  53  54  55  56  57  58  59  60
                          W   Y   K   Q   E   P   G   A   G   L   Q   L   L   T   Y   I   F   S
AE000659,TRAV5*01        TGG TAT AAG CAA GAA CCT GGA GCA GGT CTC CAG TTG CTG ACG TAT ATT TTT TCA ... ...

M27376  ,TRAV5*01        --- --- --- --- --- --- --- --- --- --- --- --- --- --- --- --- --- --- ... ...

                         IMGT_______
                         61  62  63  64  65  66  67  68  69  70  71  72  73  74  75  76  77  78  79  80
                                                  N   M   D   M   K   Q   D       Q   R   L   T   V   L   L
AE000659,TRAV5*01        ... ... ... ... ... AAT ATG GAC ATG AAA CAA GAC ... CAA AGA CTC ACT GTT CTA TTG

M27376  ,TRAV5*01        ... ... ... ... ... --- --- --- --- --- --- --- ... --- --- --- --- --- --- ---

                         81  82  83  84  85  86  87  88  89  90  91  92  93  94  95  96  97  98  99 100
                          N   K   K   D   K   H   L   S   L   R   I   A   D   T   Q   T   G   D   S   A
AE000659,TRAV5*01        AAT AAA AAG GAT AAA CAT CTG TCT CTG CGC ATT GCA GAC ACC CAG ACT GGG GAC TCA GCT

M27376  ,TRAV5*01        --- --- --- --- --- --- --- --- --- --- --- --- --- --- --- --- --- --- --- ---

                             _CDR3-IMGT_
                        101 102 103 104 105 106 107
                          I   Y   F   C   A   E   S
AE000659,TRAV5*01        ATC TAC TTC TGT GCA GAG AGT A

M27376  ,TRAV5*01        --- --- --- --- --- --- ---        #c
```

#c: Rearranged cDNA

Framework and complementarity determining regions

FR1-IMGT: 25 (-1 aa: 8)   CDR1-IMGT: 6
FR2-IMGT: 17   CDR2-IMGT: 3
FR3-IMGT: 38 (-1 aa: 73)   CDR3-IMGT: 3

Collier de Perles for human TRAV5*01

Accession number: IMGT AE000659   EMBL/GenBank/DDBJ: AE000659

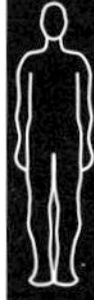

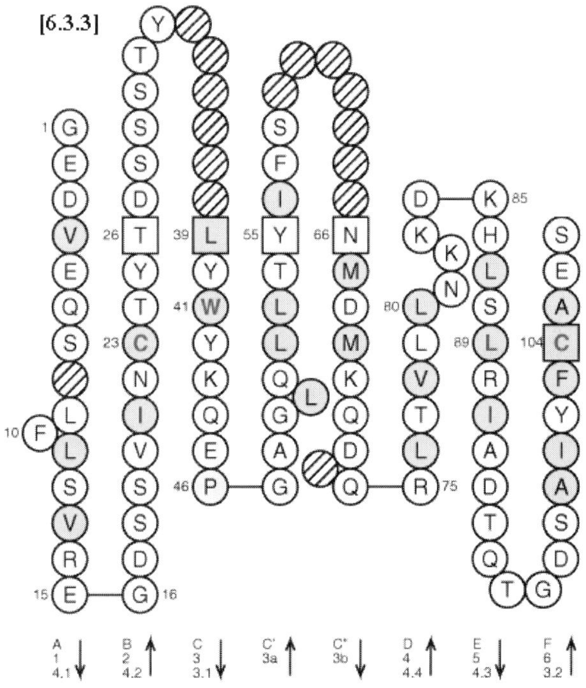

Genome database accession numbers
GDB:9953931   LocusLink: 28688

TRAV6

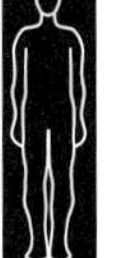

Nomenclature

TRAV6: T cell receptor alpha variable 6.

Definition and functionality

TRAV6 is the unique functional gene of the TRAV6 subgroup which only comprises this mapped gene.

Gene location

TRAV6 is in the TRA/TRD locus on chromosome 14 at 14q11.2.

Nucleotide and amino acid sequences for human TRAV6

```
                            1   2   3   4   5   6   7   8   9  10  11  12  13  14  15  16  17  18  19  20
                            S   Q   K   I   E   Q   N   S   E   A   L   N   I   Q   E   G   K   T   A   T
AE000659,TRAV6*01     [6]  AGC CAA AAG ATA GAA CAG AAT TCC GAG GCC CTG AAC ATT CAG GAG GGT AAA ACG GCC ACC
X58747  ,TRAV6*02    [28]  --- --- --- --- --- --- --- --- --- --- --- --- --- --- --- --- --- --- --- ---
Z49060  ,TRAV6*03    [13]                          --- --- --- --- --- --- --- --- --- --- --- --- --- ---
Y10409  ,TRAV6*04    [14]                          --- --- --- --- --- --- --- --- --- --- --- --- --- ---
Y10410  ,TRAV6*05    [14]                          --- --- --- --- --- --- --- --- --- --- --- --- --- ---
U32542  ,TRAV6*06     [5]  --- --- --- --- --- --- --- --- --- --- --- --- --- --- --- --- --- --- --- ---

                                                                              CDR1-IMGT
                           21  22  23  24  25  26  27  28  29  30  31  32  33  34  35  36  37  38  39  40
                            L   T   C   N   Y   T   N   Y   S   P   A   Y                           L   Q
AE000659,TRAV6*01          CTG ACC TGC AAC TAT ACA AAC TAT TCC CCA GCA TAC ... ... ... ... ... ... TTA CAG
X58747  ,TRAV6*02          --- --- --- --- --- --- --- --- --T --- --- --- ... ... ... ... ... ... --- ---
Z49060  ,TRAV6*03          --- --- --- --- --- --- --- --- --T --- --- --- ... ... ... ... ... ... --- ---
Y10409  ,TRAV6*04          --- --- --- --- --- --- --- --- --T --- --- --- ... ... ... ... ... ... --- ---
Y10410  ,TRAV6*05          --- --- --- --- --- --G --- --- --T --- --- --- ... ... ... ... ... ... --- ---
U32542  ,TRAV6*06          --- --- --- --- --- --- --- --- --T --- --- --- ... ... ... ... ... ... --- ---

                                                                                              CDR2-
                           41  42  43  44  45  46  47  48  49  50  51  52  53  54  55  56  57  58  59  60
                            W   Y   R   Q   D   P   G   R   G   P   V   F   L   L   L   I   R   E
AE000659,TRAV6*01          TGG TAC CGA CAA GAT CCA GGA AGA GGC CCT GTT TTC TTG CTA CTC ATA CGT GAA ... ...
X58747  ,TRAV6*02          --- --- --- --- --- --- --- --- --- --- --- --- --- --- --- --- --- --- ... ...
Z49060  ,TRAV6*03          --- --- --- --- --- --- --- --- --- --- --- --- --- --- --T --- --- --- ... ...
Y10409  ,TRAV6*04          --- --- --- --- --- --- --- --- --- --- --- --- --- --- --- --- --- --- ... ...
Y10410  ,TRAV6*05          --- --- --- --- --- --- --- --- --- --- --- --- --- --- --- --- --- --- ... ...
U32542  ,TRAV6*06          --- --- --- --- --- --- --- --- --- --- --- --- --- --- --- --- --- --- ... ...

                           IMGT
                           61  62  63  64  65  66  67  68  69  70  71  72  73  74  75  76  77  78  79  80
                                                    N   E   K   R   K       E   R   L   K   V   T   F
AE000659,TRAV6*01          ... ... ... ... ... AAT GAG AAA GAA AAA AGG AAA ... GAA AGA CTG AAG GTC ACC TTT
X58747  ,TRAV6*02          ... ... ... ... ... --- --- --- --- --- --- --- ... --- --- --- --- --- --- ---
Z49060  ,TRAV6*03          ... ... ... ... ... --- --- --- --- --- --- --- ... --- --- --- --- --- --- ---
Y10409  ,TRAV6*04          ... ... ... ... ... --- --- --- --- --- --- --- ... --- --- --- --- --- --- ---
Y10410  ,TRAV6*05          ... ... ... ... ... --- --- --- --- --- --- --- ... --- --- --- --- --- --- ---
U32542  ,TRAV6*06          ... ... ... ... ... --- --- --- --- --- --- --- ... --- --- --- --- --- --- ---

                           81  82  83  84  85  86  87  88  89  90  91  92  93  94  95  96  97  98  99 100
                            D   T   T   L   K   Q   S   L   F   H   I   T   A   S   Q   P   A   D   S   A
AE000659,TRAV6*01          GAT ACC ACC CTT AAA CAG AGT TTG TTT CAT ATC ACA GCC TCC CAG CCT GCA GAC TCA GCT
X58747  ,TRAV6*02          --- --- --- --- --- --- --- --- --- --- --- --- --- --- --- --- --- --- --- ---
Z49060  ,TRAV6*03          --- --- --- --- --- --- --- --- --- --- --- --- --- --- --- --- --- --- --- ---
                                                                        V
Y10409  ,TRAV6*04          --- --- --- --- --- --- --- --- --- --- G-- --- --- --- --- --- --- --- --- ---
Y10410  ,TRAV6*05          --- --- --- --- --- --- --- --- --- --- --- --- --- --- --- --- --- --- --- ---
                                               N
U32542  ,TRAV6*06          --- --- --- --C --- -

                                  CDR3-IMGT
                          101 102 103 104 105 106 107
                            T   Y   L   C   A   L   D
AE000659,TRAV6*01          ACC TAC CTC TGT GCT CTA GAC A
X58747  ,TRAV6*02          --- --- --- --- ---              #c
Z49060  ,TRAV6*03          --- --- --- --- ---              °
Y10409  ,TRAV6*04          --- --- --- --- ---              °
Y10410  ,TRAV6*05          --- --- --- --- ---              °
U32542  ,TRAV6*06                                           °
```

#c: Rearranged cDNA
°: Genomic DNA, but not known as being germline or rearranged

Framework and complementarity determining regions

FR1-IMGT: 26
FR2-IMGT: 17
FR3-IMGT: 38 (-1 aa: 73)

CDR1-IMGT: 6
CDR2-IMGT: 3
CDR3-IMGT: 3

Collier de Perles for human TRAV6*01

Accession number: IMGT AE000659   EMBL/GenBank/DDBJ: AE000659

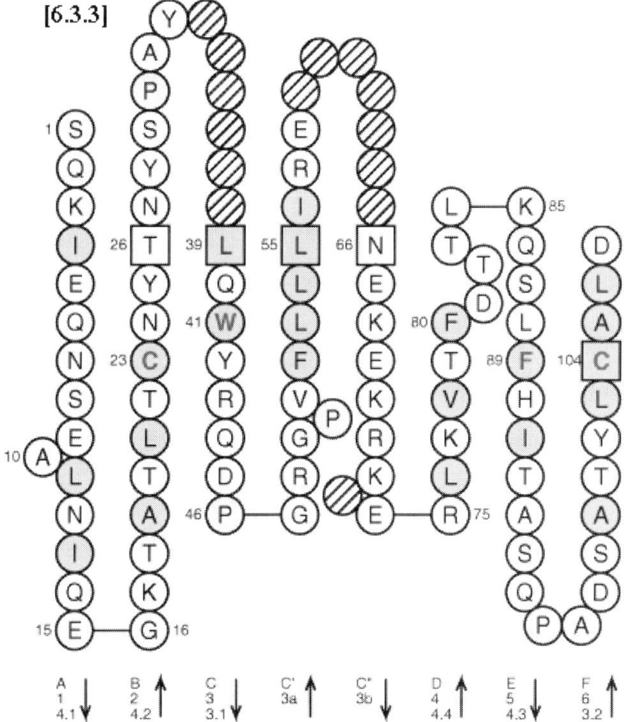

Genome database accession numbers

GDB:9953933   LocusLink: 28687

Nomenclature

TRAV7: T cell receptor alpha variable 7.

Definition and functionality

TRAV7 is the unique functional gene of the TRAV7 subgroup which only comprises this mapped gene.

Gene location

TRAV7 is in the TRA/TRD locus on chromosome 14 at 14q11.2.

Nucleotide and amino acid sequences for human TRAV7

```
                      1    2    3    4    5    6    7    8    9   10   11   12   13   14   15   16   17   18   19   20
                      E    N    Q    V    E    H    S    P    H    F    L    G    P    Q    Q    G    D    V    A    S
AE000659,TRAV7*01  [6] GAA  AAC  CAG  GTG  GAG  CAC  AGC  CCT  CAT  TTT  CTG  GGA  CCC  CAG  CAG  GGA  GAC  GTT  GCC  TCC

                                                                    ________________________CDR1-IMGT________________________
                     21   22   23   24   25   26   27   28   29   30   31   32   33   34   35   36   37   38   39   40
                      M    S    C    T    Y    S    V    S    R    F    N    N                                    L    Q
AE000659,TRAV7*01    ATG  AGC  TGC  ACG  TAC  TCT  GTC  AGT  CGT  TTT  AAC  AAT  ...  ...  ...  ...  ...  ...  TTG  CAG

                                                                                           ________________CDR2-
                     41   42   43   44   45   46   47   48   49   50   51   52   53   54   55   56   57   58   59   60
                      W    Y    R    Q    N    T    G    M    G    P    K    H    L    L    S    M    Y    S
AE000659,TRAV7*01    TGG  TAC  AGG  CAA  AAT  ACA  GGG  ATG  GGT  CCC  AAA  CAC  CTA  TTA  TCC  ATG  TAT  TCA  ...  ...

                     IMGT________________
                     61   62   63   64   65   66   67   68   69   70   71   72   73   74   75   76   77   78   79   80
                                              A    G    Y    E    K    Q    K         G    R    L    N    A    T    L
AE000659,TRAV7*01    ...  ...  ...  ...  ...  GCT  GGA  TAT  GAG  AAG  CAG  AAA  ...  GGA  AGA  CTA  AAT  GCT  ACA  TTA

                     81   82   83   84   85   86   87   88   89   90   91   92   93   94   95   96   97   98   99  100
                                L    K    N    G    S    S    L    Y    I    T    A    V    Q    P    E    D    S    A
AE000659,TRAV7*01    ...  ...  CTG  AAG  AAT  GGA  AGC  AGC  TTG  TAC  ATT  ACA  GCC  GTG  CAG  CCT  GAA  GAT  TCA  GCC

                          _CDR3-IMGT_
                    101  102  103  104  105  106  107
                      T    Y    F    C    A    V    D
AE000659,TRAV7*01    ACC  TAT  TTC  TGT  GCT  GTA  GAT  G
```

Framework and complementarity determining regions

FR1-IMGT: 26	CDR1-IMGT: 6
FR2-IMGT: 17	CDR2-IMGT: 3
FR3-IMGT: 36 (-3 aa: 73,81,82)	CDR3-IMGT: 3

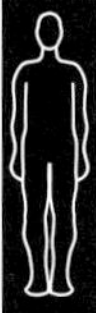

Collier de Perles for human TRAV7*01

Accession number: IMGT AE000659   EMBL/GenBank/DDBJ: AE000659

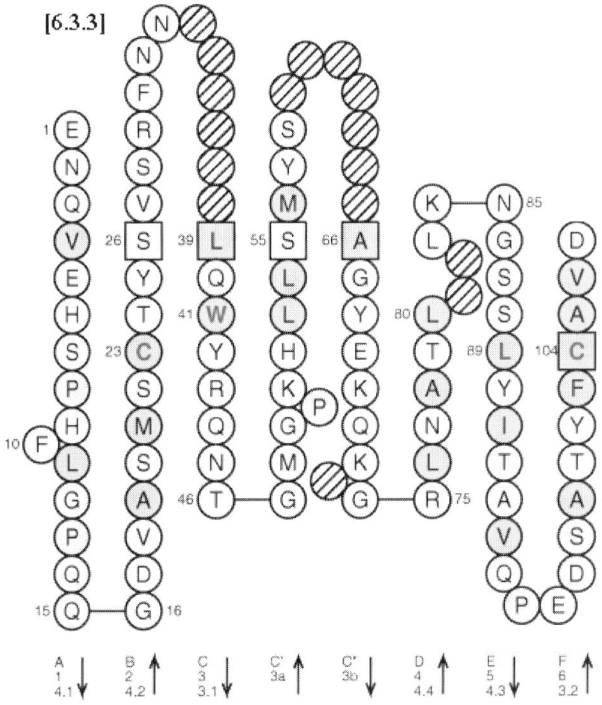

Genome database accession numbers
GDB:9953935   LocusLink: 28686

TRAV8-1

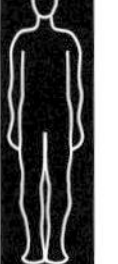

Nomenclature

TRAV8-1: T cell receptor alpha variable 8-1.

Definition and functionality

TRAV8-1 is one of the six functional genes of the TRAV8 subgroup which comprises seven mapped genes.

Gene location

TRAV8-1 is in the TRA/TRD locus on chromosome 14 at 14q11.2.

Nucleotide and amino acid sequences for human TRAV8-1

```
                          1    2    3    4    5    6    7    8    9    10   11   12   13   14   15   16   17   18   19   20
                          A    Q    S    V    S    Q    H    N    H    H    V    I    L    S    E    A    A    S    L    E
AE000659,TRAV8-1*01  [6]  GCC  CAG  TCT  GTG  AGC  CAG  CAT  AAC  CAC  CAC  GTA  ATT  CTC  TCT  GAA  GCA  GCC  TCA  CTG  GAG

X04949  ,TRAV8-1*01 [38]  ---  ---  ---  ---  ---  ---  ---  ---  ---  ---  ---  ---  ---  ---  ---  ---  ---  ---  ---  ---

U32520  ,TRAV8-1*02  [5]  ---  ---  ---  ---  ---  ---  ---  ---  ---  ---  ---  ---  ---  ---  ---  ---  ---  ---  ---  ---


                                                                          ____________________CDR1-IMGT____________________
                          21   22   23   24   25   26   27   28   29   30   31   32   33   34   35   36   37   38   39   40
                          L    G    C    N    Y    S    Y    G    G    T    V    N                                  L    F
AE000659,TRAV8-1*01       TTG  GGA  TGC  AAC  TAT  TCC  TAT  GGT  GGA  ACT  GTT  AAT  ...  ...  ...  ...  ...  ...  CTC  TTC

X04949  ,TRAV8-1*01       ---  ---  ---  ---  ---  ---  ---  ---  ---  ---  ---  ---  ...  ...  ...  ...  ...  ...  ---  ---

U32520  ,TRAV8-1*02       ---  ---  ---  ---  ---  ---  ---  ---  ---  ---  ---  ---  ...  ...  ...  ...  ...  ...  ---  ---


                                                                                                    ____________________CDR2-
                          41   42   43   44   45   46   47   48   49   50   51   52   53   54   55   56   57   58   59   60
                          W    Y    V    Q    Y    P    G    Q    H    L    Q    L    L    L    K    Y    F    S    G
AE000659,TRAV8-1*01       TGG  TAT  GTC  CAG  TAC  CCT  GGT  CAA  CAC  CTT  CAG  CTT  CTC  CTC  AAG  TAC  TTT  TCA  GGG  ...

X04949  ,TRAV8-1*01       ---  ---  ---  ---  ---  ---  ---  ---  ---  ---  ---  ---  ---  ---  ---  ---  ---  ---  ---  ...

U32520  ,TRAV8-1*02       ---  ---  ---  ---  ---  ---  ---  ---  ---  ---  ---  ---  ---  ---  ---  ---  ---  ---  ---  ...


                          IMGT________________
                          61   62   63   64   65   66   67   68   69   70   71   72   73   74   75   76   77   78   79   80
                                                   D    P    L    V    K    G    I         K    G    F    E    A    E    F
AE000659,TRAV8-1*01       ...  ...  ...  ...  ...  GAT  CCA  CTG  GTT  AAA  GGC  ATC  ...  AAG  GGC  TTT  GAG  GCT  GAA  TTT

X04949  ,TRAV8-1*01       ...  ...  ...  ...  ...  ---  ---  ---  ---  ---  ---  ---  ...  ---  ---  ---  ---  ---  ---  ---
                                                                                                    V
U32520  ,TRAV8-1*02       ...  ...  ...  ...  ...  ---  ---  ---  ---  ---  ---  ---  ...  ---  ---  G--  ---  ---  ---  ---


                          81   82   83   84   85   86   87   88   89   90   91   92   93   94   95   96   97   98   99  100
                          I    K    S    K    F    S    F    N    L    R    K    P    S    V    Q    W    S    D    T    A
AE000659,TRAV8-1*01       ATA  AAG  AGT  AAA  TTC  TCC  TTT  AAT  CTG  AGG  AAA  CCC  TCT  GTG  CAG  TGG  AGT  GAC  ACA  GCT

X04949  ,TRAV8-1*01       ---  ---  ---  ---  ---  ---  ---  ---  ---  ---  ---  ---  ---  ---  ---  ---  ---  ---  ---  ---

U32520  ,TRAV8-1*02       ---  ---  ---  ---  ---  ---  ---  ---  ---  ---  ---  ---  ---  ---  ---  ---  ---  ---  ---  ---  -


                                        _CDR3-IMGT_
                          101  102  103  104  105  106  107
                          E    Y    F    C    A    V    N
AE000659,TRAV8-1*01       GAG  TAC  TTC  TGT  GCC  GTG  AAT  GC

X04949  ,TRAV8-1*01       ---  ---  ---  ---  ---  ---  ---          #c

U32520  ,TRAV8-1*02                                                  °
```

#c: Rearranged cDNA
°: Genomic DNA, but not known as being germline or rearranged

Framework and complementarity determining regions

FR1-IMGT: 26

FR2-IMGT: 17

FR3-IMGT: 38 (-1 aa: 73)

CDR1-IMGT: 6

CDR2-IMGT: 4

CDR3-IMGT: 3

Collier de Perles for human TRAV8-1*01

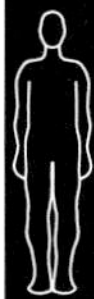

Accession number: IMGT AE000659   EMBL/GenBank/DDBJ: AE000659

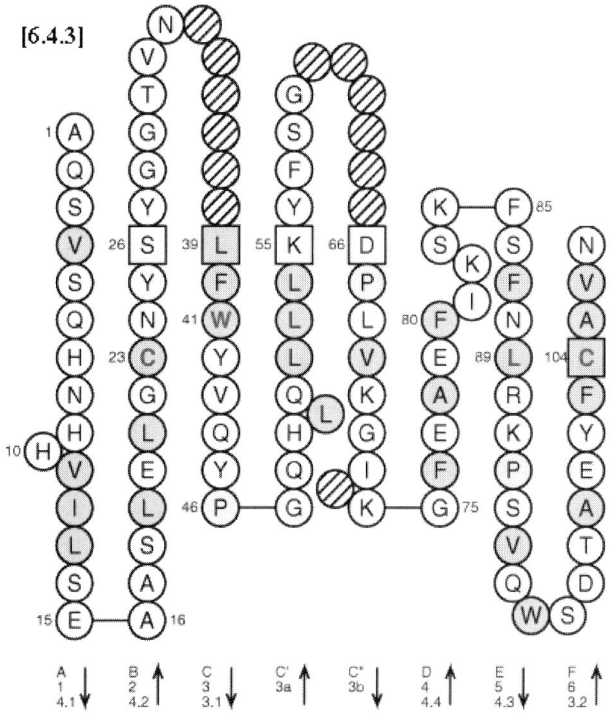

Genome database accession numbers
GDB:9953937   LocusLink: 28685

TRAV8-2

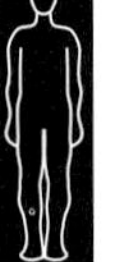

Nomenclature

TRAV8-2: T cell receptor alpha variable 8-2.

Definition and functionality

TRAV8-2 is one of the six functional genes of the TRAV8 subgroup which comprises seven mapped genes.

Gene location

TRAV8-2 is in the TRA/TRD locus on chromosome 14 at 14q11.2.

Nucleotide and amino acid sequences for human TRAV8-2

```
                        1   2   3   4   5   6   7   8   9   10  11  12  13  14  15  16  17  18  19  20
                        A   Q   S   V   T   Q   L   D   S   H   V   S   V   S   E   G   T   P   V   L
AE000659,TRAV8-2*01 [6] GCC CAG TCG GTG ACC CAG CTT GAC AGC CAC GTC TCT GTC TCT GAA GGA ACC CCG GTG CTG
                                                        S
M17650   ,TRAV8-2*02 [17] --- --- --- --- --- --- --- AG- --- --- --- --- --- --- --- --- --- --- --- ---

                                                             ________________________CDR1-IMGT_________________________
                        21  22  23  24  25  26  27  28  29  30  31  32  33  34  35  36  37  38  39  40
                        L   R   C   N   Y   S   S   S   Y   S   P   S                           L   F
AE000659,TRAV8-2*01     CTG AGG TGC AAC TAC TCA TCT TCT TAT TCA CCA TCT ... ... ... ... ... ... CTC TTC
M17650   ,TRAV8-2*02    --- --- --- --- --- --- --- --- --- --- --- --- ... ... ... ... ... ... --- ---

                                                                                            ________________CDR2-
                        41  42  43  44  45  46  47  48  49  50  51  52  53  54  55  56  57  58  59  60
                        W   Y   V   Q   H   P   N   K   G   L   Q   L   L   L   K   Y   T   S   A
AE000659,TRAV8-2*01     TGG TAT GTG CAA CAC CCC AAC AAA GGA CTC CAG CTT CTC CTG AAG TAC ACA TCA GCG ...
M17650   ,TRAV8-2*02    --- --- --- --- --- --- --- --- --- --- --- --- --- --- --- --- --- --- --- ...

                        IMGT________
                        61  62  63  64  65  66  67  68  69  70  71  72  73  74  75  76  77  78  79  80
                                                A   T   L   V   K   G   I       N   G   F   E   A   E   F
AE000659,TRAV8-2*01     ... ... ... ... ... GCC ACC CTG GTT AAA GGC ATC ... AAC GGT TTT GAG GCT GAA TTT
M17650   ,TRAV8-2*02    ... ... ... ... ... --- --- --- --- --- --- --- ... --- --- --- --- --- --- ---

                        81  82  83  84  85  86  87  88  89  90  91  92  93  94  95  96  97  98  99  100
                        K   K   S   E   T   S   F   H   L   T   K   P   S   A   H   M   S   D   A   A
AE000659,TRAV8-2*01     AAG AAG AGT GAA ACC TCC TTC CAC CTG ACG AAA CCC TCA GCC CAT ATG AGC GAC GCG GCT
M17650   ,TRAV8-2*02    --- --- --- --- --- --- --- --- --- --- --- --- --- --- --- --- --- --- --- ---

                                        ___CDR3-IMGT___
                        101 102 103 104 105 106 107
                        E   Y   F   C   V   V   S
AE000659,TRAV8-2*01     GAG TAC TTC TGT GTT GTG AGT GA
M17650   ,TRAV8-2*02    --- --- --- --- --- ---            #c
#c: Rearranged cDNA
```

Framework and complementarity determining regions

FR1-IMGT: 26   CDR1-IMGT: 6
FR2-IMGT: 17   CDR2-IMGT: 4
FR3-IMGT: 38 (-1 aa: 73)   CDR3-IMGT: 3

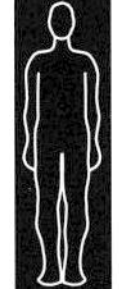

Collier de Perles for human TRAV8-2*01

Accession number: IMGT AE000659   EMBL/GenBank/DDBJ: AE000659

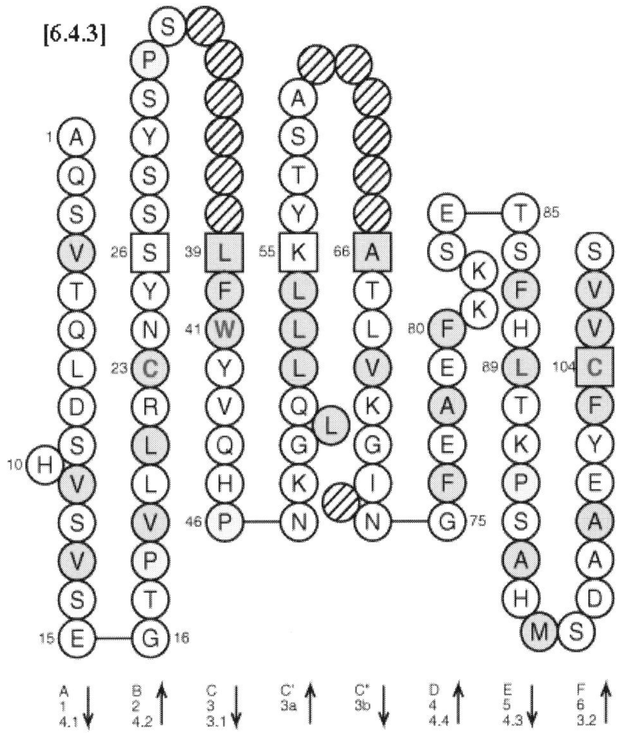

Genome database accession numbers
GDB:9953939   LocusLink: 28684

TRAV8-3

Nomenclature

TRAV8-3: T cell receptor alpha variable 8-3.

Definition and functionality

TRAV8-3 is one of the six functional genes of the TRAV8 subgroup which comprises seven mapped genes.

Gene location

TRAV8-3 is in the TRA/TRD locus on chromosome 14 at 14q11.2.

Nucleotide and amino acid sequences for human TRAV8-3

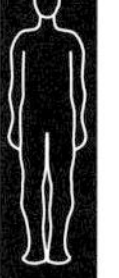

```
                             1   2   3   4   5   6   7   8   9  10  11  12  13  14  15  16  17  18  19  20
                             A   Q   S   V   T   Q   P   D   I   H   I   T   V   S   E   G   A   S   L   E
   AE000659,TRAV8-3*01  [6] GCC CAG TCA GTG ACC CAG CCT GAC ATC CAC ATC ACT GTC TCT GAA GGA GCC TCA CTG GAG

   M35617  ,TRAV8-3*02  [2] --- --- --- --- --- --- --- --- --- --- --- --- --- --- --- --- --- --- --- ---

   L06885  ,TRAV8-3*03 [29] --- --- --- --- --- --- --- --- --- --- --- --- --- --- --- --- --- --- --- ---

                                                                       ____________CDR1-IMGT______________________
                            21  22  23  24  25  26  27  28  29  30  31  32  33  34  35  36  37  38  39  40
                             L   R   C   N   Y   S   Y   G   A   T   P   Y                           L   F
   AE000659,TRAV8-3*01      TTG AGA TGT AAC TAT TCC TAT GGG GCA ACA CCT TAT ... ... ... ... ... ... CTC TTC

   M35617  ,TRAV8-3*02      --- --- --- --- --- --- --- --- --- --- --- --- ... ... ... ... ... ... --- ---

   L06885  ,TRAV8-3*03      --- --- --- --- --- --- --- --- --- --- --- --- ... ... ... ... ... ... --- ---

                                                                               ________________CDR2-
                            41  42  43  44  45  46  47  48  49  50  51  52  53  54  55  56  57  58  59  60
                             W   Y   V   Q   S   P   G   Q   G   L   Q   L   L   L   K   Y   F   S   G
   AE000659,TRAV8-3*01      TGG TAT GTC CAG TCC CCC GGC CAA GGC CTC CAG CTG CTC CTG AAG TAC TTT TCA GGA ...

   M35617  ,TRAV8-3*02      --- --- --- --- --- --- --- --- --- --- --- --- --- --- --- --- --- --- --- ...

   L06885  ,TRAV8-3*03      --- --- --- --- --- --- --- --- --- --- --- --- --- --- --- --- --- --- --- ...

                           IMGT________________
                            61  62  63  64  65  66  67  68  69  70  71  72  73  74  75  76  77  78  79  80
                                                 D   T   L   V   Q   G   I       K   G   F   E   A   E   F
   AE000659,TRAV8-3*01      ... ... ... ... ... GAC ACT CTG GTT CAA GGC ATT ... AAA GGC TTT GAG GCT GAA TTT

   M35617  ,TRAV8-3*02      ... ... ... ... ... --- --- --- --- --- --- --- ... --- --- --- --- --- --- ---

   L06885  ,TRAV8-3*03      ... ... ... ... ... --- --- --- --- --- --T --- ... --- --- --- --- --- --- ---

                            81  82  83  84  85  86  87  88  89  90  91  92  93  94  95  96  97  98  99 100
                             K   R   S   Q   S   S   F   N   L   R   K   P   S   V   H   W   S   D   A   A
   AE000659,TRAV8-3*01      AAG AGG AGT CAA TCT TCC TTC AAT CTG AGG AAA CCC TCT GTG CAT TGG AGT GAT GCT GCT

   M35617  ,TRAV8-3*02      --- --- --- --- --- --- --- --C --- --- --- --- --- --- --- --- --- --- --- ---

                                                                                                          S
   L06885  ,TRAV8-3*03      --- --- --- --- --- --- --- --- --- --- --- --- --- --- --- --- --- --- --G T--

                                    _CDR3-IMGT_
                           101 102 103 104 105 106 107
                             E   Y   F   C   A   V   G
   AE000659,TRAV8-3*01      GAG TAC TTC TGT GCT GTG GGT GC

                                                 V
   M35617  ,TRAV8-3*02      --- --- --- --- --- --- -T-      #g

   L06885  ,TRAV8-3*03      --- --- --- --- ---              #c
```

#c: Rearranged cDNA
#g: Rearranged genomic DNA

Framework and complementarity determining regions

FR1-IMGT: 26

FR2-IMGT: 17

FR3-IMGT: 38 (-1 aa: 73)

CDR1-IMGT: 6

CDR2-IMGT: 4

CDR3-IMGT: 3

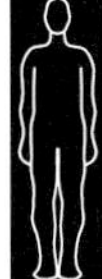

Collier de Perles for human TRAV8-3*01

Accession number: IMGT AE000659   EMBL/GenBank/DDBJ: AE000659

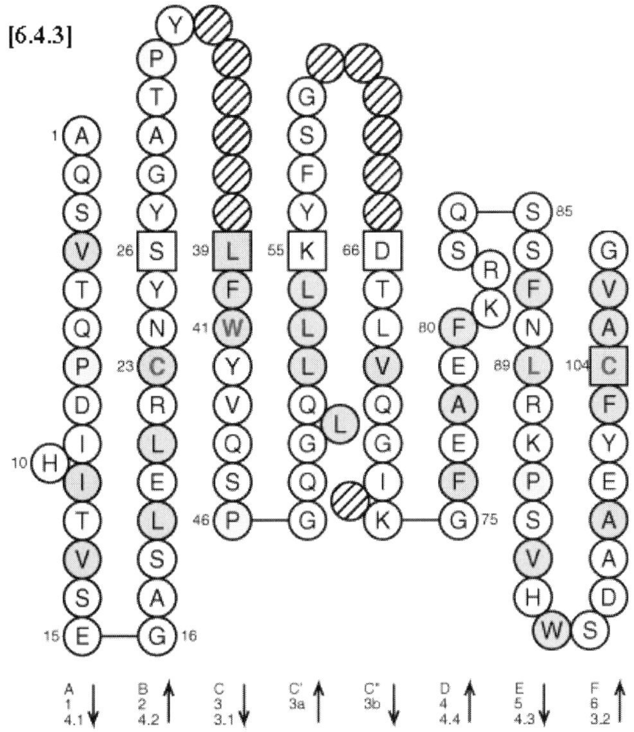

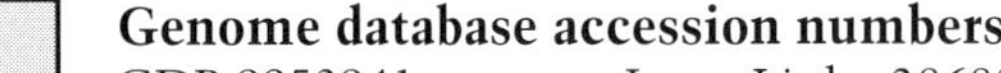

Genome database accession numbers
GDB:9953941   LocusLink: 28683

Nomenclature

TRAV8-4: T cell receptor alpha variable 8-4.

Definition and functionality

TRAV8-4 is one of the six functional genes of the TRAV8 subgroup which comprises seven mapped genes.

Gene location

TRAV8-4 is in the TRA/TRD locus on chromosome 14 at 14q11.2.

Nucleotide and amino acid sequences for human TRAV8-4

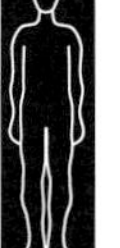

```
                          1   2   3   4   5   6   7   8   9  10  11  12  13  14  15  16  17  18  19  20
                          A   Q   S   V   T   Q   L   G   S   H   V   S   V   S   E   G   A   L   V   L
AE000659,TRAV8-4*01  [6]  GCC CAG TCG GTG ACC CAG CTT GGC AGC CAC GTC TCT GTC TCT GAA GGA GCC CTG GTT CTG
X02592  ,TRAV8-4*01 [26]  --- --- --- --- --- --- --- --- --- --- --- --- --- --- --- --- --- --- --- ---
M12423  ,TRAV8-4*02 [35]  --- --- --- --- --- --- --- --- --- --- --- --- --- --- --- --- --- --- --- ---
D13077  ,TRAV8-4*03 [23]  --- --- --- --- --- --- --- --- --- --- --- --- --- --- --- --G --- --- --- ---
                                                                                       R
M12959  ,TRAV8-4*04 [26]  --- --- --- --- --- --- --- --- --- --- --- --- --- --- --- C-- --- --- --- ---
X63455  ,TRAV8-4*05 [11]  --- --- --- --- --- --- --- --- --- --- --- --- --- --- --- --- --- --- --- ---
K02777  ,TRAV8-4*06  [9]
M17665  ,TRAV8-4*07 [17]


                                                                      CDR1-IMGT
                         21  22  23  24  25  26  27  28  29  30  31  32  33  34  35  36  37  38  39  40
                          L   R   C   N   Y   S   S   S   V   P   P   Y                           L   F
AE000659,TRAV8-4*01      CTG AGG TGC AAC TAC TCA TCG TCT GTT CCA CCA TAT ... ... ... ... ... ... CTC TTC
X02592  ,TRAV8-4*01      --- --- --- --- --- --- --- --- --- --- --- --- ... ... ... ... ... ... --- ---
M12423  ,TRAV8-4*02      --- --- --- --- --- --- --- --- --- --- --- --- ... ... ... ... ... ... --- ---
D13077  ,TRAV8-4*03      --- --- --- --- --- --- --- --- --- --- --- --- ... ... ... ... ... ... --- ---
M12959  ,TRAV8-4*04      --- --- --- --- --- --- --- --- --- --- --- --- ... ... ... ... ... ... --- ---
X63455  ,TRAV8-4*05      --- --- --- --- --- --- --- --- --- --- --- --- ... ... ... ... ... ... --- ---
K02777  ,TRAV8-4*06                                                                                  --- ---
M17665  ,TRAV8-4*07                                          E
                         --- --- --- --- --- --- --- GA- --- --- ... ... ... ... ... ... --- ---


                                                                                                 CDR2-
                         41  42  43  44  45  46  47  48  49  50  51  52  53  54  55  56  57  58  59  60
                          W   Y   V   Q   Y   P   N   Q   G   L   Q   L   L   L   K   Y   T   S   A
AE000659,TRAV8-4*01      TGG TAT GTG CAA TAC CCC AAC CAA GGA CTC CAG CTT CTC CTG AAG TAC ACA TCA GCG ...
X02592  ,TRAV8-4*01      --- --- --- --- --- --- --- --- --- --- --- --- --- --- --- --- --- --- --- ...
M12423  ,TRAV8-4*02      --- --- --- --- --- --- --- --- --- --- --- --- --- --- --- --- --- --- --- ...
D13077  ,TRAV8-4*03                                                                          T   G
                         --- --- --- --- --- --- --- --- --- --- --- --- --- --- --- --- --- A-- -G- ...
M12959  ,TRAV8-4*04      --- --- --- --- --- --- --- --- --- --- --- --- --- --- --- --- --- --- --- ...
X63455  ,TRAV8-4*05      --- --- --- --- --- --- --- --- --- --- --- --- --- --- --- --- --- --- --- ...
K02777  ,TRAV8-4*06      --- --- --- --- --- --- --- --- --- --- --- --- --- --- --- --- --- --- --- ...
M17665  ,TRAV8-4*07                                                                          T   G
                         --- --- --- --- --- --- --- --- --- --- --- --- --- --- --- --- --- A-- -G- ...


                         IMGT
                         61  62  63  64  65  66  67  68  69  70  71  72  73  74  75  76  77  78  79  80
                                                  A   T   L   V   K   G   I       N   G   F   E   A   E   F
AE000659,TRAV8-4*01      ... ... ... ... ... GCC ACC CTG GTT AAA GGC ATC ... AAC GGT TTT GAG GCT GAA TTT
X02592  ,TRAV8-4*01      ... ... ... ... ... --- --- --- --- --- --- --- ... --- --- --- --- --- ---
M12423  ,TRAV8-4*02      ... ... ... ... ... --- --- --- --- --- --- --- ... --- --- --- --- --- ---
D13077  ,TRAV8-4*03      ... ... ... ... ... --- --- --- --- --- --- --- ... --- --- --- --- --- ---
M12959  ,TRAV8-4*04      ... ... ... ... ... --- --- --- --- --- --- --- ... --- --- --- --- --- ---
X63455  ,TRAV8-4*05      ... ... ... ... ... --- --- --- --- --- --A --- ... --- --- --- --- --- ---
K02777  ,TRAV8-4*06      ... ... ... ... ... --- --- --- --- --- --- --- ... --- --- --- --- --- ---
M17665  ,TRAV8-4*07      ... ... ... ... ... --- --- --- --- --- --- --- ... --- --- --- --- --- ---


                         81  82  83  84  85  86  87  88  89  90  91  92  93  94  95  96  97  98  99 100
                          K   K   S   E   T   S   F   H   L   T   K   P   S   A   H   M   S   D   A   A
AE000659,TRAV8-4*01      AAG AAG AGT GAA ACC TCC TTC CAC CTG ACG AAA CCC TCA GCC CAT ATG AGC GAC GCG GCT
X02592  ,TRAV8-4*01      --- --- --- --- --- --- --- --- --- --- --- --- --- --- --- --- --- --- --- ---
M12423  ,TRAV8-4*02      --- --- --- --- --- --- --- --- --- --A --- --- --- --- --- --- --- --- --- ---
D13077  ,TRAV8-4*03      --- --- --- --- --- --- --- --- --- --- --- --- --- --- --- --- --- --- --- ---
M12959  ,TRAV8-4*04      --- --- --- --- --- --- --- --- --- --- --- --- --- --- --- --- --- --- --- ---
X63455  ,TRAV8-4*05      --- --- --- --- --- --- --- --- --- --- --- --- --- --- --- --- --- --- --- ---
K02777  ,TRAV8-4*06                                                          A
                         --- --- --- --- --- --- --- --- --- --- --- G-- --- --- --- --- --- --- --- ---
M17665  ,TRAV8-4*07                                                                              T       P
                         --A --- --- --- --- --- --- --- --- --- --- --- --- --- --- --- -C- --- C-- ---
```

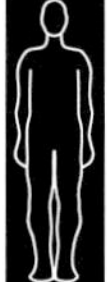

```
                                      _CDR3-IMGT_
                         101 102 103 104 105 106 107
                          E   Y   F   C   A   V   S
    AE000659 ,TRAV8-4*01  GAG TAC TTC TGT GCT GTG AGT GA

    X02592   ,TRAV8-4*01  --- --- --- --- --- --- ---       #c
    M12423   ,TRAV8-4*02  --- --- --- --- --- --- ---       #c
    D13077   ,TRAV8-4*03  --- --- --- --- ---               #c
    M12959   ,TRAV8-4*04  --- --- --- ---                   #c
    X63455   ,TRAV8-4*05  --- --- --- --- --- --- ---       #c
    K02777   ,TRAV8-4*06  --- --- --- --- --- --- ---       #c
                                                      R
    M17665   ,TRAV8-4*07  --- --- --- --- --- --- -GG       #c

#c: Rearranged cDNA
```

Framework and complementarity determining regions

FR1-IMGT: 26   CDR1-IMGT: 6
FR2-IMGT: 17   CDR2-IMGT: 4
FR3-IMGT: 38 (-1 aa: 73)   CDR3-IMGT: 3

Collier de Perles for human TRAV8-4*01

Accession number: IMGT AE000659   EMBL/GenBank/DDBJ: AE000659

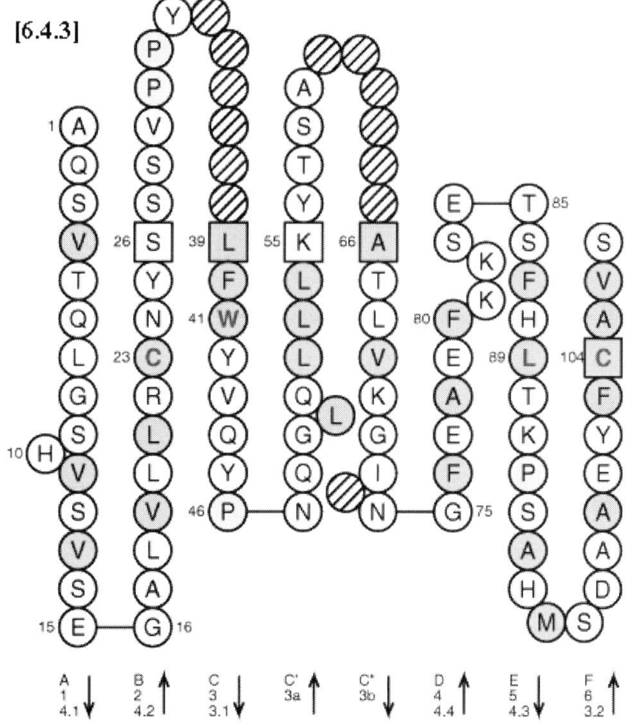

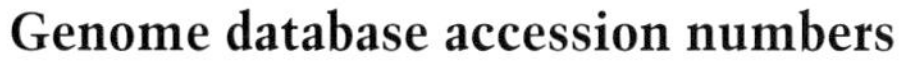

Genome database accession numbers
GDB:9953943   LocusLink: 28682

TRAV8-6

Nomenclature

TRAV8-6: T cell receptor alpha variable 8-6.

Definition and functionality

TRAV8-6 is one of the six functional genes of the TRAV8 subgroup which comprises seven mapped genes.

Gene location

TRAV8-6 is in the TRA/TRD locus on chromosome 14 at 14q11.2.

Nucleotide and amino acid sequences for human TRAV8-6

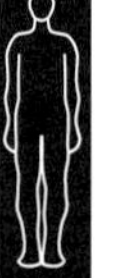

```
                      1   2   3   4   5   6   7   8   9   10  11  12  13  14  15  16  17  18  19  20
                      A   Q   S   V   T   Q   L   D   S   Q   V   P   V   F   E   E   A   P   V   E
X02850   ,TRAV8-6*01  [37] GCC CAG TCT GTG ACC CAG CTT GAC AGC CAA GTC CCT GTC TTT GAA GAA GCC CCT GTG GAG
AE000659,TRAV8-6*02   [6]  --- --- --- --- --- --- --- --- --- --- --- --- --- --- --- --- --- --- --- ---
M86361   ,TRAV8-6*02  [18] --- --- --- --- --- --- --- --- --- --- --- --- --- --- --- --- --- --- --- ---

                                                                  ________________CDR1-IMGT________
                      21  22  23  24  25  26  27  28  29  30  31  32  33  34  35  36  37  38  39  40
                      L   R   C   N   Y   S   S   S   V   S   V   Y                           L   F
X02850   ,TRAV8-6*01  CTG AGG TGC AAC TAC TCA TCG TCT GTT TCA GTG TAT ... ... ... ... ... ... CTC TTC
AE000659,TRAV8-6*02   --- --- --- --- --- --- --- --- --- --- --- --- ... ... ... ... ... ... --- ---
M86361   ,TRAV8-6*02  --- --- --- --- --- --- --- --- --- --- --- --- ... ... ... ... ... ... --- ---

                                                                                          ______CDR2-
                      41  42  43  44  45  46  47  48  49  50  51  52  53  54  55  56  57  58  59  60
                      W   Y   V   Q   Y   P   N   Q   G   L   Q   L   L   L   K   Y   L   S   G
X02850   ,TRAV8-6*01  TGG TAT GTG CAA TAC CCC AAC CAA GGA CTC CAG CTT CTC CTG AAG TAT TTA TCA GGA ...
AE000659,TRAV8-6*02   --- --- --- --- --- --- --- --- --- --- --- --- --- --- --- --- --- --- --- ...
M86361   ,TRAV8-6*02  --- --- --- --- --- --- --- --- --- --- --- --- --- --- --- --- --- --- --- ...

                      IMGT________
                      61  62  63  64  65  66  67  68  69  70  71  72  73  74  75  76  77  78  79  80
                                          S   T   L   V   E   S   I       N   G   F   E   A   E   F
X02850   ,TRAV8-6*01  ... ... ... ... ... TCC ACC CTG GTT GAA AGC ATC ... AAC GGT TTT GAG GCT GAA TTT
                                                              K   G
AE000659,TRAV8-6*02   ... ... ... ... ... --- --- --- --- A-- G-- --- ... --- --- --- --- --- --- ---
                                                              K   G
M86361   ,TRAV8-6*02  ... ... ... ... ... --- --- --- --- A-- G-- --- ... --- --- --- --- --- --- ---

                      81  82  83  84  85  86  87  88  89  90  91  92  93  94  95  96  97  98  99  100
                      N   K   S   Q   T   S   F   H   L   R   K   P   S   V   H   I   S   D   T   A
X02850   ,TRAV8-6*01  AAC AAG AGT CAA ACT TCC TTC CAC TTG AGG AAA CCC TCA GTC CAT ATA AGC GAC ACG GCT
AE000659,TRAV8-6*02   --- --- --- --- --- --- --- --- --- --- --- --- --- --- --- --- --- --- --- ---
M86361   ,TRAV8-6*02  --- --- --- --- --- --- --- --- --- --- --- --- --- --- --- --- --- --- --- ---

                            ___CDR3-IMGT___
                      101 102 103 104 105 106 107 108
                      E   Y   F   C   A   V   S
X02850   ,TRAV8-6*01  GAG TAC TTC TGT GCT GTG AGT GA
AE000659,TRAV8-6*02   --- --- --- --- --- --- --- --
                                                  R
M86361   ,TRAV8-6*02  --- --- --- --- --- --- --G       #c
```

#c: Rearranged cDNA

Framework and complementarity determining regions

FR1-IMGT: 26

FR2-IMGT: 17

FR3-IMGT: 38 (-1 aa: 73)

CDR1-IMGT: 6

CDR2-IMGT: 4

CDR3-IMGT: 3

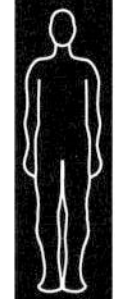

Collier de Perles for human TRAV8-6*01

Accession number: IMGT X02850   EMBL/GenBank/DDBJ: X02850

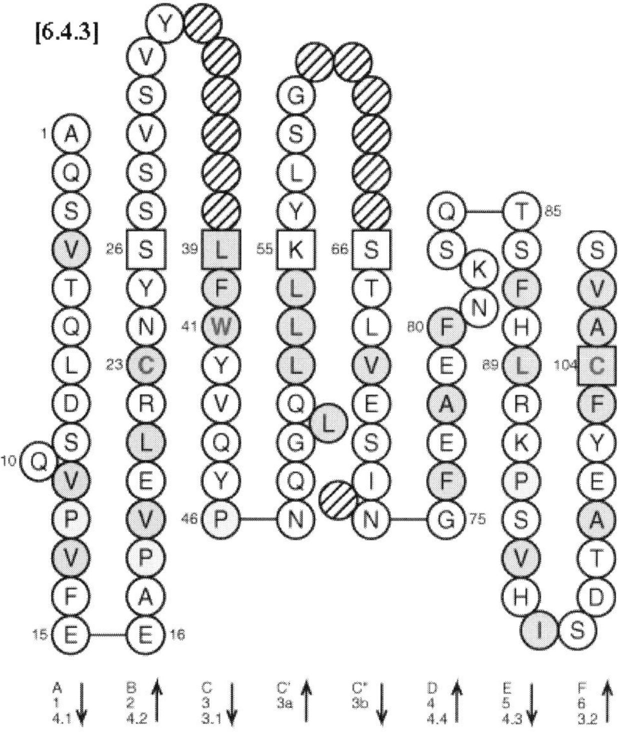

Genome database accession numbers
GDB:9953947   LocusLink: 28680

Nomenclature

TRAV8-7: T cell receptor alpha variable 8-7.

Definition and functionality

TRAV8-7 is one of the six functional genes of the TRAV8 subgroup which comprises seven mapped genes.

Gene location

TRAV8-7 is in the TRA/TRD locus on chromosome 14 at 14q11.2.

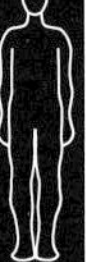

Nucleotide and amino acid sequences for human TRAV8-7

```
                          1    2    3    4    5    6    7    8    9   10   11   12   13   14   15   16   17   18   19   20
                          T    Q    S    V    T    Q    L    D    G    H    I    T    V    S    E    E    A    P    L    E
AE000660,TRAV8-7*01  [6]  ACC  CAG  TCG  GTG  ACC  CAG  CTT  GAT  GGC  CAC  ATC  ACT  GTC  TCT  GAA  GAA  GCC  CCT  CTG  GAA

                                                                                  ____________CDR1-IMGT____________
                         21   22   23   24   25   26   27   28   29   30   31   32   33   34   35   36   37   38   39   40
                          L    K    C    N    Y    S    Y    S    G    V    P    S                             L    F
AE000660,TRAV8-7*01       CTG  AAG  TGC  AAC  TAT  TCC  TAT  AGT  GGA  GTT  CCT  TCT  ...  ...  ...  ...  ...  ...  CTC  TTC

                                                                                            ____________CDR2-
                         41   42   43   44   45   46   47   48   49   50   51   52   53   54   55   56   57   58   59   60
                          W    Y    V    Q    Y    S    S    Q    S    L    Q    L    L    L    K    D    L    T    E
AE000660,TRAV8-7*01       TGG  TAT  GTC  CAA  TAC  TCT  AGC  CAA  AGC  CTC  CAG  CTT  CTC  CTC  AAA  GAC  CTA  ACA  GAG  ...

                         IMGT____
                         61   62   63   64   65   66   67   68   69   70   71   72   73   74   75   76   77   78   79   80
                                                        A    T    Q    V    K    G    I         R    G    F    E    A    E    F
AE000660,TRAV8-7*01       ...  ...  ...  ...  ...  GCC  ACC  CAG  GTT  AAA  GGC  ATC  ...  AGA  GGT  TTT  GAG  GCT  GAA  TTT

                         81   82   83   84   85   86   87   88   89   90   91   92   93   94   95   96   97   98   99  100
                          K    K    S    E    T    S    F    Y    L    R    K    P    S    T    H    V    S    D    A    A
AE000660,TRAV8-7*01       AAG  AAG  AGC  GAA  ACC  TCC  TTC  TAC  CTG  AGG  AAA  CCA  TCA  ACC  CAT  GTG  AGT  GAT  GCT  GCT

                                                   ______CDR3-IMGT______
                        101  102  103  104  105  106  107  108  109
                          E    Y    F    C    A    V    G    D    R
AE000660,TRAV8-7*01       GAG  TAC  TTC  TGT  GCT  GTG  GGT  GAC  AGG  AG
```

Framework and complementarity determining regions

FR1-IMGT: 26	CDR1-IMGT: 6
FR2-IMGT: 17	CDR2-IMGT: 4
FR3-IMGT: 38 (-1 aa: 73)	CDR3-IMGT: 5

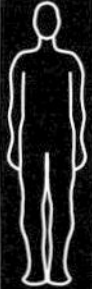

Collier de Perles for human TRAV8-7*01

Accession number: IMGT AE000660   EMBL/GenBank/DDBJ: AE000660

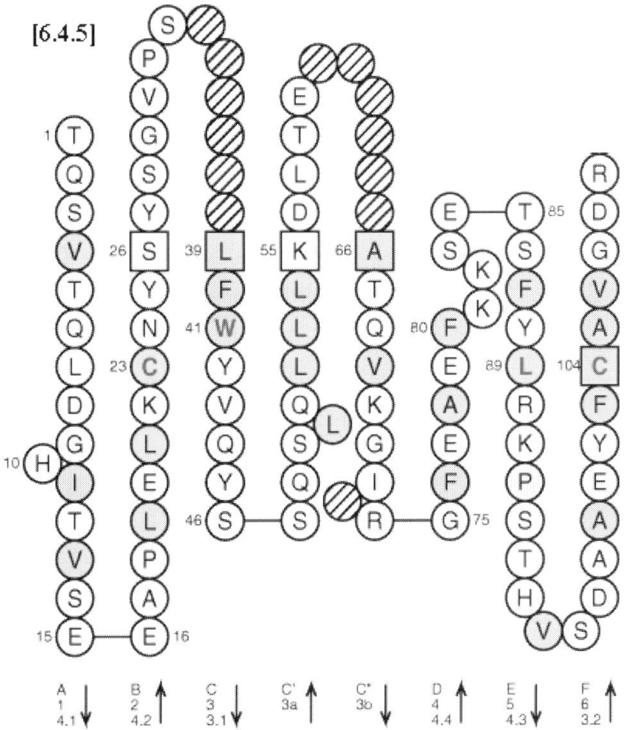

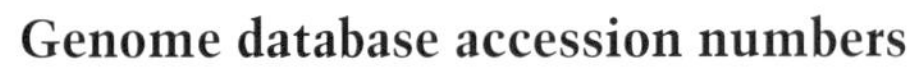

Genome database accession numbers
GDB:9953949   LocusLink: 28679

TRAV9-1

Nomenclature

TRAV9-1: T cell receptor alpha variable 9-1.

Definition and functionality

TRAV9-1 is one of the two functional genes of the TRAV9 subgroup which comprises two mapped genes.

Gene location

TRAV9-1 is in the TRA/TRD locus on chromosome 14 at 14q11.2.

Nucleotide and amino acid sequences for human TRAV9-1

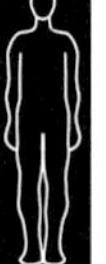

```
                       1    2    3    4    5    6    7    8    9   10   11   12   13   14   15   16   17   18   19   20
                       G    D    S    V    V    Q    T    E    G    Q    V    L    P    S    E    G    D    S    L    I
   AE000659,TRAV9-1*01   [6]  GGA  GAT  TCA  GTG  GTC  CAG  ACA  GAA  GGC  CAA  GTG  CTC  CCC  TCT  GAA  GGG  GAT  TCC  CTG  ATT

                                                             ________________________CDR1-IMGT____________________
                      21   22   23   24   25   26   27   28   29   30   31   32   33   34   35   36   37   38   39   40
                       V    N    C    S    Y    E    T    T    Q    Y    P    S                                  L    F
   AE000659,TRAV9-1*01  GTG  AAC  TGC  TCC  TAT  GAA  ACC  ACA  CAG  TAC  CCT  TCC  ...  ...  ...  ...  ...  ...  CTT  TTT

                                                                                      ___________________CDR2-
                      41   42   43   44   45   46   47   48   49   50   51   52   53   54   55   56   57   58   59   60
                       W    Y    V    Q    Y    P    G    E    G    P    Q    L    H    L    K    A    M    K
   AE000659,TRAV9-1*01  TGG  TAT  GTC  CAA  TAT  CCT  GGA  GAA  GGT  CCA  CAG  CTC  CAC  CTG  AAA  GCC  ATG  AAG  ...  ...

                      IMGT________________
                      61   62   63   64   65   66   67   68   69   70   71   72   73   74   75   76   77   78   79   80
                                                  A    N    D    K    G    R    N         K    G    F    E    A    M    Y
   AE000659,TRAV9-1*01  ...  ...  ...  ...  ...  GCC  AAT  GAC  AAG  GGA  AGG  AAC  ...  AAA  GGT  TTT  GAA  GCC  ATG  TAC

                      81   82   83   84   85   86   87   88   89   90   91   92   93   94   95   96   97   98   99  100
                       R    K    E    T    T    S    F    H    L    E    K    D    S    V    Q    E    S    D    S    A
   AE000659,TRAV9-1*01  CGT  AAA  GAA  ACC  ACT  TCT  TTC  CAC  TTG  GAG  AAA  GAC  TCA  GTT  CAA  GAG  TCA  GAC  TCC  GCT

                                           _CDR3-IMGT_
                     101  102  103  104  105  106  107
                       V    Y    F    C    A    L    S
   AE000659,TRAV9-1*01  GTG  TAC  TTC  TGT  GCT  CTG  AGT  GA
```

Framework and complementarity determining regions

FR1-IMGT: 26

FR2-IMGT: 17

FR3-IMGT: 38 (-1 aa: 73)

CDR1-IMGT: 6

CDR2-IMGT: 3

CDR3-IMGT: 3

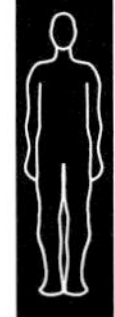

Collier de Perles for human TRAV9-1*01

Accession number: IMGT AE000659   EMBL/GenBank/DDBJ: AE000659

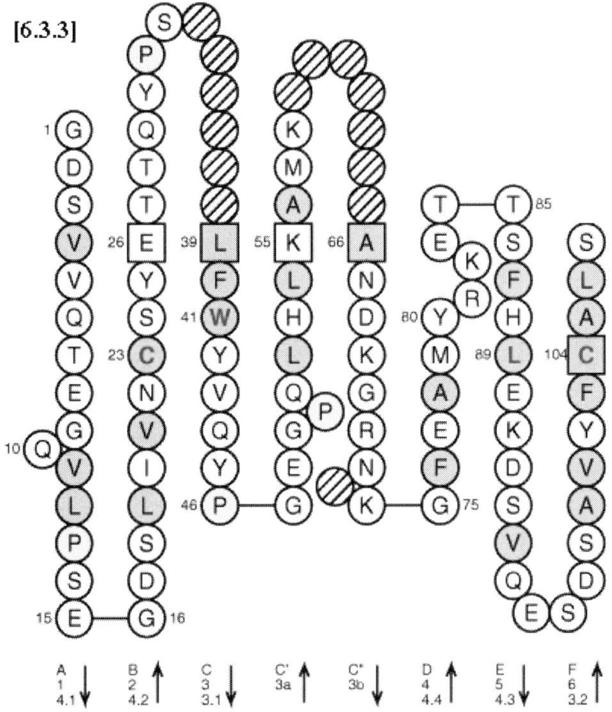

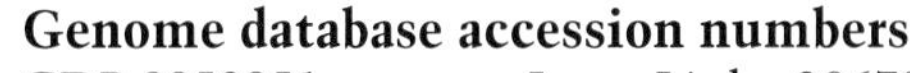

Genome database accession numbers

GDB:9953951   LocusLink: 28678

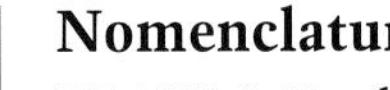

Nomenclature

TRAV9-2: T cell receptor alpha variable 9-2.

Definition and functionality

TRAV9-2 is one of the two functional genes of the TRAV9 subgroup which comprises two mapped genes.

Gene location

TRAV9-2 is in the TRA/TRD locus on chromosome 14 at 14q11.2.

Nucleotide and amino acid sequences for human TRAV9-2

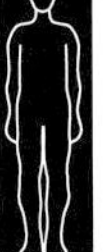

```
                           1   2   3   4   5   6   7   8   9  10  11  12  13  14  15  16  17  18  19  20
                           G   N   S   V   T   Q   M   E   G   P   V   T   L   S   E   E   A   F   L   T
AE000659,TRAV9-2*01   [6]  GGA AAT TCA GTG ACC CAG ATG GAA GGG CCA GTG ACT CTC TCA GAA GAG GCC TTC CTG ACT
D13072  ,TRAV9-2*01  [23]  --- --- --- --- --- --- --- --- --- --- --- --- --- --- --- --- --- --- --- ---
                               D
X58745  ,TRAV9-2*02  [28]  --- G-- --- --- --- --- --- --- --- --- --- --- --- --- --- --- --- --- --- ---
                               D
U32530  ,TRAV9-2*02   [5]  --- G-- --- --- --- --- --- --- --- --- --- --- --- --- --- --- --- --- --- ---
                               D
L06881  ,TRAV9-2*03  [29]  --- G-- --- --- --- --- --- --- --- --- --- --- --- --- --- --- --- --- --- ---
L06882  ,TRAV9-2*04  [29]  --- --- --- --- --- --- --- --- --- --- --- --- --- --- --- --- --- --- --- ---

                                                              ____________________CDR1-IMGT____________________
                          21  22  23  24  25  26  27  28  29  30  31  32  33  34  35  36  37  38  39  40
                           I   N   C   T   Y   T   A   T   G   Y   P   S                           L   F
AE000659,TRAV9-2*01       ATA AAC TGC ACG TAC ACA GCC ACA GGA TAC CCT TCC ... ... ... ... ... ... CTT TTC
D13072  ,TRAV9-2*01       --- --- --- --- --- --- --- --- --- --- --- --- ... ... ... ... ... ... --- ---
X58745  ,TRAV9-2*02       --- --- --- --- --- --- --- --- --- --- --- --- ... ... ... ... ... ... --- ---
U32530  ,TRAV9-2*02       --- --- --- --- --- --- --- --- --- --- --- --- ... ... ... ... ... ... --- ---
L06881  ,TRAV9-2*03       --- --- --- --- --- --- --- --- --- --- --- --- ... ... ... ... ... ... --- ---
L06882  ,TRAV9-2*04       --- --- --- --- --- --- --- --- --- --- --- --- ... ... ... ... ... ... --- ---

                                                                                          ________________CDR2-
                          41  42  43  44  45  46  47  48  49  50  51  52  53  54  55  56  57  58  59  60
                           W   Y   V   Q   Y   P   G   E   G   L   Q   L   L   L   K   A   T   K
AE000659,TRAV9-2*01       TGG TAT GTC CAA TAT CCT GGA GAA GGT CTA CAG CTC CTC CTG AAA GCC ACG AAG ... ...
D13072  ,TRAV9-2*01       --- --- --- --- --- --- --- --- --- --- --- --- --- --- --- --- --- --- ... ...
X58745  ,TRAV9-2*02       --- --- --- --- --- --- --- --- --- --- --- --- --- --- --- --- --- --- ... ...
U32530  ,TRAV9-2*02       --- --- --- --- --- --- --- --- --- --- --- --- --- --- --- --- --- --- ... ...
L06881  ,TRAV9-2*03       --- --- --- --- --- --- --- --- --- --- --- --- --- --- --- --- --- --- ... ...
L06882  ,TRAV9-2*04       --- --- --- --- --- --- --- --- --- --- --- --- --- --- --- --- --- --- ... ...

                          IMGT____________________
                          61  62  63  64  65  66  67  68  69  70  71  72  73  74  75  76  77  78  79  80
                                                   A   D   D   K   G   S   N       K   G   F   E   A   T   Y
AE000659,TRAV9-2*01       ... ... ... ... ... GCT GAT GAC AAG GGA AGC AAC ... AAA GGT TTT GAA GCC ACA TAC
D13072  ,TRAV9-2*01       ... ... ... ... ... --- --- --- --- --- --- --- ... --- --- --- --- --- --- ---
X58745  ,TRAV9-2*02       ... ... ... ... ... --- --- --- --- --- --- --- ... --- --- --- --- --- --- ---
U32530  ,TRAV9-2*02       ... ... ... ... ... --- --- --- --- --- --- --- ... --- --- --- --- --- --- ---
L06881  ,TRAV9-2*03       ... ... ... ... ... --- --- --- --- --- --- --- ... --- --- --- --- --- --- ---
L06882  ,TRAV9-2*04       ... ... ... ... ... --- --- --- --- --- --- --- ... --- --- --- --- --- --- ---

                          81  82  83  84  85  86  87  88  89  90  91  92  93  94  95  96  97  98  99 100
                           R   K   E   T   T   S   F   H   L   E   K   G   S   V   Q   V   S   D   S   A
AE000659,TRAV9-2*01       CGT AAA GAA ACC ACT TCT TTC CAC TTG GAG AAA GGC TCA GTT CAA GTG TCA GAC TCA GCG
D13072  ,TRAV9-2*01       --- --- --- --- --- --- --- --- --- --- --- --- --- --- --- --- --- --- --- ---
X58745  ,TRAV9-2*02       --- --- --- --- --- --- --- --- --- --- --- --- --- --- --- --- --- --- --- ---
U32530  ,TRAV9-2*02       --- --- --- --- --- --- --- --- --- --- --- --- --- --- --- --- --- --- --- --
L06881  ,TRAV9-2*03       --- --G --- --- --- --- --- --- --- --- --- --- --- --- --- --- --- --- --- ---
L06882  ,TRAV9-2*04       --- --G --- --- --- --- --- --- --- --- --- --- --- --- --- --- --- --- --- ---

                              _CDR3-IMGT_
                         101 102 103 104 105 106 107
                           V   Y   F   C   A   L   S
AE000659,TRAV9-2*01       GTG TAC TTC TGT GCT CTG AGT GA
D13072  ,TRAV9-2*01       --- --- --- --- --- ---          #c
X58745  ,TRAV9-2*02       --- --- --- --- ---              #c
U32530  ,TRAV9-2*02                                        o
L06881  ,TRAV9-2*03       --- --- --- --- ---              #c
L06882  ,TRAV9-2*04       --- --- --- --- ---              #c
```

#c: Rearranged cDNA
o: Genomic DNA, but not known as being germline or rearranged

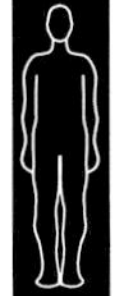

Framework and complementarity determining regions

FR1-IMGT: 26
FR2-IMGT: 17
FR3-IMGT: 38 (-1 aa: 73)

CDR1-IMGT: 6
CDR2-IMGT: 3
CDR3-IMGT: 3

Collier de Perles for human TRAV9-2*01

Accession number: IMGT AE000659   EMBL/GenBank/DDBJ: AE000659

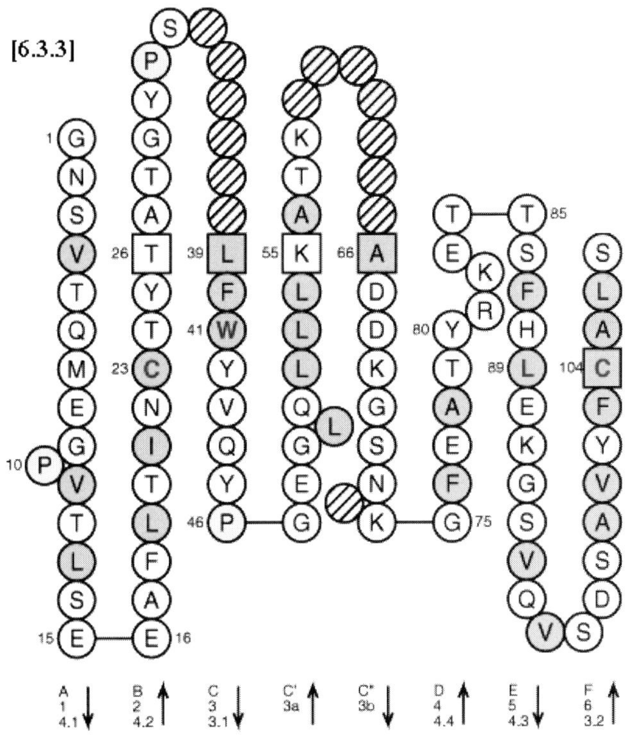

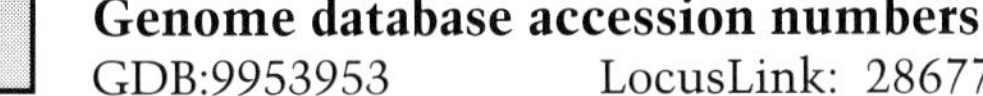

Genome database accession numbers
GDB:9953953   LocusLink: 28677

TRAV10

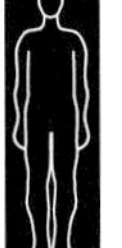

Nomenclature

TRAV10: T cell receptor alpha variable 10.

Definition and functionality

TRAV10 is the unique functional gene of the TRAV10 subgroup which only comprises this mapped gene.

Gene location

TRAV10 is in the TRA/TRD locus on chromosome 14 at 14q11.2.

Nucleotide and amino acid sequences for human TRAV10

```
                      1   2   3   4   5   6   7   8   9  10  11  12  13  14  15  16  17  18  19  20
                      K   N   Q   V   E   Q   S   P   Q   S   L   I   I   L   E   G   K   N   C   T
AE000659,TRAV10*01 [6] AAA AAC CAA GTG GAG CAG AGT CCT CAG TCC CTG ATC ATC CTG GAG GGA AAG AAC TGC ACT

X58737  ,TRAV10*01 [28] --- --- --- --- --- --- --- --- --- --- --- --- --- --- --- --- --- --- --- ---

U32532  ,TRAV10*01 [5]  --- --- --- --- --- --- --- --- --- --- --- --- --- --- --- --- --- --- --- ---


                                                                      ____________CDR1-IMGT__________
                     21  22  23  24  25  26  27  28  29  30  31  32  33  34  35  36  37  38  39  40
                      L   Q   C   N   Y   T   V   S   P   F   S   N                           L   R
AE000659,TRAV10*01   CTT CAA TGC AAT TAT ACA GTG AGC CCC TTC AGC AAC ... ... ... ... ... ... TTA AGG

X58737  ,TRAV10*01   --- --- --- --- --- --- --- --- --- --- --- --- ... ... ... ... ... ... --- ---

U32532  ,TRAV10*01   --- --- --- --- --- --- --- --- --- --- --- --- ... ... ... ... ... ... --- ---


                                                                              ________________CDR2-
                     41  42  43  44  45  46  47  48  49  50  51  52  53  54  55  56  57  58  59  60
                      W   Y   K   Q   D   T   G   R   G   P   V   S   L   T   I   M   T   F
AE000659,TRAV10*01   TGG TAT AAG CAA GAT ACT GGG AGA GGT CCT GTT TCC CTG ACA ATC ATG ACT TTC ... ...

X58737  ,TRAV10*01   --- --- --- --- --- --- --- --- --- --- --- --- --- --- --- --- --- --- ... ...

U32532  ,TRAV10*01   --- --- --- --- --- --- --- --- --- --- --- --- --- --- --- --- --- --- ... ...


IMGT______________
  61  62  63  64  65  66  67  68  69  70  71  72  73  74  75  76  77  78  79  80
                      S   E   N   T   K   S   N       G   R   Y   T   A   T   L
AE000659,TRAV10*01   ... ... ... ... ... AGT GAG AAC ACA AAG TCG AAC ... GGA AGA TAT ACA GCA ACT CTG

X58737  ,TRAV10*01   ... ... ... ... ... --- --- --- --- --- --- --- ... --- --- --- --- --- --- ---

U32532  ,TRAV10*01   ... ... ... ... ... --- --- --- --- --- --- --- ... --- --- --- --- --- --- ---


                     81  82  83  84  85  86  87  88  89  90  91  92  93  94  95  96  97  98  99 100
                      D   A   D   T   K   Q   S   S   L   H   I   T   A   S   Q   L   S   D   S   A
AE000659,TRAV10*01   GAT GCA GAC ACA AAG CAA AGC TCT CTG CAC ATC ACA GCC TCC CAG CTC AGC GAT TCA GCC

X58737  ,TRAV10*01   --- --- --- --- --- --- --- --- --- --- --- --- --- --- --- --- --- --- --- ---

U32532  ,TRAV10*01   --- --- --- --- --- --- --- --- --- --- --- --- ---


                       _CDR3-IMGT_
                     101 102 103 104 105 106 107
                      S   Y   I   C   V   V   S
AE000659,TRAV10*01   TCC TAC ATC TGT GTG GTG AGC G

X58737  ,TRAV10*01   --- --- --- --- ---                        #c

U32532  ,TRAV10*01                                              o

#c: Rearranged cDNA
o: Genomic DNA, but not known as being germline or rearranged
```

Framework and complementarity determining regions

FR1-IMGT: 26

FR2-IMGT: 17

FR3-IMGT: 38 (-1 aa: 73)

CDR1-IMGT: 6

CDR2-IMGT: 3

CDR3-IMGT: 3

Collier de Perles for human TRAV10*01

Accession number: IMGT AE000659   EMBL/GenBank/DDBJ: AE000659

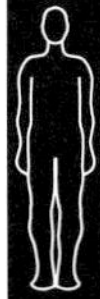

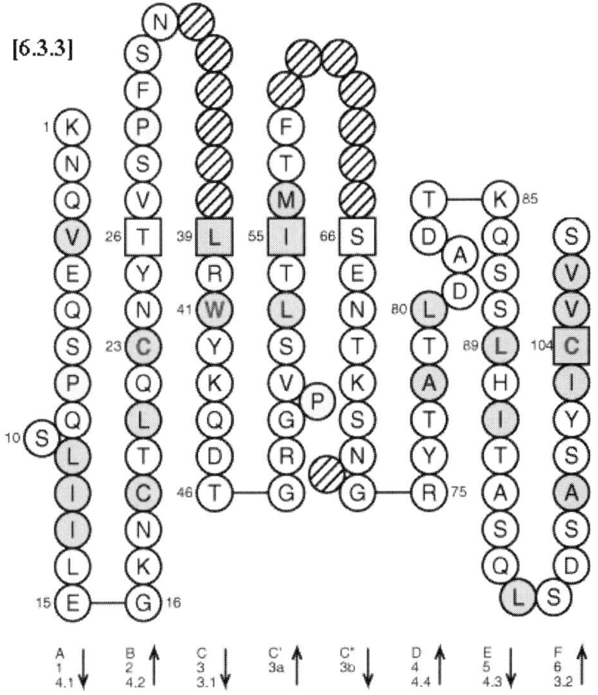

Genome database accession numbers
GDB:9953955   LocusLink: 28676

TRAV12-1

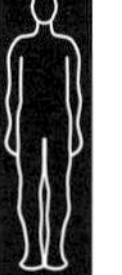

Nomenclature

TRAV12-1: T cell receptor alpha variable 12-1.

Definition and functionality

TRAV12-1 is one of the three functional genes of the TRAV12 subgroup which comprises three mapped genes.

Gene location

TRAV12-1 is in the TRA/TRD locus on chromosome 14 at 14q11.2.

Nucleotide and amino acid sequences for human TRAV12-1

```
                               1   2   3   4   5   6   7   8   9  10  11  12  13  14  15  16  17  18  19  20
                               R   K   E   V   E   Q   D   P   G   P   F   N   V   P   E   G   A   T   V   A
AE000659,TRAV12-1*01    [6]   CGG AAG GAG GTG GAG CAG GAT CCT GGA CCC TTC AAT GTT CCA GAG GGA GCC ACT GTC GCT
D13078  ,TRAV12-1*01   [23]   --- --- --- --- --- --- --- --- --- --- --- --- --- --- --- --- --- --- --- ---
M17657  ,TRAV12-1*02   [17]   --- --- --- --- --- --- --- --- --- --- --- --- --- --- --- --- --- --- --- ---

                                                                            __________________CDR1-IMGT________________
                              21  22  23  24  25  26  27  28  29  30  31  32  33  34  35  36  37  38  39  40
                               F   N   C   T   Y   S   N   S   A   S   Q   S                               F   F
AE000659,TRAV12-1*01          TTC AAC TGT ACT TAC AGC AAC AGT GCT TCT CAG TCT ... ... ... ... ... ... TTC TTC
D13078  ,TRAV12-1*01          --- --- --- --- --- --- --- --- --- --- --- --- ... ... ... ... ... ... --- ---
M17657  ,TRAV12-1*02          --- --- --- --- --- --- --- --- --- --- --- --- ... ... ... ... ... ... --- ---

                                                                                            _________________CDR2-
                              41  42  43  44  45  46  47  48  49  50  51  52  53  54  55  56  57  58  59  60
                               W   Y   R   Q   D   C   R   K   E   P   K   L   L   M   S   V   Y
AE000659,TRAV12-1*01          TGG TAC AGA CAG GAT TGC AGG AAA GAA CCT AAG TTG CTG ATG TCC GTA TAC ... ... ...
D13078  ,TRAV12-1*01          --- --- --- --- --- --- --- --- --- --- --- --- --- --- --- --- --- ... ... ...
M17657  ,TRAV12-1*02          --- --- --- --- --- --- --- --- --- --- --- --- --- --- --- --- --- ... ... ...

                              IMGT________________
                              61  62  63  64  65  66  67  68  69  70  71  72  73  74  75  76  77  78  79  80
                                               S   S   G   N       E   D       G   R   F   T   A   Q   L
AE000659,TRAV12-1*01          ... ... ... ... ... TCC AGT GGT AAT ... GAA GAT ... GGA AGG TTT ACA GCA CAG CTC
D13078  ,TRAV12-1*01          ... ... ... ... ... --- --- --- --- ... --- --- ... --- --- --- --- --- --- ---
                                                                                                        H   V
M17657  ,TRAV12-1*02          ... ... ... ... ... --- --- --- --- ... --- --- ... --- --- --- --- --- --C G--

                              81  82  83  84  85  86  87  88  89  90  91  92  93  94  95  96  97  98  99 100
                               N   R   A   S   Q   Y   I   S   L   L   I   R   D   S   K   L   S   D   S   A
AE000659,TRAV12-1*01          AAT AGA GCC AGC CAG TAT ATT TCC CTG CTC ATC AGA GAC TCC AAG CTC AGT GAT TCA GCC
D13078  ,TRAV12-1*01          --- --- --- --- --- --- --- --- --- --- --- --- --- --- --- --- --- --- --- ---
M17657  ,TRAV12-1*02          --- --- --- --- --- --- --- --- --- --- --- --- --- --- --- --- --- --- --- ---

                              _CDR3-IMGT_
                             101 102 103 104 105 106 107
                               T   Y   L   C   V   V   N
AE000659,TRAV12-1*01          ACC TAC CTC TGT GTG GTG AAC A
D13078  ,TRAV12-1*01          --- --- --- --- ---             #c
M17657  ,TRAV12-1*02          --- --- --- --- --- --- ---     #c

#c: Rearranged cDNA
```

Framework and complementarity determining regions

FR1-IMGT: 26	CDR1-IMGT: 6
FR2-IMGT: 17	CDR2-IMGT: 2
FR3-IMGT: 37 (-2 aa: 70,73)	CDR3-IMGT: 3

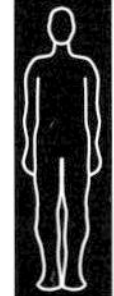

Collier de Perles for human TRAV12-1*01

Accession number: IMGT AE000659   EMBL/GenBank/DDBJ: AE000659

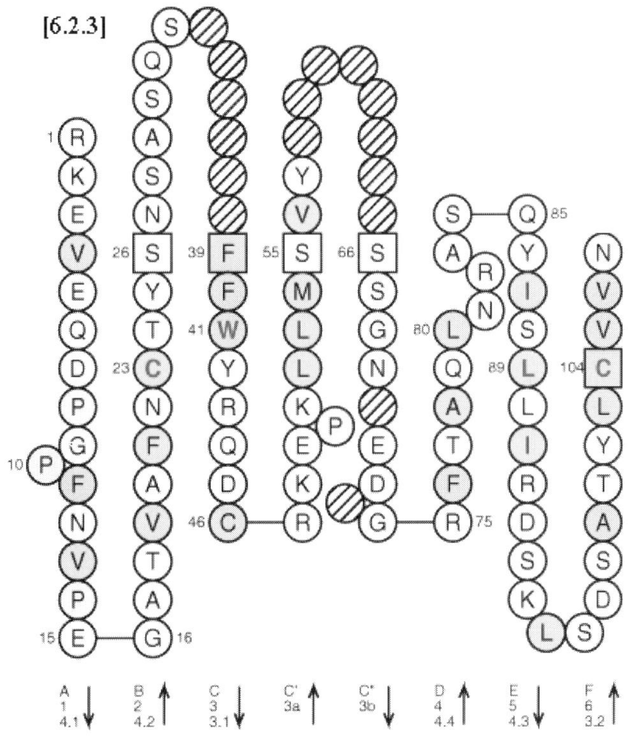

Genome database accession numbers
GDB:9953959   LocusLink: 28674

TRAV12-2

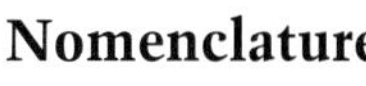

Nomenclature

TRAV12-2: T cell receptor alpha variable 12-2.

Definition and functionality

TRAV12-2 is one of the three functional genes of the TRAV12 subgroup which comprises three mapped genes.

Gene location

TRAV12-2 is in the TRA/TRD locus on chromosome 14 at 14q11.2.

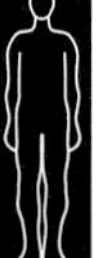

Nucleotide and amino acid sequences for human TRAV12-2

```
                          1   2   3   4   5   6   7   8   9  10  11  12  13  14  15  16  17  18  19  20
                          Q   K   E   V   E   Q   N   S   G   P   L   S   V   P   E   G   A   I   A   S
AE000659,TRAV12-2*01  [6] CAG AAG GAG GTG GAG CAG AAT TCT GGA CCC CTC AGT GTT CCA GAG GGA GCC ATT GCC TCT

M27369  ,TRAV12-2*01 [16]                         --- --- --- --- --- --- --- --- --- --- --- ---

M81774  ,TRAV12-2*02 [31] --- --- --- --- --- --- --- --- --- --- --- --- --- --- --- --- --- --- --- ---

L11159  ,TRAV12-2*02  [7] --- --- --- --- --- --- --- --- --- --- --- --- --- --- --- --- --- --- --- ---

X04946  ,TRAV12-2*03 [38] --- --- --- --- --- --- --- --- --- --- --- --- --- --- --- --- --- --- --- ---


                                                              ________________CDR1-IMGT________________
                         21  22  23  24  25  26  27  28  29  30  31  32  33  34  35  36  37  38  39  40
                          L   N   C   T   Y   S   D   R   G   S   Q   S                           F   F
AE000659,TRAV12-2*01      CTC AAC TGC ACT TAC AGT GAC CGA GGT TCC CAG TCC ... ... ... ... ... ... TTC TTC

M27369  ,TRAV12-2*01      --- --- --- --- --- --- --- --- --- --- --- --- ... ... ... ... ... ... --- ---

M81774  ,TRAV12-2*02      --- --- --- --- --- --- --- --- --- --- --- --- ... ... ... ... ... ... --- ---

L11159  ,TRAV12-2*02      --- --- --- --- --- --- --- --- --- --- --- --- ... ... ... ... ... ... --- ---
                                                              V
X04946  ,TRAV12-2*03      --- --- --- --- --- --- --- --- -T- --- --- --- ... ... ... ... ... ... --- ---


                                                                                  ____________________CDR2-
                         41  42  43  44  45  46  47  48  49  50  51  52  53  54  55  56  57  58  59  60
                          W   Y   R   Q   Y   S   G   K   S   P   E   L   I   M   F   I   Y
AE000659,TRAV12-2*01      TGG TAC AGA CAA TAT TCT GGG AAA AGC CCT GAG TTG ATA ATG TTC ATA TAC ... ... ...

M27369  ,TRAV12-2*01      --- --- --- --- --- --- --- --- --- --- --- --- --- --- --- --- --- ... ... ...
                                                                                      S
M81774  ,TRAV12-2*02      --- --- --- --- --- --- --- --- --- --- --- --- --- --- -C- --- --- ... ... ...
                                                                                      S
L11159  ,TRAV12-2*02      --- --- --- --- --- --- --- --- --- --- --- --- --- --- -C- --- --- ... ... ...

X04946  ,TRAV12-2*03      --- --- --- --- --- --- --- --- --- --- --- --- --- --- --- --- --- ... ... ...


                         IMGT________________
                         61  62  63  64  65  66  67  68  69  70  71  72  73  74  75  76  77  78  79  80
                                                  S   N   G   D   K   E   D       G   R   F   T   A   Q   L
AE000659,TRAV12-2*01      ... ... ... ... ... TCC AAT GGT GAC AAA GAA GAT ... GGA AGG TTT ACA GCA CAG CTC

M27369  ,TRAV12-2*01      ... ... ... ... ... --- --- --- --- --- --- --- ... --- --- --- --- --- --- ---

M81774  ,TRAV12-2*02      ... ... ... ... ... --- --- --- --- --- --- --- ... --- --- --- --- --- --- ---

L11159  ,TRAV12-2*02      ... ... ... ... ... --- --- --- --- --- --- --- ... --- --- --- --- --- --- ---

X04946  ,TRAV12-2*03      ... ... ... ... ... --- --- --- --- --- --- --- ... --- --- --- --- --- --- ---


                         81  82  83  84  85  86  87  88  89  90  91  92  93  94  95  96  97  98  99 100
                          N   K   A   S   Q   Y   V   S   L   L   I   R   D   S   Q   P   S   D   S   A
AE000659,TRAV12-2*01      AAT AAA GCC AGC CAG TAT GTT TCT CTG CTC ATC AGA GAC TCC CAG CCC AGT GAT TCA GCC

M27369  ,TRAV12-2*01      --- --- --- --- --- --- --- --- --- --- --- --- --- --- --- --- --- --- --- ---

M81774  ,TRAV12-2*02      --- --- --- --- --- --- --- --- --- --- --- --- --- --- --- --- --- --- --- ---

L11159  ,TRAV12-2*02      --- --- --- --- --- --- --- --- --- -

X04946  ,TRAV12-2*03      --- --- --- --- --- --- --- --- --- --- --- --- --- --- --- --- --- --- --- ---


                                     _CDR3-IMGT_
                        101 102 103 104 105 106 107
                          T   Y   L   C   A   V   N
AE000659,TRAV12-2*01      ACC TAC CTC TGT GCC GTG AAC A

M27369  ,TRAV12-2*01      --- --- --- --- --- --         #c

M81774  ,TRAV12-2*02      --- --- --- --- ---            #c

L11159  ,TRAV12-2*02                                     °

X04946  ,TRAV12-2*03      --- --- --- --- --- --- ---    #c
```

#c: Rearranged cDNA
°: Genomic DNA, but not known as being germline or rearranged

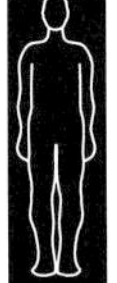

Framework and complementarity determining regions

FR1-IMGT: 26
FR2-IMGT: 17
FR3-IMGT: 38 (-1 aa: 73)

CDR1-IMGT: 6
CDR2-IMGT: 2
CDR3-IMGT: 3

Collier de Perles for human TRAV12-2*01

Accession number: IMGT AE000659   EMBL/GenBank/DDBJ: AE000659

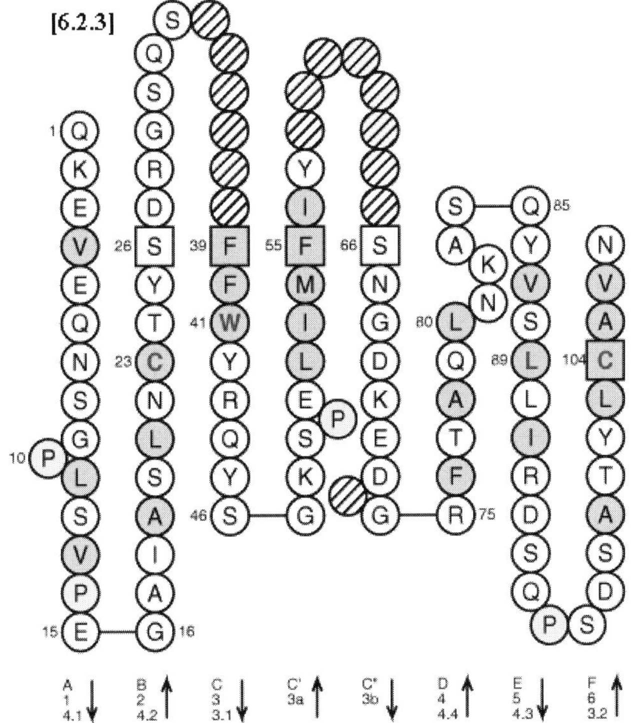

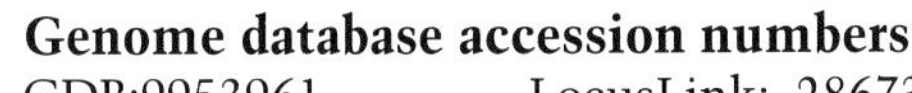

Genome database accession numbers
GDB:9953961   LocusLink: 28673

TRAV12-3

Nomenclature

TRAV12-3: T cell receptor alpha variable 12-3.

Definition and functionality

TRAV12-3 is one of the three functional genes of the TRAV12 subgroup which comprises three mapped genes.

Gene location

TRAV12-3 is in the TRA/TRD locus on chromosome 14 at 14q11.2.

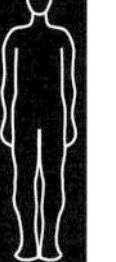

Nucleotide and amino acid sequences for human TRAV12-3

```
                         1   2   3   4   5   6   7   8   9  10  11  12  13  14  15  16  17  18  19  20
                         Q   K   E   V   E   Q   D   P   G   P   L   S   V   P   E   G   A   I   V   S
X06193   ,TRAV12-3*01 [21] CAG AAG GAG GTG GAG CAG GAT CCT GGA CCA CTC AGT GTT CCA GAG GGA GCC ATT GTT TCT
AE000659,TRAV12-3*01  [6] --- --- --- --- --- --- --- --- --- --- --- --- --- --- --- --- --- --- --- ---
U32538   ,TRAV12-3*01 [5] --- --- --- --- --- --- --- --- --- --- --- --- --- --- --- --- --- --- --- ---
M17656   ,TRAV12-3*02 [17] --- --- --- --- --- --- --- --- --- --- --- --- --- --- --- --- --- --- --- ---

                                                        ________________CDR1-IMGT__________________
                        21  22  23  24  25  26  27  28  29  30  31  32  33  34  35  36  37  38  39  40
                         L   N   C   T   Y   S   N   S   A   F   Q   Y                           F   M
X06193   ,TRAV12-3*01   CTC AAC TGC ACT TAC AGC AAC AGT GCT TTT CAA TAC ... ... ... ... ... ... TTC ATG
AE000659,TRAV12-3*01    --- --- --- --- --- --- --- --- --- --- --- --- ... ... ... ... ... ... --- ---
U32538   ,TRAV12-3*01   --- --- --- --- --- --- --- --- --- --- --- --- ... ... ... ... ... ... --- ---
M17656   ,TRAV12-3*02   --- --- --- --- --- --- --- --- --- --- --- --- ... ... ... ... ... ... --- ---

                                                                        ________________CDR2-
                        41  42  43  44  45  46  47  48  49  50  51  52  53  54  55  56  57  58  59  60
                         W   Y   R   Q   Y   S   R   K   G   P   E   L   L   M   Y   T   Y
X06193   ,TRAV12-3*01   TGG TAC AGA CAG TAT TCC AGA AAA GGC CCT GAG TTG CTG ATG TAC ACA TAC ... ... ...
AE000659,TRAV12-3*01    --- --- --- --- --- --- --- --- --- --- --- --- --- --- --- --- --- --- ... ... ...
U32538   ,TRAV12-3*01   --- --- --- --- --- --- --- --- --- --- --- --- --- --- --- --- --- --- ... ... ...
M17656   ,TRAV12-3*02   --- --- --- --- --- --- --- I-- --- --- --- --- --- --- --- --- --- --- ... ... ...
                                                    -T-

IMGT________________
                        61  62  63  64  65  66  67  68  69  70  71  72  73  74  75  76  77  78  79  80
                                                 S   S   G   N   K   E   D       G   R   F   T   A   Q   V
X06193   ,TRAV12-3*01   ... ... ... ... ... TCC AGT GGT AAC AAA GAA GAT ... GGA AGG TTT ACA GCA CAG GTC
AE000659,TRAV12-3*01    ... ... ... ... ... --- --- --- --- --- --- --- ... --- --- --- --- --- --- ---
U32538   ,TRAV12-3*01   ... ... ... ... ... --- --- --- --- --- --- --- ... --- --- --- --- --- --- ---
M17656   ,TRAV12-3*02   ... ... ... ... ... --- --- --- --- --- --- --- ... --- --- --- --- --- --- ---

                        81  82  83  84  85  86  87  88  89  90  91  92  93  94  95  96  97  98  99 100
                         D   K   S   S   K   Y   I   S   L   F   I   R   D   S   Q   P   S   D   S   A
X06193   ,TRAV12-3*01   GAT AAA TCC AGC AAG TAT ATC TCC TTG TTC ATC AGA GAC TCA CAG CCC AGT GAT TCA GCC
AE000659,TRAV12-3*01    --- --- --- --- --- --- --- --- --- --- --- --- --- --- --- --- --- --- --- ---
U32538   ,TRAV12-3*01   --
M17656   ,TRAV12-3*02   --- --- --- --- --- --- --- --- --- --- --- --- --- --- --- --- --- --- --- ---

                                ___CDR3-IMGT___
                       101 102 103 104 105 106 107 108
                         T   Y   L   C   A   M   S
X06193   ,TRAV12-3*01   ACC TAC CTC TGT GCA ATG AGC G
AE000659,TRAV12-3*01    --- --- --- --- --- --- --- -
U32538   ,TRAV12-3*01                                °
M17656   ,TRAV12-3*02   --- --- --- --- --- --- ---   #c
```

#c: Rearranged cDNA
°: Genomic DNA, but not known as being rearranged or germline

Framework and complementarity determining regions

FR1-IMGT: 26
FR2-IMGT: 17
FR3-IMGT: 38 (-1 aa: 73)

CDR1-IMGT: 6
CDR2-IMGT: 2
CDR3-IMGT: 3

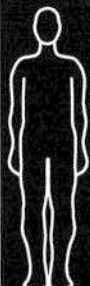

Collier de Perles for human TRAV12-3*01

Accession number: IMGT X06193   EMBL/GenBank/DDBJ: X06193

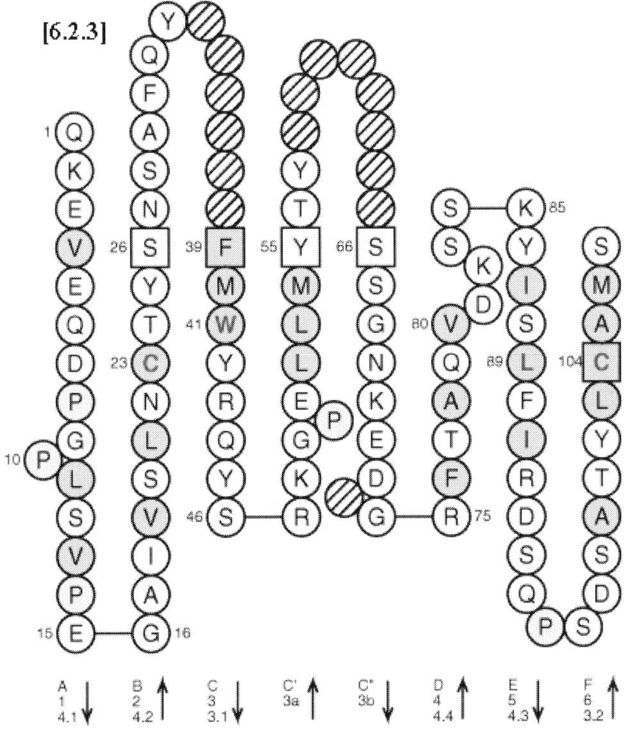

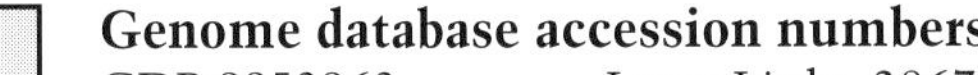

Genome database accession numbers
GDB:9953963   LocusLink: 28672

Nomenclature

TRAV13-1: T cell receptor alpha variable 13-1.

Definition and functionality

TRAV13-1 is one of the two functional genes of the TRAV13 subgroup which comprises two mapped genes.

Gene location

TRAV13-1 is in the TRA/TRD locus on chromosome 14 at 14q11.2.

Nucleotide and amino acid sequences for human TRAV13-1

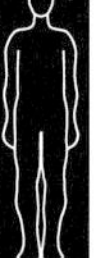

```
                         1   2   3   4   5   6   7   8   9  10  11  12  13  14  15  16  17  18  19  20
                         G   E   N   V   E   Q   H   P   S   T   L   S   V   Q   E   G   D   S   A   V
AE000659,TRAV13-1*01 [6] GGA GAG AAT GTG GAG CAG CAT CCT TCA ACC CTG AGT GTC CAG GAG GGA GAC AGC GCT GTT
D13079  ,TRAV13-1*01 [23] --- --- --- --- --- --- --- --- --- --- --- --- --- --- --- --- --- --- --- ---
M99570  ,TRAV13-1*01 [8]      --- --- --- --- --- --- --- --- --- --- --- --- --- --- --- --- --- --- ---
X04954  ,TRAV13-1*02 [38] --- --- --- --- --- --- --- --- --- --- --- --- --- --- --- --- --- --- --- ---
L11162  ,TRAV13-1*03 [7]  --- --- --- --- --- --- --- --- --- --- --- --- --- --- --- --- --- --- --- ---

                                                                   ________CDR1-IMGT________
                        21  22  23  24  25  26  27  28  29  30  31  32  33  34  35  36  37  38  39  40
                         I   K   C   T   Y   S   D   S   A   S   N   Y                           F   P
AE000659,TRAV13-1*01    ATC AAG TGT ACT TAT TCA GAC AGT GCC TCA AAC TAC ... ... ... ... ... ... TTC CCT
D13079  ,TRAV13-1*01    --- --- --- --- --- --- --- --- --- --- --- --- ... ... ... ... ... ... --- ---
M99570  ,TRAV13-1*01    --- --- --- --- --- --- --- --- --- --- --- --- ... ... ... ... ... ... --- ---
X04954  ,TRAV13-1*02    --- --- --- --- --- --- --- --- --- --- --- --- ... ... ... ... ... ... --- ---
L11162  ,TRAV13-1*03    --- --- --- --- --- --- --- --- --- --- --- --- ... ... ... ... ... ... --- ---

                                                                                       ________CDR2-
                        41  42  43  44  45  46  47  48  49  50  51  52  53  54  55  56  57  58  59  60
                         W   Y   K   Q   E   L   G   K   G   P   Q   L   I   I   D   I   R   S
AE000659,TRAV13-1*01    TGG TAT AAG CAA GAA CTT GGA AAA GGA CCT CAG CTT ATT ATA GAC ATT CGT TCA ... ...
D13079  ,TRAV13-1*01    --- --- --- --- --- --- --- --- --- --- --- --- --- --- --- --- --- --- ... ...
M99570  ,TRAV13-1*01    --- --- --- --- --- --- --- --- --- --- --- --- --- --- --- --- --- --- ... ...
                                                             R
X04954  ,TRAV13-1*02    --- --- --- --- --- --- --- --- A-- --- --- --- --- --- --- --- --- --- ... ...
L11162  ,TRAV13-1*03    --- --- --- --- --- --- --- --- --- --- --- --- --- --- --- --- --- --- ... ...

                        IMGT________
                        61  62  63  64  65  66  67  68  69  70  71  72  73  74  75  76  77  78  79  80
                                             N   V   G   E   K   K   D       Q   R   I   A   V   T   L
AE000659,TRA13-11*01    ... ... ... ... ... AAT GTG GGC GAA AAG AAA GAC ... CAA CGA ATT GCT GTT ACA TTG
D13079  ,TRAV13-1*01    ... ... ... ... ... --- --- --- --- --- --- --- ... --- --- --- --- --- --- ---
M99570  ,TRAV13-1*01    ... ... ... ... ... --- --- --- --- --- --- --- ... --- --- --- --- --- --- ---
X04954  ,TRAV13-1*02    ... ... ... ... ... --- --- --- --- --- --- --- ... --- --- --- --- --- --- ---
L11162  ,TRAV13-1*03    ... ... ... ... ... --- --- --- --- --- --- --- ... --- --- --- --- --- --- ---

                        81  82  83  84  85  86  87  88  89  90  91  92  93  94  95  96  97  98  99 100
                         N   K   T   A   K   H   F   S   L   H   I   T   E   T   Q   P   E   D   S   A
AE000659,TRAV13-1*01    AAC AAG ACA GCC AAA CAT TTC TCC CTG CAC ATC ACA GAG ACC CAA CCT GAA GAC TCG GCT
D13079  ,TRAV13-1*01    --- --- --- --- --- --- --- --- --- --- --- --- --- --- --- --- --- --- --- ---
M99570  ,TRAV13-1*01    --- --- --- --- --- --- --- --- --- --- --- --- --- --- --- --- --- --- --- ---
X04954  ,TRAV13-1*02    --- --- --- --- --- --- --- --- --- --- --- --- --- --- --- --- --- --- --- ---
                                                                          Q
L11162  ,TRAV13-1*03    --- --- --- --- --- --- --- --- --- --G --- ---

                                     _CDR3-IMGT_
                        101 102 103 104 105 106 107
                         V   Y   F   C   A   A   S
AE000659,TRAV13-1*01    GTC TAC TTC TGT GCA GCA AGT A
D13079  ,TRAV13-1*01    --- --- --- --- ---              #c
M99570  ,TRAV13-1*01    --- --- --- --- ---
X04954  ,TRAV13-1*02    --- --- --- --- --- --- ---      #c
L11162  ,TRAV13-1*03                                     °
```

#c: Rearranged cDNA
°: Genomic DNA, but not known as being germline or rearranged

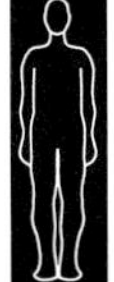

Framework and complementarity determining regions

FR1-IMGT: 26
FR2-IMGT: 17
FR3-IMGT: 38 (-1 aa: 73)

CDR1-IMGT: 6
CDR2-IMGT: 3
CDR3-IMGT: 3

Collier de Perles for human TRAV13-1*01

Accession number: IMGT AE000659   EMBL/GenBank/DDBJ: AE000659

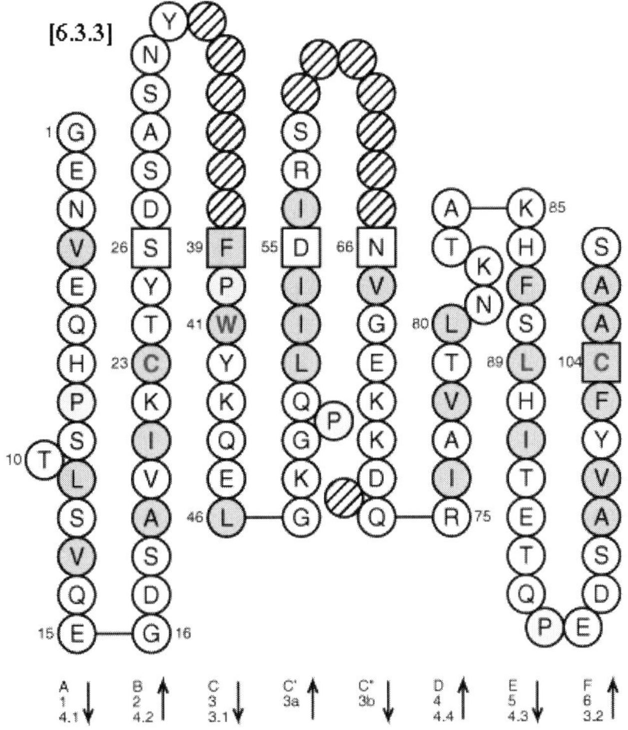

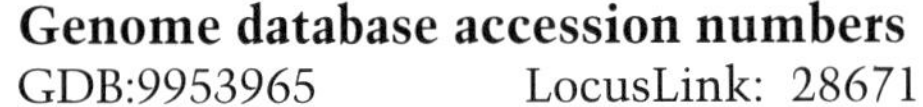

Genome database accession numbers

GDB:9953965   LocusLink: 28671

TRAV13-2

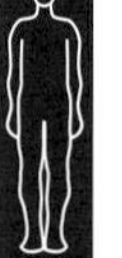

Nomenclature

TRAV13-2: T cell receptor alpha variable 13-2.

Definition and functionality

TRAV13-2 is one of the two functional genes of the TRAV13 subgroup which comprises two mapped genes.

Gene location

TRAV13-2 is in the TRA/TRD locus on chromosome 14 at 14q11.2.

Nucleotide and amino acid sequences for human TRAV13-2

```
                        1   2   3   4   5   6   7   8   9  10  11  12  13  14  15  16  17  18  19  20
                        G   E   S   V   G   L   H   L   P   T   L   S   V   Q   E   G   D   N   S   I
AE000659,TRAV13-2*01 [6]  GGA GAG AGT GTG GGG CTG CAT CTT CCT ACC CTG AGT GTC CAG GAG GGT GAC AAC TCT ATT

X04956  ,TRAV13-2*01 [38] --- --- --- --- --- --- --- --- --- --- --- --- --- --- --- --- --- --- --- ---

U32545  ,TRAV13-2*01 [5]  --- --- --- --- --- --- --- --- --- --- --- --- --- --- --- --- --- --- --- ---

M17658  ,TRAV13-2*02 [17] --- --- --- --- --- --- --- --- --- --- --- --- --- --- --- --- --- --- --- ---


                                                                  ___________CDR1-IMGT____________
                       21  22  23  24  25  26  27  28  29  30  31  32  33  34  35  36  37  38  39  40
                        I   N   C   A   Y   S   N   S   A   S   D   Y                           F   I
AE000659,TRAV13-2*01    ATC AAC TGT GCT TAT TCA AAC AGC GCC TCA GAC TAC ... ... ... ... ... ... TTC ATT

X04956  ,TRAV13-2*01    --- --- --- --- --- --- --- --- --- --- --- --- ... ... ... ... ... ... --- ---

U32545  ,TRAV13-2*01    --- --- --- --- --- --- --- --- --- --- --- --- ... ... ... ... ... ... --- ---

M17658  ,TRAV13-2*02    --- --- --- --- --- --- --- --- --- --- --- --- ... ... ... ... ... ... --- ---


                                                                                      _________CDR2-
                       41  42  43  44  45  46  47  48  49  50  51  52  53  54  55  56  57  58  59  60
                        W   Y   K   Q   E   S   G   K   G   P   Q   F   I   I   D   I   R   S
AE000659,TRAV13-2*01    TGG TAC AAG CAA GAA TCT GGA AAA GGT CCT CAA TTC ATT ATA GAC ATT CGT TCA ... ...

X04956  ,TRAV13-2*01    --- --- --- --- --- --- --- --- --- --- --- --- --- --- --- --- --- --- ... ...

U32545  ,TRAV13-2*01    --- --- --- --- --- --- --- --- --- --- --- --- --- --- --- --- --- --- ... ...

M17658  ,TRAV13-2*02    --- --- --A --- --- --- --- --- --- --- --- --- --- --- --- --- --- --- ... ...


                       IMGT__________________
                       61  62  63  64  65  66  67  68  69  70  71  72  73  74  75  76  77  78  79  80
                                            N   M   D   K   R   Q   G       Q   R   V   T   V   L   L
AE000659,TRAV13-2*01   ... ... ... ... ... AAT ATG GAC AAA AGG CAA GGC ... CAA AGA GTC ACC GTT TTA TTG

X04956  ,TRAV13-2*01   ... ... ... ... ... --- --- --- --- --- --- --- ... --- --- --- --- --- --- ---

U32545  ,TRAV13-2*01   ... ... ... ... ... --- --- --- --- --- --- --- ... --- --- --- --- --- --- ---

M17658  ,TRAV13-2*02   ... ... ... ... ... --- --- --- --- --- --- --- ... --- --- --- --- --- --- ---


                       81  82  83  84  85  86  87  88  89  90  91  92  93  94  95  96  97  98  99 100
                        N   K   T   V   K   H   L   S   L   Q   I   A   A   T   Q   P   G   D   S   A
AE000659,TRAV13-2*01   AAT AAG ACA GTG AAA CAT CTC TCT CTG CAA ATT GCA GCT ACT CAA CCT GGA GAC TCA GCT

X04956  ,TRAV13-2*01   --- --- --- --- --- --- --- --- --- --- --- --- --- --- --- --- --- --- --- ---

U32545  ,TRAV13-2*01   --- --- --- --- --- --- --- --- -

M17658  ,TRAV13-2*02   --- --- --- --- --- --- --- --- --- --- --- --- --- --- --- --- --- --- --- ---


                          _CDR3-IMGT_
                      101 102 103 104 105 106 107
                        V   Y   F   C   A   E   N
AE000659,TRAV13-2*01   GTC TAC TTT TGT GCA GAG AAT A

X04956  ,TRAV13-2*01   --- --- --- --- --- ---              #c

U32545  ,TRAV13-2*01                                         o

M17658  ,TRAV13-2*02   --- --- --- --- --- ---              #c
```

#c: Rearranged cDNA
o: Genomic DNA, but not known as being germline or rearranged

Framework and complementarity determining regions

FR1-IMGT: 26   CDR1-IMGT: 6
FR2-IMGT: 17   CDR2-IMGT: 3
FR3-IMGT: 38 (-1 aa: 73)   CDR3-IMGT: 3

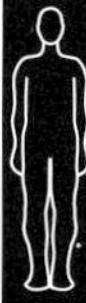

Collier de Perles for human TRAV13-2*01

Accession number: IMGT AE000659   EMBL/GenBank/DDBJ: AE000659

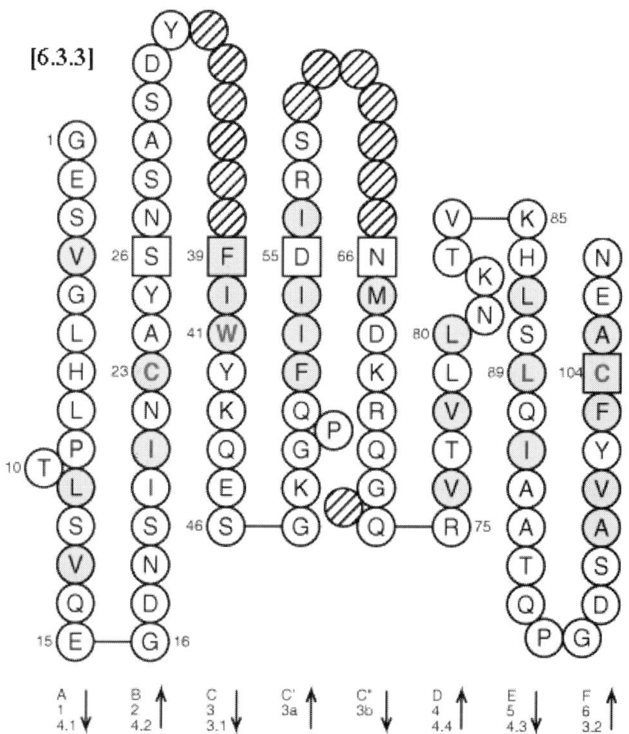

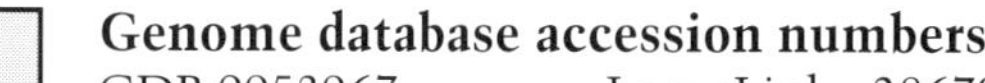

Genome database accession numbers
GDB:9953967   LocusLink: 28670

TRAV14/DV4

Nomenclature

TRAV14/DV4: T cell receptor alpha variable 14/delta variable 4.

Definition and functionality

TRAV14/DV4 is the unique functional gene of the TRAV14 subgroup which only comprises this mapped gene.

TRAV14/DV4 has been found rearranged to both (D)J genes of the TRD locus and TRAJ genes, the TRD locus being embedded in the TRA locus. This gene can therefore be used for the synthesis of both delta and alpha chains.

Gene location

TRAV14/DV4 is in the TRA/TRD locus on chromosome 14 at 14q11.2.

Nucleotide and amino acid sequences for human TRAV14/DV4

```
                        1   2   3   4   5   6   7   8   9   10  11  12  13  14  15  16  17  18  19  20
                        A   Q   K   I   T   Q   T   Q   P   G   M   F   V   Q   E   K   E   A   V   T
  M21626   ,TRAV14*01  [10] GCC CAG AAG ATA ACT CAA ACC CAA CCA GGA ATG TTC GTG CAG GAA AAG GAG GCT GTG ACT
  AE000659 ,TRAV14*02  [6]  --- --- --- --- --- --- --- --- --- --- --- --- --- --- --- --- --- --- --- ---
  S51029   ,TRAV14*02  [36] --- --- --- --- --- --- --- --- --- --- --- --- --- --- --- --- --- --- --- ---
  M21624   ,TRAV14*03  [10] --- --- --- --- --- --- --- --- --- --- --- --- --- --- --- --- --- --- --- ---
  L09758   ,TRAV14*04  [27]     --- --- --- --- --- --- --- --- --- --- --- --- --- --- --- --- --- --- ---

                                                                    ____________CDR1-IMGT________________
                        21  22  23  24  25  26  27  28  29  30  31  32  33  34  35  36  37  38  39  40
                        L   D   C   T   Y   D   T   S   D   P   S   Y   G                   L   F
  M21626   ,TRAV14*01  CTG GAC TGC ACA TAT GAC ACC AGT GAT CCA AGT TAT GGT ... ... ... ... ... CTA TTC
                                                          Q
  AE000659 ,TRAV14*02  --- --- --- --- --- --- --- --- --- -A- --- --- --- ... ... ... ... ... --- ---
                                                          Q
  S51029   ,TRAV14*02  --- --- --- --- --- --- --- --- --- -A- --- --- --- ... ... ... ... ... --- ---
  M21624   ,TRAV14*03  --- --- --- --- --- --- --- --- --- --- --- --- --- ... ... ... ... ... --- ---
                                                          Q
  L09758   ,TRAV14*04  --- --- --- --- --- --- --- --- --- -A- --- --- --- ... ... ... ... ... --C ---

                                                                                ________________CDR2-
                        41  42  43  44  45  46  47  48  49  50  51  52  53  54  55  56  57  58  59  60
                        W   Y   K   Q   P   S   S   G   E   M   I   F   L   I   Y   Q   G   S   Y
  M21626   ,TRAV14*01  TGG TAC AAG CAG CCC AGC AGT GGG GAA ATG ATT TTT CTT ATT TAT CAG GGG TCT TAT ...
  AE000659 ,TRAV14*02  --- --- --- --- --- --- --- --- --- --- --- --- --- --- --- --- --- --- --- ...
  S51029   ,TRAV14*02  --- --- --- --- --- --- --- --- --- --- --- --- --- --- --- --- --- --- --- ...
  M21624   ,TRAV14*03  --- --- --- --- --- --- --- --- --- --- --- --- --- --- --- --- --- --- --- ...
  L09758   ,TRAV14*04  --- --- --- --- --- --- --- --- --- --- --- --- --- --- --- --- --- --- --- ...

                        IMGT________________
                        61  62  63  64  65  66  67  68  69  70  71  72  73  74  75  76  77  78  79  80
                                                D   Q   Q   N   A   T   E       G   R   Y   S   L   N   F
  M21626   ,TRAV14*01  ... ... ... ... ... GAC CAG CAA AAT GCA ACA GAA ... GGT CGC TAC TCA TTG AAT TTC
                                                E
  AE000659 ,TRAV14*02  ... ... ... ... ... --- G-- --- --- --- --- --- ... --- --- --- --- --- --- ---
                                                E
  S51029   ,TRAV14*02  ... ... ... ... ... --- G-- --- --- --- --- --- ... --- --- --- --- --- --- ---
  M21624   ,TRAV14*03  ... ... ... ... ... --- --- --- --- --- --- --- ... --- --- --- --- --- --- ---
                                                E
  L09758   ,TRAV14*04  ... ... ... ... ... --- G-- --- --- --- --- --- ... --- --- --- --- --- --- ---

                        81  82  83  84  85  86  87  88  89  90  91  92  93  94  95  96  97  98  99  100
                        Q   K   A   R   K   S   A   N   L   V   I   S   A   S   Q   L   G   D   S   A
  M21626   ,TRAV14*01  CAG AAG GCA AGA AAA TCC GCC AAC CTT GTC ATC TCC GCT TCA CAA CTG GGG GAC TCA GCA
  AE000659 ,TRAV14*02  --- --- --- --- --- --- --- --- --- --- --- --- --- --- --- --- --- --- --- ---
  S51029   ,TRAV14*02  --- --- --- --- --- --- --- --- --- --- --- --- --- --- --- --- --- --- --- ---
  M21624   ,TRAV14*03  --- --- --- --- --- --- --- --- --- --- --- --- --- --- --- --- --- --- --- ---
  L09758   ,TRAV14*04  --- --- --- --- --- --- --- --- --- --- --- --- --- --- --- --- --- --- --- ---
```

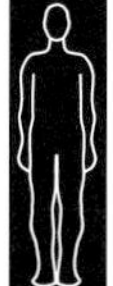

```
                                      ____CDR3-IMGT____
                         101 102 103 104 105 106 107 108 109
                          M   Y   F   C   A   M   R   E
   M21626   ,TRAV14*01   ATG TAC TTC TGT GCA ATG AGA GAG GG

   AE000659,TRAV14*02    --- --T --- --- --- --- --- --- --

   S51029   ,TRAV14*02   --- --T --- --- --- --- --- ---      #c

   M21624   ,TRAV14*03   --- --T --- --- --- --- --- ---      #c

   L09758   ,TRAV14*04   --- --- --- -                         °
```

#c:Rearranged cDNA
°: Genomic DNA, but not known as being germline or rearranged

Framework and complementarity determining regions

FR1-IMGT: 26   CDR1-IMGT: 7
FR2-IMGT: 17   CDR2-IMGT: 4
FR3-IMGT: 38 (-1 aa: 73)   CDR3-IMGT: 4

Collier de Perles for human TRAV14/DV4*01

Accession number: IMGT M21626   EMBL/GenBank/DDBJ: M21626

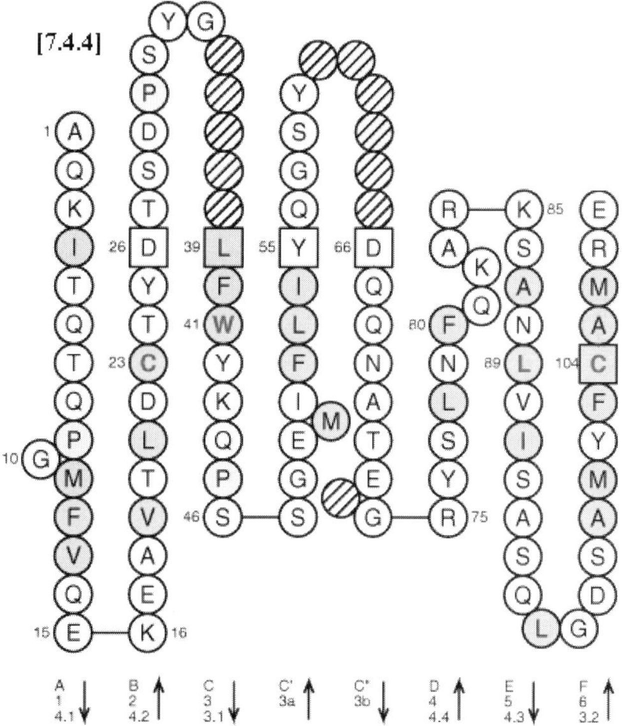

Genome database accession numbers
GDB:9953969   LocusLink: 28669

Nomenclature

TRAV16: T cell receptor alpha variable 16.

Definition and functionality

TRAV16 is the unique functional gene of the TRAV16 subgroup which only comprises this mapped gene.

Gene location

TRAV16 is in the TRA/TRD locus on chromosome 14 at 14q11.2.

Nucleotide and amino acid sequences for human TRAV16

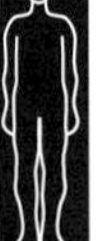

```
                      1    2    3    4    5    6    7    8    9   10   11   12   13   14   15   16   17   18   19   20
                      A    Q    R    V    T    Q    P    E    K    L    L    S    V    F    K    G    A    P    V    E
AE000659,TRAV16*01  [6] GCC  CAG  AGA  GTG  ACT  CAG  CCC  GAG  AAG  CTC  CTC  TCT  GTC  TTT  AAA  GGG  GCC  CCA  GTG  GAG
X04942  ,TRAV16*01 [38] ---  ---  ---  ---  ---  ---  ---  ---  ---  ---  ---  ---  ---  ---  ---  ---  ---  ---  ---  ---
U32546  ,TRAV16*01  [5] ---  ---  ---  ---  ---  ---  ---  ---  ---  ---  ---  ---  ---  ---  ---  ---  ---  ---  ---  ---

                                                           ____________________CDR1-IMGT____________________
                     21   22   23   24   25   26   27   28   29   30   31   32   33   34   35   36   37   38   39   40
                      L    K    C    N    Y    S    Y    S    G    S    P    E                             L    F
AE000659,TRAV16*01  CTG  AAG  TGC  AAC  TAT  TCC  TAT  TCT  GGG  AGT  CCT  GAA  ...  ...  ...  ...  ...  ...  CTC  TTC
X04942  ,TRAV16*01  ---  ---  ---  ---  ---  ---  ---  ---  ---  ---  ---  ---            ...  ...  ...  ---  ---
U32546  ,TRAV16*01  ---  ---  ---  ---  ---  ---  ---  ---  ---  ---  ---  ---            ...  ...  ...  ---  ---

                                                                                             __________________CDR2-
                     41   42   43   44   45   46   47   48   49   50   51   52   53   54   55   56   57   58   59   60
                      W    Y    V    Q    Y    S    R    Q    R    L    Q    L    L    L    R
AE000659,TRAV16*01  TGG  TAT  GTC  CAG  TAC  TCC  AGA  CAA  CGC  CTC  CAG  TTA  CTC  TTG  AGA  ...  ...  ...  ...  ...
X04942  ,TRAV16*01  ---  ---  ---  ---  ---  ---  ---  ---  ---  ---  ---  ---  ---  ---  ---  ...  ...  ...  ...  ...
U32546  ,TRAV16*01  ---  ---  ---  ---  ---  ---  ---  ---  ---  ---  ---  ---  ---  ---  ---  ...  ...  ...  ...  ...

                    IMGT_________________
                     61   62   63   64   65   66   67   68   69   70   71   72   73   74   75   76   77   78   79   80
                                          H    I    S    R    E    S    I         K    G    F    T    A    D    L
AE000659,TRAV16*01  ...  ...  ...  ...  ...  CAC  ATC  TCT  AGA  GAG  AGC  ATC  ...  AAA  GGC  TTC  ACT  GCT  GAC  CTT
X04942  ,TRAV16*01  ...  ...  ...  ...  ...  ---  ---  ---  ---  ---  ---  ---  ...  ---  ---  ---  ---  ---  ---  ---
U32546  ,TRAV16*01  ...  ...  ...  ...  ...  ---  ---  ---  ---  ---  ---  ---  ...  ---  ---  ---  ---  ---  ---  ---

                     81   82   83   84   85   86   87   88   89   90   91   92   93   94   95   96   97   98   99  100
                      N    K    G    E    T    S    F    H    L    K    K    P    F    A    Q    E    E    D    S    A
AE000659,TRAV16*01  AAC  AAA  GGC  GAG  ACA  TCT  TTC  CAC  CTG  AAG  AAA  CCA  TTT  GCT  CAA  GAG  GAA  GAC  TCA  GCC
X04942  ,TRAV16*01  ---  ---  ---  ---  ---  ---  ---  ---  ---  ---  ---  ---  ---  ---  ---  ---  ---  ---  ---  ---
U32546  ,TRAV16*01  ---  ---  ---  ---  ---  ---  ---  ---  ---  ---  ---  ---  ---  ---  ---  ---  ---  ---  ---  --

                                   -CDR3-IMGT-
                    101  102  103  104  105  106  107
                      M    Y    Y    C    A    L    S
AE000659,TRAV16*01  ATG  TAT  TAC  TGT  GCT  CTA  AGT  GG
X04942  ,TRAV16*01  ---  ---  ---  ---  ---  ---  ---        #c
U32546  ,TRAV16*01                                          °

#c: Rearranged cDNA
°: Genomic DNA, but not known as being germline or rearranged
```

Framework and complementarity determining regions

FR1-IMGT: 26	CDR1-IMGT: 6
FR2-IMGT: 17	CDR2-IMGT: 0
FR3-IMGT: 38 (-1 aa: 73)	CDR3-IMGT: 3

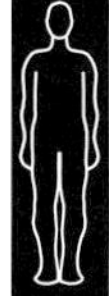

Collier de Perles for human TRAV16*01

Accession number: IMGT AE000659   EMBL/GenBank/DDBJ: AE000659

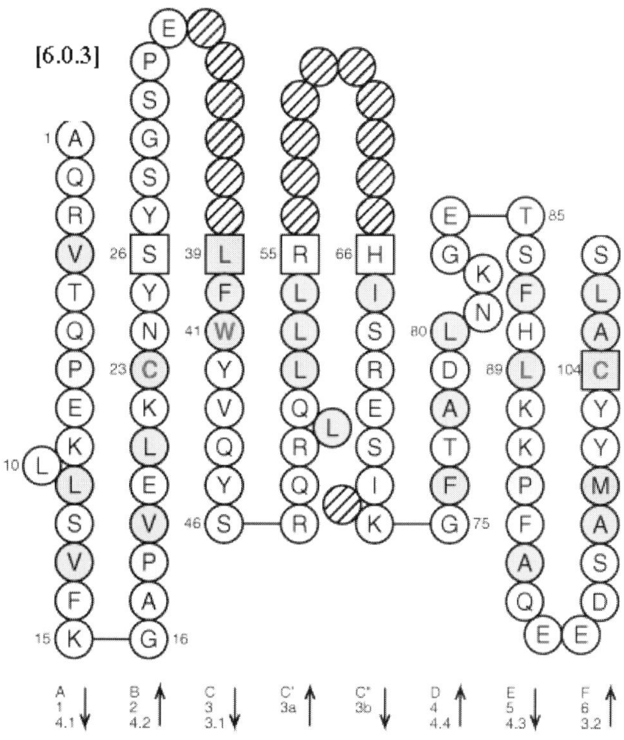

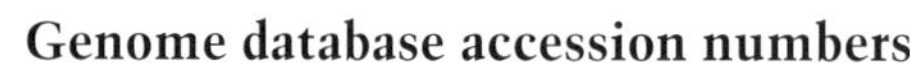

Genome database accession numbers
GDB:9953973   LocusLink: 28667

Nomenclature

TRAV17: T cell receptor alpha variable 17.

Definition and functionality

TRAV17 is the unique functional gene of the TRAV17 subgroup which only comprises this mapped gene.

Gene location

TRAV17 is in the TRA/TRD locus on chromosome 14 at 14q11.2.

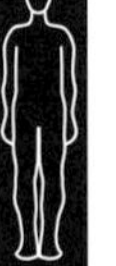

Nucleotide and amino acid sequences for human TRAV17

```
                       1   2   3   4   5   6   7   8   9  10  11  12  13  14  15  16  17  18  19  20
                       S   Q   Q   G   E   E   D   P   Q   A   L   S   I   Q   E   G   E   N   A   T
AE000660,TRAV17*01 [6] AGT CAA CAG GGA GAA GAG GAT CCT CAG GCC TTG AGC ATC CAG GAG GGT GAA AAT GCC ACC

X04955  ,TRAV17*01 [38] --- --- --- --- --- --- --- --- --- --- --- --- --- --- --- --- --- --- --- ---

U32540  ,TRAV17*01 [5]  --- --- --- --- --- --- --- --- --- --- --- --- --- --- --- --- --- --- --- ---


                                                          ____________________CDR1-IMGT____________________
                       21  22  23  24  25  26  27  28  29  30  31  32  33  34  35  36  37  38  39  40
                       M   N   C   S   Y   K   T   S   I   N   N                               L   Q
AE000660,TRAV17*01     ATG AAC TGC AGT TAC AAA ACT AGT ATA AAC AAT ... ... ... ... ... ... ... TTA CAG

X04955  ,TRAV17*01     --- --- --- --- --- --- --- --- --- --- --- ... ... ... ... ... ... ... --- ---

U32540  ,TRAV17*01     --- --- --- --- --- --- --- --- --- --- --- ... ... ... ... ... ... ... --- ---


                                                                              ________________________CDR2-
                       41  42  43  44  45  46  47  48  49  50  51  52  53  54  55  56  57  58  59  60
                       W   Y   R   Q   N   S   G   R   G   L   V   H   L   I   L   I   R   S
AE000660,TRAV17*01     TGG TAT AGA CAA AAT TCA GGT AGA GGC CTT GTC CAC CTA ATT TTA ATA CGT TCA ... ...

X04955  ,TRAV17*01     --- --- --- --- --- --- --- --- --- --- --- --- --- --- --- --- --- --- ... ...

U32540  ,TRAV17*01     --- --- --- --- --- --- --- --- --- --- --- --- --- --- --- --- --- --- ... ...


                       IMGT________________
                       61  62  63  64  65  66  67  68  69  70  71  72  73  74  75  76  77  78  79  80
                                               N   E   R   E   K   H   S       G   R   L   R   V   T   L
AE000660,TRAV17*01     ... ... ... ... ... AAT GAA AGA GAG AAA CAC AGT ... GGA AGA TTA AGA GTC ACG CTT

X04955  ,TRAV17*01     ... ... ... ... ... --- --- --- --- --- --- --- ... --- --- --- --- --- --- ---

U32540  ,TRAV17*01     ... ... ... ... ... --- --- --- --- --- --- --- ... --- --- --- ---


                       81  82  83  84  85  86  87  88  89  90  91  92  93  94  95  96  97  98  99 100
                       D   T   S   K   K   S   S   S   L   L   I   T   A   S   R   A   A   D   T   A
AE000660,TRAV17*01     GAC ACT TCC AAG AAA AGC AGT TCC TTG TTG ATC ACG GCT TCC CGG GCA GCA GAC ACT GCT

X04955  ,TRAV17*01     --- --- --- --- --- --- --- --- --- --- --- --- --- --- --- --- --- --- --- ---

U32540  ,TRAV17*01


                              _CDR3-IMGT_
                      101 102 103 104 105 106 107
                       S   Y   F   C   A   T   D
AE000660,TRAV17*01     TCT TAC TTC TGT GCT ACG GAC G

X04955  ,TRAV17*01     --- --- --- --- ---              #c

U32540  ,TRAV17*01                                       o
```

#c: Rearranged cDNA
o: Genomic DNA, but not known as being germline or rearranged

Framework and complementarity determining regions

FR1-IMGT: 26   CDR1-IMGT: 5
FR2-IMGT: 17   CDR2-IMGT: 3
FR3-IMGT: 38 (-1 aa: 73)   CDR3-IMGT: 3

Collier de Perles for human TRAV17*01

Accession number: IMGT AE000660   EMBL/GenBank/DDBJ: AE000660

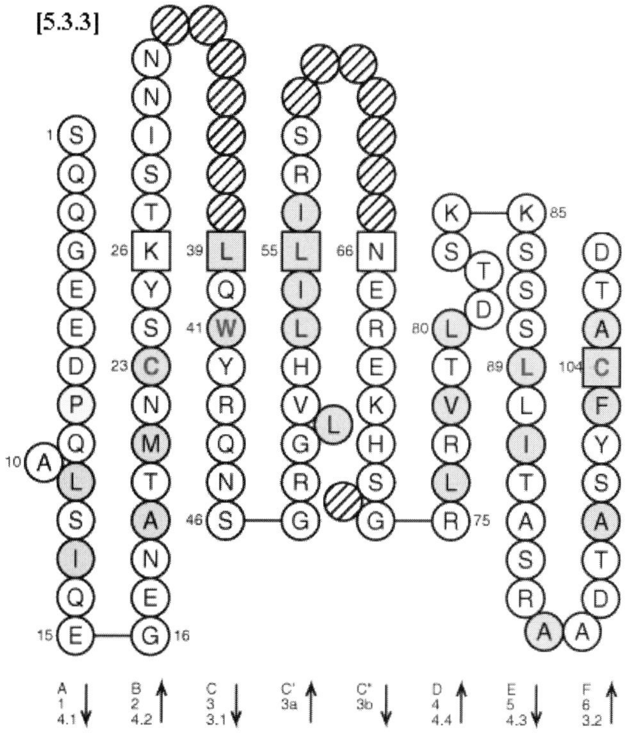

Genome database accession numbers
GDB:9953975   LocusLink: 28666

TRAV18

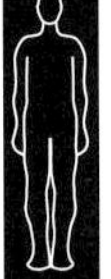

Nomenclature

TRAV18: T cell receptor alpha variable 18.

Definition and functionality

TRAV18 is the unique functional gene of the TRAV18 subgroup which only comprises this mapped gene.

Gene location

TRAV18 is in the TRA/TRD locus on chromosome 14 at 14q11.2.

Nucleotide and amino acid sequences for human TRAV18

```
                          1   2   3   4   5   6   7   8   9  10  11  12  13  14  15  16  17  18  19  20
                          G   D   S   V   T   Q   T   E   G   P   V   T   L   P   E   R   A   A   L   T
AE000660,TRAV18*01   [6] GGA GAC TCG GTT ACC CAG ACA GAA GGC CCA GTT ACC CTC CCT GAG AGG GCA GCT CTG ACA

                                                                       ______________CDR1-IMGT________________
                         21  22  23  24  25  26  27  28  29  30  31  32  33  34  35  36  37  38  39  40
                          L   N   C   T   Y   Q   S   S   Y   S   T   F                           L   F
AE000660,TRAV18*01       TTA AAC TGC ACT TAT CAG TCC AGC TAT TCA ACT TTT ... ... ... ... ... ... CTA TTC

                                                                               ________________CDR2-
                         41  42  43  44  45  46  47  48  49  50  51  52  53  54  55  56  57  58  59  60
                          W   Y   V   Q   Y   L   N   K   E   P   E   L   L   L   K   S   S
AE000660,TRAV18*01       TGG TAT GTC CAG TAT CTA AAC AAA GAG CCT GAG CTC CTC CTG AAA AGT TCA ... ... ...

                         IMGT________________
                         61  62  63  64  65  66  67  68  69  70  71  72  73  74  75  76  77  78  79  80
                                                  E   N   Q   E   T   D   S       R   G   F   Q   A   S   P
AE000660,TRAV18*01       ... ... ... ... ... GAA AAC CAG GAG ACG GAC AGC ... AGA GGT TTT CAG GCC AGT CCT

                         81  82  83  84  85  86  87  88  89  90  91  92  93  94  95  96  97  98  99 100
                          I   K   S   D   S   S   F   H   L   E   K   P   S   V   Q   L   S   D   S   A
AE000660,TRAV18*01       ATC AAG AGT GAC AGT TCC TTC CAC CTG GAG AAG CCC TCG GTG CAG CTG TCG GAC TCT GCC

                                             _CDR3-IMGT_
                        101 102 103 104 105 106 107
                          V   Y   Y   C   A   L   R
AE000660,TRAV18*01       GTG TAC TAC TGC GCT CTG AGA GA
```

Framework and complementarity determining regions

FR1-IMGT: 26   CDR1-IMGT: 6
FR2-IMGT: 17   CDR2-IMGT: 2
FR3-IMGT: 38 (-1 aa: 73)   CDR3-IMGT: 3

Collier de Perles for human TRAV18*01

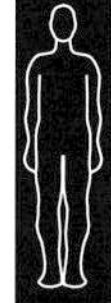

Accession number: IMGT AE000660   EMBL/GenBank/DDBJ: AE000660

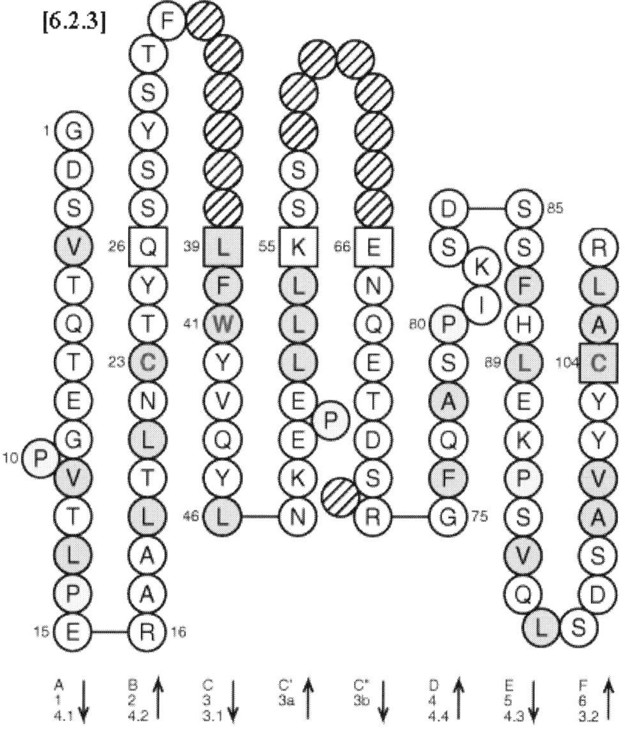

Genome database accession numbers
GDB:9953977   LocusLink: 28665

TRAV19

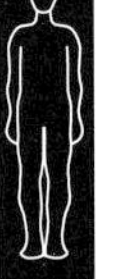

Nomenclature

TRAV19: T cell receptor alpha variable 19.

Definition and functionality

TRAV19 is the unique functional gene of the TRAV19 subgroup which only comprises this mapped gene.

Gene location

TRAV19 is in the TRA/TRD locus on chromosome 14 at 14q11.2.

Nucleotide and amino acid sequences for human TRAV19

```
                          1   2   3   4   5   6   7   8   9   10  11  12  13  14  15  16  17  18  19  20
                          A   Q   K   V   T   Q   A   Q   T   E   I   S   V   V   E   K   E   D   V   T
AE000660,TRAV19*01   [6]  GCT CAG AAG GTA ACT CAA GCG CAG ACT GAA ATT TCT GTG GTG GAG AAG GAG GAT GTG ACC

X01403  ,TRAV19*01  [32]  --- --- --- --- --- --- --- --- --- --- --- --- --- --- --- --- --- --- --- ---


                                                              _____________________CDR1-IMGT_____________________
                          21  22  23  24  25  26  27  28  29  30  31  32  33  34  35  36  37  38  39  40
                          L   D   C   V   Y   E   T   R   D   T   T   Y   Y                       L   F
AE000660,TRAV19*01        TTG GAC TGT GTG TAT GAA ACC CGT GAT ACT ACT TAT TAC ... ... ... ... ... TTA TTC

X01403  ,TRAV19*01        --- --- --- --- --- --- --- --- --- --- --- --- --- ... ... ... ... ... --- ---


                                                                                      _________________CDR2-
                          41  42  43  44  45  46  47  48  49  50  51  52  53  54  55  56  57  58  59  60
                          W   Y   K   Q   P   P   S   G   E   L   V   F   L   I   R   R   N   S   F
AE000660,TRAV19*01        TGG TAC AAG CAA CCA CCA AGT GGA GAA TTG GTT TTC CTT ATT CGT CGG AAC TCT TTT ...

X01403  ,TRAV19*01        --- --- --- --- --- --- --- --- --- --- --- --- --- --- --- --- --- --- --- ...


                          IMGT_________________
                          61  62  63  64  65  66  67  68  69  70  71  72  73  74  75  76  77  78  79  80
                                                  D   E   Q   N   E   I   S       G   R   Y   S   W   N   F
AE000660,TRAV19*01        ... ... ... ... ... GAT GAG CAA AAT GAA ATA AGT ... GGT CGG TAT TCT TGG AAC TTC

X01403  ,TRAV19*01        ... ... ... ... ... --- --- --- --- --- --- --- ... --- --- --- --- --- --- ---


                          81  82  83  84  85  86  87  88  89  90  91  92  93  94  95  96  97  98  99  100
                          Q   K   S   T   S   S   F   N   F   T   I   T   A   S   Q   V   V   D   S   A
AE000660,TRAV19*01        CAG AAA TCC ACC AGT TCC TTC AAC TTC ACC ATC ACA GCC TCA CAA GTC GTG GAC TCA GCA

X01403  ,TRAV19*01        --- --- --- --- --- --- --- --- --- --- --- --- --- --- --- --- --- --- --- ---


                              ___CDR3-IMGT___
                          101 102 103 104 105 106 107 108
                          V   Y   F   C   A   L   S   E
AE000660,TRAV19*01        GTA TAC TTC TGT GCT CTG AGT GAG GC

X01403  ,TRAV19*01        --- --- --- --- --- ---               #c

#c: Rearranged cDNA
```

Framework and complementarity determining regions

FR1-IMGT: 26	CDR1-IMGT: 7
FR2-IMGT: 17	CDR2-IMGT: 4
FR3-IMGT: 38 (-1 aa: 73)	CDR3-IMGT: 4

Collier de Perles for human TRAV19*01

Accession number: IMGT AE000660   EMBL/GenBank/DDBJ: AE000660

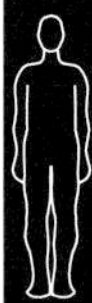

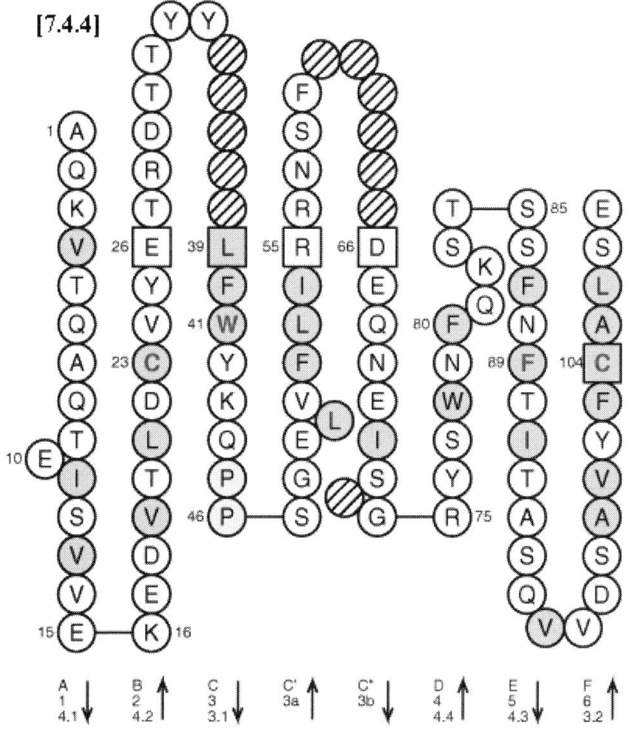

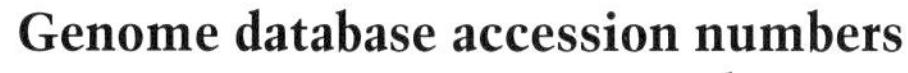

Genome database accession numbers
GDB:9953979   LocusLink: 28664

TRAV20

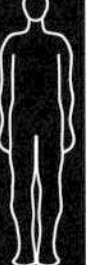

Nomenclature

TRAV20: T cell receptor alpha variable 20.

Definition and functionality

TRAV20 is the unique functional gene of the TRAV20 subgroup which only comprises this mapped gene.

Gene location

TRAV20 is in the TRA/TRD locus on chromosome 14 at 14q11.2.

Nucleotide and amino acid sequences for human TRAV20

```
                          1   2   3   4   5   6   7   8   9   10  11  12  13  14  15  16  17  18  19  20
                          E   D   Q   V   T   Q   S   P   E   A   L   R   L   Q   E   G   E   S   S   S
AE000660,TRAV20*01   [6]  GAA GAC CAG GTG ACG CAG AGT CCC GAG GCC CTG AGA CTC CAG GAG GGA GAG AGT AGC AGT
X68696  ,TRAV20*02  [26]  --- --- --- --- --- --- --- --- --- --- --- --- --- --- --- --- --- --- --- ---
                                                                                                      R
S60789  ,TRAV20*03  [33]  --- --- --- --- --- --- --- --- --- --- --- --- --- --- --- --- --- C-- ---
X70305  ,TRAV20*04  [24]  --- --- --- --- --- --- --- --- --- --- --- --- --- --- --- --- --- --- --- ---


                                                                        ________CDR1-IMGT_________
                          21  22  23  24  25  26  27  28  29  30  31  32  33  34  35  36  37  38  39  40
                          L   N   C   S   Y   T   V   S   G   L   R   G                           L   F
AE000660,TRAV20*01        CTT AAC TGC AGT TAC ACA GTC AGC GGT TTA AGA GGG ... ... ... ... ... ... CTG TTC
X68696  ,TRAV20*02        --C --- --- --- --- --- --- --- --- --- --- --- ... ... ... ... ... ... --- ---
S60789  ,TRAV20*03        --C --- --- --- --- --- --- --- --- --- --- --- ... ... ... ... ... ... --- ---
                                              C
X70305  ,TRAV20*04        --C --- --- --- -G- --- --- --- --- --- --- --- ... ... ... ... ... ... --- ---


                                                                                            ________CDR2-
                          41  42  43  44  45  46  47  48  49  50  51  52  53  54  55  56  57  58  59  60
                          W   Y   R   Q   D   P   G   K   G   P   E   F   L   F   T   L   Y   S
AE000660,TRAV20*01        TGG TAT AGG CAA GAT CCT GGG AAA GGC CCT GAA TTC CTC TTC ACC CTG TAT TCA ... ...
X68696  ,TRAV20*02        --- --- --- --- --- --- --- --- --- --- --- --- --- --- --- --- --- --- ... ...
S60789  ,TRAV20*03        --- --- --- --- --- --- --- --- --- --- --- --- --- --- --- --- --- --- ... ...
X70305  ,TRAV20*04        --- --- --- --- --- --- --- --- --- --- --- --- --- --- --- --- --- --- ... ...


                          IMGT________________
                          61  62  63  64  65  66  67  68  69  70  71  72  73  74  75  76  77  78  79  80
                                            A   G   E   E   K   E   K       E   R   L   K   A   T   L
AE000660,TRAV20*01        ... ... ... ... ... GCT GGG GAA GAA AAG GAG AAA ... GAA AGG CTA AAA GCC ACA TTA
X68696  ,TRAV20*02        ... ... ... ... ... --- --- --- --- --- --- --- ... --- --- --- --- --- --- ---
S60789  ,TRAV20*03        ... ... ... ... ... --- --- --- --- --- --- --- ... --- --- --- --- --- --- ---
X70305  ,TRAV20*04        ... ... ... ... ... --- --- --- --- --- --- --- ... --- --- --- --- --- --- ---


                          81  82  83  84  85  86  87  88  89  90  91  92  93  94  95  96  97  98  99  100
                                  T   K   K   E   S   F   L   H   I   T   A   P   K   P   E   D   S   A
AE000660,TRAV20*01        ... ... ACA AAG AAG GAA AGC TTT CTG CAC ATC ACA GCC CCT AAA CCT GAA GAC TCA GCC
X68696  ,TRAV20*02        ... ... --- --- --- --- --- --- --- --- --- --- --- --- --- --- --- --- --- ---
S60789  ,TRAV20*03        ... ... --- --- --- --- --- --- --- --- --- --- --- --- --- --- --- --- --- ---
X70305  ,TRAV20*04        ... ... --- --- --- --- --- --- --- --- --- --- --- --- --- --- --- --- --- ---


                          _CDR3-IMGT_
                          101 102 103 104 105 106 107
                          T   Y   L   C   A   V   Q
AE000660,TRAV20*01        ACT TAT CTC TGT GCT GTG CAG G
X68696  ,TRAV20*02        --- --- --- --- ---            #c
S60789  ,TRAV20*03        --- --- --- ---                #c
X70305  ,TRAV20*04        --- --- --- --- ---            #c

#c: Rearranged cDNA
```

Framework and complementarity determining regions

FR1-IMGT: 26   CDR1-IMGT: 6
FR2-IMGT: 17   CDR2-IMGT: 3
FR3-IMGT: 36 (-3 aa: 73,81,82)   CDR3-IMGT: 3

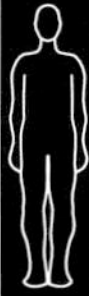

Collier de Perles for human TRAV20*01

Accession number: IMGT AE000660   EMBL/GenBank/DDBJ: AE000660

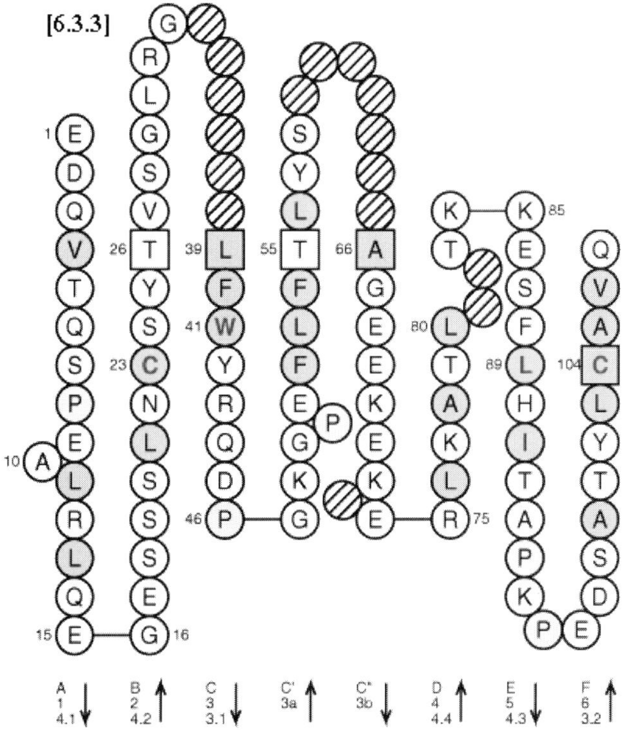

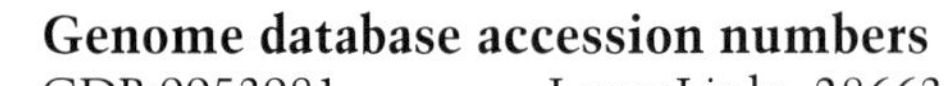

Genome database accession numbers
GDB:9953981   LocusLink: 28663

Nomenclature

TRAV21: T cell receptor alpha variable 21.

Definition and functionality

TRAV21 is the unique functional gene of the TRAV21 subgroup which only comprises this mapped gene.

Gene location

TRAV21 is in the TRA/TRD locus on chromosome 14 at 14q11.2.

Nucleotide and amino acid sequences for human TRAV21

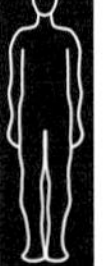

```
                          1   2   3   4   5   6   7   8   9  10  11  12  13  14  15  16  17  18  19  20
                          K   Q   E   V   T   Q   I   P   A   A   L   S   V   P   E   G   E   N   L   V
AE000660,TRAV21*01   [6]  AAA CAG GAG GTG ACG CAG ATT CCT GCA GCT CTG AGT GTC CCA GAA GGA GAA AAC TTG GTT

X58736  ,TRAV21*02  [28]  --- --- --- --- --A --- --- --- --- --- --- --- --- --- --- --- --- --- --- ---


                                                              ______________CDR1-IMGT___________________
                         21  22  23  24  25  26  27  28  29  30  31  32  33  34  35  36  37  38  39  40
                          L   N   C   S   F   T   D   S   A   I   Y   N                           L   Q
AE000660,TRAV21*01       CTC AAC TGC AGT TTC ACT GAT AGC GCT ATT TAC AAC ... ... ... ... ... ... CTC CAG

X58736  ,TRAV21*02       --- --- --- --- --- --- --- --- --- --- --- --- ... ... ... ... ... ... --- ---


                                                                              ________________CDR2-
                         41  42  43  44  45  46  47  48  49  50  51  52  53  54  55  56  57  58  59  60
                          W   F   R   Q   D   P   G   K   G   L   T   S   L   L   L   I   Q   S
AE000660,TRAV21*01       TGG TTT AGG CAG GAC CCT GGG AAA GGT CTC ACA TCT CTG TTG CTT ATT CAG TCA ... ...

X58736  ,TRAV21*02       --- --- --- --- --- --- --- --- --- --- --- --- --- --- --- --- --- --- ... ...


                         IMGT________________
                         61  62  63  64  65  66  67  68  69  70  71  72  73  74  75  76  77  78  79  80
                                                  S   Q   R   E   P   T   S       G   R   L   N   A   S   L
AE000660,TRAV21*01       ... ... ... ... ... AGT CAG AGA GAG CCA ACA AGT ... GGA AGA CTT AAT GCC TCG CTG

X58736  ,TRAV21*02       ... ... ... ... ... --- --- --- --- --- --- --- ... --- --- --- --- --- --- ---


                         81  82  83  84  85  86  87  88  89  90  91  92  93  94  95  96  97  98  99 100
                          D   K   S   S   G   R   S   T   L   Y   I   A   A   S   Q   P   G   D   S   A
AE000660,TRAV21*01       GAT AAA TCA TCA GGA CGT AGT ACT TTA TAC ATT GCA GCT TCT CAG CCT GGT GAC TCA GCC

X58736  ,TRAV21*02       --- --- --- --- --- --- --- --- --- --- --- --- --- --- --- --- --- --- --- ---


                                     _CDR3-IMGT_
                        101 102 103 104 105 106 107
                          T   Y   L   C   A   V   R
AE000660,TRAV21*01       ACC TAC CTC TGT GCT GTG AGG

X58736  ,TRAV21*02       --- --- --- --- ---                #c
```
#c: Rearranged cDNA

Framework and complementarity determining regions

FR1-IMGT: 26	CDR1-IMGT: 6
FR2-IMGT: 17	CDR2-IMGT: 3
FR3-IMGT: 38 (-1 aa: 73)	CDR3-IMGT: 3

Collier de Perles for human TRAV21*01

Accession number: IMGT AE000660   EMBL/GenBank/DDBJ: AE000660

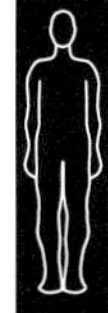

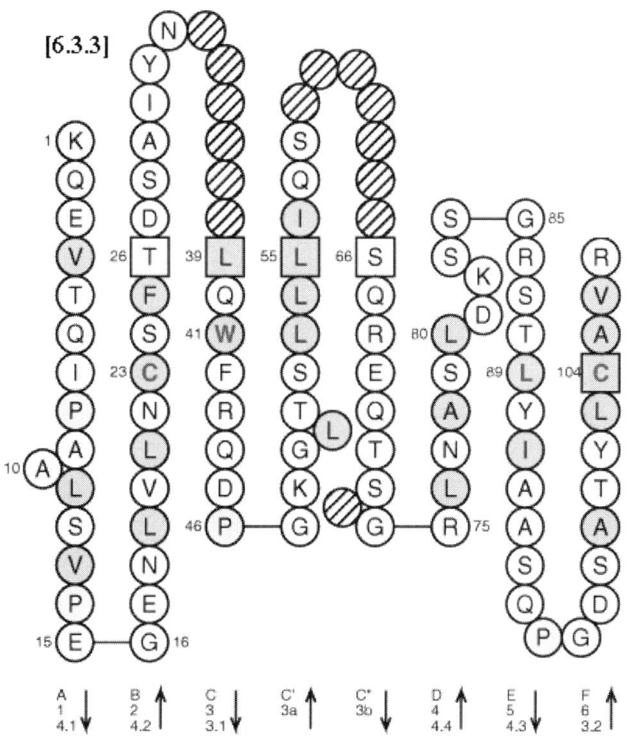

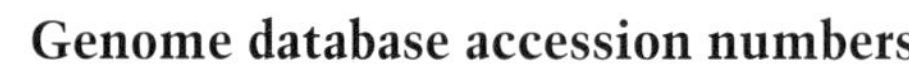

Genome database accession numbers
GDB:9953983   LocusLink: 28662

TRAV22

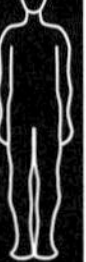

Nomenclature

TRAV22: T cell receptor alpha variable 22.

Definition and functionality

TRAV22 is the unique functional gene of the TRAV22 subgroup which only comprises this mapped gene.

Gene location

TRAV22 is in the TRA/TRD locus on chromosome 14 at 14q11.2.

Nucleotide and amino acid sequences for human TRAV22

```
                        1    2    3    4    5    6    7    8    9   10   11   12   13   14   15   16   17   18   19   20
                        G    I    Q    V    E    Q    S    P    P    D    L    I    L    Q    E    G    A    N    S    T
AE000660,TRAV22*01  [6] GGA  ATA  CAA  GTG  GAG  CAG  AGT  CCT  CCA  GAC  CTG  ATT  CTC  CAG  GAG  GGA  GCC  AAT  TCC  ACG

M27374  ,TRAV22*01 [16] ---  ---  ---  ---  ---  ---  ---  ---  ---  ---  ---  ---  ---  ---  ---  ---  ---  ---  ---  ---


                                                                        ________CDR1-IMGT________
                       21   22   23   24   25   26   27   28   29   30   31   32   33   34   35   36   37   38   39   40
                        L    R    C    N    F    S    D    S    V    N    N                                    L    Q
AE000660,TRAV22*01     CTG  CGG  TGC  AAT  TTT  TCT  GAC  TCT  GTG  AAC  AAT  ...  ...  ...  ...  ...  ...  ...  TTG  CAG

M27374  ,TRAV22*01     ---  ---  ---  ---  ---  ---  ---  ---  ---  ---  ---  ...  ...  ...  ...  ...  ...  ...  ---  ---


                                                                                            ________CDR2-
                       41   42   43   44   45   46   47   48   49   50   51   52   53   54   55   56   57   58   59   60
                        W    F    H    Q    N    P    W    G    Q    L    I    N    L    F    Y    I
AE000660,TRAV22*01     TGG  TTT  CAT  CAA  AAC  CCT  TGG  GGA  CAG  CTC  ATC  AAC  CTG  TTT  TAC  ATT  ...  ...  ...  ...

M27374  ,TRAV22*01     ---  ---  ---  ---  ---  ---  ---  ---  ---  ---  ---  ---  ---  ---  ---  ...  ...  ...  ...


                       IMGT________
                       61   62   63   64   65   66   67   68   69   70   71   72   73   74   75   76   77   78   79   80
                                                 P    S    G    T    K    Q    N         G    R    L    S    A    T    T
AE000660,TRAV22*01     ...  ...  ...  ...  ...  CCC  TCA  GGG  ACA  AAA  CAG  AAT  ...  GGA  AGA  TTA  AGC  GCC  ACG  ACT

M27374  ,TRAV22*01     ...  ...  ...  ...  ...  ---  ---  ---  ---  ---  ---  ---  ...  ---  ---  ---  ---  ---  ---  ---


                       81   82   83   84   85   86   87   88   89   90   91   92   93   94   95   96   97   98   99  100
                        V    A    T    E    R    Y    S    L    L    Y    I    S    S    S    Q    T    T    D    S    G
AE000660,TRAV22*01     GTC  GCT  ACG  GAA  CGC  TAC  AGC  TTA  TTG  TAC  ATT  TCC  TCT  TCC  CAG  ACC  ACA  GAC  TCA  GGC

M27374  ,TRAV22*01     ---  ---  ---  ---  ---  ---  ---  ---  ---  ---  ---  ---  ---  ---  ---  ---  ---  ---  ---  ---


                             _CDR3-IMGT_
                       101  102  103  104  105  106  107
                        V    Y    F    C    A    V    E
AE000660,TRAV22*01     GTT  TAT  TTC  TGT  GCT  GTG  GAG  C

M27374  ,TRAV22*01     ---  ---  ---  ---  ---            #c
```

#c: Rerranged cDNA

Framework and complementarity determining regions

FR1-IMGT: 26

FR2-IMGT: 17

FR3-IMGT: 38 (-1 aa: 73)

CDR1-IMGT: 5

CDR2-IMGT: 1

CDR3-IMGT: 3

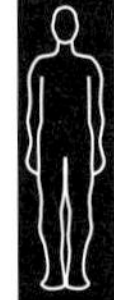

Collier de Perles for human TRAV22*01

Accession number: IMGT AE000660   EMBL/GenBank/DDBJ: AE000660

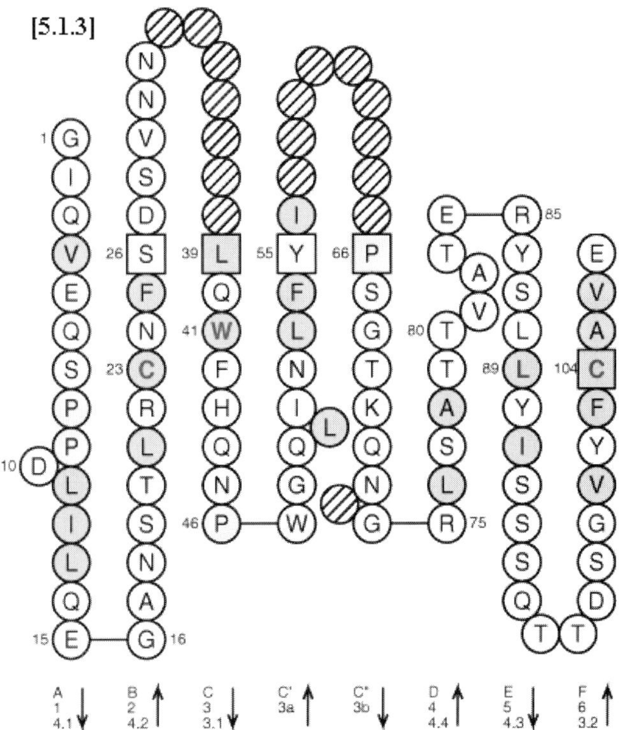

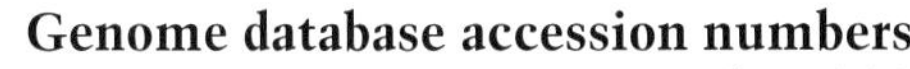

Genome database accession numbers
GDB:9953985   LocusLink: 28661

TRAV23/DV6

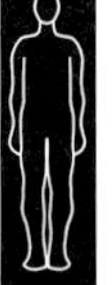

Nomenclature

TRAV23/DV6: T cell receptor alpha variable 23/delta variable 6.

Definition and functionality

TRAV23/DV6 is the unique functional gene of the TRAV23 subgroup which only comprises this mapped gene.

TRAV23/DV6 has been found rearranged to both (D)J genes of the TRD locus and TRAJ genes, the TRD locus being embedded in the TRA locus. This gene can therefore be used for the synthesis of both delta and alpha chains.

Gene location

TRAV23/DV6 is in the TRA/TRD locus on chromosome 14 at 14q11.2.

Nucleotide and amino acid sequences for human TRAV23/DV6

```
                             1   2   3   4   5   6   7   8   9  10  11  12  13  14  15  16  17  18  19  20
                             Q   Q   Q   V   K   Q   S   P   Q   S   L   I   V   Q   K   G   G   I   S   I
AE000660,TRAV23*01       [6] CAG CAG CAG GTG AAA CAA AGT CCT CAA TCT TTG ATA GTC CAG AAA GGA GGG ATT TCA ATT
X70309  ,TRAV23*01      [24] --- --- --- --- --- --- --- --- --- --- --- --- --- --- --- --- --- --- --- ---
U32526  ,TRAV23*01       [5] --- --- --- --- --- --- --- --- --- --- --- --- --- --- --- --- --- --- --- ---
                                                                                                     P
M17660  ,TRAV23*02      [17] --- --- --- --- --- --- --- --- --- --- --- --- --- --- --- --- --- --- C-- ---
M22936  ,TRAV23*01/*02 (1)[30]
M97704  ,TRAV23*03      [12] --- --- --- --- --- --- --- --- --- --- --- --- --- --- --- --- --- --- --- ---
Z49057  ,TRAV23*03      [13]     --- --- --- --- --- --- --- --- --- --- --- --- --- --- --- --- --- --- ---
Y10411  ,TRAV23*04      [14]     --- --- --- --- --- --- --- --- --- --- --- --- --- --- --- --- --- --- ---


                                                                       ___________CDR1-IMGT___________
                            21  22  23  24  25  26  27  28  29  30  31  32  33  34  35  36  37  38  39  40
                             I   N   C   A   Y   E   N   T   A   F   D   Y                           F   P
AE000660,TRAV23*01          ATA AAC TGT GCT TAT GAG AAC ACT GCG TTT GAC TAC ... ... ... ... ... ... TTT CCA
X70309  ,TRAV23*01          --- --- --- --- --- --- --- --- --- --- --- --- ... ... ... ... ... ... --- ---
U32526  ,TRAV23*01          --- --- --- --- --- --- --- --- --- --- --- --- ... ... ... ... ... ... --- ---
M17660  ,TRAV23*02          --- --- --- --- --- --- --- --- --- --- --- --- ... ... ... ... ... ... --- ---
M22936  ,TRAV23*01/*02 (1)
M97704  ,TRAV23*03          --- --- --- --- --- --- --- --- --- --- --- --- ... ... ... ... ... ... --- ---
Z49057  ,TRAV23*03          --- --- --- --- --- --- --- --- --- --- --- --- ... ... ... ... ... ... --- ---
Y10411  ,TRAV23*04          --- --- --- --- --- --- --- --- --- --- --- --- ... ... ... ... ... ... --- ---


                                                                                       ___________CDR2-
                            41  42  43  44  45  46  47  48  49  50  51  52  53  54  55  56  57  58  59  60
                             W   Y   Q   Q   F   P   G   K   G   P   A   L   L   I   A   I   R   P
AE000660,TRAV23*01          TGG TAC CAA CAA TTC CCT GGG AAA GGC CCT GCA TTA TTG ATA GCC ATA CGT CCA ... ...
X70309  ,TRAV23*01          --- --- --- --- --- --- --- --- --- --- --- --- --- --- --- --- --- --- ... ...
U32526  ,TRAV23*01          --- --- --- --- --- --- --- --- --- --- --- --- --- --- --- --- --- --- ... ...
M17660  ,TRAV23*02          --- --- --- --- --- --- --- --- --- --- --- --- --- --- --- --- --- --- ... ...
M22936  ,TRAV23*01/*02 (1)  --- --- --- --- --- --- --- --- --- --- --- --- --- --- --- --- --- --- ... ...
M97704  ,TRAV23*03          --- --- --- --G --- --- --- --- --- --- --- --- --- --- --- --- --- --- ... ...
Z49057  ,TRAV23*03          --- --- --- --G --- --- --- --- --- --- --- --- --- --- --- --- --- --- ... ...
Y10411  ,TRAV23*04          --- --- --G --- --- --- --- --- --- --- --- --- --- --- --- --- --- --- ... ...
```

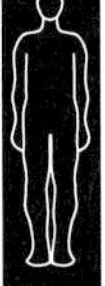

```
                             IMGT________________
                             61  62  63  64  65  66  67  68  69  70  71  72  73  74  75  76  77  78  79  80
                                                 D   V   S   E   K   K   E       G   R   F   T   I   S   F
AE000660,TRAV23*01           ... ... ... ... ... GAT GTG AGT GAA AAG AAA GAA ... GGA AGA TTC ACA ATC TCC TTC

X70309 ,TRAV23*01            ... ... ... ... ... --- --- --- --- --- --- --- ... --- --- --- --- --- --- ---

U32526 ,TRAV23*01            ... ... ... ... ... --- --- --- --- --- --- --- ... --- --- --- --- --- --- ---

M17660 ,TRAV23*02            ... ... ... ... ... --- --- --- --- --- --- --- ... --- --- --- --- --- --- ---

M22936 ,TRAV23*01/*02 (1)    ... ... ... ... ... --- --- --- --- --- --- --- ... --- --- --- --- --- --- ---

M97704 ,TRAV23*03            ... ... ... ... ... --- --- --- --- --- --- --- ... --- --- --- --- --- --- ---

Z49057 ,TRAV23*03            ... ... ... ... ... --- --- --- --- --- --- --- ... --- --- --- --- --- --- ---

Y10411 ,TRAV23*04            ... ... ... ... ... --- --- --- --- --- --- --- ... --- --- --- --- --- --- ---


                             81  82  83  84  85  86  87  88  89  90  91  92  93  94  95  96  97  98  99 100
                             N   K   S   A   K   Q   F   S   L   H   I   M   D   S   Q   P   G   D   S   A
AE000660,TRAV23*01           AAT AAA AGT GCC AAG CAG TTC TCA TTG CAT ATC ATG GAT TCC CAG CCT GGA GAC TCA GCC

X70309 ,TRAV23*01            --- --- --- --- --- --- --- --- --- --- --- --- --- --- --- --- --- --- --- ---

U32526 ,TRAV23*01            --- --- --- --- --- --- --- --- --- --- --- --- --- --- --- --- --- --- --- -

M17660 ,TRAV23*02            --- --- --- --- --- --- --- --- --- --- --- --- --- --- --- --- --- --- --- ---

M22936 ,TRAV23*01/*02 (1)    --- --- --- --- --- --- --- --- --- --- --- --- --- --- --- --- --- --- --- ---

M97704 ,TRAV23*03            --- --- --- --- --- --- --- --- --- --- --- --- --- --- --- --- --- --- --- ---

Z49057 ,TRAV23*03            --- --- --- --- --- --- --- --- --- --- --- --- --- --- --- --- --- --- --- ---

Y10411 ,TRAV23*04            --- --- --- --- --- --- --- --- --- --- --- --- --- --- --- --- --- --- --- ---


                                             _CDR3-IMGT_
                             101 102 103 104 105 106 107
                             T   Y   F   C   A   A   S
AE000660,TRAV23*01           ACC TAC TTC TGT GCA GCA AGC A

X70309 ,TRAV23*01            --- --- --- --- ---              #c

U32526 ,TRAV23*01                                            o

M17660 ,TRAV23*02            --- --- --- --- --- ---          #c
                                                     R
M22936 ,TRAV23*01/*02 (1)    --- --- --- --- --- --- --A      o

M97704 ,TRAV23*03            --- --- --- --- --- ---          #c

Z49057 ,TRAV23*03            --- --- --- ---                  o

Y10411 ,TRAV23*04            --- --- --- ---                  o
```

#c: Rearranged cDNA
o: Genomic DNA, but not known to be germline or rearranged

Note:

(1) Partial sequence which could not be assigned to a given allele.

Framework and complementarity determining regions

FR1-IMGT: 26

FR2-IMGT: 17

FR3-IMGT: 38 (-1 aa: 73)

CDR1-IMGT: 6

CDR2-IMGT: 3

CDR3-IMGT: 3

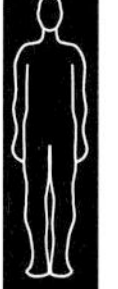

Collier de Perles for human TRAV23/DV6*01

Accession number: IMGT AE000660   EMBL/GenBank/DDBJ: AE000660

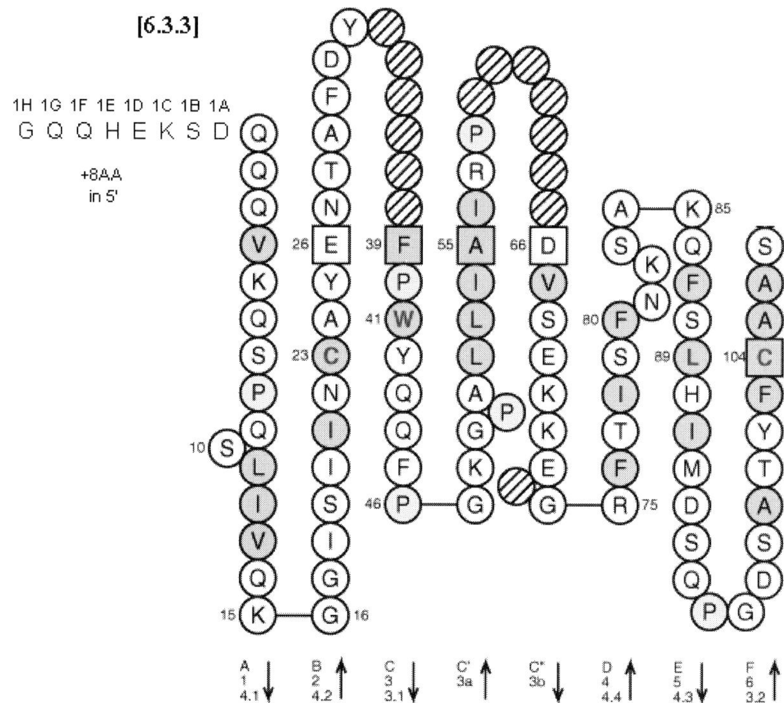

Note:

The 8 additional amino acids, predicted by the program SIGSEQ2 and described by Wülfing, C. and Plückthun, A. (1995) Immunology Today 16, 405–406, are numbered 1A to 1H.

Genome database accession numbers

GDB:9953987   LocusLink: 28660

TRAV24

Nomenclature

TRAV24: T cell receptor alpha variable 24.

Definition and functionality

TRAV24 is the unique functional gene of the TRAV24 subgroup which only comprises this mapped gene.

Gene location

TRAV24 is in the TRA/TRD locus on chromosome 14 at 14q11.2.

Nucleotide and amino acid sequences for human TRAV24

```
                         1   2   3   4   5   6   7   8   9  10  11  12  13  14  15  16  17  18  19  20
                         I   L   N   V   E   Q   S   P   Q   S   L   H   V   Q   E   G   D   S   T   N
AE000660,TRAV24*01   [6] ATA CTG AAC GTG GAA CAA AGT CCT CAG TCA CTG CAT GTT CAG GAG GGA GAC AGC ACC AAT
                                                     G
M17661  ,TRAV24*02  [17] --- --- --- --- --- --- G-- --- --- --- --- --- --- --- --- --- --- --- --- ---


                                                           __________________CDR1-IMGT__________________
                         21  22  23  24  25  26  27  28  29  30  31  32  33  34  35  36  37  38  39  40
                         F   T   C   S   F   P   S   S   N   F   Y   A                           L   H
AE000660,TRAV24*01       TTC ACC TGC AGC TTC CCT TCC AGC AAT TTT TAT GCC ... ... ... ... ... ... TTA CAC
M17661  ,TRAV24*02       --- --- --- --- --- --- --- --- --- --- --- --- ... ... ... ... ... ... --- ---


                                                                                   ___________CDR2-
                         41  42  43  44  45  46  47  48  49  50  51  52  53  54  55  56  57  58  59  60
                         W   Y   R   W   E   T   A   K   S   P   E   A   L   F   V   M   T   L
AE000660,TRAV24*01       TGG TAC AGA TGG GAA ACT GCA AAA AGC CCC GAG GCC TTG TTT GTA ATG ACT TTA ... ...
                                                     T
M17661  ,TRAV24*02       --- --- --- --- --- --- --C --- -CA --- --- --- --- --- --- --- --- --- ... ...


                         IMGT________________
                         61  62  63  64  65  66  67  68  69  70  71  72  73  74  75  76  77  78  79  80
                                                 N   G   D   E   K   K   K       G   R   I   S   A   T   L
AE000660,TRAV24*01       ... ... ... ... ... AAT GGG GAT GAA AAG AAG AAA ... GGA CGA ATA AGT GCC ACT CTT
M17661  ,TRAV24*02       ... ... ... ... ... --- --- --- --- --- --- --- ... --- --- --- --- --- --- ---


                         81  82  83  84  85  86  87  88  89  90  91  92  93  94  95  96  97  98  99 100
                         N   T   K   E   G   Y   S   Y   L   Y   I   K   G   S   Q   P   E   D   S   A
AE000660,TRAV24*01       AAT ACC AAG GAG GGT TAC AGC TAT TTG TAC ATC AAA GGA TCC CAG CCT GAA GAC TCA GCC
M17661  ,TRAV24*02       --- --- --- --- --- --- --- --- --- --- --- --- --- --- --- --- --- --T --- ---


                                         _CDR3-IMGT_
                         101 102 103 104 105 106 107
                         T   Y   L   C   A   F
AE000660,TRAV24*01       ACA TAC CTC TGT GCC TTT A
M17661  ,TRAV24*02       --- --- --- --- --- ---         #c

#c: Rearranged cDNA
```

Framework and complementarity determining regions

FR1-IMGT: 26   CDR1-IMGT: 6
FR2-IMGT: 17   CDR2-IMGT: 3
FR3-IMGT: 38 (-1 aa: 73) CDR3-IMGT: 2

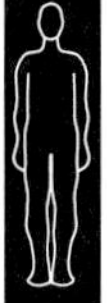

Collier de Perles for human TRAV24*01

Accession number: IMGT AE000660   EMBL/GenBank/DDBJ: AE000660

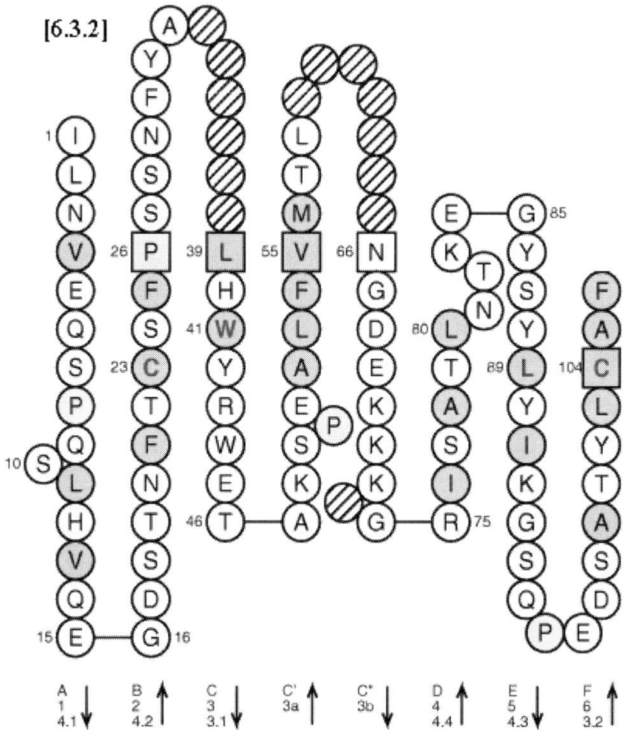

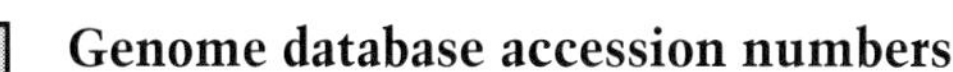

Genome database accession numbers
GDB:9953989   LocusLink: 28659

Nomenclature

TRAV25: T cell receptor alpha variable 25.

Definition and functionality

TRAV25 is the unique functional gene of the TRAV25 subgroup which only comprises this mapped gene.

Gene location

TRAV25 is in the TRA/TRD locus on chromosome 14 at 14q11.2.

Nucleotide and amino acid sequences for human TRAV25

```
                        1   2   3   4   5   6   7   8   9  10  11  12  13  14  15  16  17  18  19  20
                        G   Q   Q   V   M   Q   I   P   Q   Y   Q   H   V   Q   E   G   E   D   F   T
AE000660,TRAV25*01  [6] GGA CAA CAG GTA ATG CAA ATT CCT CAG TAC CAG CAT GTA CAA GAA GGA GAG GAC TTC ACC

M64350  ,TRAV25*01  [4] --- --- --- --- --- --- --- --- --- --- --- --- --- --- --- --- --- --- --- ---


                                                                  ______________CDR1-IMGT________________
                        21  22  23  24  25  26  27  28  29  30  31  32  33  34  35  36  37  38  39  40
                        T   Y   C   N   S   S   T   T   L   S   N                               I   Q
AE000660,TRAV25*01      ACG TAC TGC AAT TCC TCA ACT ACT TTA AGC AAT ... ... ... ... ... ... ... ATA CAG

M64350  ,TRAV25*01      --- --- --- --- --- --- --- --- --- --- --- ... ... ... ... ... ... ... --- ---


                                                                                      ______________CDR2-
                        41  42  43  44  45  46  47  48  49  50  51  52  53  54  55  56  57  58  59  60
                        W   Y   K   Q   R   P   G   G   H   P   V   F   L   I   Q   L   V   K
AE000660,TRAV25*01      TGG TAT AAG CAA AGG CCT GGT GGA CAT CCC GTT TTT TTG ATA CAG TTA GTG AAG ... ...

M64350  ,TRAV25*01      --- --- --- --- --- --- --- --- --- --- --- --- --- --- --- --- --- --- ... ...


                        IMGT______________
                        61  62  63  64  65  66  67  68  69  70  71  72  73  74  75  76  77  78  79  80
                                                S   G   E   V   K   K   Q       K   R   L   T   F   Q   F
AE000660,TRAV25*01      ... ... ... ... ... AGT GGA GAA GTG AAG AAG CAG ... AAA AGA CTG ACA TTT CAG TTT

M64350  ,TRAV25*01      ... ... ... ... ... --- --- --- --- --- --- --- ... --- --- --- --- --- --- ---


                        81  82  83  84  85  86  87  88  89  90  91  92  93  94  95  96  97  98  99 100
                        G   E   A   K   K   N   S   S   L   H   I   T   A   T   Q   T   T   D   V   G
AE000660,TRAV25*01      GGA GAA GCA AAA AAG AAC AGC TCC CTG CAC ATC ACA GCC ACC CAG ACT ACA GAT GTA GGA

M64350  ,TRAV25*01      --- --- --- --- --- --- --- --- --- --- --- --- --- --- --- --- --- --- --- ---


                        _CDR3-IMGT_
                       101 102 103 104 105 106
                        T   Y   F   C   A   G
AE000660,TRAV25*01      ACC TAC TTC TGT GCA GGG

M64350  ,TRAV25*01      --- --- --- --- --- ---      #c
```

#c: Rearranged cDNA

Framework and complementarity determining regions

FR1-IMGT: 26
FR2-IMGT: 17
FR3-IMGT: 38 (-1 aa: 73)

CDR1-IMGT: 5
CDR2-IMGT: 3
CDR3-IMGT: 2

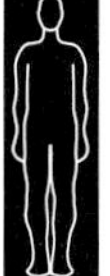

Collier de Perles for human TRAV25*01

Accession number: IMGT AE000660   EMBL/GenBank/DDBJ: AE000660

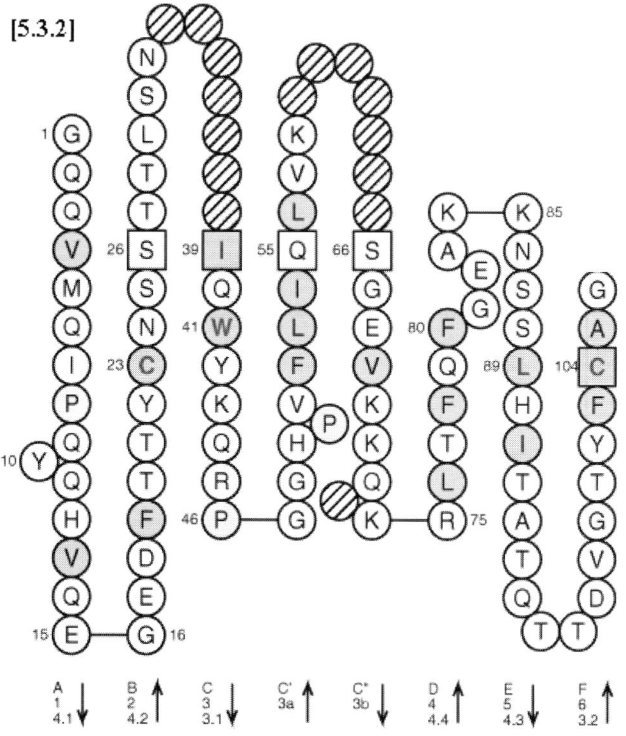

Genome database accession numbers
GDB:9953991   LocusLink: 28658

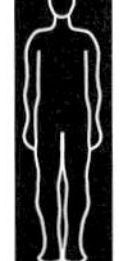

Nomenclature

TRAV26-1: T cell receptor alpha variable 26-1.

Definition and functionality

TRAV26-1 is one of the two functional genes of the TRAV26 subgroup which comprises two mapped genes.

Gene location

TRAV26-1 is in the TRA/TRD locus on chromosome 14 at 14q11.2.

Nucleotide and amino acid sequences for human TRAV26-1

```
                          1   2   3   4   5   6   7   8   9  10  11  12  13  14  15  16  17  18  19  20
                          D   A   K   T   T   Q       P   P   S   M   D   C   A   E   G   R   A   A   N
AE000660,TRAV26-1*01  [6] GAT GCT AAG ACC ACC CAG ... CCC CCC TCC ATG GAT TGC GCT GAA GGA AGA GCT GCA AAC

M27370  ,TRAV26-1*01 [16] --- --- --- --- --- --- ... --- --- --- --- --- --- --- --- --- --- --- --- ---
                                                                T
M27371  ,TRAV26-1*02 [16] --- --- --- --- --- --- ... --- A-- --- --- --- --- --- --- --- --- --- --- ---
                                                                T
U32541  ,TRAV26-1*02  [5] --- --- --- --- --- --- ... --- A-- --- --- --- --- --- --- --- --- --- --- ---
                                                                T
L06886  ,TRAV26-1*03 [29] --- --- --- --- --- --- ... --- A-- --- --- --- --- --- --- --- --- --- --- ---


                                                                      ________CDR1-IMGT________
                         21  22  23  24  25  26  27  28  29  30  31  32  33  34  35  36  37  38  39  40
                          L   P   C   N   H   S   T   I   S   G   N   E   Y                       V   Y
AE000660,TRAV26-1*01     CTG CCT TGT AAT CAC TCT ACC ATC AGT GGA AAT GAG TAT ... ... ... ... ... GTG TAT

M27370  ,TRAV26-1*01     --- --- --- --- --- --- --- --- --- --- --- --- --- ... ... ... ... ... --- ---

M27371  ,TRAV26-1*02     --- --- --- --- --- --- --- --- --- --- --- --- --- ... ... ... ... ... --- ---

U32541  ,TRAV26-1*02     --- --- --- --- --- --- --- --- --- --- --- --- --- ... ... ... ... ... --- ---

L06886  ,TRAV26-1*03     --- --- --- --- --- --- --- --- --- --- --- --- --- ... ... ... ... ... --- ---


                                                                             ________________CDR2-
                         41  42  43  44  45  46  47  48  49  50  51  52  53  54  55  56  57  58  59  60
                          W   Y   R   Q   I   H   S   Q   G   P   Q   Y   I   I   H   G
AE000660,TRAV26-1*01     TGG TAT CGA CAG ATT CAC TCC CAG GGG CCA CAG TAT ATC ATT CAT GGT ... ... ... ...

M27370  ,TRAV26-1*01     --- --- --- --- --- --- --- --- --- --- --- --- --- --- --- ... ... ... ...

M27371  ,TRAV26-1*02     --- --- --- --- --- --- --- --- --- --- --- --- --- --- --- ... ... ... ...

U32541  ,TRAV26-1*02     --- --- --- --- --- --- --- --- --- --- --- --- --- --- --- ... ... ... ...
                                                                          N
L06886  ,TRAV26-1*03     --- --- --- --- --- --- --- --- --- --- --- A-- --- --- --- ... ... ... ...


                         IMGT________________
                         61  62  63  64  65  66  67  68  69  70  71  72  73  74  75  76  77  78  79  80
                                              L   K   N   N   E   T   N       E   M   A   S   L   I   I
AE000660,TRAV26-1*01     ... ... ... ... ... CTA AAA AAC AAT GAA ACC AAT ... GAA ATG GCC TCT CTG ATC ATC

M27370  ,TRAV26-1*01     ... ... ... ... ... --- --- --- --- --- --- --- ... --- --- --- --- --- --- ---

M27371  ,TRAV26-1*02     ... ... ... ... ... --- --- --- --- --- --- --- ... --- --- --- --- --- --- ---

U32541  ,TRAV26-1*02     ... ... ... ... ... --- --- --- --- --- --- --- ... --- --- --- --- --- --- ---

L06886  ,TRAV26-1*03     ... ... ... ... ... --- --- --- --- --- --- --- ... --- --- --- --- --- --- ---


                         81  82  83  84  85  86  87  88  89  90  91  92  93  94  95  96  97  98  99 100
                          T   E   D   R   K   S   S   T   L   I   L   P   H   A   T   L   R   D   T   A
AE000660,TRAV26-1*01     ACA GAA GAC AGA AAG TCC AGC ACC TTG ATC CTG CCC CAC GCT ACG CTG AGA GAC ACT GCT

M27370  ,TRAV26-1*01     --- --- --- --- --- --- --- --- --- --- --- --- --- --- --- --- --- --- --- ---

M27371  ,TRAV26-1*02     --- --- --- --- --- --- --- --- --- --- --- --- --- --- --- --- --- --- --- ---

U32541  ,TRAV26-1*02     --- --- --- --

L06886  ,TRAV26-1*03     --- --- --- --- --- --- --- --- --- --- --- --- --- --- --- --- --- --- --- ---


                               ___CDR3-IMGT___
                        101 102 103 104 105 106 107 108
                          V   Y   Y   C   I   V   R   V
AE000660,TRAV26-1*01     GTG TAC TAT TGC ATC GTC AGA GTC G

M27370  ,TRAV26-1*01     --- --- --- --- --- --- ---          #c

M27371  ,TRAV26-1*02     --- --- --- --- --- --- ---          #c

U32541  ,TRAV26-1*02                                          °

L06886  ,TRAV26-1*03     --- --- --- --- ---                  #c
```

#c: Rearranged cDNA
°: Genomic DNA, but not known as being germline or rearranged

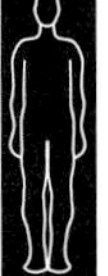

Framework and complementarity determining regions

FR1-IMGT: 25 (-1 aa: 7)   CDR1-IMGT: 7
FR2-IMGT: 17   CDR2-IMGT: 1
FR3-IMGT: 38 (-1 aa: 73)   CDR3-IMGT: 4

Collier de Perles for human TRAV26-1*01

Accession number: IMGT AE000660   EMBL/GenBank/DDBJ: AE000660

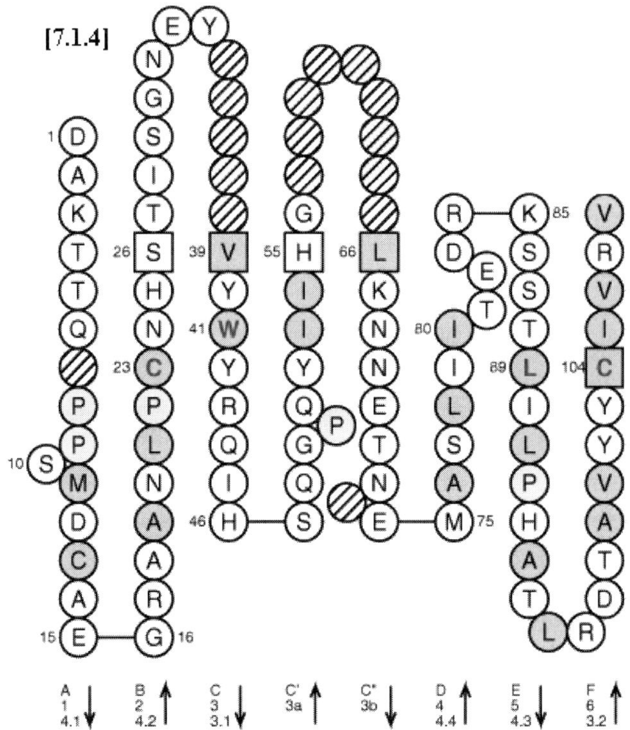

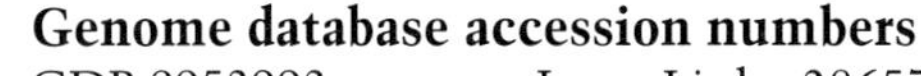

Genome database accession numbers
GDB:9953993   LocusLink: 28657

TRAV26-2

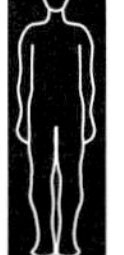

Nomenclature

TRAV26-2: T cell receptor alpha variable 26-2.

Definition and functionality

TRAV26-2 is one of the two functional genes of the TRAV26 subgroup which comprises two mapped genes.

Gene location

TRAV26-2 is in the TRA/TRD locus on chromosome 14 at 14q11.2.

Nucleotide and amino acid sequences for human TRAV26-2

```
                          1   2   3   4   5   6   7   8   9  10  11  12  13  14  15  16  17  18  19  20
                          D   A   K   T   T   Q       P   N   S   M   E   S   N   E   E   E   P   V   H
AE000660,TRAV26-2*01  [6] GAT GCT AAG ACC ACA CAG ... CCA AAT TCA ATG GAG AGT AAC GAA GAA GAG CCT GTT CAC

X04937  ,TRAV26-2*01 [38] --- --- --- --- --- --- ... --- --- --- --- --- --- --- --- --- --- --- --- ---

L11160  ,TRAV26-2*02  [7] --- --- --- --- --- --- ... --- --- --- --- --- --- --- --- --- --- --- --- ---


                                                         __________________CDR1-IMGT__________________
                         21  22  23  24  25  26  27  28  29  30  31  32  33  34  35  36  37  38  39  40
                          L   P   C   N   H   S   T   I   S   G   T   D   Y                       I   H
AE000660,TRAV26-2*01     TTG CCT TGT AAC CAC TCC ACA ATC AGT GGA ACT GAT TAC ... ... ... ... ... ATA CAT

X04937  ,TRAV26-2*01     --- --- --- --- --- --- --- --- --- --- --- --- --- ... ... ... ... ... --- ---

L11160  ,TRAV26-2*02     --- --- --- --- --- --- --- --- --- --- --- --- --- ... ... ... ... ... --- ---


                                                                             ___________________CDR2-
                         41  42  43  44  45  46  47  48  49  50  51  52  53  54  55  56  57  58  59  60
                          W   Y   R   Q   L   P   S   Q   G   P   E   Y   V   I   H   G
AE000660,TRAV26-2*01     TGG TAT CGA CAG CTT CCC TCC CAG GGT CCA GAG TAC GTG ATT CAT GGT ... ... ... ...

X04937  ,TRAV26-2*01     --- --- --- --- --- --- --- --- --- --- --- --- --- --- --- --- ... ... ... ...

L11160  ,TRAV26-2*02     --- --- --- --- --- --- --- --- --- --- --- --- --- --- --- --- ... ... ... ...


                         IMGT________________
                         61  62  63  64  65  66  67  68  69  70  71  72  73  74  75  76  77  78  79  80
                                                  L   T   S   N   V   N   N       R   M   A   S   L   A   I
AE000660,TRAV26-2*01     ... ... ... ... ... CTT ACA AGC AAT GTG AAC AAC ... AGA ATG GCC TCT CTG GCA ATC

X04937  ,TRAV26-2*01     ... ... ... ... ... --- --- --- --- --- --- --- ... --- --- --- --- --- --- ---

                                                                                     C   V
L11160  ,TRAV26-2*02     ... ... ... ... ... --- --- --- --- --- --- --- ... --- --- --- -G- G-- --- ---


                         81  82  83  84  85  86  87  88  89  90  91  92  93  94  95  96  97  98  99 100
                          A   E   D   R   K   S   S   T   L   I   L   H   R   A   T   L   R   D   A   A
AE000660,TRAV26-2*01     GCT GAA GAC AGA AAG TCC AGT ACC TTG ATC CTG CAC CGT GCT ACC TTG AGA GAT GCT GCT

X04937  ,TRAV26-2*01     --- --- --- --- --- --- --- --- --- --- --- --- --- --- --- --- --- --- --- ---

L11160  ,TRAV26-2*02     --- --- --- --- --- --- --- --- -


                                         ___CDR3-IMGT___
                        101 102 103 104 105 106 107 108
                          V   Y   Y   C   I   L   R   D
AE000660,TRAV26-2*01     GTG TAC TAC TGC ATC CTG AGA GAC

X04937  ,TRAV26-2*01     --- --- --- --- ---                    #c

L11160  ,TRAV26-2*02                                            °

#c: Rearranged cDNA
°: Genomic DNA ,but not known as being germline or rearranged
```

Framework and complementarity determining regions

FR1-IMGT: 25 (-1 aa: 7)	CDR1-IMGT: 7
FR2-IMGT: 17	CDR2-IMGT: 1
FR3-IMGT: 38 (-1 aa: 73)	CDR3-IMGT: 4

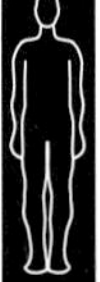

Collier de Perles for human TRAV26-2*01

Accession number: IMGT AE000660   EMBL/GenBank/DDBJ: AE000660

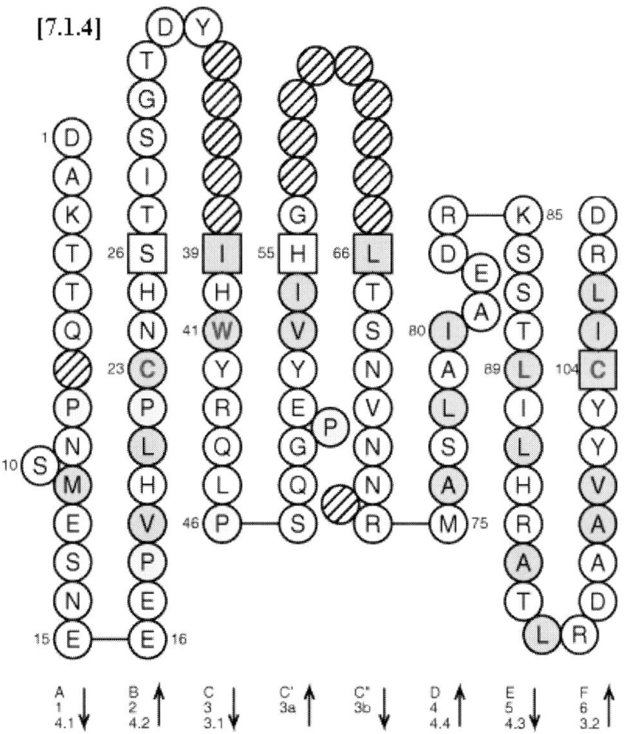

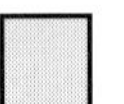

Genome database accession numbers
GDB:9953995   LocusLink: 28656

Nomenclature

TRAV27: T cell receptor alpha variable 27.

Definition and functionality

TRAV27 is the unique functional gene of the TRAV27 subgroup which only comprises this mapped gene.

Gene location

TRAV27 is in the TRA/TRD locus on chromosome 14 at 14q11.2.

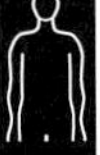

Nucleotide and amino acid sequences for human TRAV27

```
                        1    2    3    4    5    6    7    8    9   10   11   12   13   14   15   16   17   18   19   20
                        T    Q    L    L    E    Q    S    P    Q    F    L    S    I    Q    E    G    E    N    L    T
AE000660,TRAV27*01  [6] ACC  CAG  CTG  CTG  GAG  CAG  AGC  CCT  CAG  TTT  CTA  AGC  ATC  CAA  GAG  GGA  GAA  AAT  CTC  ACT

L09760  ,TRAV27*01 [27]      ---  ---  ---  ---  ---  ---  ---  ---  ---  ---  ---  ---  ---  ---  ---  ---  ---  ---  ---

X04957  ,TRAV27*02 [38] ---  ---  ---  ---  ---  ---  ---  ---  ---  ---  ---  ---  ---  ---  ---  ---  ---  ---  ---  ---

D13075  ,TRAV27*03 [23] ---  ---  ---  ---  ---  ---  ---  ---  ---  ---  ---  ---  ---  ---  ---  ---  ---  ---  ---  ---

L09759  ,TRAV27*03 [27]      ---  ---  ---  ---  ---  ---  ---  ---  ---  ---  ---  ---  ---  ---  ---  ---  ---  ---  ---

U32521  ,TRAV27*02/*03 (1)[5] ---  ---  ---  ---  ---  ---  ---  ---  ---  ---  ---  ---  ---  ---  ---  ---  ---  ---  ---
```

```
                                                        ________________________CDR1-IMGT_____________________
                        21   22   23   24   25   26   27   28   29   30   31   32   33   34   35   36   37   38   39   40
                        V    Y    C    N    S    S    S    V    F    S    S                                      L    Q
AE000660,TRAV27*01      GTG  TAC  TGC  AAC  TCC  TCA  AGT  GTT  TTT  TCC  AGC  ...  ...  ...  ...  ...  ...  ...  TTA  CAA

L09760  ,TRAV27*01      ---  ---  ---  ---  ---  ---  ---  ---  ---  ---  ---  ...  ...  ...  ...  ...  ...  ...  ---  ---

X04957  ,TRAV27*02      ---  ---  ---  ---  ---  ---  ---  ---  ---  ---  ---  ...  ...  ...  ...  ...  ...  ...  ---  ---

D13075  ,TRAV27*03      ---  ---  ---  ---  ---  ---  ---  ---  ---  ---  ---  ...  ...  ...  ...  ...  ...  ...  ---  ---

L09759  ,TRAV27*03      ---  ---  ---  ---  ---  ---  ---  ---  ---  ---  ---  ...  ...  ...  ...  ...  ...  ...  ---  ---

U32521  ,TRAV27*02/*03 (1) ---  ---  ---  ---  ---  ---  ---  ---  ---  ---  ---  ...  ...  ...  ...  ...  ...  ...  ---  ---
```

```
                                                                                            ____________CDR2-
                        41   42   43   44   45   46   47   48   49   50   51   52   53   54   55   56   57   58   59   60
                        W    Y    R    Q    E    P    G    E    G    P    V    L    L    V    T    V    V    T
AE000660,TRAV27*01      TGG  TAC  AGA  CAG  GAG  CCT  GGG  GAA  GGT  CCT  GTC  CTC  CTG  GTG  ACA  GTA  GTT  ACG  ...  ...

L09760  ,TRAV27*01      ---  ---  ---  ---  ---  ---  ---  ---  ---  ---  ---  ---  ---  ---  ---  ---  ---  ---  ...  ...

X04957  ,TRAV27*02      ---  ---  --G  ---  ---  ---  ---  ---  ---  ---  ---  ---  ---  ---  ---  ---  ---  ---  ...  ...

D13075  ,TRAV27*03      ---  ---  --G  ---  ---  ---  ---  ---  ---  ---  ---  ---  ---  ---  ---  ---  ---  ---  ...  ...

L09759  ,TRAV27*03      ---  ---  --G  ---  ---  ---  ---  ---  ---  ---  ---  ---  ---  ---  ---  ---  ---  ---  ...  ...

U32521  ,TRAV27*02/*03 (1) ---  ---  --G  ---  ---  ---  ---  ---  ---  ---  ---  ---  ---  ---  ---  ---  ---  ---  ...  ...
```

```
                        IMGT________
                        61   62   63   64   65   66   67   68   69   70   71   72   73   74   75   76   77   78   79   80
                                                       G    G    E    V    K    K    L         K    R    L    T    F    Q    F
AE000660,TRAV27*01      ...  ...  ...  ...  ...  GGT  GGA  GAA  GTG  AAG  AAG  CTG  ...  AAG  AGA  CTA  ACC  TTT  CAG  TTT

L09760  ,TRAV27*01      ...  ...  ...  ...  ...  ---  ---  ---  ---  ---  ---  ---  ...  ---  ---  ---  ---  ---  ---  ---

X04957  ,TRAV27*02      ...  ...  ...  ...  ...  ---  ---  ---  ---  ---  ---  ---  ...  ---  ---  ---  ---  ---  ---  ---

D13075  ,TRAV27*03      ...  ...  ...  ...  ...  ---  ---  ---  ---  ---  ---  ---  ...  ---  ---  ---  ---  ---  ---  ---

L09759  ,TRAV27*03      ...  ...  ...  ...  ...  ---  ---  ---  ---  ---  ---  ---  ...  ---  ---  ---  ---  ---  ---  ---

U32521  ,TRAV27*02/*03 (1) ...  ...  ...  ...  ...  ---  ---  ---  ---  ---  ---  ---  ...  ---  ---  ---  ---  ---  ---  ---
```

```
                        81   82   83   84   85   86   87   88   89   90   91   92   93   94   95   96   97   98   99  100
                        G    D    A    R    K    D    S    S    L    H    I    T    A    A    Q    P    G    D    T    G
AE000660,TRAV27*01      GGT  GAT  GCA  AGA  AAG  GAC  AGT  TCT  CTC  CAC  ATC  ACT  GCA  GCC  CAG  CCT  GGT  GAT  ACA  GGC

L09760  ,TRAV27*01      ---  ---  ---  ---  ---  ---  ---  ---  ---  ---  ---  ---  ---  ---  ---  ---  ---  ---  ---  ---

X04957  ,TRAV27*02      ---  ---  ---  ---  ---  ---  ---  ---  ---  ---  ---  ---  --G  ---  ---  ---  ---  ---  ---  ---
                                                                                                       T
D13075  ,TRAV27*03      ---  ---  ---  ---  ---  ---  ---  ---  ---  ---  ---  ---  --G  ---  ---  A--  ---  ---  ---  ---
                                                                                                       T
L09759  ,TRAV27*03      ---  ---  ---  ---  ---  ---  ---  ---  ---  ---  ---  ---  --G  ---  ---  A--  ---  ---  ---  ---

U32521  ,TRAV27*02/*03 (1)
```

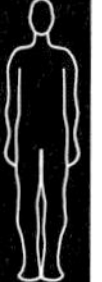

```
                                          -CDR3-IMGT-
                              101 102 103 104 105 106
                               L   Y   L   C   A   G
    AE000660,TRAV27*01       CTC TAC CTC TGT GCA GGA G

    L09760  ,TRAV27*01       --- --- --- ---                    o
                              H
    X04957  ,TRAV27*02       -A- --- --- --- --- --C            #c
                              H
    D13075  ,TRAV27*03       -A- --- --- --- ---                #c
                              H
    L09759  ,TRAV27*03       -A- --- --- ---

    U32521  ,TRAV27*02/*03 (1)                                  o

#c: Rearranged cDNA sequence
o: Genomic DNA, but not known as being germline or rearranged
```

Note:

(1) Partial sequence which could not be assigned to a given allele.

Framework and complementarity determining regions

FR1-IMGT: 26

FR2-IMGT: 17

FR3-IMGT: 38 (-1 aa: 73)

CDR1-IMGT: 5

CDR2-IMGT: 3

CDR3-IMGT: 2

Collier de Perles for human TRAV27*01

Accession number: IMGT AE000660   EMBL/GenBank/DDBJ: AE000660

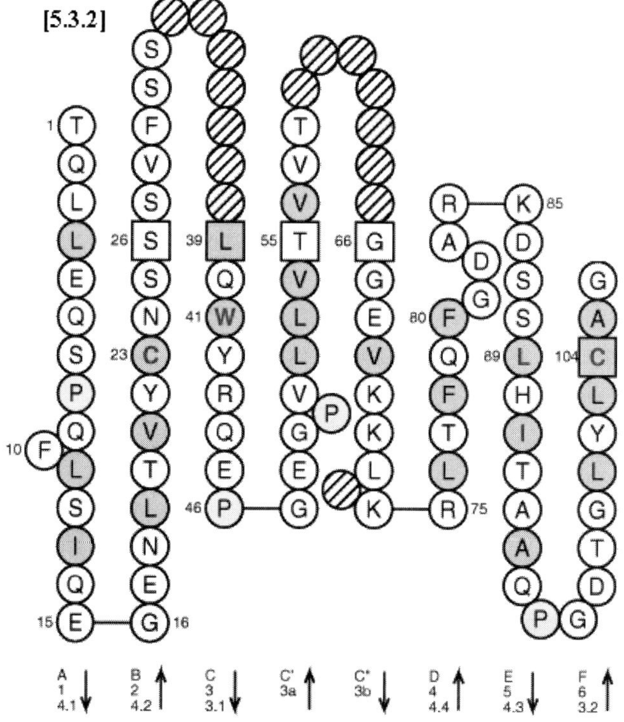

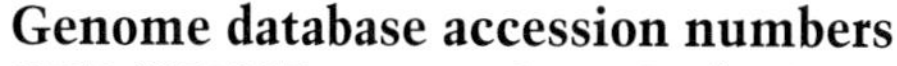

Genome database accession numbers

GDB:9953997   LocusLink: 28655

Nomenclature

TRAV29/DV5: T cell receptor alpha variable 29/delta variable 5.

Definition and functionality

TRAV29/DV5 is a functional gene (alleles *01 and *02) or a pseudogene (allele *03). TRAV29/DV5 belongs to the TRAV29 subgroup which only comprises this mapped gene.

TRAV29/DV5*03 is a pseudogene due to a 1 nt DELETION in codon 42 leading to a frameshift in FR2-IMGT.

TRAV29/DV5 has been found rearranged to both (D)J genes of the TRD locus and TRAJ genes, the TRD locus being embedded in the TRA locus. This gene can therefore be used for the synthesis of both delta and alpha chains.

Gene location

TRAV29/DV5 is in the TRA/TRD locus on chromosome 14 at 14q11.2.

Nucleotide and amino acid sequences for human TRAV29/DV5

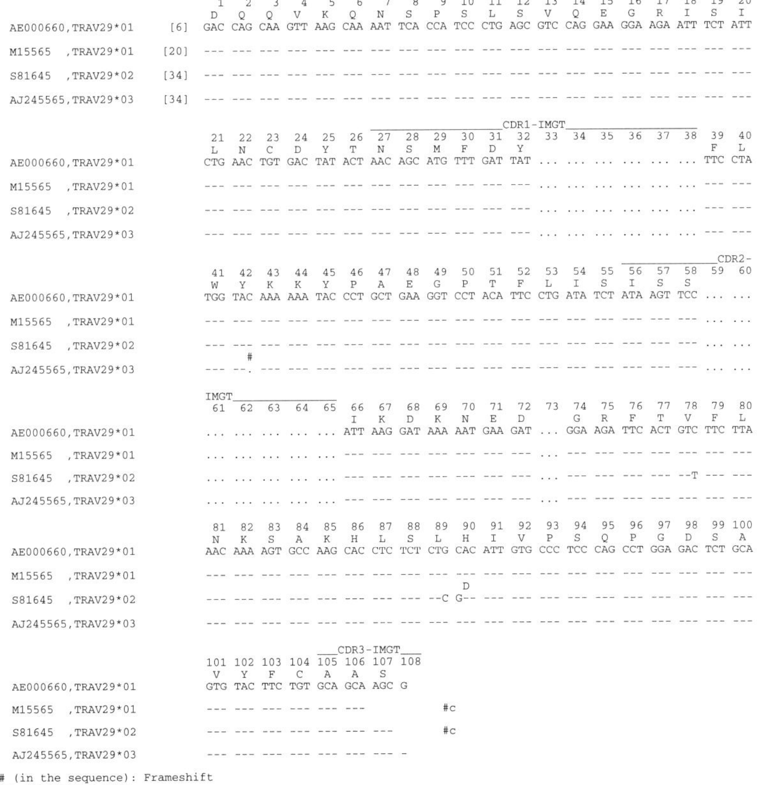

```
                                  1   2   3   4   5   6   7   8   9  10  11  12  13  14  15  16  17  18  19  20
                                  D   Q   Q   V   K   Q   N   S   P   S   L   S   V   Q   E   G   R   I   S   I
  AE000660,TRAV29*01      [6]   GAC CAG CAA GTT AAG CAA AAT TCA CCA TCC CTG AGC GTC CAG GAA GGA AGA ATT TCT ATT
  M15565  ,TRAV29*01     [20]   --- --- --- --- --- --- --- --- --- --- --- --- --- --- --- --- --- --- --- ---
  S81645  ,TRAV29*02     [34]   --- --- --- --- --- --- --- --- --- --- --- --- --- --- --- --- --- --- --- ---
  AJ245565,TRAV29*03     [34]   --- --- --- --- --- --- --- --- --- --- --- --- --- --- --- --- --- --- --- ---

                                                                       ______________________CDR1-IMGT__________
                                 21  22  23  24  25  26  27  28  29  30  31  32  33  34  35  36  37  38  39  40
                                  L   N   C   D   Y   T   N   S   M   F   D   Y                           F   L
  AE000660,TRAV29*01            CTG AAC TGT GAC TAT ACT AAC AGC ATG TTT GAT TAT ... ... ... ... ... ... TTC CTA
  M15565  ,TRAV29*01            --- --- --- --- --- --- --- --- --- --- --- --- ... ... ... ... ... ... --- ---
  S81645  ,TRAV29*02            --- --- --- --- --- --- --- --- --- --- --- --- ... ... ... ... ... ... --- ---
  AJ245565,TRAV29*03            --- --- --- --- --- --- --- --- --- --- --- --- ... ... ... ... ... ... --- ---

                                                                                               ________________CDR2-
                                 41  42  43  44  45  46  47  48  49  50  51  52  53  54  55  56  57  58  59  60
                                  W   Y   K   K   Y   P   A   E   G   P   T   F   L   I   S   I   S   S
  AE000660,TRAV29*01            TGG TAC AAA AAA TAC CCT GCT GAA GGT CCT ACA TTC CTG ATA TCT ATA AGT TCC ... ...
  M15565  ,TRAV29*01            --- --- --- --- --- --- --- --- --- --- --- --- --- --- --- --- --- --- ... ...
  S81645  ,TRAV29*02            --- --- --- --- --- --- --- --- --- --- --- --- --- --- --- --- --- --- ... ...
                                       #
  AJ245565,TRAV29*03            --- --. --- --- --- --- --- --- --- --- --- --- --- --- --- --- --- --- ... ...

                                IMGT______________________
                                 61  62  63  64  65  66  67  68  69  70  71  72  73  74  75  76  77  78  79  80
                                                  I   K   D   K   N   E   D       G   R   F   T   V   F   L
  AE000660,TRAV29*01            ... ... ... ... ... ATT AAG GAT AAA AAT GAA GAT ... GGA AGA TTC ACT GTC TTC TTA
  M15565  ,TRAV29*01            ... ... ... ... ... --- --- --- --- --- --- --- ... --- --- --- --- --- --- ---
  S81645  ,TRAV29*02            ... ... ... ... ... --- --- --- --- --- --- --- ... --- --- --- --- --T --- ---
  AJ245565,TRAV29*03            ... ... ... ... ... --- --- --- --- --- --- --- ... --- --- --- --- --- --- ---

                                 81  82  83  84  85  86  87  88  89  90  91  92  93  94  95  96  97  98  99 100
                                  N   K   S   A   K   H   L   S   L   H   I   V   P   S   Q   P   G   D   S   A
  AE000660,TRAV29*01            AAC AAA AGT GCC AAG CAC CTC TCT CTG CAC ATT GTG CCC TCC CAG CCT GGA GAC TCT GCA
  M15565  ,TRAV29*01            --- --- --- --- --- --- --- --- --- --- --- --- --- --- --- --- --- --- --- ---
                                                                      D
  S81645  ,TRAV29*02            --- --- --- --- --- --- --- --- --C G-- --- --- --- --- --- --- --- --- --- ---
  AJ245565,TRAV29*03            --- --- --- --- --- --- --- --- --- --- --- --- --- --- --- --- --- --- --- ---

                                       ____CDR3-IMGT____
                                101 102 103 104 105 106 107 108
                                  V   Y   F   C   A   A   S
  AE000660,TRAV29*01            GTG TAC TTC TGT GCA GCA AGC G
  M15565  ,TRAV29*01            --- --- --- --- --- ---           #c
  S81645  ,TRAV29*02            --- --- --- --- --- --- ---       #c
  AJ245565,TRAV29*03            --- --- --- --- --- --- --- -
```

\# (in the sequence): Frameshift
\#c: Rearranged cDNA

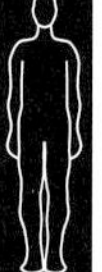

Framework and complementarity determining regions

FR1-IMGT: 26
FR2-IMGT: 17
FR3-IMGT: 38 (-1 aa: 73)

CDR1-IMGT: 6
CDR2-IMGT: 3
CDR3-IMGT: 3

Collier de Perles for human TRAV29/DV5*01

Accession number: IMGT AE000660   EMBL/GenBank/DDBJ: AE000660

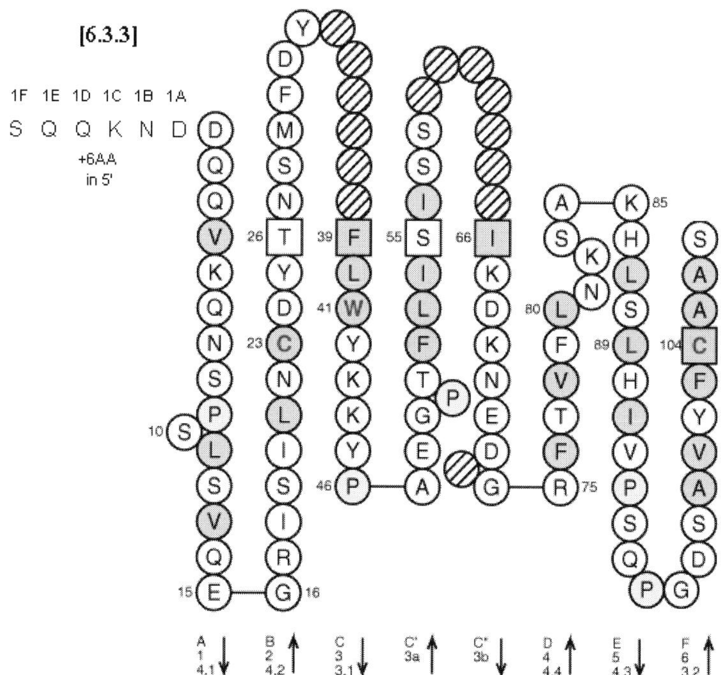

Note:
The 6 additional amino acids, predicted by the program SIGSEQ2 and described by Wülfing, C. and Plückthun, A. (1995) Immunology Today 16, 405–406, are numbered 1A to 1F.

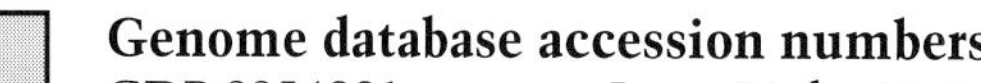

Genome database accession numbers
GDB:9954001   LocusLink: 28653

TRAV30

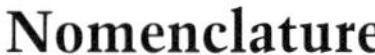

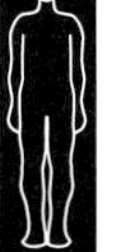

Nomenclature

TRAV30: T cell receptor alpha variable 30.

Definition and functionality

TRAV30 is the unique functional gene of the TRAV30 subgroup which only comprises this mapped gene.

Gene location

TRAV30 is in the TRA/TRD locus on chromosome 14 at 14q11.2.

Nucleotide and amino acid sequences for human TRAV30

```
                           1   2   3   4   5   6   7   8   9  10  11  12  13  14  15  16  17  18  19  20
                           Q   Q   P   V       Q   S   P   Q   A   V   I   L   R   E   G   E   D   A   V
AE000660,TRAV30*01   [6]  CAA CAA CCA GTG ... CAG AGT CCT CAA GCC GTG ATC CTC CGA GAA GGG GAA GAT GCT GTC
S63879  ,TRAV30*01  [20]  --- --- --- --- ... --- --- --- --- --- --- --- --- --- --- --- --- --- --- ---
X58768  ,TRAV30*02  [28]  --- --- --- --- ... --- --- --- --- --- --- --- --- --- --- --- --- --- --- ---
L06883  ,TRAV30*03  [29]  --- --- --- --- ... --- --- --- --- --- --- --- --- --- --- --- --- --- --- ---
U32537  ,TRAV30*04   [5]  --- --- --- --- ... --- --- --- --- --- --- --- --- --- --- --- --- --- --- ---

                                                                      ___________________CDR1-IMGT_____________________
                          21  22  23  24  25  26  27  28  29  30  31  32  33  34  35  36  37  38  39  40
                           I   N   C   S   S   S   K   A   L   Y   S                               V   H
AE000660,TRAV30*01        ATC AAC TGC AGT TCC TCC AAG GCT TTA TAT TCT ... ... ... ... ... ... ... GTA CAC
S63879  ,TRAV30*01        --- --- --- --- --- --- --- --- --- --- --- ... ... ... ... ... ... ... --- ---
                           T
X58768  ,TRAV30*02        -C- --- --- --- --- --- --- --- --- --- --- ... ... ... ... ... ... ... --- ---
L06883  ,TRAV30*03        --- --- --- --- --- --- --- --- --- --- --- ... ... ... ... ... ... ... --- ---
U32537  ,TRAV30*04        --- --- --- --- --- --- --- --- --- --- --- ... ... ... ... ... ... ... --- ---

                                                                                              _______________CDR2-
                          41  42  43  44  45  46  47  48  49  50  51  52  53  54  55  56  57  58  59  60
                           W   Y   R   Q   K   H   G   E   A   P   V   F   L   M   I   L   L   K
AE000660,TRAV30*01        TGG TAC AGG CAG AAG CAT GGT GAA GCA CCC GTC TTC CTG ATG ATA TTA CTG AAG ... ...
S63879  ,TRAV30*01        --- --- --- --- --- --- --- --- --- --- --- --- --- --- --- --- --- --- ... ...
X58768  ,TRAV30*02        --- --- --- --- --- --- --- --- --- --- --- --- --- --- --- --- --- --- ... ...
L06883  ,TRAV30*03        --- --- --- --- --- --- --- --- --- --- --- --- --- --- --- --- --- --- ... ...
U32537  ,TRAV30*04        --- --- --- --- --- --- --- --- --- --- --- --- --- --- --- --- --- --- ... ...

                          IMGT________________
                          61  62  63  64  65  66  67  68  69  70  71  72  73  74  75  76  77  78  79  80
                                                   G   G   E   Q   K   G   H       E   K   I   S   A   S   F
AE000660,TRAV30*01        ... ... ... ... ... GGT GGA GAA CAG AAG GGT CAT ... GAA AAA ATA TCT GCT TCA TTT
S63879  ,TRAV30*01        ... ... ... ... ... --- --- --- --- --- --- --- ... --- --- --- --- --- --- ---
                                                               M   R   R
X58768  ,TRAV30*02        ... ... ... ... ... --- --- --- --- -T- C-- -G- ... --- --- --- --- --- --- ---
L06883  ,TRAV30*03        ... ... ... ... ... --- --- --- --- --- --- --- ... --- --- --- --- --- --- ---
                                                                   R
U32537  ,TRAV30*04        ... ... ... ... ... --- --- --- --- --- C-- --- ... --- --- --- --- --- --- ---

                          81  82  83  84  85  86  87  88  89  90  91  92  93  94  95  96  97  98  99 100
                           N   E   K   K   Q   Q   S   S   L   Y   L   T   A   S   Q   L   S   Y   S   G
AE000660,TRAV30*01        AAT GAA AAA AAG CAG CAA AGC TCC CTG TAC CTT ACG GCC TCC CAG CTC AGT TAC TCA GGA
S63879  ,TRAV30*01        --- --- --- --- --- --- --- --- --- --- --- --- --- --- --- --- --- --- --- ---
X58768  ,TRAV30*02        --- --- --- --- --- --- --- --- --- --- --- --- --- --- --- --- --- --- --- ---
                                               R
L06883  ,TRAV30*03        --- --- --- --- -G- --- --- --- --- --- --- --- --- --- --- --- --- --- --- ---
U32537  ,TRAV30*04        --- --- --- --- --- --- --- --- --- --- --- --- --- --- --- --- --

                                       ___CDR3-IMGT____
                         101 102 103 104 105 106 107 108
                           T   Y   F   C   G   T   E
AE000660,TRAV30*01        ACC TAC TTC TGC GGC ACA GAG A
S63879  ,TRAV30*01        --- --- --- --- --- ---        #g
X58768  ,TRAV30*02        --- --- --- --- --G            #c
L06883  ,TRAV30*03        --- --- --- --- ---            #c
U32537  ,TRAV30*04                                       °

#c: Rearranged cDNA
#g: Rearranged genomic DNA
°: Genomic DNA, but not known as being germline or rearranged
```

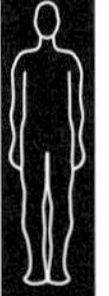

Framework and complementarity determining regions

FR1-IMGT: 25 (-1 aa: 5)   CDR1-IMGT: 5
FR2-IMGT: 17   CDR2-IMGT: 3
FR3-IMGT: 38 (-1 aa: 73)   CDR3-IMGT: 3

Collier de Perles for human TRAV30*01

Accession number: IMGT AE000660   EMBL/GenBank/DDBJ: AE000660

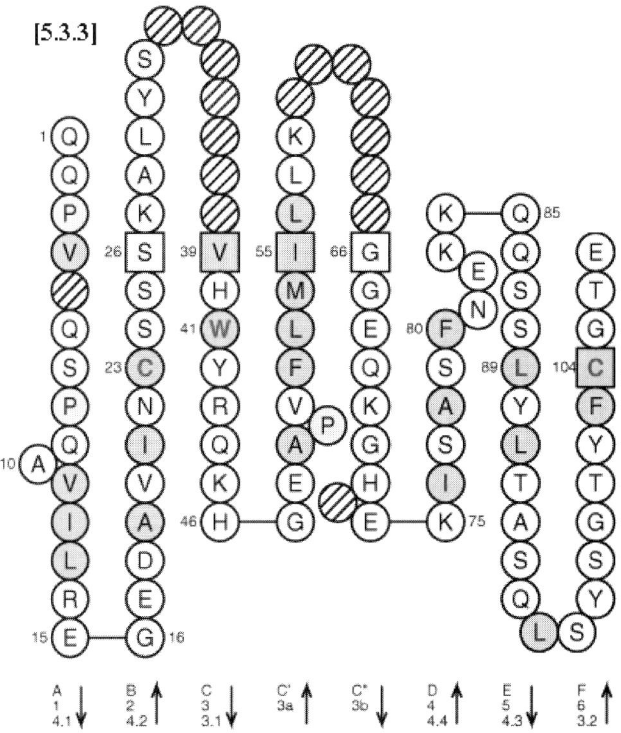

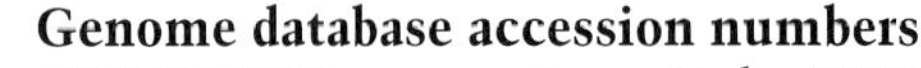

Genome database accession numbers
GDB:9954003   LocusLink: 28652

TRAV34

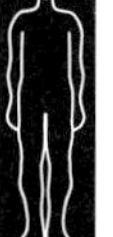

Nomenclature

TRAV34: T cell receptor alpha variable 34.

Definition and functionality

TRAV34 is the unique functional gene of the TRAV34 subgroup which only comprises this mapped gene.

Gene location

TRAV34 is in the TRA/TRD locus on chromosome 14 at 14q11.2.

Nucleotide and amino acid sequences for human TRAV34

```
                          1    2    3    4    5    6    7    8    9   10   11   12   13   14   15   16   17   18   19   20
                          S    Q    E    L    E    Q    S    P    Q    S    L    I    V    Q    E    G    K    N    L    T
AE000660,TRAV34*01   [6]  AGC  CAA  GAA  CTG  GAG  CAG  AGT  CCT  CAG  TCC  TTG  ATC  GTC  CAA  GAG  GGA  AAG  AAT  CTC  ACC

X58739  ,TRAV34*01  [28]  ---  ---  ---  ---  ---  ---  ---  ---  ---  ---  ---  ---  ---  ---  ---  ---  ---  ---  ---  ---

U32534  ,TRAV34*01   [5]  ---  ---  ---  ---  ---  ---  ---  ---  ---  ---  ---  ---  ---  ---  ---  ---  ---  ---  ---  ---


                                                              ________________________CDR1-IMGT________________________
                          21   22   23   24   25   26   27   28   29   30   31   32   33   34   35   36   37   38   39   40
                          I    N    C    T    S    S    K    T    L    Y    G                                  L    Y
AE000660,TRAV34*01        ATA  AAC  TGC  ACG  TCA  TCA  AAG  ACG  TTA  TAT  GGC  ...  ...  ...  ...  ...  ...  ...  TTA  TAC

X58739  ,TRAV34*01        ---  ---  ---  ---  ---  ---  ---  ---  ---  ---  ---  ...  ...  ...  ...  ...  ...  ...  ---  ---

U32534  ,TRAV34*01        ---  ---  ---  ---  ---  ---  ---  ---  ---  ---  ---  ...  ...  ...  ...  ...  ...  ...  ---  ---


                                                                                          ____________________CDR2-
                          41   42   43   44   45   46   47   48   49   50   51   52   53   54   55   56   57   58   59   60
                          W    Y    K    Q    K    Y    G    E    G    L    I    F    L    M    M    L    Q    K
AE000660,TRAV34*01        TGG  TAT  AAG  CAA  AAG  TAT  GGT  GAA  GGT  CTT  ATC  TTC  TTG  ATG  ATG  CTA  CAG  AAA  ...  ...

X58739  ,TRAV34*01        ---  ---  ---  ---  ---  ---  ---  ---  ---  ---  ---  ---  ---  ---  ---  ---  ---  ---  ...  ...

U32534  ,TRAV34*01        ---  ---  ---  ---  ---  ---  ---  ---  ---  ---  ---  ---  ---  ---  ---  ---  ---  ---  ---  ...  ...


                          IMGT________________
                          61   62   63   64   65   66   67   68   69   70   71   72   73   74   75   76   77   78   79   80
                                                    G    G    E    E    K    S    H         E    K    I    T    A    K    L
AE000660,TRAV34*01        ...  ...  ...  ...  ...  GGT  GGG  GAA  GAG  AAA  AGT  CAT  ...  GAA  AAG  ATA  ACT  GCC  AAG  TTG

X58739  ,TRAV34*01        ...  ...  ...  ...  ...  ---  ---  ---  ---  ---  ---  ---  ...  ---  ---  ---  ---  ---  ---  ---

U32534  ,TRAV34*01        ...  ...  ...  ...  ...  ---  ---  ---  ---  ---  ---  ---  ...  ---  ---  ---  ---  ---  ---  ---


                          81   82   83   84   85   86   87   88   89   90   91   92   93   94   95   96   97   98   99  100
                          D    E    K    K    Q    S    S    L    H    I    T    A    S    Q    P    S    H    A    G
AE000660,TRAV34*01        GAT  GAG  AAA  AAG  CAG  CAA  AGT  TCC  CTG  CAT  ATC  ACA  GCC  TCC  CAG  CCC  AGC  CAT  GCA  GGC

X58739  ,TRAV34*01        ---  ---  ---  ---  ---  ---  ---  ---  ---  ---  ---  ---  ---  ---  ---  ---  ---  ---  ---  ---

U32534  ,TRAV34*01        ---  ---  ---  ---  ---  ---  ---  ---  ---  ---  ---  ---  ---  -


                          ____CDR3-IMGT_
                          101  102  103  104  105  106  107
                          I    Y    L    C    G    A    D
AE000660,TRAV34*01        ATC  TAC  CTC  TGT  GGA  GCA  GAC  A

X58739  ,TRAV34*01        ---  ---  ---  ---  ---                 #c

U32534  ,TRAV34*01                                              o
```

#c: Rearranged cDNA
o: Genomic DNA, but not known as being germline or rearranged

Framework and complementarity determining regions

FR1-IMGT: 26	CDR1-IMGT: 5
FR2-IMGT: 17	CDR2-IMGT: 3
FR3-IMGT: 38 (-1 aa: 73)	CDR3-IMGT: 3

Collier de Perles for human TRAV34*01

Accession number: IMGT AE000660   EMBL/GenBank/DDBJ: AE000660

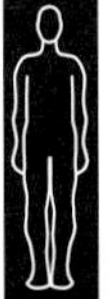

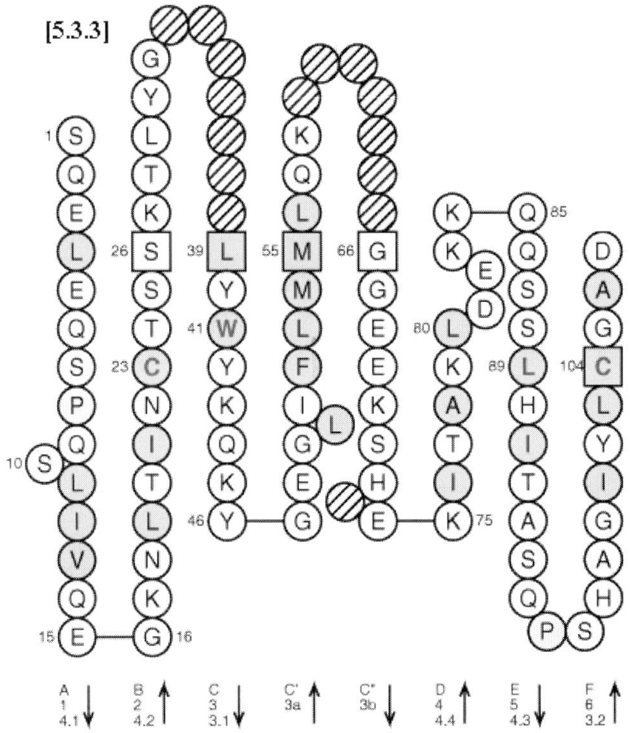

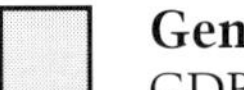

Genome database accession numbers
GDB:9954011   LocusLink: 28648

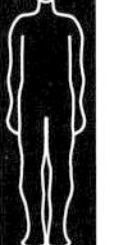

Nomenclature

TRAV35: T cell receptor alpha variable 35.

Definition and functionality

TRAV35 is the unique functional gene of the TRAV35 subgroup which only comprises this mapped gene.

Gene location

TRAV35 is in the TRA/TRD locus on chromosome 14 at 14q11.2.

Nucleotide and amino acid sequences for human TRAV35

```
                          1   2   3   4   5   6   7   8   9  10  11  12  13  14  15  16  17  18  19  20
                          G   Q   Q   L   N   Q   S   P   Q   S   M   F   I   Q   E   G   E   D   V   S
AE000660,TRAV35*01   [6]  GGT CAA CAG CTG AAT CAG AGT CCT CAA TCT ATG TTT ATC CAG GAA GGA GAA GAT GTC TCC

X58738  ,TRAV35*02  [28]  --- --- --- --- --- --- --- --- --- --- --- --- --- --- --- --- --- --- --- ---

U32533  ,TRAV35*02   [5]  --- --- --- --- --- --- --- --- --- --- --- --- --- --- --- --- --- --- --- ---


                                                         ___________________CDR1-IMGT___________________
                         21  22  23  24  25  26  27  28  29  30  31  32  33  34  35  36  37  38  39  40
                          M   N   C   T   S   S   S   I   F   N   T                               W   L
AE000660,TRAV35*01       ATG AAC TGC ACT TCT TCA AGC ATA TTT AAC ACC ... ... ... ... ... ... ... TGG CTA

X58738  ,TRAV35*02       --- --- --- --- --- --- --- --- --- --- --- ... ... ... ... ... ... ... --- ---

U32533  ,TRAV35*02       --- --- --- --- --- --- --- --- --- --- --- ... ... ... ... ... ... ... --- ---


                                                                                 _________________CDR2-
                         41  42  43  44  45  46  47  48  49  50  51  52  53  54  55  56  57  58  59  60
                          W   Y   K   Q   E   P   G   E   G   P   V   L   L   I   A   L   Y   K
AE000660,TRAV35*01       TGG TAC AAG CAG GAA CCT GGG GAA GGT CCT GTC CTC TTG ATA GCC TTA TAT AAG ... ...
                                          D
X58738  ,TRAV35*02       --- --- --- --- --C --- --- --- --- --- --- --- --- --- --- --- --- --- ... ...
                                          D
U32533  ,TRAV35*02       --- --- --- --- --C --- --- --- --- --- --- --- --- --- --- --- --- --- ... ...


                         IMGT________________
                         61  62  63  64  65  66  67  68  69  70  71  72  73  74  75  76  77  78  79  80
                                              A   G   E   L   T   S   N       G   R   L   T   A   Q   F
AE000660,TRAV35*01       ... ... ... ... ... GCT GGT GAA TTG ACC TCA AAT ... GGA AGA CTG ACT GCT CAG TTT

X58738  ,TRAV35*02       ... ... ... ... ... --- --- --- --- --- --- --- ... --- --- --- --- --- --- ---

U32533  ,TRAV35*02       ... ... ... ... ... --- --- --- --- --- --- --- ... --- --- --- --- --- --- ---


                         81  82  83  84  85  86  87  88  89  90  91  92  93  94  95  96  97  98  99 100
                          G   I   T   R   K   D   S   F   L   N   I   S   A   S   I   P   S   D   V   G
AE000660,TRAV35*01       GGT ATA ACC AGA AAG GAC AGC TTC CTG AAT ATC TCA GCA TCC ATA CCT AGT GAT GTA GGC

X58738  ,TRAV35*02       --- --- --- --- --- --- --- --- --- --- --- --- --- --- --- --- --- --- --- ---

U32533  ,TRAV35*02       --- --- --- --- --- --- --- --- --- --- --- --- --- --- --- --- --- --- --- ---


                              _CDR3-IMGT_
                         101 102 103 104 105 106 107
                          I   Y   F   C   A   G   Q
AE000660,TRAV35*01       ATC TAC TTC TGT GCT GGG CAG

X58738  ,TRAV35*02       --- --- --- --- ---         #c

U32533  ,TRAV35*02                                   o
```

#c Rearranged cDNA
o: Genomic DNA, but not known as being germline or rearranged

Framework and complementarity determining regions

FR1-IMGT: 26	CDR1-IMGT: 5
FR2-IMGT: 17	CDR2-IMGT: 3
FR3-IMGT: 38 (-1 aa: 73)	CDR3-IMGT: 3

Collier de Perles for human TRAV35*01

Accession number: IMGT AE000660   EMBL/GenBank/DDBJ: AE000660

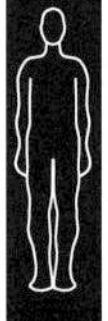

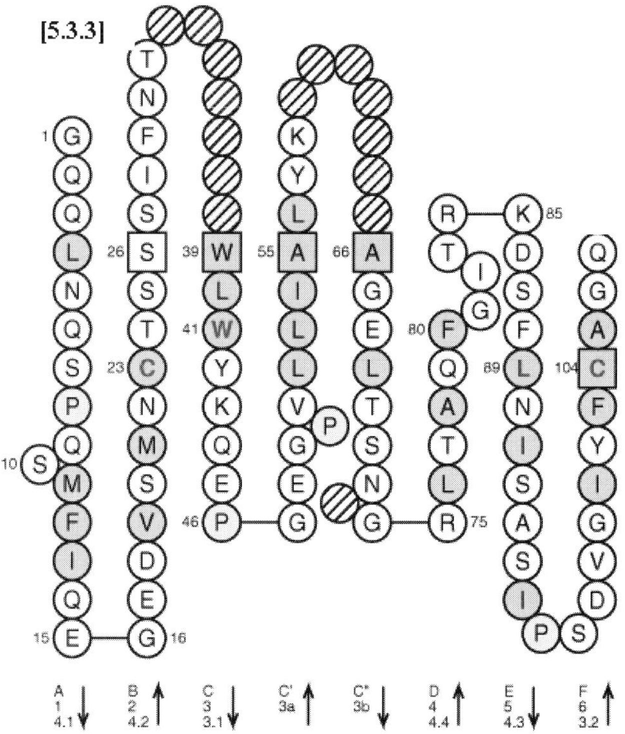

Genome database accession numbers
GDB:9954013   LocusLink: 28647

TRAV36/DV7

Nomenclature

TRAV36/DV7: T cell receptor alpha variable 36/delta variable 7.

Definition and functionality

TRAV36/DV7 is the unique functional gene of the TRAV36 subgroup which only comprises this mapped gene.

TRAV36/DV7 has been found rearranged to both (D)J genes of the TRD locus and TRAJ genes, the TRD locus being embedded in the TRA locus. This gene can therefore be used for the synthesis of both delta and alpha chains.

Gene location

TRAV36/DV7 is in the TRA/TRD locus on chromosome 14 at 14q11.2.

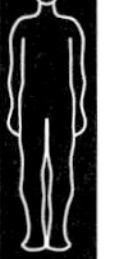

Nucleotide and amino acid sequences for human TRAV36/DV7

```
                            1   2   3   4   5   6   7   8   9   10  11  12  13  14  15  16  17  18  19  20
                            E   D   K   V   V   Q   S   P   L   S   L   V   V   H   E   G   D   T   V   T
AE000660,TRAV36*01   [6]   GAA GAC AAG GTG GTA CAA AGC CCT CTA TCT CTG GTT GTC CAC GAG GGA GAC ACC GTA ACT
                                                            Q
X61070  ,TRAV36*02  [28]   --- --- --- --- --- --- --- --- -A- --- --- --- --- --- --- --- --- --T --- ---
X58767  ,TRAV36*03  [28]   --- --- --- --- --- --- --- --- --- --- --- --- --- --- --- --- --- --T --- ---
Z46643  ,TRAV36*04  [22]   --- --- --- --- --- --- --- --- --- --- --- --- --- --- --- --- --- --T --- ---
U32536  ,TRAV36*04   [5]   --- --- --- --- --- --- --- --- --- --- --- --- --- --- --- --- --- --T --- ---


                                                           __________________CDR1-IMGT___________________
                            21  22  23  24  25  26  27  28  29  30  31  32  33  34  35  36  37  38  39  40
                            L   N   C   S   Y   E   V   T   N   F   R   S                           L   L
AE000660,TRAV36*01         CTC AAT TGC AGT TAT GAA GTG ACT AAC TTT CGA AGC ... ... ... ... ... ... CTA CTA
                                                        M                                               Q
X61070  ,TRAV36*02         --- --- --- --- --- --- A-- --- --- --- --- --- ... ... ... ... ... ... --- -A-
                            P
X58767  ,TRAV36*03         -C- --- --- --- --- --- --- --- --- --- --- --- ... ... ... ... ... ... --- ---
Z46643  ,TRAV36*04         --- --- --- --- --- --- --- --- --- --- --- --- ... ... ... ... ... ... --- ---
U32536  ,TRAV36*04         --- --- --- --- --- --- --- --- --- --- --- --- ... ... ... ... ... ... --- ---


                                                                                           ____________CDR2-
                            41  42  43  44  45  46  47  48  49  50  51  52  53  54  55  56  57  58  59  60
                            W   Y   K   Q   E   K   K   A   P       T   F   L   F   M   L   T   S
AE000660,TRAV36*01         TGG TAC AAG CAG GAA AAG AAA GCT CCC ... ACA TTT CTA TTT ATG CTA ACT TCA ... ...
X61070  ,TRAV36*02         --- --- --- --- --- --- --- --- --- ... --- --- --- --- --- --- --- --- ... ...
X58767  ,TRAV36*03         --- --- --- --- --- --- --- --- --- ... --- --- --- --- --- --- --- --- ... ...
Z46643  ,TRAV36*04         --- --- --- --- --- --- --- --- --- ... --- --- --- --- --- --- --- --- ... ...
U32536  ,TRAV36*04         --- --- --- --- --- --- --- --- --- ... --- --- --- --- --- --- --- --- ... ...


                            IMGT______________________
                            61  62  63  64  65  66  67  68  69  70  71  72  73  74  75  76  77  78  79  80
                                                        S   G   I   E   K   K   S       G   R   L   S   S   I   L
AE000660,TRAV36*01         ... ... ... ... ... AGT GGA ATT GAA AAG AAG TCA ... GGA AGA CTA AGT AGC ATA TTA
X61070  ,TRAV36*02         ... ... ... ... ... --- --- --- --- --- --- --- ... --- --- --- --- --- --- ---
X58767  ,TRAV36*03         ... ... ... ... ... --- --- --- --- --- --- --- ... --- --- --- --- --- --- ---
Z46643  ,TRAV36*04         ... ... ... ... ... --- --- --- --- --- --- --- ... --- --- --- --- --- --- ---
U32536  ,TRAV36*04         ... ... ... ... ... --- --- --- --- --- --- --- ... --- --- --- --- --- --- ---


                            81  82  83  84  85  86  87  88  89  90  91  92  93  94  95  96  97  98  99  100
                            D   K   K   E   L   S   S   I   L   N   I   T   A   T   Q   T   G   D   S   A
AE000660,TRAV36*01         GAT AAG AAA GAA CTT TCC AGC ATC CTG AAC ATC ACA GCC ACC CAG ACC GGA GAC TCG GCC
                                                        F
X61070  ,TRAV36*02         --- --- --- --- --- -T- --- --- --- --- --- --- --- --- --- --- --- --- --- ---
                                                        F
X58767  ,TRAV36*03         --- --- --- --- --- -T- --- --- --- --- --- --- --- --- --- --- --- --- --- ---
                                                        F
Z46643  ,TRAV36*04         --- --- --- --- --- -T- --- --- --- --- --- --- --- --- --- --- --- --- --- ---
                                                        F
U32536  ,TRAV36*04         --- --- --- --- --- -T- --- --- --- --- --- --- --- --- --- --- --- --- --- --
```

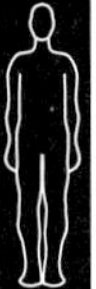

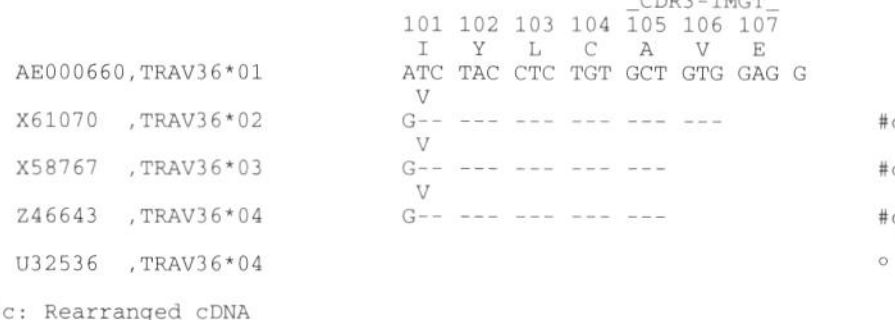

```
                                     _CDR3-IMGT_
                    101 102 103 104 105 106 107
                     I   Y   L   C   A   V   E
    AE000660,TRAV36*01  ATC TAC CTC TGT GCT GTG GAG G
                     V
    X61070  ,TRAV36*02  G-- --- --- --- --- ---        #c
                     V
    X58767  ,TRAV36*03  G-- --- --- --- ---            #c
                     V
    Z46643  ,TRAV36*04  G-- --- --- --- ---            #c

    U32536  ,TRAV36*04                                 o

#c: Rearranged cDNA
o: Genomic DNA, but not known as being germline or rearranged
```

Framework and complementarity determining regions

FR1-IMGT: 26   CDR1-IMGT: 6
FR2-IMGT: 16 (-1 aa: 50)   CDR2-IMGT: 3
FR3-IMGT: 38 (-1 aa: 73)   CDR3-IMGT: 3

Collier de Perles for human TRAV36/DV7*01

Accession number: IMGT AE000660   EMBL/GenBank/DDBJ: AE000660

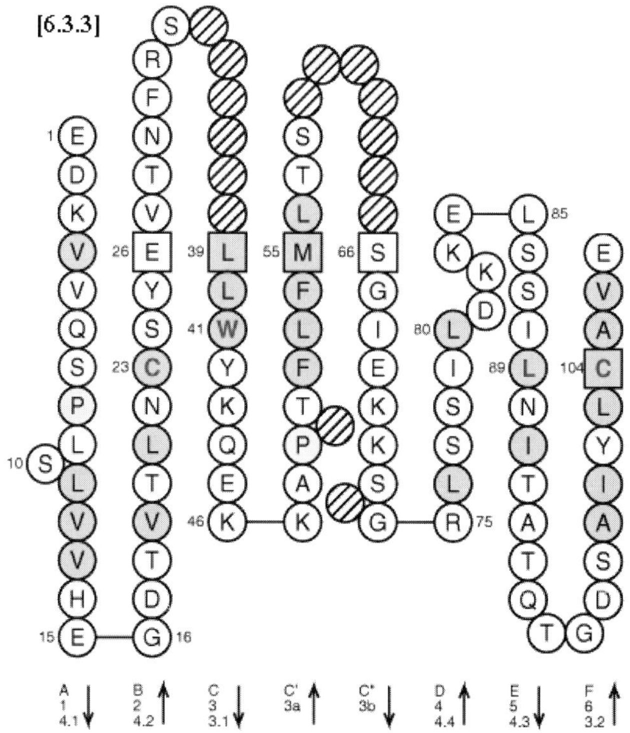

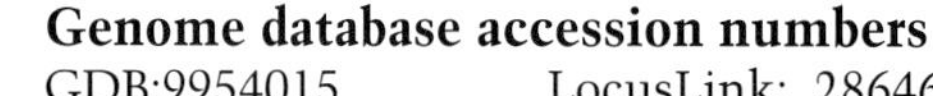

Nomenclature

TRAV38-1: T cell receptor alpha variable 38-1.

Definition and functionality

TRAV38-1 is one of the two functional genes of the TRAV38 subgroup which comprises two mapped genes.

Gene location

TRAV38-1 is in the TRA/TRD locus on chromosome 14 at 14q11.2.

Nucleotide and amino acid sequences for human TRAV38-1

```
                        1   2   3   4   5   6   7   8   9  10  11  12  13  14  15  16  17  18  19  20
                        A   Q   T   V   T   Q   S   Q   P   E   M   S   V   Q   E   A   E   T   V   T
AE000661,TRAV38-1*01 [6] GCC CAG ACA GTC ACT CAG TCT CAA CCA GAG ATG TCT GTG CAG GAG GCA GAG ACT GTG ACC

D13074  ,TRAV38-1*01 [23] --- --- --- --- --- --- --- --- --- --- --- --- --- --- --- --- --- --- --- ---

M64355  ,TRAV38-1*02  [4] --- --- --- --- --- --- --- --- --- --- --- --- --- --- --- --- --- --- --- ---

M95394  ,TRAV38-1*03 [19] --- --- --- --- --- --- --- --- --- --- --- --- --- --- --- --- --- --- --- ---

L06880  ,TRAV38-1*04 [29] --- --- --- --- --- --- --C --G --- --- --- --- --- --- --- --- --- --- --- ---


                                                            _______________CDR1-IMGT________________
                       21  22  23  24  25  26  27  28  29  30  31  32  33  34  35  36  37  38  39  40
                        L   S   C   T   Y   D   T   S   E   N   N   Y   Y                       L   F
AE000661,TRAV38-1*01    CTG AGT TGC ACA TAT GAC ACC AGT GAG AAT AAT TAT TAT ... ... ... ... ... TTG TTC

D13074  ,TRAV38-1*01    --- --- --- --- --- --- --- --- --- --- --- --- --- ... ... ... ... ... --- ---
                                                                    D
M64355  ,TRAV38-1*02    --- --- --- --- --- --- --- --- --- --- G-- --- --- ... ... ... ... ... --- ---
                                                                S
M95394  ,TRAV38-1*03    --- --- --- --- --- --- --- --- --- --- -G- --- --- ... ... ... ... ... --- ---

L06880  ,TRAV38-1*04    --- --- --- --- --- --- --- --- --- --- --- --- --- ... ... ... ... ... --- ---


                                                                                     ________________CDR2-
                       41  42  43  44  45  46  47  48  49  50  51  52  53  54  55  56  57  58  59  60
                        W   Y   K   Q   P   P   S   R   Q   M   I   L   V   I   R   Q   E   A   Y
AE000661,TRAV38-1*01    TGG TAC AAG CAG CCT CCC AGC AGG CAG ATG ATT CTC GTT ATT CGC CAA GAA GCT TAT ...

D13074  ,TRAV38-1*01    --- --- --- --- --- --- --- --- --- --- --- --- --- --- --- --- --- --- --- ...

M64355  ,TRAV38-1*02    --- --- --- --- --- --- --- --- --- --- --- --- --- --- --- --- --- --- --- ...

M95394  ,TRAV38-1*03    --- --- --A --- --- --- --- --- --- --- --- --- --- --- --- --- --- --- --- ...

L06880  ,TRAV38-1*04    --- --- --- --- --- --- --- --- --- --- --- --- --- --- --- --- --- --- --- ...


                       IMGT________________
                       61  62  63  64  65  66  67  68  69  70  71  72  73  74  75  76  77  78  79  80
                                            K   Q   Q   N   A   T   E       N   R   F   S   V   N   F
AE000661,TRAV38-1*01    ... ... ... ... ... AAG CAA CAG AAT GCA ACG GAG ... AAT CGT TTC TCT GTG AAC TTC

D13074  ,TRAV38-1*01    ... ... ... ... ... --- --- --- --- --- --- --- ... --- --- --- --- --- --- ---

M64355  ,TRAV38-1*02    ... ... ... ... ... --- --- --- --- --- --- --- ... --- --- --- --- --- --- ---

M95394  ,TRAV38-1*03    ... ... ... ... ... --- --- --- --- --- --- --- ... --- --- --- --- --- --- ---

L06880  ,TRAV38-1*04    ... ... ... ... ... --- --- --- --- --- --- --- ... --- --- --- --- --- --- ---


                       81  82  83  84  85  86  87  88  89  90  91  92  93  94  95  96  97  98  99 100
                        Q   K   A   A   K   S   F   S   L   K   I   S   D   S   Q   L   G   D   T   A
AE000661,TRAV38-1*01    CAG AAA GCA GCC AAA TCC TTC AGT CTC AAG ATC TCA GAC TCA CAG CTG GGG GAC ACT GCG

D13074  ,TRAV38-1*01    --- --- --- --- --- --- --- --- --- --- --- --- --- --- --- --- --- --- --- ---

M64355  ,TRAV38-1*02    --- --- --- --- --- --- --- --- --- --- --- --- --- --- --- --- --- --- --- ---

M95394  ,TRAV38-1*03    --- --- --- --- --- --- --- --- --- --- --- --- --- --- --- --- --- --- --- ---

L06880  ,TRAV38-1*04    --- --- --- --- --- --- --- --- --- --- --- --- --- --- --- --- --- --- --- ---


                             ____CDR3-IMGT____
                      101 102 103 104 105 106 107 108
                        M   Y   F   C   A   F   M   K
AE000661,TRAV38-1*01    ATG TAT TTC TGT GCT TTC ATG AAG CA

D13074  ,TRAV38-1*01    --- --- --- --- ---                 #c

M64355  ,TRAV38-1*02    --- --- --- --- ---                 #c

M95394  ,TRAV38-1*03    --- --- --- --- --- ---             #c

L06880  ,TRAV38-1*04    --- --- --- --- --                  #c

#c: Rearranged cDNA
```

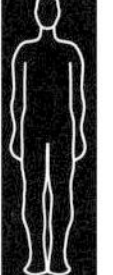

Framework and complementarity determining regions

FR1-IMGT: 26
FR2-IMGT: 17
FR3-IMGT: 38 (-1 aa: 73)

CDR1-IMGT: 7
CDR2-IMGT: 4
CDR3-IMGT: 4

Collier de Perles for human TRAV38-1*01

Accession number: IMGT AE000661   EMBL/GenBank/DDBJ: AE000661

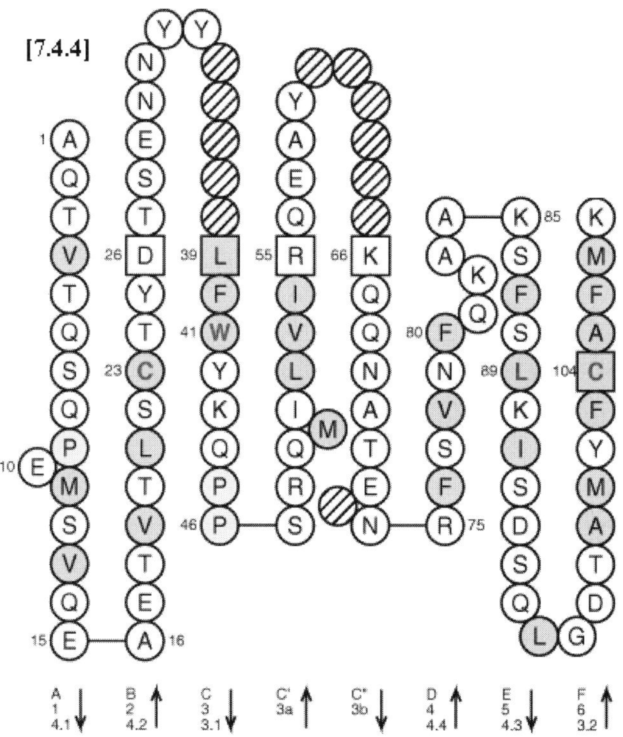

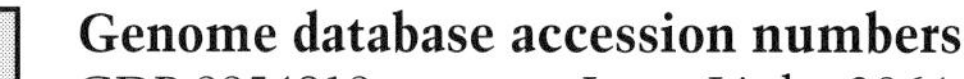

Genome database accession numbers
GDB:9954019   LocusLink: 28644

TRAV38-2/DV8

Nomenclature

TRAV38-2/DV8: T cell receptor alpha variable 38-2/delta variable 8.

Definition and functionality

TRAV38-2/DV8 is one of the two functional genes of the TRAV38 subgroup which comprises two mapped genes.

TRAV38-2/DV8 has been found rearranged to both (D)J genes of the TRD locus and TRAJ genes, the TRD locus being embedded in the TRA locus. This gene can therefore be used for the synthesis of both delta and alpha chains.

Gene location

TRAV38-2/DV8 is in the TRA/TRD locus on chromosome 14 at 14q11.2.

Nucleotide and amino acid sequences for human TRAV38-2/DV8

```
                              1    2    3    4    5    6    7    8    9   10   11   12   13   14   15   16   17   18   19   20
                              A    Q    T    V    T    Q    S    Q    P    E    M    S    V    Q    E    A    E    T    V    T
AE000661,TRAV38-2*01   [6]   GCT  CAG  ACA  GTC  ACT  CAG  TCT  CAA  CCA  GAG  ATG  TCT  GTG  CAG  GAG  GCA  GAG  ACC  GTG  ACC

Z29614   ,TRAV38-2*01  [15]  ---  ---  ---  ---  ---  ---  ---  ---  ---  ---  ---  ---  ---  ---  ---  ---  ---  ---  ---  ---

Z46644   ,TRAV38-2*01  [22]  ---  ---  ---  ---  ---  ---  ---  ---  ---  ---  ---  ---  ---  ---  ---  ---  ---  ---  ---  ---

U32524   ,TRAV38-2*01   [5]  ---  ---  ---  ---  ---  ---  ---  ---  ---  ---  ---  ---  ---  ---  ---  ---  ---  ---  ---  ---

X58158   ,TRAV38-2*01  [25]  ---  ---  ---  ---  ---  ---  ---  ---  ---  ---  ---  ---  ---  ---  ---  ---  ---  ---  ---  ---  ---


                                                                    _____________________CDR1-IMGT_________________________
                             21   22   23   24   25   26   27   28   29   30   31   32   33   34   35   36   37   38   39   40
                              L    S    C    T    Y    D    T    S    E    S    D    Y    Y                             L    F
AE000661,TRAV38-2*01         CTG  AGC  TGC  ACA  TAT  GAC  ACC  AGT  GAG  AGT  GAT  TAT  TAT  ...  ...  ...  ...  ...  TTA  TTC

Z29614   ,TRAV38-2*01        ---  ---  ---  ---  ---  ---  ---  ---  ---  ---  ---  ---  ---  ...  ...  ...  ...  ...  ---  ---

Z46644   ,TRAV38-2*01        ---  ---  ---  ---  ---  ---  ---  ---  ---  ---  ---  ---  ---  ...  ...  ...  ...  ...  ---  ---

U32524   ,TRAV38-2*01        ---  ---  ---  ---  ---  ---  ---  ---  ---  ---  ---  ---  ---  ...  ...  ...  ...  ...  ---  ---

X58158   ,TRAV38-2*01        ---  ---  ---  ---  ---  ---  ---  ---  ---  ---  ---  ---  ---  ...  ...  ...  ...  ...  ---  ---


                                                                                                   _________________CDR2-
                             41   42   43   44   45   46   47   48   49   50   51   52   53   54   55   56   57   58   59   60
                              W    Y    K    Q    P    P    S    R    Q    M    I    L    V    I    R    Q    E    A    Y
AE000661,TRAV38-2*01         TGG  TAC  AAG  CAG  CCT  CCC  AGC  AGG  CAG  ATG  ATT  CTC  GTT  ATT  CGC  CAA  GAA  GCT  TAT  ...

Z29614   ,TRAV38-2*01        ---  ---  ---  ---  ---  ---  ---  ---  ---  ---  ---  ---  ---  ---  ---  ---  ---  ---  ---  ...

Z46644   ,TRAV38-2*01        ---  ---  ---  ---  ---  ---  ---  ---  ---  ---  ---  ---  ---  ---  ---  ---  ---  ---  ---  ...

U32524   ,TRAV38-2*01        ---  ---  ---  ---  ---  ---  ---  ---  ---  ---  ---  ---  ---  ---  ---  ---  ---  ---  ---

X58158   ,TRAV38-2*01        ---  ---  ---  ---  ---  ---  ---  ---  ---  ---  ---  ---  ---  ---  ---  ---  ---  ---  ---  -


                             IMGT_________________
                             61   62   63   64   65   66   67   68   69   70   71   72   73   74   75   76   77   78   79   80
                                                     K    Q    Q    N    A    T    E         N    R    F    S    V    N    F
AE000661,TRAV38-2*01         ...  ...  ...  ...  ...  AAG  CAA  CAG  AAT  GCA  ACA  GAG  ...  AAT  CGT  TTC  TCT  GTG  AAC  TTC

Z29614   ,TRAV38-2*01        ...  ...  ...  ...  ...  ---  ---  ---  ---  ---  ---  ---  ...  ---  ---  ---  ---  ---  ---  ---

Z46644   ,TRAV38-2*01        ...  ...  ...  ...  ...  ---  ---  ---  ---  ---  ---  ---  ...  ---  ---  ---  ---  ---  ---  ---

U32524   ,TRAV38-2*01

X58158   ,TRAV38-2*01


                             81   82   83   84   85   86   87   88   89   90   91   92   93   94   95   96   97   98   99  100
                              Q    K    A    A    K    S    F    S    L    K    I    S    D    S    Q    L    G    D    A    A
AE000661,TRAV38-2*01         CAG  AAA  GCA  GCC  AAA  TCC  TTC  AGT  CTC  AAG  ATC  TCA  GAC  TCA  CAG  CTG  GGG  GAT  GCC  GCG

Z29614   ,TRAV38-2*01        ---  ---  ---  ---  ---  ---  ---  ---  ---  ---  ---  ---  ---  ---  ---  ---  ---  ---  ---  ---

Z46644   ,TRAV38-2*01        ---  ---  ---  ---  ---  ---  ---  ---  ---  ---  ---  ---  ---  ---  ---  ---  ---  ---  ---  ---

U32524   ,TRAV38-2*01

X58158   ,TRAV38-2*01
```

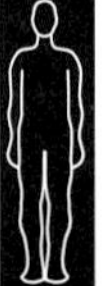

```
                                        ___CDR3-IMGT___
                         101 102 103 104 105 106 107 108
                          M   Y   F   C   A   Y   R   S
   AE000661,TRAV38-2*01  ATG TAT TTC TGT GCT TAT AGG AGC G
                                                         T
   Z29614  ,TRAV38-2*01  --- --- --- --- --- --- --- -CG    #c

   Z46644  ,TRAV38-2*01  --- --- --- --- --- --- --- --- -  #g

   U32524  ,TRAV38-2*01                                  o

   X58158  ,TRAV38-2*01
```

```
#c: Rearranged cDNA
#g: Rearranged genomic DNA
o: Genomic DNA sequence but not known as being germline or rearranged
```

Framework and complementarity determining regions

FR1-IMGT: 26	CDR1-IMGT: 7
FR2-IMGT: 17	CDR2-IMGT: 4
FR3-IMGT: 38 (-1 aa: 73)	CDR3-IMGT: 4

Collier de Perles for human TRAV38-2/DV8*01

Accession number: IMGT AE000661   EMBL/GenBank/DDBJ: AE000661

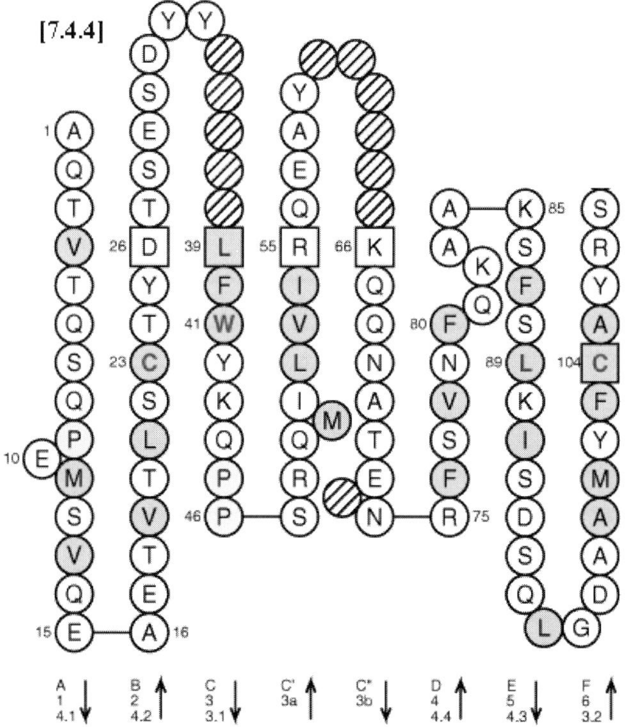

Genome database accession numbers

GDB:9954021   LocusLink: 28643

TRAV39

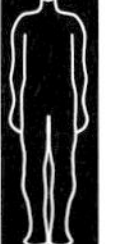

Nomenclature

TRAV39: T cell receptor alpha variable 39.

Definition and functionality

TRAV39 is the unique functional gene of the TRAV39 subgroup which only comprises this mapped gene.

Gene location

TRAV39 is in the TRA/TRD locus on chromosome 14 at 14q11.2.

Nucleotide and amino acid sequences for human TRAV39

```
                         1   2   3   4   5   6   7   8   9  10  11  12  13  14  15  16  17  18  19  20
                         E   L   K   V   E   Q   N   P   L   F   L   S   M   Q   E   G   K   N   Y   T
AE000661,TRAV39*01  [6]  GAG CTG AAA GTG GAA CAA AAC CCT CTG TTC CTG AGC ATG CAG GAG GGA AAA AAC TAT ACC

X58740  ,TRAV39*01 [28]  --- --- --- --- --- --- --- --- --- --- --- --- --- --- --- --- --- --- --- ---


                                                                 _____________CDR1-IMGT________________
                        21  22  23  24  25  26  27  28  29  30  31  32  33  34  35  36  37  38  39  40
                         I   Y   C   N   Y   S   T   T   S   D   R                           L   Y
AE000661,TRAV39*01      ATC TAC TGC AAT TAT TCA ACC ACT TCA GAC AGA ... ... ... ... ... ... ... CTG TAT

X58740  ,TRAV39*01      --- --- --- --- --- --- --- --- --- --- --- ... ... ... ... ... ... ... --- ---


                                                                                  ________________CDR2-
                        41  42  43  44  45  46  47  48  49  50  51  52  53  54  55  56  57  58  59  60
                         W   Y   R   Q   D   P   G   K   S   L   E   S   L   F   V   L   L   S
AE000661,TRAV39*01      TGG TAC AGG CAG GAT CCT GGG AAA AGT CTG GAA TCT CTG TTT GTG TTG CTA TCA ... ...

X58740  ,TRAV39*01      --- --- --- --- --- --- --- --- --- --- --- --- --- --- --- --- --- --- ... ...


                        IMGT________________
                        61  62  63  64  65  66  67  68  69  70  71  72  73  74  75  76  77  78  79  80
                                                 N   G   A   V   K   Q   E       G   R   L   M   A   S   L
AE000661,TRAV39*01      ... ... ... ... ... AAT GGA GCA GTG AAG CAG GAG ... GGA CGA TTA ATG GCC TCA CTT

X58740  ,TRAV39*01      ... ... ... ... ... --- --- --- --- --- --- --- ... --- --- --- --- --- --- ---


                        81  82  83  84  85  86  87  88  89  90  91  92  93  94  95  96  97  98  99 100
                         D   T   K   A   R   L   S   T   L   H   I   T   A   A   V   H   D   L   S   A
AE000661,TRAV39*01      GAT ACC AAA GCC CGT CTC AGC ACC CTC CAC ATC ACA GCT GCC GTG CAT GAC CTC TCT GCC

X58740  ,TRAV39*01      --- --- --- --- --- --- --- --- --- --- --- --- --- --- --- --- --- --- --- ---


                                 __CDR3-IMGT__
                       101 102 103 104 105 106 107
                         T   Y   F   C   A   V   D
AE000661,TRAV39*01      ACC TAC TTC TGT GCC GTG GAC A

X58740  ,TRAV39*01      --- --- --- --- ---              #c

#c: Rearranged cDNA
```

Framework and complementarity determining regions

FR1-IMGT: 26   CDR1-IMGT: 5
FR2-IMGT: 17   CDR2-IMGT: 3
FR3-IMGT: 38 (-1 aa: 73)   CDR3-IMGT: 3

Collier de Perles for human TRAV39*01

Accession number: IMGT AE000661   EMBL/GenBank/DDBJ: AE000661

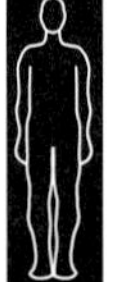

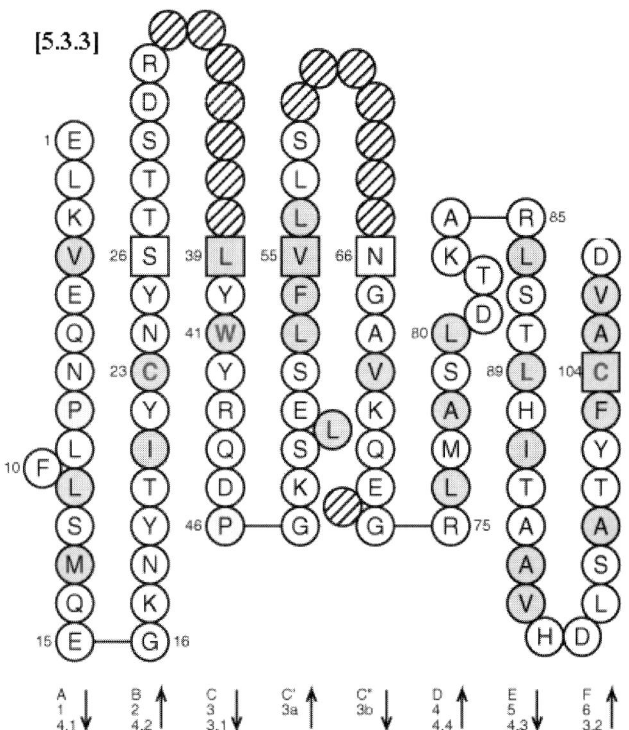

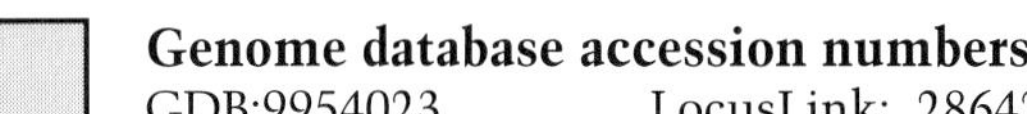

Genome database accession numbers
GDB:9954023   LocusLink: 28642

TRAV40

Nomenclature

TRAV40: T cell receptor alpha variable 40.

Definition and functionality

TRAV40 is the unique functional gene of the TRAV40 subgroup which only comprises this mapped gene.

Gene location

TRAV40 is in the TRA/TRD locus on chromosome 14 at 14q11.2.

Nucleotide and amino acid sequences for human TRAV40

```
                  1   2   3   4   5   6   7   8   9  10  11  12  13  14  15  16  17  18  19  20
                  S   N   S   V   K   Q   T       G   Q   I   T   V   S   E   G   A   S   V   T
X73521   ,TRAV40*01  [3] AGC AAT TCA GTC AAG CAG ACG ... GGC CAA ATA ACC GTC TCG GAG GGA GCA TCT GTG ACT

AE000661,TRAV40*01  [6] --- --- --- --- --- --- --- ... --- --- --- --- --- --- --- --- --- --- --- ---


                                                          ________________CDR1-IMGT________________
                 21  22  23  24  25  26  27  28  29  30  31  32  33  34  35  36  37  38  39  40
                  M   N   C   T   Y   T   S   T   G   Y   P   T                           L   F
X73521   ,TRAV40*01  ATG AAC TGC ACA TAC ACA TCC ACG GGG TAC CCT ACC ... ... ... ... ... ... CTT TTC

AE000661,TRAV40*01  --- --- --- --- --- --- --- --- --- --- --- --- ... ... ... ... ... ... --- ---


                                                                              ________________CDR2-
                 41  42  43  44  45  46  47  48  49  50  51  52  53  54  55  56  57  58  59  60
                  W   Y   V   E   Y   P   S   K   P   L   Q   L   L   Q   R
X73521   ,TRAV40*01  TGG TAT GTG GAA TAC CCC AGC AAA CCT CTG CAG CTT CTT CAG AGA ... ... ... ... ...

AE000661,TRAV40*01  --- --- --- --- --- --- --- --- --- --- --- --- --- --- --- ... ... ... ... ...


                 IMGT________________
                 61  62  63  64  65  66  67  68  69  70  71  72  73  74  75  76  77  78  79  80
                                          E   T   M   E   N   S       K   N   F   G   G   G   N
X73521   ,TRAV40*01  ... ... ... ... ... ... GAG ACA ATG GAA AAC AGC ... AAA AAC TTC GGA GGC GGA AAT

AE000661,TRAV40*01  ... ... ... ... ... ... --- --- --- --- --- --- ... --- --- --- --- --- --- ---


                 81  82  83  84  85  86  87  88  89  90  91  92  93  94  95  96  97  98  99 100
                  I       K   D   K   N   S   P   I   V   K   Y   S   V   Q   V   S   D   S   A
X73521   ,TRAV40*01  ATT ... AAA GAC AAA AAC TCC CCC ATT GTG AAA TAT TCA GTC CAG GTA TCA GAC TCA GCC

AE000661,TRAV40*01  --- ... --- --- --- --- --- --- --- --- --- --- --- --- --- --- --- --- --- ---


                             ____CDR3-IMGT____
                101 102 103 104 105 106 107 108
                  V   Y   Y   C   L   L   G
X73521   ,TRAV40*01  GTG TAC TAC TGT CTT CTG GGA GA

AE000661,TRAV40*01  --- --- --- --- --- --- --- --
```

Framework and complementarity determining regions

FR1-IMGT: 25 (-1 aa: 8)   CDR1-IMGT: 6
FR2-IMGT: 17   CDR2-IMGT: 0
FR3-IMGT: 36 (-3 aa: 66,73,82)   CDR3-IMGT: 3

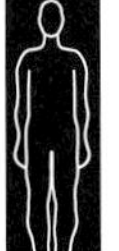

Collier de Perles for human TRAV40*01

Accession number: IMGT X73521   EMBL/GenBank/DDBJ: X73521

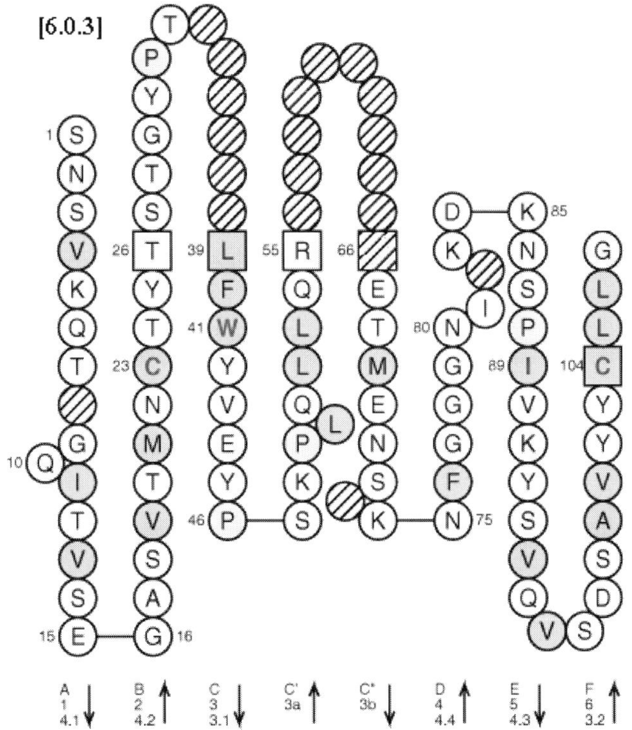

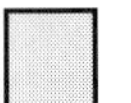

Genome database accession numbers
GDB:9954025   LocusLink: 28641

TRAV41

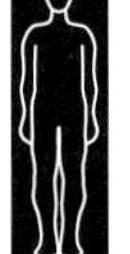

Nomenclature

TRAV41: T cell receptor alpha variable 41.

Definition and functionality

TRAV41 is the unique functional gene of the TRAV41 subgroup which only comprises this mapped gene.

Gene location

TRAV41 is in the TRA/TRD locus on chromosome 14 at 14q11.2.

Nucleotide and amino acid sequences for human TRAV41

```
                        1   2   3   4   5   6   7   8   9  10  11  12  13  14  15  16  17  18  19  20
                        K   N   E   V   E   Q   S   P   Q   N   L   T   A   Q   E   G   E   F   I   T
AE000661,TRAV41*01  [6] AAA AAT GAA GTG GAG CAG AGT CCT CAG AAC CTG ACT GCC CAG GAA GGA GAA TTT ATC ACA

M17662  ,TRAV41*01 [17] --- --- --- --- --- --- --- --- --- --- --- --- --- --- --- --- --- --- --- ---

U32528  ,TRAV41*01  [5] --- --- --- --- --- --- --- --- --- --- --- --- --- --- --- --- --- --- --- ---


                                                                     ________________CDR1-IMGT__________________
                       21  22  23  24  25  26  27  28  29  30  31  32  33  34  35  36  37  38  39  40
                        I   N   C   S   Y   S   V   G   I   S   A                               L   H
AE000661,TRAV41*01     ATC AAC TGC AGT TAC TCG GTA GGA ATA AGT GCC ... ... ... ... ... ... ... TTA CAC

M17662  ,TRAV41*01     --- --- --- --- --- --- --- --- --- --- --- ... ... ... ... ... ... ... --- ---

U32528  ,TRAV41*01     --- --- --- --- --- --- --- --- --- --- --- ... ... ... ... ... ... ... --- ---


                                                                                     _______________CDR2-
                       41  42  43  44  45  46  47  48  49  50  51  52  53  54  55  56  57  58  59  60
                        W   L   Q   Q   H   P   G   G   G   I   V   S   L   F   M   L
AE000661,TRAV41*01     TGG CTG CAA CAG CAT CCA GGA GGA GGC ATT GTT TCC TTG TTT ATG CTG ... ... ... ...

M17662  ,TRAV41*01     --- --- --- --- --- --- --- --- --- --- --- --- --- --- --- --- ... ... ... ...

U32528  ,TRAV41*01     --- --- --- --- --- --- --- --- --- --- --- --- --- --- --- --- ... ... ... ...


                       IMGT_________________
                       61  62  63  64  65  66  67  68  69  70  71  72  73  74  75  76  77  78  79  80
                                            S   S   G   K   K   K   H       G   R   L   I   A   T   I
AE000661,TRAV41*01     ... ... ... ... ... AGC TCA GGG AAG AAG AAG CAT ... GGA AGA TTA ATT GCC ACA ATA

M17662  ,TRAV41*01     ... ... ... ... ... --- --- --- --- --- --- --- ... --- --- --- --- --- --- ---

U32528  ,TRAV41*01     ... ... ... ... ... --- --- --- --- --- --- --- ... --- --- --- --- --- --- ---


                       81  82  83  84  85  86  87  88  89  90  91  92  93  94  95  96  97  98  99 100
                        N   I   Q   E   K   H   S   S   L   H   I   T   A   S   H   P   R   D   S   A
AE000661,TRAV41*01     AAC ATA CAG GAA AAG CAC AGC TCC CTG CAC ATC ACA GCC TCC CAT CCC AGA GAC TCT GCC

M17662  ,TRAV41*01     --- --- --- --- --- --- --- --- --- --- --- --- --- --- --- --- --- --- --- ---

U32528  ,TRAV41*01     --- --- --- --- -


                                       _CDR3-IMGT_
                      101 102 103 104 105 106 107
                        V   Y   I   C   A   V   R
AE000661,TRAV41*01     GTC TAC ATC TGT GCT GTC ACA
                                                T
M17662  ,TRAV41*01     --- --- --- --- --- --- --G        #c

U32528  ,TRAV41*01                                °
```

#c: Rearranged cDNA
°: Genomic DNA, but not known as being germline or rearranged

Framework and complementarity determining regions

FR1-IMGT: 26   CDR1-IMGT: 5

FR2-IMGT: 17   CDR2-IMGT: 1

FR3-IMGT: 38 (-1 aa: 73)   CDR3-IMGT: 3

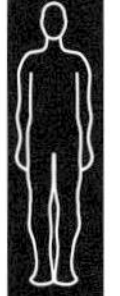

Collier de Perles for human TRAV41*01

Accession number: IMGT AE000661   EMBL/GenBank/DDBJ: AE000661

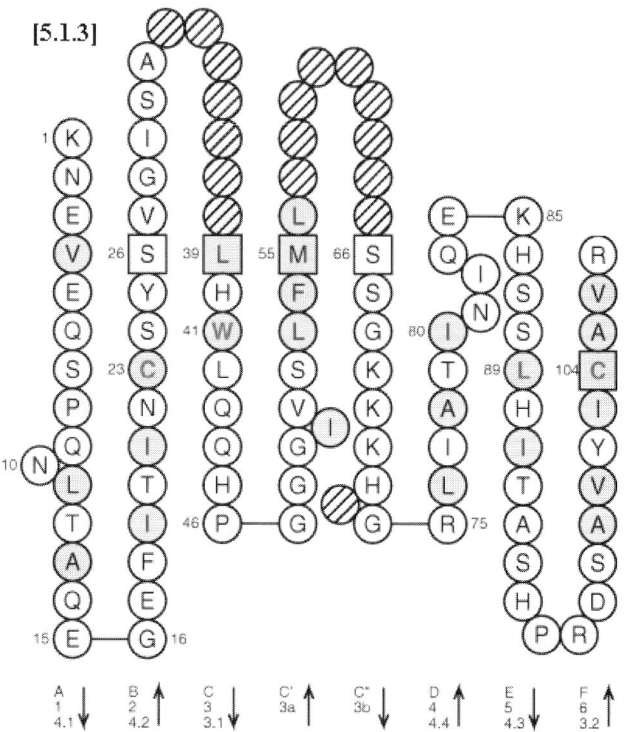

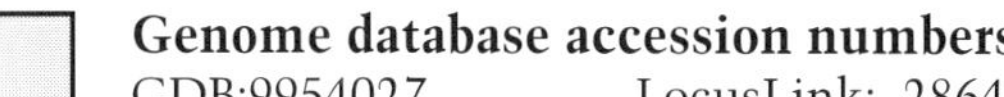

Genome database accession numbers
GDB:9954027   LocusLink: 28640

TRAV protein display

Protein display of the human TRA V-REGIONs

*Only the *01 allele of each functional or ORF V-REGION is shown. TRAV genes are listed, for each subgroup, according to their position from 5' to 3' in the locus. N-glycosylation sites (NXS/T, where X is different from P) are underlined.*

TRAV gene	FR1-IMGT (1-26)	CDR1-IMGT (27-38)	FR2-IMGT (39-55)	CDR2-IMGT (56-65)	FR3-IMGT (66-104)	CDR3-IMGT (105-115)
	1 .... 10 20	30	40 50	60	70 ..... 80 ..... 90 100	110
AE000658,TRAV1-1	GQSLEQ.PSEVTAVEGAIVQINCTYQ	TSGFYG......	LSWYQQHDGGAPTFLSY	NA........	LDGLEET.GRFSSFLSRSDSYGYLLLQELQMKDSASYFC	AVR........
AE000658,TRAV1-2	GQNIDQ.PTEMTATEGAIVQINCTYQ	TSGFNG......	LFWYQQHAGEAPTFLSY	NV........	LDGLEEK.GRFSSFLSRSKGYSYLLLKELQMKDSASYLC	AVR........
AE000658,TRAV2	KDQVFQ.PSTVASSEGAVVEIFCNHS	VSNAYN......	FFWYLHFPGCAPRLLVK	....	GSKPSQQ.GRYNMTY..ERFSSSLLILQVREADAAVYYC	AVE........
AE000658,TRAV3	AQSVAQPEDQVNVAEGNPLTVKCTYS	VSGNPY......	LFWYVQYPNRGLQFLLK	YITG......	DNLVKGS.YGFEAEFNKSQTSFHLKKPSALVSDSALYFC	AVRD.......
AE000658,TRAV4	LAKTTQ.PISMDSYEGQEVNITCSHN	NIATNDY.....	ITWYQQFPSQGPRFIIQ	G.........	YKTKVTN.EVASLFIPADRKSSTLSLPRVSLSDTAVYYC	LVGD.......
AE000659,TRAV5	GEDVEQS.LFLSVREGDSSVINCTYT	DSSSTY......	LYWYKQEPGAGLQLLTY	IFS.......	NMDMKQD.QRLTVLLNKKDKHLSLRIADTQTGDSAIYFC	AES........
AE000659,TRAV6	SQKIEQNSEALNIQEGKTATLTCNYT	NYSPAY......	LQWYRQDPGRGPVFLLL	IRE.......	NEKEKRK.ERLKVTFDTTLKQSLFHITASQPADSATYLC	ALD........
AE000659,TRAV7	ENQVEHSPHFLGPQQGDVASMSCTYS	VSRFNN......	LQWYRQNTGMGPKHLLS	MYS.......	AGYEKQK.GRLNATL..LKNGSLYITAVQPEDSATYFC	AVD........
AE000659,TRAV8-1	AQSVSQHNHHVILSEAASLELGCNYS	YGGTVN......	LFWYVQYPGQHLQLLLK	YFSG......	DPLVKGI.KGFEAEFIKSKFSFNLRKPSVQWSDTAEYFC	AVN........
AE000659,TRAV8-2	AQSVTQLDSHVSVSEGTPVLLRCNYS	SSYSPS......	LFWYVQHPNKGLQLLLK	YTSA......	ATLVKGI.NGFEAEFKKSETSFHLTKPSAHMSDAAEYFC	VVS........
AE000659,TRAV8-3	AQSVTQPDIHITVSEGASLELRCNYS	YGATPY......	LFWYVQSPGQGLQLLLK	YFSG......	DTLVQGI.KGFEAEFKRSQSSFNLRKPSVHWSDAAEYFC	AVG........
AE000659,TRAV8-4	AQSVTQLGSHVSVSEGALVLLRCNYS	SSVPPY......	LFWYVQYPNQGLQLLLK	YTSA......	ATLVKGI.NGFEAEFKKSETSFHLTKPSAHMSDAAEYFC	AVS........
X02850 ,TRAV8-6	AQSVTQLDSQVPVFEEAPVELRCNYS	SSVSVY......	LFWYVQYPNQGLQLLLK	YLSG......	STLVESI.NGFEAEFNKSQTSFHLRKPSVHISDTAEYFC	AVS........
AE000660,TRAV8-7	TQSVTQLDGHITVSEEAPLELKCNYS	YSGVPS......	LFWYVQYSSQSLQLLLK	DLTE......	ATQVKGI.RGFEAEFKKSETSFYLRKPSTHVSDAAEYFC	AVGDR......
AE000659,TRAV9-1	GDSVVQTEGQVLPSEGDSLIVNCSYE	TTQYPS......	LFWYVQYPGEGPQLHLK	AMK.......	ANDKGRN.KGFEAMYRKETTSFHLEKDSVQESDSAVYFC	ALS........
AE000659,TRAV9-2	GNSVTQMEGPVTLSEEAFLTINCTYT	ATGYPS......	LFWYVQYPGEGLQLLLK	ATK.......	ADDKGSN.KGFEATYRKETTSFHLEKGSVQVSDSAVYFC	ALS........
AE000659,TRAV10	KNQVEQSPQSLIILEGKNCTLQCNYT	VSPFSN......	LRWYKQDTGRGPVSLTI	MTF.......	SENTKSN.GRYTATLDADTKQSSLHITASQLSDSASYIC	VVS........
AE000659,TRAV12-1	RKEVEQDPGPFNVPEGATVAFNCTYS	NSASQS......	FFWYRQDCRKEPKLLMS	VY........	SSGN.ED.GRFTAQLNRASQYISLLIRDSKLSDSATYLC	VVN........
AE000659,TRAV12-2	QKEVEQNSGPLSVPEGAIASLNCTYS	DRGSQS......	FFWYRQYSGKSPELIMF	IY........	SNGDKED.GRFTAQLNKASQYVSLLIRDSQPSDSATYLC	AVN........
X06193 ,TRAV12-3	QKEVEQDPGPLSVPEGAIVSLNCTYS	NSAFQY......	FMWYRQYSRKGPELLMY	TY........	SSGNKED.GRFTAQVDKSSKYISLFIRDSQPSDSATYLC	AMS........
AE000659,TRAV13-1	GENVEQHPSTLSVQEGDSAVIKCTYS	DSASNY......	FPWYKQELGKGPQLIID	IRS.......	NVGEKKD.QRIAVTLNKTAKHFSLHITETQPEDSAVYFC	AAS........
AE000659,TRAV13-2	GESVGLHLPTLSVQEGDNSIINCAYS	NSASDY......	FIWYKQESGKGPQFIID	IRS.......	NMDKRQG.QRVTVLLNKTVKHLSLQIAATQPGDSAVYFC	AEN........
M21626 ,TRAV14/DV4	AQKITQTQPGMFVQEKEAVTLDCTYD	TSDPSYG.....	LFWYKQPSSGEMIFLIY	QGSY......	DQQNATE.GRYSLNFQKARKSANLVISASQLGDSAMYFC	AMRE.......
AE000660,TRAV17	SQQGEEDPQALSIQEGENATMNCSYK	TSINN.......	LQWYRQNSGRGLVHLIL	IRS.......	NEREKHS.GRLRVTLDTSKKSSSLLITASRAADTASYFC	ATD........
AE000659,TRAV16	AQRVTQPEKLLSVFKGAPVELKCNYS	YSGSPE......	LFWYVQYSRQRLQLLLR	....	HISRESI.KGFTADLNKGETSFHLKKPFAQEEDSAMYYC	ALS........

TRAV gene	FR1-IMGT (1-26)	CDR1-IMGT (27-38)	FR2-IMGT (39-55)	CDR2-IMGT (56-65)	FR3-IMGT (66-104)	CDR3-IMGT (105-115)
AE000660,TRAV17	SQQGEEDPQALSIQEGENATMNCSYK	TSINN.......	LQWYRQNSGRGLVHLIL	IRS.......	NEREKHS.GRLRVTLDTSKKSSSLLITASRAADTASYFC	ATD........
AE000660,TRAV18	GDSVTQTEGPVTLPERAALTLNCTYQ	SSYSTF......	LFWYVQYLNKEPELLLK	SS........	ENQETDS.RGFQASPIKSDSSFHLEKPSVQLSDSAVYYC	ALR.......
AE000660,TRAV19	AQKVTQAQTEISVVEKEDVTLDCVYE	TRDTTYY.....	LFWYKQPPSGELVFLIR	RNSF......	DEQNEIS.GRYSWNFQKSTSSFNFTITASQVVDSAVYFC	ALSE......
AE000660,TRAV20	EDQVTQSPEALRLQEGESSSLNCSYT	VSGLRG......	LFWYRQDPGKGPEFLFT	LYS......	AGEEKEK.ERLKATL..TKKESFLHITAPKPEDSATYLC	AVQ......
AE000660,TRAV21	KQEVTQIPAALSVPEGENLVLNCSFT	DSAIYN......	LQWFRQDPGKGLTSLLL	IQS.......	SQREQTS.GRLNASLDKSSGRSTLYIAASQPGDSATYLC	AVR.......
AE000660,TRAV22	GIQVEQSPPDLILQEGANSTLRCNFS	DSVNN.......	LQWFHQNPWGQLINLFY	I.........	PSGTKQN.GRLSATTVATERYSLLYISSSQTTDSGVYFC	AVE.......
AE000660,TRAV23/DV6	QQQVKQSPQSLIVQKGGISIINCAYE	NTAFDY......	FPWYQQFPGKGPALLIA	IRP.......	DVSEKKE.GRFTISFNKSAKQFSLHIMDSQPGDSATYFC	AAS.......
AE000660,TRAV24	ILNVEQSPQSLHVQEGDSTNFTCSFP	SSNFYA......	LHWYRWETAKSPEALFV	MTL.......	NGDEKKK.GRISATLNTKEGYSYLYIKGSQPEDSATYLC	AF........
AE000660,TRAV25	GQQVMQIPQYQHVQEGEDFTTYCNSS	TTLSN.......	IQWYKQRPGGHPVFLIQ	LVK.......	SGEVKKQ.KRLTFQFGEAKKNSSLHITATQTTDVGTYFC	AG........
AE000660,TRAV26-1	DAKTTQ.PPSMDCAEGRAANLPCNHS	TISGNEY.....	VYWYRQIHSQGPQYIIH	G.........	LKNNETN.EMASLIITEDRKSSTLILPHATLRDTAVYYC	IVRV......
AE000660,TRAV26-2	DAKTTQ.PNSMESNEEEPVHLPCNHS	TISGTDY.....	IHWYRQLPSQGPEYVIH	G.........	LTSNVNN.RMASLAIAEDRKSSTLILHRATLRDAAVYYC	ILRD......
AE000660,TRAV27	TQLLEQSPQFLSIQEGENLTVYCNSS	SVFSS.......	LQWYRQEPGEGPVLLVT	VVT.......	GGEVKKL.KRLTFQFGDARKDSSLHITAAQPGDTGLYLC	AG........
AE000660,TRAV29/DV5	DQQVKQNSPSLSVQEGRISILNCDYT	NSMFDY......	FLWYKKYPAEGPTFLIS	ISS.......	IKDKNED.GRFTVFLNKSAKHLSLHIVPSQPGDSAVYFC	AAS.......
AE000660,TRAV30	QQPV.QSPQAVILREGEDAVINCSSS	KALYS.......	VHWYRQKHGEAPVFLMI	LLK.......	GGEQKGH.EKISASFNEKKQQSSLYLTASQLSYSGTYFC	GTE.......
AE000660,TRAV34	SQELEQSPQSLIVQEGKNLTINCTSS	KTLYG.......	LYWYKQKYGEGLIFLMM	LQK.......	GGEEKSH.EKITAKLDEKKQQSSLHITASQPSHAGIYLC	GAD.......
AE000660,TRAV35	GQQLNQSPQSMFIQEGEDVSMNCTSS	SIFNT.......	WLWYKQEPGEGPVLLIA	LYK.......	AGELTSN.GRLTAQFGITRKDSFLNISASIPSDVGIYFC	AGQ.......
AE000660,TRAV36/DV7	EDKVVQSPLSLVVHEGDTVTLNCSYE	VTNFRS......	LLWYKQEKKAP.TFLFM	LTS.......	SGIEKKS.GRLSSILDKKELSSILNITATQTGDSAIYLC	AVE.......
AE000661,TRAV38-1	AQTVTQSQPEMSVQEAETVTLSCTYD	TSENNYY.....	LFWYKQPPSRQMILVIR	QEAY......	KQQNATE.NRFSVNFQKAAKSFSLKISDSQLGDTAMYFC	AFMK......
AE000661,TRAV38-2/DV8	AQTVTQSQPEMSVQEAETVTLSCTYD	TSESDYY.....	LFWYKQPPSRQMILVIR	QEAY......	KQQNATE.NRFSVNFQKAAKSFSLKISDSQLGDAAMYFC	AYRS......
AE000661,TRAV39	ELKVEQNPLFLSMQEGKNYTIYCNYS	TTSDR.......	LYWYRQDPGKSLESLFV	LLS.......	NGAVKQE.GRLMASLDTKARLSTLHITAAVHDLSATYFC	AVD.......
X73521 ,TRAV40	SNSVKQT.GQITVSEGASVTMNCTYT	STGYPT......	LFWYVEYPSKPLQLLQR	....	.ETMENS.KNFGGGNI.KDKNSPIVKYSVQVSDSAVYYC	LLG.......
AE000661,TRAV41	KNEVEQSPQNLTAQEGEFITINCSYS	VGISA.......	LHWLQQHPGGGIVSLFM	L.........	SSGKKKH.GRLIATINIQEKHSSLHITASHPRDSAVYIC	AVR.......

Recombination signals

Only the recombination signals of the allele *01 of each functional TRA V-REGION are shown.

TRAV gene name	V-HEPTAMER	(bp)	V-NONAMER
TRAV1-1	CACAGTG	23	CCAAAATTC
TRAV1-2	CACGGTG	23	CCAAAATTC
TRAV2	CACAGAG	23	ACAGAAACA
TRAV3	CACACTG	23	ACACAAACT
TRAV4	CACAGTG	23	CCGTTTTCC
TRAV5	CACATTG	23	ACCCAAACC
TRAV6	CACAGTA	23	ACCCAAACT
TRAV7	CACAGTA	23	ATCCAAACA
TRAV8-1	CACAGTG	23	ACACAAACT
TRAV8-2	CACAGTG	22	ACACAAGCC
TRAV8-3	CACAGTG	23	ACACAAACT
TRAV8-4	CACAGTG	22	ACATAAACC
TRAV8-6	CACAGTG	22	ACACAAACT
TRAV8-7	GACTGTG	23	ACACAAACT
TRAV9-1	CACAGTG	23	GCACAAACT
TRAV9-2	CACAGTG	23	GCACAAACT
TRAV10	CACTGTG	23	ATGCAAACC
TRAV12-1	CACAGTG	23	ACCCAAACC
TRAV12-2	CACAGTG	23	ACCCAAACC
TRAV12-3	CACAGTG	27/23	ACCCAAACC
TRAV13-1	CACATTG	23	ACACAAACC
TRAV13-2	CACATTG	23	ACCCAAACC
TRAV14/DV4	CACAGTG	23	ACAAAAGCC
TRAV16	CACAGTA	22	ACACAAACC
TRAV17	CACAGTG	23	ACGCAAACC
TRAV18	CAGAGTG	23	GCACAAACC
TRAV19	CACAGTG	23	ACAAAAACC
TRAV20	CACAGCG	23	ATCAAAACC
TRAV21	CACAGTG	23	ACCCAAACT
TRAV22	CACAGTG	23	ACACAAACC
TRAV23/DV6	CACAGTG	23	ACCCAAACC
TRAV24	CACAGTG	23	ACGCAAACC
TRAV25	CACAGTG	23	CTCCAAATC
TRAV26-1	CACACTG	23	CAATATCTC
TRAV26-2	CACAGTG	23	CAATATCTC
TRAV27	CACAGTG	23	ACCCAAACC
TRAV29/DV5	CACAGTG	23	ACTCAAACC
TRAV30	CACAGTG	23	ACTCAAACC
TRAV34	CACAGCG	23	CTCCAAACC
TRAV35	CACAGTG	23	ACTCAAACT
TRAV36/DV7	CACAGTG	23	ACTCAAATT
TRAV38-1	CACAATG	23	ACAGAAACC
TRAV38-2/DV8	CACAGTG	23	ACAGAAACC
TRAV39	CACAGTG	23	ACCCAAACC
TRAV40	CACTGTG	22	ACAAAAACC
TRAV41	CACAGTG	23	ACCTAAACT

References

[1] Baer, R. et al. (1985) Cell 43, 705–713.
[2] Baer, R. et al. (1988) EMBO J. 7, 1661–1668.
[3] Bernard, O. et al. (1993) Leukemia 7, 1645–1653.
[4] Bortel, B. et al. (1992) J. Exp. Med. 175, 765–777.
[5] Boysen, C. et al. (1996) Immunogenetics 44, 121–127.
[6] Boysen, C. et al. (1997) unpublished.
[7] Charmley, P. et al. (1994) Immunogenetics 39, 138–145.
[8] Cornelis, F. (1992) unpublished.
[9] Croce, C.M. et al. (1985) Science 227, 1044–1047.
[10] Guglielmi, P. et al. (1988) Proc. Natl Acad. Sci. USA 85, 5634–5638.
[11] Hewitt, C.R.A. et al. (1992) J. Exp. Med. 175, 1493–1499.
[12] Hurley, C.K. et al. (1993) J. Immunol. 150, 1314–1324.
[13] Ibberson, M.R. et al. (1995) Genomics 28, 131–139.
[14] Ibberson, M.R. et al. (1998) Immunogenetics 47, 124–130.
[15] Kalams, S.A. et al. (1994) J. Exp. Med. 179, 1261–1271.
[16] Kimura, N. et al. (1987) Eur. J. Immunol. 17, 375–383.
[17] Klein, M.H. et al. (1987) Proc. Natl Acad. Sci. USA 84, 6884–6888.
[18] Korthäuer, U. et al. (1992) Scand. J. Immunol. 36, 855–863.
[19] Lauzurica, P. et al. (1992) unpublished.
[20] Leiden, J.M. et al. (1986) Immunogenetics 24, 17–23.
[21] Luria, S. et al. (1987) EMBO J. 6, 3307–3312.
[22] Migone, N. et al. (1995) Immunogenetics 42, 323–332.
[23] Obata, F. et al. (1993) Immunogenetics 38, 67–70.
[24] Plaza, P. et al. (1993) unpublished.
[25] Pluschke, G. et al. (1991) Eur. J. Immunol. 21, 2749–2754.
[26] Rabbitts, T.H. et al. (1985) EMBO J. 4, 1461–1465.
[27] Reyburn, H. et al. (1993) Immunogenetics 38, 287–291.
[28] Roman-Roman, S. et al. (1991) Eur. J. Immunol. 21, 927–933.
[29] Santamaria, P. et al. (1993) Immunogenetics 38, 163–163.
[30] Satyanarayana, K. et al. (1988) Proc. Natl Acad. Sci. USA 85, 8166–8170.
[31] Sensi, M. et al. (1991) Melanoma Res. 1, 261–271.
[32] Sim, G. K. et al. (1984) Nature 312, 771–775.
[33] Tsuruta, Y. et al. (1993) J. Immunol. Methods 161, 721–721.
[34] Wright, J.A. et al. (1991) Hum. Immunol. 32, 277–283.
[35] Yanagi, Y. et al. (1985) Proc. Natl Acad. Sci. USA 82, 3430–3434.
[36] Yassai, M. et al. (1992) Hum. Immunol. 34, 279–283.
[37] Yoshikai, Y. et al. (1985) Nature 316, 837–840.
[38] Yoshikai, Y. et al. (1986) J. Exp. Med. 164, 90–103.

THE HUMAN
T CELL RECEPTOR
TRB GENES

TRBC

Nomenclature

TRBC1: T cell receptor beta constant 1.

Definition and functionality

TRBC1 is one of the two functional genes of the TRBC group which comprises two mapped genes. TRBC1 and TRBC2 result from a recent duplication.

Gene location

TRBC1 is in the TRB locus on chromosome 7 at 7q34.

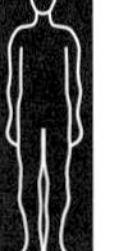

Nucleotide and amino acid sequences for human TRBC1

The nucleotide between parentheses at the beginning of exons comes from a DONOR–SPLICE (n from ngt).

The Cysteines involved in the intrachain disulfide bridges are shown with their number and letter **C** in bold.

N-Glycosylation sites (NXS/T, where X is different from P) are underlined.

```
                         1    2    3    4    5    6    7    8    9   10   11   12   13   14   15   16   17   18   19   20
                         E    D    L    N    K    V    F    P    P    E    V    A    V    F    E    P    S    E    A    E
 M12887  ,TRBC1*01, (EX1)  [1] (G)AG  GAC  CTG  AAC  AAG  GTG  TTC  CCA  CCC  GAG  GTC  GCT  GTG  TTT  GAG  CCA  TCA  GAA  GCA  GAG

 M14157  ,TRBC1*01        [2] (-)--  ---  ---  ---  ---  ---  ---  ---  ---  ---  ---  ---  ---  ---  ---  ---  ---  ---  ---  ---

(1)L36092,U66061,TRBC1*02 [3] (-)--  ---  ---  ---  ---  ---  ---  ---  ---  ---  ---  ---  ---  ---  ---  ---  ---  ---  ---  ---


                        21   22   23   24   25   26   27   28   29   30   31   32   33   34   35   36   37   38   39   40
                         I    S    H    T    Q    K    A    T    L    V    C    L    A    T    G    F    F    P    D    H
 M12887  ,TRBC1*01        ATC  TCC  CAC  ACC  CAA  AAG  GCC  ACA  CTG  GTG  TGC  CTG  GCC  ACA  GGC  TTC  TTC  CCC  GAC  CAC

 M14157  ,TRBC1*01        ---  ---  ---  ---  ---  ---  ---  ---  ---  ---  ---  ---  ---  ---  ---  ---  ---  ---  ---  ---

(1)L36092,U66061,TRBC1*02 ---  ---  ---  ---  ---  ---  ---  ---  ---  ---  ---  ---  ---  ---  ---  ---  ---  ---  ---  ---


                        41   42   43   44   45   46   47   48   49   50   51   52   53   54   55   56   57   58   59   60
                         V    E    L    S    W    W    V    N    G    K    E    V    H    S    G    V    S    T    D    P
 M12887  ,TRBC1*01        GTG  GAG  CTG  AGC  TGG  TGG  GTG  AAT  GGG  AAG  GAG  GTG  CAC  AGT  GGG  GTC  AGC  ACG  GAC  CCG

 M14157  ,TRBC1*01        ---  ---  ---  ---  ---  ---  ---  ---  ---  ---  ---  ---  ---  ---  ---  ---  ---  ---  ---  ---

(1)L36092,U66061,TRBC1*02 ---  ---  ---  ---  ---  ---  ---  ---  ---  ---  ---  ---  ---  ---  ---  ---  -A-  ---  ---


                        61   62   63   64   65   66   67   68   69   70   71   72   73   74   75   76   77   78   79   80
                         Q    P    L    K    E    Q    P    A    L    N    D    S    R    Y    C    L    S    S    R    L
 M12887  ,TRBC1*01        CAG  CCC  CTC  AAG  GAG  CAG  CCC  GCC  CTC  AAT  GAC  TCC  AGA  TAC  TGC  CTG  AGC  AGC  CGC  CTG

 M14157  ,TRBC1*01        ---  ---  ---  ---  ---  ---  ---  ---  ---  ---  ---  ---  ---  ---  ---  ---  ---  ---  ---  ---

(1)L36092,U66061,TRBC1*02 ---  ---  ---  ---  ---  ---  ---  ---  ---  ---  ---  ---  ---  ---  ---  ---  ---  ---  ---  ---


                        81   82   83   84   85   86   87   88   89   90   91   92   93   94   95   96   97   98   99  100
                         R    V    S    A    T    F    W    Q    N    P    R    N    H    F    R    C    Q    V    Q    F
 M12887  ,TRBC1*01        AGG  GTC  TCG  GCC  ACC  TTC  TGG  CAG  AAC  CCC  CGC  AAC  CAC  TTC  CGC  TGT  CAA  GTC  CAG  TTC

 M14157  ,TRBC1*01        ---  ---  ---  ---  ---  ---  ---  ---  ---  ---  ---  ---  ---  ---  ---  ---  ---  ---  ---  ---

(1)L36092,U66061,TRBC1*02 ---  ---  ---  ---  ---  ---  ---  ---  ---  ---  ---  ---  ---  ---  ---  ---  ---  ---  ---  ---


                       101  102  103  104  105  106  107  108  109  110  111  112  113  114  115  116  117  118  119  120
                         Y    G    L    S    E    N    D    E    W    T    Q    D    R    A    K    P    V    T    Q    I
 M12887  ,TRBC1*01        TAC  GGG  CTC  TCG  GAG  AAT  GAC  GAG  TGG  ACC  CAG  GAT  AGG  GCC  AAA  CCC  GTC  ACC  CAG  ATC

 M14157  ,TRBC1*01        ---  ---  ---  ---  ---  ---  ---  ---  ---  ---  ---  ---  ---  ---  ---  ---  ---  ---  ---  ---

(1)L36092,U66061,TRBC1*02 ---  ---  ---  ---  ---  ---  ---  ---  ---  ---  ---  ---  ---  ---  ---  ---  ---  ---  ---  ---


                       121  122  123  124  125  126  127  128  129
                         V    S    A    E    A    W    G    R    A
 M12887  ,TRBC1*01        GTC  AGC  GCC  GAG  GCC  TGG  GGT  AGA  GCA  G

 M14157  ,TRBC1*01        ---  ---  ---  ---  ---  ---  ---  ---  -

(1)L36092,U66061,TRBC1*02 ---  ---  ---  ---  ---  ---  ---  ---  -


                         1    2    3    4    5    6
                         D    C    G    F    T    S
 M12887  ,TRBC1*01, (EX2)  AC   TGT  GGC  TTT  ACC  TCG  G

 M14157  ,TRBC1*01        --   ---  ---  ---  ---  ---  -

(1)L36092,U66061,TRBC1*01 --   ---  ---  ---  ---  ---  -
```

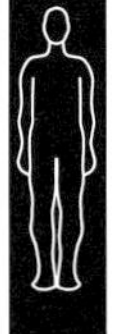

```
                1    2    3    4    5    6    7    8    9    10   11   12   13   14   15   16   17   18   19   20
                V    S    Y    Q    Q    G    V    L    S    A    T    I    L    Y    E    I    L    L    G    K
  M12887  ,TRBC1*01, (EX3)  TG  TCC  TAC  CAG  CAA  GGG  GTC  CTG  TCT  GCC  ACC  ATC  CTC  TAT  GAG  ATC  CTG  CTA  GGG  AAG

  M14157  ,TRBC1*01         --   ---  ---  ---  ---  ---  ---  ---  ---  ---  ---  ---  ---  ---  ---  ---  ---  ---  ---  ---

(1)L36092,U66061,TRBC1*01   --   ---  ---  ---  ---  ---  ---  ---  ---  ---  ---  ---  ---  ---  ---  ---  ---  ---  ---  ---


                21   22   23   24   25   26   27   28   29   30   31   32   33   34   35   36
                A    T    L    Y    A    V    L    V    S    A    L    V    L    M    A    M
  M12887  ,TRBC1*01          GCC  ACC  CTG  TAT  GCT  GTG  CTG  GTC  AGC  GCC  CTT  GTG  TTG  ATG  GCC  ATG

  M14157  ,TRBC1*01          ---  ---  ---  ---  ---  ---  ---  ---  ---  ---  ---  ---  ---  ---  ---  ---

(1)L36092,U66061,TRBC1*01    ---  ---  ---  ---  ---  ---  ---  ---  ---  ---  ---  ---  ---  ---  ---  ---


                1    2    3    4    5    6
                V    K    R    K    D    F    *
  M12887  ,TRBC1*01, (EX4)   GTC  AAG  AGA  AAG  GAT  TTC

  M14157  ,TRBC1*01          ---  ---  ---  ---  ---  ---

(1)L36092,U66061,TRBC1*01    ---  ---  ---  ---  ---  ---
```

Note:

(1) The original L36092 sequence (684 973 bp) has been split in EMBL into three sequences of 267 156 bp (U66059), 215 422 bp (U66060), and 232 650 bp (U66061); L36092 has become the secondary accession number of U66059, U66060, and U66061. In IMGT, the original sequence L36092, which is fully annotated, has also been kept as primary accession number, in addition to U66059, U66060, and U66061.

Genome database accession numbers

GDB:9954029   LocusLink: 28639

References

[1] Tunnacliffe, A. et al. (1985) Proc. Natl Acad. Sci. USA 82, 5068–5072.
[2] Toyonaga, B. et al. (1985) Proc. Natl Acad. Sci. USA 82, 8624–8628.
[3] Rowen, L. et al. (1996) Science 272, 1755–1762.

Protein display

Protein display of the TRBC1 gene is shown on page 372.

Nomenclature

TRBC2: T cell receptor beta constant 2.

Definition and functionality

TRBC2 is one of the two functional genes of the TRBC group which comprises two mapped genes. TRBC1 and TRBC2 result from a recent duplication.

Gene location

TRBC2 is in the TRB locus on chromosome 7 at 7q34.

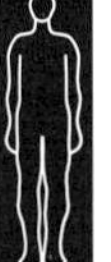

Nucleotide and amino acid sequences for human TRBC2

The nucleotide between parentheses at the beginning of exons comes from a DONOR–SPLICE (n from ngt).
The Cysteines involved in the intrachain disulfide bridges are shown with their number and letter **C** in bold.
N-Glycosylation sites (NXS/T, where X is different from P) are underlined.

```
                        1    2    3    4    5    6    7    8    9    10   11   12   13   14   15   16   17   18   19   20
                        E    D    L    K    N    V    F    P    P    E    V    A    V    F    E    P    S    E    A    E
   M12888   ,TRBC2*01, (EX1)  [1] (G)AG GAC CTG AAA AAC GTG TTC CCA CCC GAG GTC GCT GTG TTT GAG CCA TCA GAA GCA GAG

   M12510   ,TRBC2*01         [2] (-)-- --- --- --- --- --- --- --- --- --- --- --- --- --- --- --- --- --- --- ---

 (1)L36092,U66061,TRBC2*02    [3] (-)-- --- --- --- --- --- --- --- --- --- --- --- --- --- --- --- --- --- --- ---


                        21   22   23   24   25   26   27   28   29   30   31   32   33   34   35   36   37   38   39   40
                        I    S    H    T    Q    K    A    T    L    V    C    L    A    T    G    F    Y    P    D    H
   M12888   ,TRBC2*01         ATC TCC CAC ACC CAA AAG GCC ACA CTG GTG TGC CTG GCC ACA GGC TTC TAC CCC GAC CAC

   M12510   ,TRBC2*01         --- --- --- --- --- --- --- --- --- --- --- --- --- --- --- --- --- --- --- ---

 (1)L36092,U66061,TRBC2*02    --- --- --- --- --- --- --- --- --- --A --- --- --- --- --- --- --- --- --- ---


                        41   42   43   44   45   46   47   48   49   50   51   52   53   54   55   56   57   58   59   60
                        V    E    L    S    W    W    V    N    G    K    E    V    H    S    G    V    S    T    D    P
   M12888   ,TRBC2*01         GTG GAG CTG AGC TGG TGG GTG AAT GGG AAG GAG GTG CAC AGT GGG GTC AGC ACA GAC CCG

   M12510   ,TRBC2*01         --- --- --- --- --- --- --- --- --- --- --- --- --- --- --- --- --- --- --- ---

 (1)L36092,U66061,TRBC2*02    --- --- --- --- --- --- --- --- --- --- --- --- --- --- --- --- --- --- --- ---


                        61   62   63   64   65   66   67   68   69   70   71   72   73   74   75   76   77   78   79   80
                        Q    P    L    K    E    Q    P    A    L    N    D    S    R    Y    C    L    S    S    R    L
   M12888   ,TRBC2*01         CAG CCC CTC AAG GAG CAG CCC GCC CTC AAT GAC TCC AGA TAC TGC CTG AGC AGC CGC CTG

   M12510   ,TRBC2*01         --- --- --- --- --- --- --- --- --- --- --- --- --- --- --- --- --- --- --- ---

 (1)L36092,U66061,TRBC2*02    --- --- --- --- --- --- --- --- --- --- --- --- --- --- --- --- --- --- --- ---


                        81   82   83   84   85   86   87   88   89   90   91   92   93   94   95   96   97   98   99  100
                        R    V    S    A    T    F    W    Q    N    P    R    N    H    F    R    C    Q    V    Q    F
   M12888   ,TRBC2*01         AGG GTC TCG GCC ACC TTC TGG CAG AAC CCC CGC AAC CAC TTC CGC TGT CAA GTC CAG TTC

   M12510   ,TRBC2*01         --- --- --- --- --- --- --- --- --- --- --- --- --- --- --- --- --- --- --- ---

 (1)L36092,U66061,TRBC2*02    --- --- --- --- --- --- --- --- --- --- --- --- --- --- --- --- --- --- --- ---


                       101  102  103  104  105  106  107  108  109  110  111  112  113  114  115  116  117  118  119  120
                        Y    G    L    S    E    N    D    E    W    T    Q    D    R    A    K    P    V    T    Q    I
   M12888   ,TRBC2*01         TAC GGG CTC TCG GAG AAT GAC GAG TGG ACC CAG GAT AGG GCC AAA CCT GTC ACC CAG ATC

   M12510   ,TRBC2*01         --- --- --- --- --- --- --- --- --- --- --- --- --- --- --- --- --- --- --- ---

 (1)L36092,U66061,TRBC2*02    --- --- --- --- --- --- --- --- --- --- --- --- --- --- --- --C --- --- --- ---


                       121  122  123  124  125  126  127  128  129
                        V    S    A    E    A    W    G    R    A
   M12888   ,TRBC2*01         GTC AGC GCC GAG GCC TGG GGT AGA GCA G

   M12510   ,TRBC2*01         --- --- --- --- --- --- --- --- -

 (1)L36092,U66061,TRBC2*02    --- --- --- --- --- --- --- --- -


                        1    2    3    4    5    6
                        D    C    G    F    T    S
   M12888   ,TRBC2*01, (EX2)  AC TGT GGC TTC ACC TCC G

   M12510   ,TRBC2*01         -- --- --- --- --- --- -

 (1)L36092,U66061,TRBC2*01    -- --- --- --- --- --- -
```

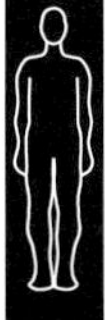

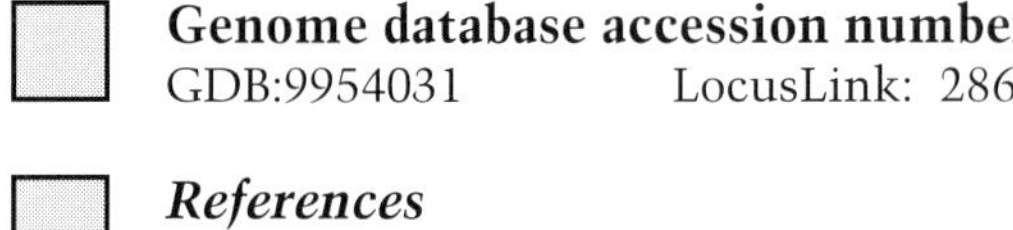

```
                          1   2   3   4   5   6   7   8   9   10  11  12  13  14  15  16  17  18  19  20
                          E   S   Y   Q   Q   G   V   L   S   A   T   I   L   Y   E   I   L   L   G   K
  M12888   ,TRBC2*01, (EX3) AG  TCT TAC CAG CAA GGG GTC CTG TCT GCC ACC ATC CTC TAT GAG ATC TTG CTA GGG AAG

  M12510   ,TRBC2*01        --  --- --- --- --- --- --- --- --- --- --- --- --- --- --- --- --- --- --- ---

(1)L36092,U66061,TRBC2*01    --  --- --- --- --- --- --- --- --- --- --- --- --- --- --- --- --- --- --- ---


                          21  22  23  24  25  26  27  28  29  30  31  32  33  34  35  36
                          A   T   L   Y   A   V   L   V   S   A   L   V   L   M   A   M
  M12888   ,TRBC2*01        GCC ACC TTG TAT GCC GTG CTG GTC AGT GCC CTC GTG CTG ATG GCC ATG

  M12510   ,TRBC2*01        --- --- --- --- --- --- --- --- --- --- --- --- --- --- --- ---

(1)L36092,U66061,TRBC2*01    --- --- --- --- --- --- --- --- --- --- --- --- --- --- --- ---


                          1   2   3   4   5   6   7   8
                          V   K   R   K   D   S   R   G   *
  M12888   ,TRBC2*01, (EX4) GTC AAG AGA AAG GAT TCC AGA GGC

  M12510   ,TRBC2*01        --- --- --- --- --- --- --- ---

(1)L36092,U66061,TRBC2*01    --- --- --- --- --- --- --- ---
```

Note:

(1) The original L36092 sequence (684 973 bp) has been split in EMBL into three sequences of 267 156 bp (U66059), 215 422 bp (U66060) and 232 650 bp (U66061); L36092 has become secondary accession number of U66059, U66060, and U66061. In IMGT, the original sequence L36092, which is fully annotated, has also been kept as primary accession number, in addition to U66059, U66060, and U66061.

Genome database accession numbers

GDB:9954031   LocusLink: 28638

References

[1] Tunnacliffe, A. et al. (1985) Proc. Natl Acad. Sci. USA 82, 5068–5072.
[2] Toyonaga, B. et al. (1985) Proc. Natl Acad. Sci. USA 82, 8624–8628.
[3] Rowen, L. et al. (1996) Science 272, 1755–1762.

Protein display

Protein display of the TRBC2 gene is shown on page 372.

Part 2

TRBD

Nomenclature

T cell receptor beta diversity group.

Definition and functionality

The human TRBD group comprises two functional mapped genes, TRBD1 and TRBD2. The TRBD1 and TRBD2 genes have two or three open reading frames in both the direct and inverted orientations.

Gene location

The human TRBD genes are located in the TRB locus on chromosome 7 at 7q34. TRBD1 is upstream from the TRBJ1-1 to TRBJ1-6 gene cluster. TRBD2 is upstream from the TRBJ2-1 to TRBJ2-7 gene cluster.

Nucleotide and amino acid sequences for the human TRBD genes with nomenclature

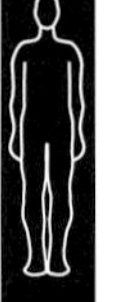

```
                                Direct 5' – 3' orientation            Inverted orientation

TRBD1
T cell receptor beta diversity 1
                                    G   T   G   G                        A   P   C   P
                                      G   Q   G                            P   P   V
                                        D   R   G                            P   L   S
X00936   ,TRBD1*01          [1]   gggacaggggggc                        gccccctgtccc


TRBD2
T cell receptor beta diversity 2
                                    G   T   S   G   G                    P   P   R   *   S
                                      G   L   A   G   G                    P   P   A   S   P
                                        D   *   R   G                      P   P   L   V
X02987   ,TRBD2*01          [3]   gggactagcggggggg                     cccccccgctagtccc


                                    G   T   S   G   R                    P   S   R   *   S
                                      G   L   A   G   G                    P   P   A   S   P
                                        D   *   R   E                      L   P   L   V
M14159   ,TRBD2*02          [2]   gggactagcgggaggg                     ccctcccgctagtccc
```

Recombination signals

5′D Recombination Signal (5′D-RS)			TRBD gene and allele name	3′D Recombination Signal (3′D-RS)		
5′D-NONAMER	(bp)	5′D-HEPTAMER		3′D-HEPTAMER	(bp)	3′D-NONAMER
TGTTTTTGT	12	CATTGTG	TRBD1*01	CACAATG	23	ACAAAAACC
CATTTTTGT	12	CATTGTG	TRBD2*01	CACGATG	23	ACAAAAAAC
CATTTTTGT	12	CATTGTG	TRBD2*02	CACGATG	23	ACAAAAAAC

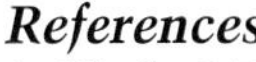

References

[1] Clark, S.P. et al. (1984) Nature 311, 387–389.
[2] Toyonaga, B. et al. (1985) Proc. Natl Acad. Sci. USA 82, 8624–8628.
[3] Tunnacliffe, A. et al. (1985) Nucleic Acids Res. 13, 6651–6661.

Part 3

TRBJ

Nomenclature

T cell receptor beta joining group.

Definition and functionality

The human TRBJ group comprises 14 mapped genes of which 12–13 are functional, and 1–2 are ORF.

TRBJ2-2P is an ORF due to J-PHE replaced by Leucine in J-SEGMENT and to missing J-NONAMER.

TRBJ2-7*02 is an ORF due to J-PHE replaced by Valine in J-SEGMENT.

Gene location

The human TRBJ genes are located in the TRB locus on chromosome 7 at 7q34, upstream from the TRBC genes. Six functional TRBJ (TRBJ1-1 to TRBJ1-6) are located upstream from TRBC1, and eight TRBJ (TRBJ2-1 to TRBJ2-7) of which 6–7 are functional, are located upstream from TRBC2.

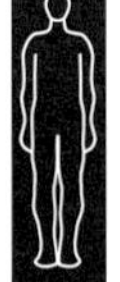

Nucleotide and amino acid sequences for the human functional or ORF TRBJ genes with nomenclature

The conserved **FGXG** motif, characteristic of the TRB J-REGION is underlined.

```
TRBJ1-1
T cell receptor beta 1-1
                                N   T   E   A   F   F   G   Q   G   T   R   L   T   V   V
   X00936  ,TRBJ1-1*01     [1]     TG AAC ACT GAA GCT TTC TTT GGA CAA GGC ACC AGA CTC ACA GTT GTA G

TRBJ1-2
T cell receptor beta 1-2
                                N   Y   G   Y   T   F   G   S   G   T   R   L   T   V   V
   X00936  ,TRBJ1-2*01     [1]     CT AAC TAT GGC TAC ACC TTC GGT TCG GGG ACC AGG TTA ACC GTT GTA G

TRBJ1-3
T cell receptor beta 1-3
                                S   G   N   T   I   Y   F   G   E   G   S   W   L   T   V   V
   M14158  ,TRBJ1-3*01     [3]   C TCT GGA AAC ACC ATA TAT TTT GGA GAG GGA AGT TGG CTC ACT GTT GTA G

TRBJ1-4
T cell receptor beta 1-4
                                T   N   E   K   L   F   F   G   S   G   T   Q   L   S   V   L
   M14158  ,TRBJ1-4*01     [3]   GA ACT AAT GAA AAA CTG TTT TTT GGC AGT GGA ACC CAG CTC TCT GTC TTG G

TRBJ1-5
T cell receptor beta 1-5
                                S   N   Q   P   Q   H   F   G   D   G   T   R   L   S   I   L
   M14158  ,TRBJ1-5*01     [3]   T AGC AAT CAG CCC CAG CAT TTT GGT GAT GGG ACT CGA CTC TCC ATC CTA G

TRBJ1-6
T cell receptor beta 1-6
                                S   Y   N   S   P   L   H   F   G   N   G   T   R   L   T   V   T
   M14158  ,TRBJ1-6*01     [3] C TCC TAT AAT TCA CCC CTC CAC TTT GGG AAT GGG ACC AGG CTC ACT GTG ACA G
L36092,U66061,TRBJ1-6*02 (1)[2]  - --- --- --- --- --- --- --- --- --- --C --- --- --- --- --- --- ---

TRBJ2-1
T cell receptor beta 2-1
                                S   Y   N   E   Q   F   F   G   P   G   T   R   L   T   V   L
   X02987  ,TRBJ2-1*01     [4]   C TCC TAC AAT GAG CAG TTC TTC GGG CCA GGG ACA CGG CTC ACC GTG CTA G

TRBJ2-2
T cell receptor beta 2-2
                                N   T   G   E   L   F   F   G   E   G   S   R   L   T   V   L
   X02987  ,TRBJ2-2*01     [4]   CG AAC ACC GGG GAG CTG TTT TTT GGA GAA GGC TCT AGG CTG ACC GTA CTG G

TRBJ2-2P
T cell receptor beta 2-2P
                                L   R   G   A   A   G   R   L   G   G   G   L   L   V   L
   X02987  ,TRBJ2-2P*01    [4]   CTG AGA GGC GCT GCT GGG CGT CTG GGC GGA GGA CTC CTG GTT CTG G

TRBJ2-3
T cell receptor beta 2-3
                                S   T   D   T   Q   Y   F   G   P   G   T   R   L   T   V   L
   X02987  ,TRBJ2-3*01     [4]   AGC ACA GAT ACG CAG TAT TTT GGC CCA GGC ACC CGG CTG ACA GTG CTC G
```

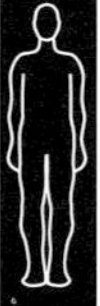

```
TRBJ2-4
T cell receptor beta 2-4
                                        A   K   N   I   Q   Y   F   G   A   G   T   R   L   S   V   L
   X02987  ,TRBJ2-4*01      [4]      A GCC AAA AAC ATT CAG TAC TTC GGC GCC GGG ACC CGG CTC TCA GTG CTG G

TRBJ2-5
T cell receptor beta 2-5
                                            Q   E   T   Q   Y   F   G   P   G   T   R   L   L   V   L
   X02987  ,TRBJ2-5*01      [4]        AC CAA GAG ACC CAG TAC TTC GGG CCA GGC ACG CGG CTC CTG GTG CTC G

TRBJ2-6
T cell receptor beta 2-6
                                        S   G   A   N   V   L   T   F   G   A   G   S   R   L   T   V   L
   X02987  ,TRBJ2-6*01      [4]      C TCT GGG GCC AAC GTC CTG ACT TTC GGG GCC GGC AGC AGG CTG ACC GTG CTG G

TRBJ2-7
T cell receptor beta 2-7
                                        S   Y   E   Q   Y   F   G   P   G   T   R   L   T   V   T
   M14159  ,TRBJ2-7*01      [3]      C TCC TAC GAG CAG TAC TTC GGG CCG GGC ACC AGG CTC ACG GTC ACA G
                                                                V
   X02987  ,TRBJ2-7*02      [4]      - --- --- --- --- --- G-- --- --- --- --- --- --- --- --- --- -
```

Note:

(1) The original L36092 sequence (684 973 bp) has been split in EMBL into three sequences of 267 156 bp (U66059), 215 422 bp (U66060), and 232 650 bp (U66061); L36092 has become secondary accession number of U66059, U66060, and U66061. In IMGT, the original sequence L36092, which is fully annotated, has also been kept as primary accession number, in addition to U66059, U66060, and U66061.

Recombination signals

J Recombination Signal (J-RS)			TRBJ gene and allele name
J-NONAMER	(bp)	J-HEPTAMER	
GATTTTCAC	12	CACTGTG	TRBJ1-1*01
CCTTTTAGA	12	TTATGTG	TRBJ1-2*01
GGTTTTGAA	12	GGCTGTG	TRBJ1-3*01
GGTTTTCCT	12	TGTTGTG	TRBJ1-4*01
GGGTTTGCC	12	CACTGTG	TRBJ1-5*01
GGGTTTTAT	12	AGCTGTG	TRBJ1-6*01
GGGTTTTAT	12	AGCTGTG	TRBJ1-6*02
GAATTCTGG	12	CACTGTG	TRBJ2-1*01
GGTTTGCGC	12	GGCTGTG	TRBJ2-2*01
del	del	GGCTGTG	TRBJ2-2P*01 (ORF)
GGTTTTTGT	12	GGCTGTG	TRBJ2-3*01
AGTTTCTGT	12	GGCTGTG	TRBJ2-4*01
GGTTTTTGT	12	GGCCGTG	TRBJ2-5*01
GGTTTTTGC	12	GGCTGTG	TRBJ2-6*01
GGTTTGCAT	12	CTCCGTG	TRBJ2-7*01
GGTTTGCAT	12	CTCCGTG	TRBJ2-7*02 (ORF)

del: deleted

References

1 Clark, S.P. et al. (1984) Nature 311, 387–389.
2 Rowen, L. et al. (1996) Science 272, 1755–1762.
3 Toyonaga, B. et al. (1985) Proc. Natl Acad. Sci. USA 82, 8624–8628.
4 Tunnacliffe, A. et al. (1985) Nucleic Acids Res. 13, 6651–6661.

Part 4

TRBV

TRBV2

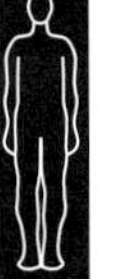

Nomenclature

TRBV2: T cell receptor beta variable 2.

Definition and functionality

TRBV2 is the unique functional gene of the TRBV2 subgroup which only comprises this mapped gene in the TRB locus.

Gene location

TRBV2 is in the TRB locus on chromosome 7 at 7q34.

Nucleotide and amino acid sequences for human TRBV2

```
                              1    2    3    4    5    6    7    8    9   10   11   12   13   14   15   16   17   18   19   20
                              E    P    E    V    T    Q    T    P    S    H    Q    V    T    Q    M    G    Q    E    V    I
L36092,U66059,TRBV2*01  [34]  GAA  CCT  GAA  GTC  ACC  CAG  ACT  CCC  AGC  CAT  CAG  GTC  ACA  CAG  ATG  GGA  CAG  GAA  GTG  ATC

M62379   ,TRBV2*02      [33]  ---  ---  ---  ---  ---  ---  ---  ---  ---  ---  ---  ---  ---  ---  ---  ---  ---  ---  ---  ---

M64351   ,TRBV2*03       [2]  ---  ---  ---  ---  ---  ---  ---  ---  ---  ---  ---  ---  ---  ---  ---  ---  ---  ---  ---  ---

                                                                        ___________________CDR1-IMGT___________________________
                             21   22   23   24   25   26   27   28   29   30   31   32   33   34   35   36   37   38   39   40
                              L    R    C    V    P    I    S    N    H    L    Y                                       F    Y
L36092,U66059,TRBV2*01       TTG  CGC  TGT  GTC  CCC  ATC  TCT  AAT  CAC  TTA  TAC  ...  ...  ...  ...  ...  ...  ...  TTC  TAT
                                   H
M62379   ,TRBV2*02           ---  -A-  ---  ---  ---  ---  ---  ---  ---  ---  ---  ...  ...  ...  ...  ...  ...  ...  ---  ---

M64351   ,TRBV2*03           ---  ---  ---  ---  ---  ---  ---  ---  ---  ---  ---  ...  ...  ...  ...  ...  ...  ...  ---  ---

                                                                                            _________________________CDR2-
                             41   42   43   44   45   46   47   48   49   50   51   52   53   54   55   56   57   58   59   60
                              W    Y    R    Q    I    L    G    Q    K    V    E    F    L    V    S    F    Y    N    N    E
L36092,U66059,TRBV2*01       TGG  TAC  AGA  CAA  ATC  TTG  GGG  CAG  AAA  GTC  GAG  TTT  CTG  GTT  TCC  TTT  TAT  AAT  AAT  GAA

M62379   ,TRBV2*02           ---  ---  ---  ---  ---  ---  ---  ---  ---  ---  ---  ---  ---  ---  ---  ---  ---  ---  ---  ---

M64351   ,TRBV2*03           ---  ---  ---  ---  ---  ---  ---  ---  ---  ---  ---  ---  ---  ---  ---  ---  ---  ---  ---  ---

                             IMGT________________________
                             61   62   63   64   65   66   67   68   69   70   71   72   73   74   75   76   77   78   79   80
                              I                        S    E    K    S    E    I    F    D    D    Q    F    S    V    E    R
L36092,U66059,TRBV2*01       ATC  ...  ...  ...  ...  TCA  GAG  AAG  TCT  GAA  ATA  TTC  GAT  GAT  CAA  TTC  TCA  GTT  GAA  AGG

M62379   ,TRBV2*02           ---  ...  ...  ...  ...  ---  ---  ---  ---  ---  ---  ---  ---  ---  ---  ---  ---  ---  ---  ---

M64351   ,TRBV2*03           ---  ...  ...  ...  ...  ---  ---  ---  ---  ---  ---  ---  ---  ---  ---  ---  ---  ---  ---  --G  ---

                             81   82   83   84   85   86   87   88   89   90   91   92   93   94   95   96   97   98   99  100
                              P         D    G    S    N    F    T    L    K    I    R    S    T    K    L    E    D    S    A
L36092,U66059,TRBV2*01       CCT  ...  GAT  GGA  TCA  AAT  TTC  ACT  CTG  AAG  ATC  CGG  TCC  ACA  AAG  CTG  GAG  GAC  TCA  GCC

M62379   ,TRBV2*02           ---  ...  ---  ---  ---  ---  ---  ---  ---  ---  ---  ---  ---  ---  ---  ---  ---  ---  ---  ---

M64351   ,TRBV2*03           ---  ...  ---  ---  ---  ---  ---  ---  ---  ---  ---  ---  ---  ---  ---  ---  ---  ---  ---  ---  ---

                                        _______CDR3-IMGT_______
                            101  102  103  104  105  106  107  108  109
                              M    Y    F    C    A    S    S    E
L36092,U66059,TRBV2*01       ATG  TAC  TTC  TGT  GCC  AGC  AGT  GAA  GC

M62379   ,TRBV2*02           ---  ---  ---  ---  ---  ---  ---              #c

M64351   ,TRBV2*03           ---  ---  ---  ---  ---  ---  ---  ---         #c

#c: Rearranged cDNA
```

Framework and complementarity determining regions

FR1-IMGT: 26   CDR1-IMGT: 5
FR2-IMGT: 17   CDR2-IMGT: 6
FR3-IMGT: 38 (-1 aa: 82)   CDR3-IMGT: 4

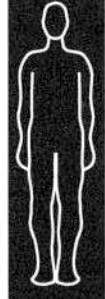

Collier de Perles for human TRBV2*01

Accession number: IMGT L36092   EMBL/GenBank/DDBJ: L36092

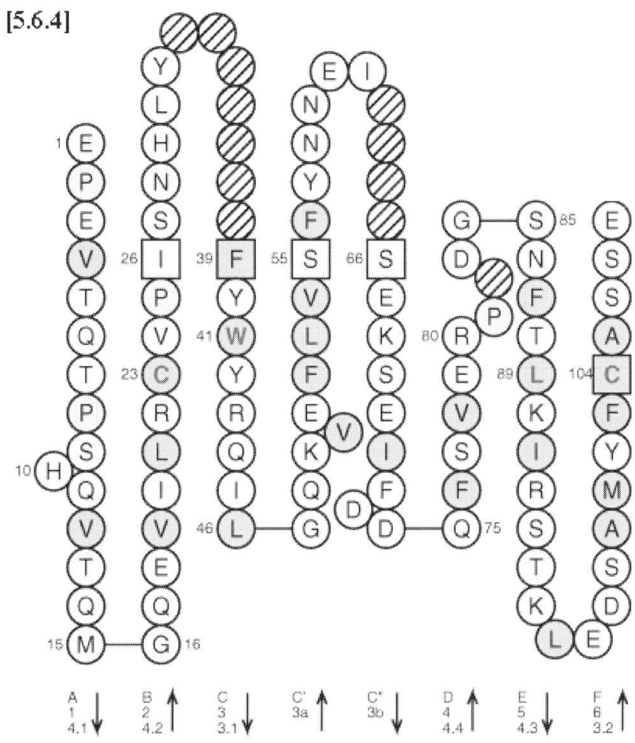

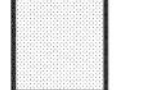

Genome database accession numbers
GDB:9954067   LocusLink: 28620

TRBV3-1

Nomenclature

TRBV3-1: T cell receptor beta variable 3-1.

Definition and functionality

TRBV3-1 is the unique functional gene of the TRBV3 subgroup which comprises one or two mapped genes, depending on the haplotypes, in the TRB locus.

Gene location

TRBV3-1 is in the TRB locus on chromosome 7 at 7q34.

Nucleotide and amino acid sequences for human TRBV3-1

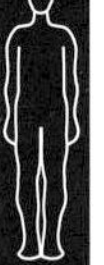

```
                            1   2   3   4   5   6   7   8   9  10  11  12  13  14  15  16  17  18  19  20
                            D   T   A   V   S   Q   T   P   K   Y   L   V   T   Q   M   G   N   D   K   S
U07977   ,TRBV3-1*01   [47] GAC ACA GCT GTT TCC CAG ACT CCA AAA TAC CTG GTC ACA CAG ATG GGA AAC GAC AAG TCC
L36092,U66059,TRBV3-1*01 [34] --- --- --- --- --- --- --- --- --- --- --- --- --- --- --- --- --- --- --- ---
L06889   ,TRBV3-1*02   [36] --- --- --- --- --- --- --- --- --- --- --- --- --- --- --- --- --- --- --- ---

                                                            ________________CDR1-IMGT________________
                           21  22  23  24  25  26  27  28  29  30  31  32  33  34  35  36  37  38  39  40
                            I   K   C   E   Q   N   L   G   H   D   T                           M   Y
U07977   ,TRBV3-1*01        ATT AAA TGT GAA CAA AAT CTG GGC CAT GAT ACT ... ... ... ... ... ... ... ATG TAT
L36092,U66059,TRBV3-1*01    --- --- --- --- --- --- --- --- --- --- --- ... ... ... ... ... ... ... --- ---
L06889   ,TRBV3-1*02        --- --- --- --- --- --- --- --- --- --- --- ... ... ... ... ... ... ... --- ---

                                                                                        ________________CDR2-
                           41  42  43  44  45  46  47  48  49  50  51  52  53  54  55  56  57  58  59  60
                            W   Y   K   Q   D   S   K   K   F   L   K   I   M   F   S   Y   N   N   K   E
U07977   ,TRBV3-1*01        TGG TAT AAA CAG GAC TCT AAG AAA TTT CTG AAG ATA ATG TTT AGC TAC AAT AAT AAG GAG
L36092,U66059,TRBV3-1*01    --- --- --- --- --- --- --- --- --- --- --- --- --- --- --- --- --- --- --- ---
L06889   ,TRBV3-1*02        --- --- --- --- --- --- --- --- --- --- --- --- --- --- --- --- --- --C --- ---

                           IMGT________________
                           61  62  63  64  65  66  67  68  69  70  71  72  73  74  75  76  77  78  79  80
                            L                   I   I   N   E   T   V   P       N   R   F   S   P   K   S
U07977   ,TRBV3-1*01        CTC ... ... ... ... ATT ATA AAT GAA ACA GTT CCA ... AAT CGC TTC TCA CCT AAA TCT
L36092,U66059,TRBV3-1*01    --- ... ... ... ... --- --- --- --- --- --- --- ... --- --- --- --- --- --- ---
                            I
L06889   ,TRBV3-1*02        A-- ... ... ... ... --- --- --- --- --- --- --- ... --- --A --- --- --- --- ---

                           81  82  83  84  85  86  87  88  89  90  91  92  93  94  95  96  97  98  99 100
                            P       D   K   A   H   L   N   L   H   I   N   S   L   E   L   G   D   S   A
U07977   ,TRBV3-1*01        CCA ... GAC AAA GCT CAC TTA AAT CTT CAC ATC AAT TCC CTG GAG CTT GGT GAC TCT GCT
L36092,U66059,TRBV3-1*01    --- ... --- --- --- --- --- --- --- --- --- --- --- --- --- --- --- --- --- ---
                                                K
L06889   ,TRBV3-1*02        --- ... --- --- --- A-A --- --- --- --- --- --- --- --- --- --- --- --- --- ---

                                           ______CDR3-IMGT______
                          101 102 103 104 105 106 107 108 109
                            V   Y   F   C   A   S   S   Q
U07977   ,TRBV3-1*01        GTG TAT TTC TGT GCC AGC AGC CAA GA
L36092,U66059,TRBV3-1*01    --- --- --- --- --- --- --- --- --
L06889   ,TRBV3-1*02        --- --- --- --- --- ---                        #c
```

#c: Rearranged cDNA

Framework and complementarity determining regions

FR1-IMGT: 26	CDR1-IMGT: 5
FR2-IMGT: 17	CDR2-IMGT: 6
FR3-IMGT: 37 (-2 aa: 73, 82)	CDR3-IMGT: 4

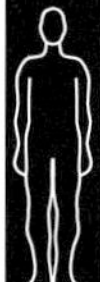

Collier de Perles for human TRBV3-1*01

Accession number: IMGT U07977   EMBL/GenBank/DDBJ: U07977

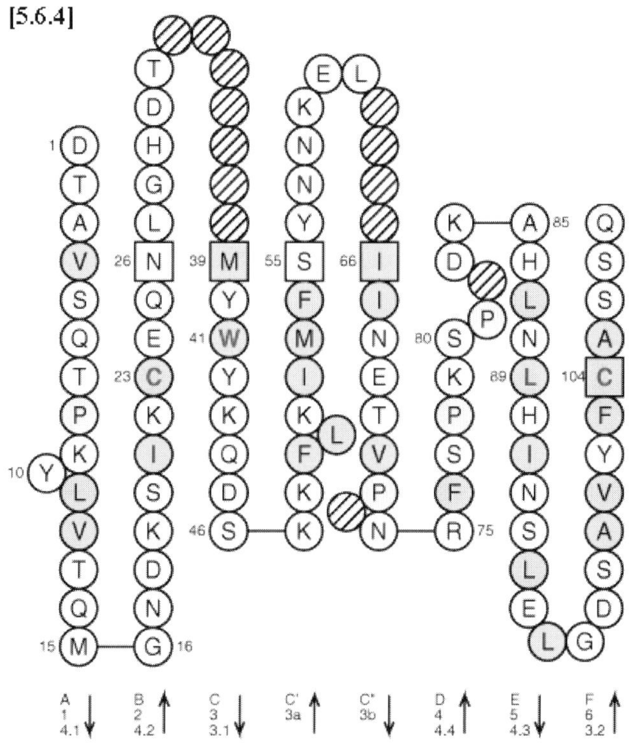

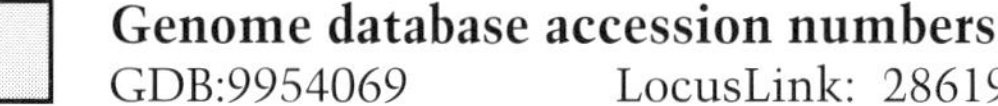

Genome database accession numbers
GDB:9954069   LocusLink: 28619

TRBV4-1

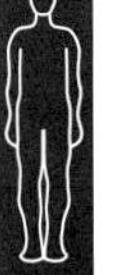

Nomenclature

TRBV4-1: T cell receptor beta variable 4-1.

Definition and functionality

TRBV4-1 is one of the 2–3 functional genes of the TRBV4 subgroup which comprises two or three mapped genes, depending on the haplotypes, in the TRB locus.

Gene location

TRBV4-1 is in the TRB locus on chromosome 7 at 7q34.

Nucleotide and amino acid sequences for human TRBV4-1

```
                           1   2   3   4   5   6   7   8   9  10  11  12  13  14  15  16  17  18  19  20
                           D   T   E   V   T   Q   T   P   K   H   L   V   M   G   M   T   N   K   K   S
U07977    ,TRBV4-1*01 [47] GAC ACT GAA GTT ACC CAG ACA CCA AAA CAC CTG GTC ATG GGA ATG ACA AAT AAG AAG TCT
L36092,U66059,TRBV4-1*01 [34] --- --- --- --- --- --- --- --- --- --- --- --- --- --- --- --- --- --- --- ---
M13855    ,TRBV4-1*02  [5]                     --- --- --- --- --- --- --- --- --- --- --- --- --- ---

                                                                                _______CDR1-IMGT________
                          21  22  23  24  25  26  27  28  29  30  31  32  33  34  35  36  37  38  39  40
                           L   K   C   E   Q   H   M   G   H   R   A                               M   Y
U07977    ,TRBV4-1*01     TTG AAA TGT GAA CAA CAT ATG GGG CAC AGG GCT ... ... ... ... ... ... ... ATG TAT
L36092,U66059,TRBV4-1*01 --- --- --- --- --- --- --- --- --- --- --- ... ... ... ... ... ... ... --- ---
M13855    ,TRBV4-1*02    --- --- --- --- --- --- --- --- --- --- --A ... ... ... ... ... ... ... --- ---

                                                                                            ______CDR2-
                          41  42  43  44  45  46  47  48  49  50  51  52  53  54  55  56  57  58  59  60
                           W   Y   K   Q   K   A   K   K   P   P   E   L   M   F   V   Y   S   Y   E   K
U07977    ,TRBV4-1*01     TGG TAC AAG CAG AAA GCT AAG AAG CCA CCG GAG CTC ATG TTT GTC TAC AGC TAT GAG AAA
L36092,U66059,TRBV4-1*01 --- --- --- --- --- --- --- --- --- --- --- --- --- --- --- --- --- --- --- ---
M13855    ,TRBV4-1*02    --- --- --- --- --- --- --- --- --- --- --- --- --- --- --- --- --- --- --- ---

                          IMGT_______________
                          61  62  63  64  65  66  67  68  69  70  71  72  73  74  75  76  77  78  79  80
                           L               S   I   N   E   S   V   P       S   R   F   S   P   E   C
U07977    ,TRBV4 1*01     CTC ... ... ... ... TCT ATA AAT GAA AGT GTG CCA ... AGT CGC TTC TCA CCT GAA TGC
L36092,U66059,TRBV4-1*01 --- ... ... ... ... --- --- --- --- --- --- --- ... --- --- --- --- --- --- ---
M13855    ,TRBV4-1*02    --- ... ... ... ... --- --- --- --- --- --- --- ... --- --- --- --- --- --- ---

                          81  82  83  84  85  86  87  88  89  90  91  92  93  94  95  96  97  98  99 100
                           P       N   S   S   L   L   N   L   H   L   H   A   L   Q   P   E   D   S   A
U07977    ,TRBV4-1*01     CCC ... AAC AGC TCT CTC TTA AAC CTT CAC CTA CAC GCC CTG CAG CCA GAA GAC TCA GCC
L36092,U66059,TRBV4-1*01 --- ... --- --- --- --- --- --- --- --- --- --- --- --- --- --- --- --- --- ---
M13855    ,TRBV4-1*02    --- ... --- --- --- --- --- --- --- --- --- --- --- --- --- --- --- --- --- ---

                                          ______CDR3-IMGT______
                         101 102 103 104 105 106 107 108 109
                           L   Y   L   C   A   S   S   Q
U07977    ,TRBV4-1*01     CTG TAT CTC TGC GCC AGC AGC CAA GA
L36092,U66059,TRBV4-1*01 --- --- --- --- --- --- --- --- --
M13855    ,TRBV4-1*02    --- --- --- --- --- --- --- ---        #c
#c: Rearranged cDNA
```

Framework and complementarity determining regions

FR1-IMGT: 26	CDR1-IMGT: 5
FR2-IMGT: 17	CDR2-IMGT: 6
FR3-IMGT: 37 (-2 aa: 73, 82)	CDR3-IMGT: 4

Collier de Perles for human TRBV4-1*01

Accession number: IMGT U07977   EMBL/GenBank/DDBJ: U07977

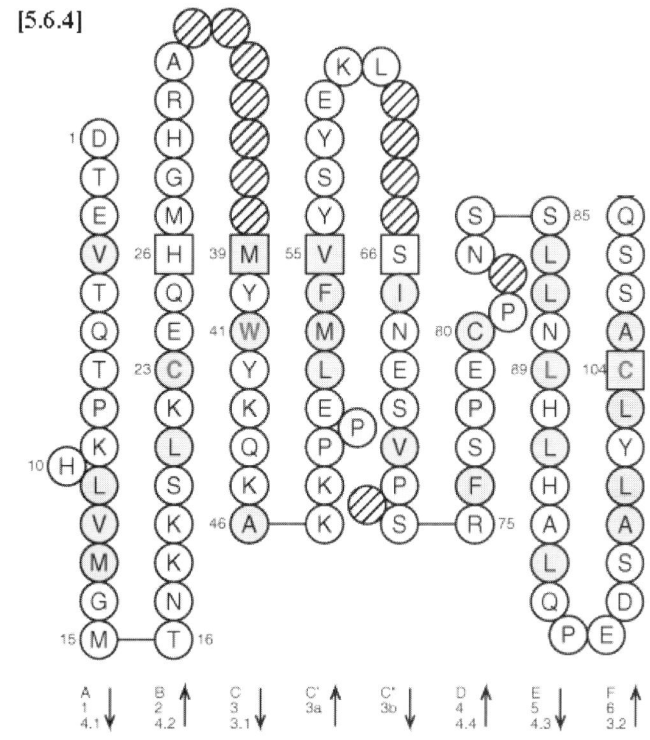

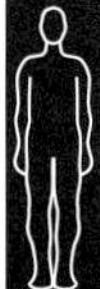

TRBV4-2

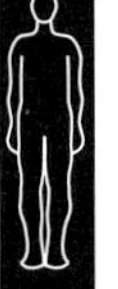

Nomenclature

TRBV4-2: T cell receptor beta variable 4-2.

Definition and functionality

TRBV4-2 is one of the 2-3 functional genes of the TRBV4 subgroup which comprises two or three mapped genes, depending on the haplotypes, in the TRB locus.

Gene location

TRBV4-2 is in the TRB locus on chromosome 7 at 7q34.

Nucleotide and amino acid sequences for human TRBV4-2

```
                          1   2   3   4   5   6   7   8   9  10  11  12  13  14  15  16  17  18  19  20
                          E   T   G   V   T   Q   T   P   R   H   L   V   M   G   M   T   N   K   K   S
U07975    ,TRBV4-2*01 [47] GAA ACG GGA GTT ACG CAG ACA CCA AGA CAC CTG GTC ATG GGA ATG ACA AAT AAG AAG TCT
U07976    ,TRBV4-2*01 [47] --- --- --- --- --- --- --- --- --- --- --- --- --- --- --- --- --- --- --- ---
U07978    ,TRBV4-2*01 [47] --- --- --- --- --- --- --- --- --- --- --- --- --- --- --- --- --- --- --- ---
L36092,U66059,TRBV4-2*01 [34] --- --- --- --- --- --- --- --- --- --- --- --- --- --- --- --- --- --- --- ---
L36190    ,TRBV4-2*01 [34] --- --- --- --- --- --- --- --- --- --- --- --- --- --- --- --- --- --- --- ---
AF009660,TRBV4-2*01   [35] --- --- --- --- --- --- --- --- --- --- --- --- --- --- --- --- --- --- --- ---
X58811    ,TRBV4-2*02 [10] --- --- --- --- --- --- --- --- --- --- --- --- --- --- --- --- --- --- --- ---

                                                            ______________CDR1-IMGT______________
                         21  22  23  24  25  26  27  28  29  30  31  32  33  34  35  36  37  38  39  40
                          L   K   C   E   Q   H   L   G   H   N   A                               M   Y
U07975    ,TRBV4-2*01     TTG AAA TGT GAA CAA CAT CTG GGG CAT AAC GCT ... ... ... ... ... ... ... ATG TAT
U07976    ,TRBV4-2*01     --- --- --- --- --- --- --- --- --- --- --- ... ... ... ... ... ... ... --- ---
U07978    ,TRBV4-2*01     --- --- --- --- --- --- --- --- --- --- --- ... ... ... ... ... ... ... --- ---
L36092,U66059,TRBV4-2*01  --- --- --- --- --- --- --- --- --- --- --- ... ... ... ... ... ... ... --- ---
L36190    ,TRBV4-2*01     --- --- --- --- --- --- --- --- --- --- --- ... ... ... ... ... ... ... --- ---
AF009660,TRBV4-2*01       --- --- --- --- --- --- --- --- --- --- --- ... ... ... ... ... ... ... --- ---
X58811    ,TRBV4-2*02     --- --- --- --- --- --- --- --- --- --- --- ... ... ... ... ... ... ... --- ---

                                                                                        ____________CDR2-
                         41  42  43  44  45  46  47  48  49  50  51  52  53  54  55  56  57  58  59  60
                          W   Y   K   Q   S   A   K   K   P   L   E   L   M   F   V   Y   N   F   K   E
U07975    ,TRBV4-2*01     TGG TAC AAG CAA AGT GCT AAG AAG CCA CTG GAG CTC ATG TTT GTC TAC AAC TTT AAA GAA
U07976    ,TRBV4-2*01     --- --- --- --- --- --- --- --- --- --- --- --- --- --- --- --- --- --- --- ---
U07978    ,TRBV4-2*01     --- --- --- --- --- --- --- --- --- --- --- --- --- --- --- --- --- --- --- ---
L36092,U66059,TRBV4-2*01  --- --- --- --- --- --- --- --- --- --- --- --- --- --- --- --- --- --- --- ---
L36190    ,TRBV4-2*01     --- --- --- --- --- --- --- --- --- --- --- --- --- --- --- --- --- --- --- ---
AF009660,TRBV4-2*01       --- --- --- --- --- --- --- --- --- --- --- --- --- --- --- --- --- --- --- ---
X58811    ,TRBV4-2*02     --- --- --- --- --- --- --- --- --- --- --- --- --- --- --- --- --- --- --- ---

                         IMGT________
                         61  62  63  64  65  66  67  68  69  70  71  72  73  74  75  76  77  78  79  80
                          Q                   T   E   N   N   S   V   P       S   R   F   S   P   E   C
U07975    ,TRBV4-2*01     CAG ... ... ... ... ACT GAA AAC AAC AGT GTG CCA ... AGT CGC TTC TCA CCT GAA TGC
U07976    ,TRBV4-2*01     --- ... ... ... ... --- --- --- --- --- --- --- ... --- --- --- --- --- --- ---
U07978    ,TRBV4-2*01     --- ... ... ... ... --- --- --- --- --- --- --- ... --- --- --- --- --- --- ---
L36092,U66059,TRBV4-2*01  --- ... ... ... ... --- --- --- --- --- --- --- ... --- --- --- --- --- --- ---
L36190    ,TRBV4-2*01     --- ... ... ... ... --- --- --- --- --- --- --- ... --- --- --- --- --- --- ---
AF009660,TRBV4-2*01       --- ... ... ... ... --- --- --- --- --- --- --- ... --- --- --- --- --- --- ---
X58811    ,TRBV4-2*02     --- ... ... ... ... --- --- --- --- --- --- --- ... --- --- --- --- --- --- ---

                         81  82  83  84  85  86  87  88  89  90  91  92  93  94  95  96  97  98  99 100
                          P       N   S   S   H   L   F   L   H   L   H   T   L   Q   P   E   D   S   A
U07975    ,TRBV4-2*01     CCC ... AAC AGC TCT CAC TTA TTC CTT CAC CTA CAC ACC CTG CAG CCA GAA GAC TCG GCC
U07976    ,TRBV4-2*01     --- ... --- --- --- --- --- --- --- --- --- --- --- --- --- --- --- --- --- ---
U07978    ,TRBV4-2*01     --- ... --- --- --- --- --- --- --- --- --- --- --- --- --- --- --- --- --- ---
L36092,U66059,TRBV4-2*01  --- ... --- --- --- --- --- --- --- --- --- --- --- --- --- --- --- --- --- ---
L36190    ,TRBV4-2*01     --- ... --- --- --- --- --- --- --- --- --- --- --- --- --- --- --- --- --- ---
AF009660,TRBV4-2*01       --- ... --- --- --- --- --- --- --- --- --- --- --- --- --- --- --- --- --- ---
                                                          C
X58811    ,TRBV4-2*02     --- ... --- --- --- --- --- -G- --- --- --- --- --- --- --- --- --- --- --- ---
```

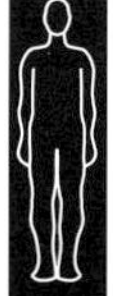

```
                                          ______CDR3-IMGT______
                          101 102 103 104 105 106 107 108 109
                           L   Y   L   C   A   S   S   Q
U07975    ,TRBV4-2*01     CTG TAT CTC TGT GCC AGC AGC CAA GA

U07976    ,TRBV4-2*01     --- --- --- --- --- --- --- --- --

U07978    ,TRBV4-2*01     --- --- --- --- --- --- --- --- --

L36092,U66059,TRBV4-2*01  --- --- --- --- --- --- --- --- --

L36190    ,TRBV4-2*01     --- --- --- --- --- --- --- --- --

AF009660,TRBV4-2*01       --- --- --- --- --- --- --- --- --
                                                  T
X58811    ,TRBV4-2*02     --- --- --- --- --- --- -C-          #c
```
#c: Rearranged cDNA

Framework and complementarity determining regions

FR1-IMGT: 26   CDR1-IMGT: 5
FR2-IMGT: 17   CDR2-IMGT: 6
FR3-IMGT: 37 (-2 aa: 73, 82)   CDR3-IMGT: 4

Collier de Perles for human TRBV4-2*01

Accession number: IMGT U07975   EMBL/GenBank/DDBJ: U07975

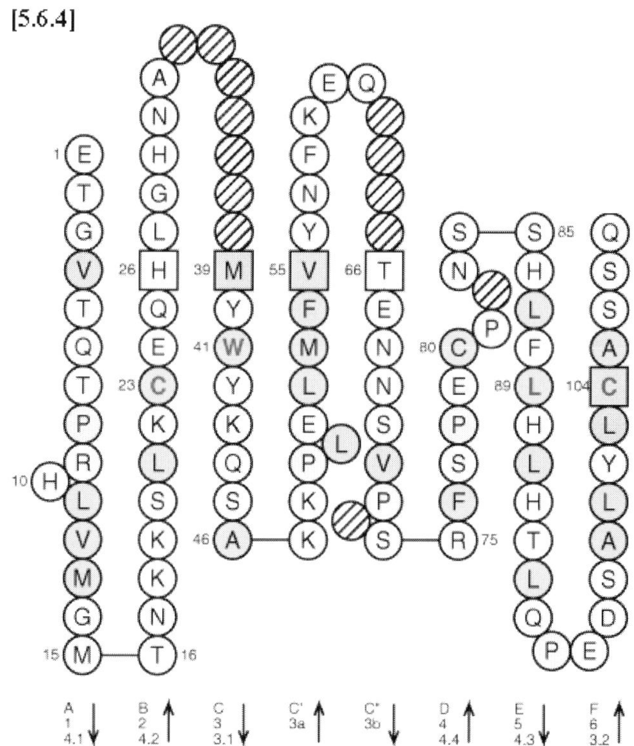

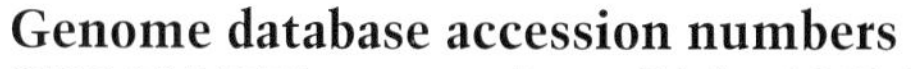

Genome database accession numbers

GDB:9954075   LocusLink: 28616

TRBV4-3

Nomenclature

TRBV4-3: T cell receptor beta variable 4-3.

Definition and functionality

TRBV4-3 is one of the 2–3 functional genes of the TRBV4 subgroup, which may, or may not, be present due to a polymorphism by insertion/deletion.TRBV4-3 belongs to the TRBV4 subgroup which comprises two or three mapped genes, depending on the haplotypes, in the TRB locus.

Gene location

TRBV4-3, in the haplotypes where it is present, is located in the TRB locus on chromosome 7 at 7q34.

Nucleotide and amino acid sequences for human TRBV4-3

```
                               1   2   3   4   5   6   7   8   9  10  11  12  13  14  15  16  17  18  19  20
                               E   T   G   V   T   Q   T   P   R   H   L   V   M   G   M   T   N   K   K   S
U07978    ,TRBV4-3*01    [44] GAA ACG GGA GTT ACG CAG ACA CCA AGA CAC CTG GTC ATG GGA ATG ACA AAT AAG AAG TCT
L36092,U66059,TRBV4-3*01 [34] --- --- --- --- --- --- --- --- --- --- --- --- --- --- --- --- --- --- --- ---
X58812    ,TRBV4-3*02    [10] --- --- --- --- --- --- --- --- --- --- --- --- --- --- --- --- --- --- --- ---
L06888    ,TRBV4-3*03    [36]     --- --- --- --- --- --- --- --- --- --- --- --- --- --- --- --- --- --- ---
X57616    ,TRBV4-3*04    [31]                                                                 --- --- ---

                                                                         CDR1-IMGT
                              21  22  23  24  25  26  27  28  29  30  31  32  33  34  35  36  37  38  39  40
                               L   K   C   E   Q   H   L   G   H   N   A                               M   Y
U07978    ,TRBV4-3*01         TTG AAA TGT GAA CAA CAT CTG GGT CAT AAC GCT ... ... ... ... ... ... ... ATG TAT
L36092,U66059,TRBV4-3*01      --- --- --- --- --- --- --- --- --- --- --- ... ... ... ... ... ... ... --- ---
X58812    ,TRBV4-3*02         --- --- --- --- --- --- --- --- --- --- --- ... ... ... ... ... ... ... --- ---
L06888    ,TRBV4-3*03         --- --- --- --- --- --- --- --- --- --- --- ... ... ... ... ... ... ... --- ---
X57616    ,TRBV4-3*04         --- --- --- --- --- --- --- --G --- --- --- ... ... ... ... ... ... ... --- ---

                                                                                         CDR2-
                              41  42  43  44  45  46  47  48  49  50  51  52  53  54  55  56  57  58  59  60
                               W   Y   K   Q   S   A   K   K   P   L   E   L   M   F   V   Y   S   L   E   E
U07978    ,TRBV4-3*01         TGG TAC AAG CAA AGT GCT AAG AAG CCA CTG GAG CTC ATG TTT GTC TAC AGT CTT GAA GAA
L36092,U66059,TRBV4-3*01      --- --- --- --- --- --- --- --- --- --- --- --- --- --- --- --- --- --- --- ---
X58812    ,TRBV4-3*02         --- --- --- --- --- --- --- --- --- --- --- --- --- --- --- --- --- --- --- ---
L06888    ,TRBV4-3*03         --- --- --- --- --- --- --- --- --- --- --- --- --- --- --- --- --- --- --- ---
X57616    ,TRBV4-3*04         --- --- --- --- --- --- --- --- --- --- --- --- --- --- --- --- --- --- --- ---

                              IMGT
                              61  62  63  64  65  66  67  68  69  70  71  72  73  74  75  76  77  78  79  80
                               R               V   E   N   N   S   V   P       S   R   F   S   P   E   C
U07978    ,TRBV4-3*01         CGG ... ... ... ... GTT GAA AAC AAC AGT GTG CCA ... AGT CGC TTC TCA CCT GAA TGC
L36092,U66059,TRBV4-3*01      --- ... ... ... ... --- --- --- --- --- --- --- ... --- --- --- --- --- --- ---
X58812    ,TRBV4-3*02         --- ... ... ... ... --- --- --- --- --- --- --- ... --- --- --- --- --- --- ---
L06888    ,TRBV4-3*03         --T ... ... ... ... --- --- --- --- --- --- --- ... --- --- --- --- --- --- ---
X57616    ,TRBV4-3*04         --- ... ... ... ... --- --- --- --- --- --- --- ... --- --- --- --- --- --- ---

                              81  82  83  84  85  86  87  88  89  90  91  92  93  94  95  96  97  98  99 100
                               P       N   S   S   H   L   F   L   H   L   H   T   L   Q   P   E   D   S   A
U07978    ,TRBV4 3*01         CCC ... AAC AGC TCT CAC TTA TTC CTT CAC CTA CAC ACC CTG CAG CCA GAA GAC TCG GCC
L36092,U66059,TRBV4-3*01      --- ... --- --- --- --- --- --- --- --- --- --- --- --- --- --- --- --- --- ---
X58812    ,TRBV4-3*02         --- ... --- --- --- --- --- --S --- --- --- --- --- --- --- --- --- --- --- ---
                                                          -C-
L06888    ,TRBV4-3*03         --- ... --- --- --- --- --- --- --- --- --- --- --- --- --- --- --- --- --- ---
X57616    ,TRBV4-3*04         --- ... --- --- --- --- --- --- --- --- --- --- --- --- --- --- --- --- --- ---

                                            CDR3-IMGT
                             101 102 103 104 105 106 107 108 109
                               L   Y   L   C   A   S   S   Q
U07978    ,TRBV4-3*01         CTG TAT CTC TGC GCC AGC AGC CAA GA
L36092,U66059,TRBV4-3*01      --- --- --- --- --- --- --- --- --
X58812    ,TRBV4-3*02         --- --- --- --- --- --- ---         #c
L06888    ,TRBV4-3*03         --- --- --- --- --- --- ---         #c
X57616    ,TRBV4-3*04         --- --- --- --- --- --- ---         #c

#c: Rearranged cDNA
```

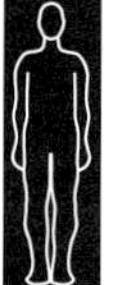

Framework and complementarity determining regions

FR1-IMGT: 26
FR2-IMGT: 17
FR3-IMGT: 37 (-2 aa: 73, 82)

CDR1-IMGT: 5
CDR2-IMGT: 6
CDR3-IMGT: 4

Collier de Perles for human TRBV4-3*01

Accession number: IMGT U07978   EMBL/GenBank/DDBJ: U07978

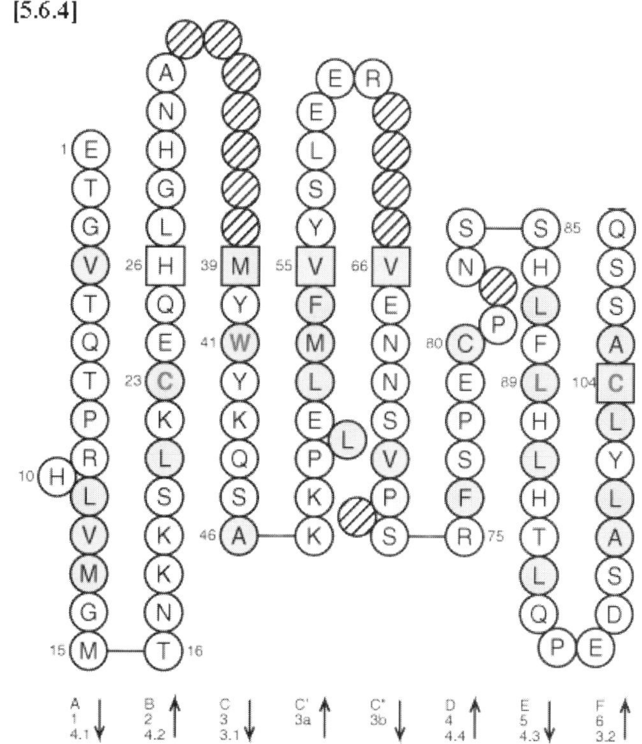

Genome database accession numbers
GDB:9954077   LocusLink: 28615

Nomenclature

TRBV5-1: T cell receptor beta variable 5-1.

Definition and functionality

TRBV5-1 is one of the five functional genes of the TRBV5 subgroup which comprises eight mapped genes in the TRB locus.

Gene location

TRBV5-1 is in the TRB locus on chromosome 7 at 7q34.

Nucleotide and amino acid sequences for human TRBV5-1

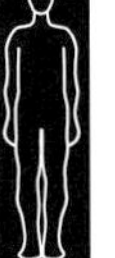

```
                                 1   2   3   4   5   6   7   8   9  10  11  12  13  14  15  16  17  18  19  20
                                 K   A   G   V   T   Q   T   P   R   Y   L   I   K   T   R   G   Q   Q   V   T
L36092,U66059,TRBV5-1*01 [34]   AAG GCT GGA GTC ACT CAA ACT CCA AGA TAT CTG ATC AAA ACG AGA GGA CAG CAA GTG ACA
                                 R                                       H
M14271   ,TRBV5-1*02            -G- --- --G --- --- --- --- --- --- C-- --- --- --- --- --- --- --- --- --- ---


                                                                    ________________CDR1-IMGT________________
                                21  22  23  24  25  26  27  28  29  30  31  32  33  34  35  36  37  38  39  40
                                 L   S   C   S   P   I   S   G   H   R   S                               V   S
L36092,U66059,TRBV5-1*01        CTG AGC TGC TCC CCT ATC TCT GGG CAT AGG AGT ... ... ... ... ... ... ... GTA TCC
                                     G
M14271   ,TRBV5-1*02            --- G-- --- --- --- --- --- --- --- --- --- ... ... ... ... ... ... ... --- ---


                                                                                            ______________CDR2-
                                41  42  43  44  45  46  47  48  49  50  51  52  53  54  55  56  57  58  59  60
                                 W   Y   Q   Q   T   P   G   Q   G   L   Q   F   L   F   E   Y   F   S   E   T
L36092,U66059,TRBV5-1*01        TGG TAC CAA CAG ACC CCA GGA CAG GGC CTT CAG TTC CTC TTT GAA TAC TTC AGT GAG ACA
                                                 L
M14271   ,TRBV5-1*02            --- --- --- --- --- -T- --- --- --- --- --- --- --- --- --- --- --- --- --- ---


                                IMGT________________
                                61  62  63  64  65  66  67  68  69  70  71  72  73  74  75  76  77  78  79  80
                                 Q                   R   N   K   G   N   F   P       G   R   F   S   G   R   Q
L36092,U66059,TRBV5-1*01        CAG ... ... ... ... AGA AAC AAA GGA AAC TTC CCT ... GGT CGA TTC TCA GGG CGC CAG
                                                                             L
M14271   ,TRBV5-1*02            --- ... ... ... ... --- --- --- --- --- --- -T- ... --- --- --- --- --- --- ---


                                81  82  83  84  85  86  87  88  89  90  91  92  93  94  95  96  97  98  99 100
                                 F       S   N   S   R   S   E   M   N   V   S   T   L   E   L   G   D   S   A
L36092,U66059,TRBV5-1*01        TTC ... TCT AAC TCT CGC TCT GAG ATG AAT GTG AGC ACC TTG GAG CTG GGG GAC TCG GCC
M14271   ,TRBV5-1*02            --- ... --- --- --- --- --- --- --- --- --- --- --- --- --- --- --- --- --- ---


                                             _______CDR3-IMGT_______
                               101 102 103 104 105 106 107 108 109
                                 L   Y   L   C   A   S   S   L
L36092,U66059,TRBV5-1*01        CTT TAT CTT TGC GCC AGC AGC TTG G
                                                             A   C
M14271   ,TRBV5-1*02            --- --- --- --- --- --- GCT TGC       #c
```

#c: Rearranged cDNA

Framework and complementarity determining regions

FR1-IMGT: 26	CDR1-IMGT: 5
FR2-IMGT: 17	CDR2-IMGT: 6
FR3-IMGT: 37 (-2 aa: 73, 82)	CDR3-IMGT: 4

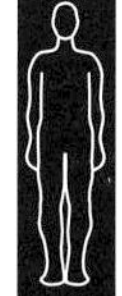

Collier de Perles for human TRBV5-1*01

Accession number: IMGT L36092   EMBL/GenBank/DDBJ: L36092

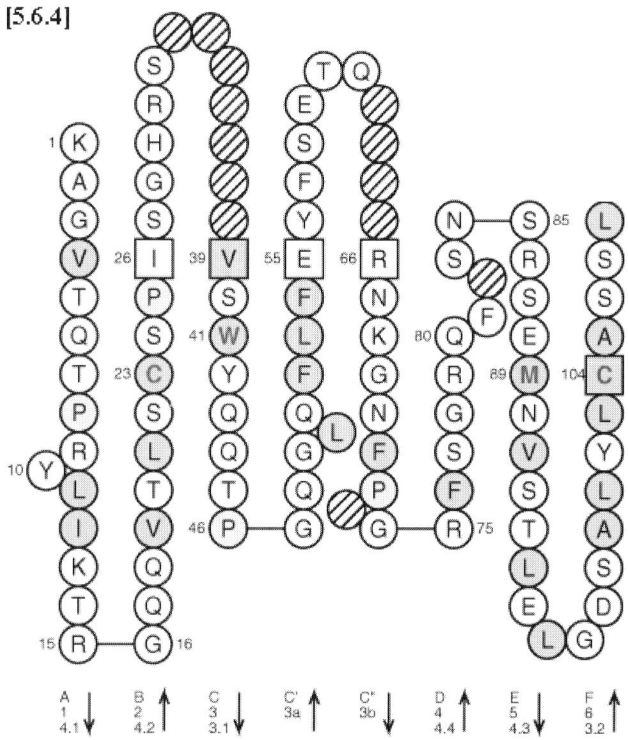

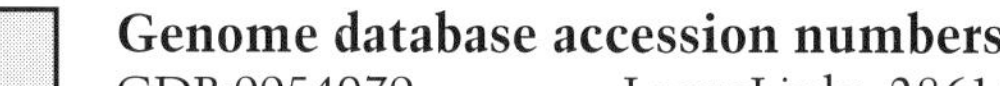

Genome database accession numbers
GDB:9954079   LocusLink: 28614

Nomenclature

TRBV5-3: T cell receptor beta variable 5-3.

Definition and functionality

TRBV5-3 is an ORF due to an unusual DONOR–SPLICE: nat instead of ngt. TRBV5-3 belongs to the TRBV5 subgroup which comprises eight mapped genes, of which five are functional in the TRB locus.

Gene location

TRBV5-3 is in the TRB locus on chromosome 7 at 7q34.

Nucleotide and amino acid sequences for human TRBV5-3

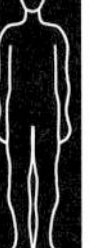

```
                              1   2   3   4   5   6   7   8   9   10  11  12  13  14  15  16  17  18  19  20
                              E   A   G   V   T   Q   S   P   T   H   L   I   K   T   R   G   Q   Q   V   T
X61439    ,TRBV5-3*01    [26] GAG GCT GGA GTC ACC CAA AGT CCC ACA CAC CTG ATC AAA ACG AGA GGA CAG CAA GTG ACT

L36092,U66059,TRBV5-3*01 [34] --- --- --- --- --- --- --- --- --- --- --- --- --- --- --- --- --- --- --- ---

AF009660,TRBV5-3*02      [35] --- --- --- --- --- --- --- --- --- --- --- --- --- --- --- --- --- --- --- ---


                                                                      ________________CDR1-IMGT_______________
                              21  22  23  24  25  26  27  28  29  30  31  32  33  34  35  36  37  38  39  40
                              L   R   C   S   P   I   S   G   H   S   S                               V   S
X61439    ,TRBV5-3*01         CTG AGA TGC TCT CCT ATC TCT GGG CAC AGC AGT ... ... ... ... ... ... ... GTG TCC

L36092,U66059,TRBV5-3*01      --- --- --- --- --- --- --- --- --- --- --- ... ... ... ... ... ... ... --- ---

AF009660,TRBV5-3*02           --- --- --- --- --- --- --- --- --- --- --- ... ... ... ... ... ... ... --- ---


                                                                                          ________________CDR2-
                              41  42  43  44  45  46  47  48  49  50  51  52  53  54  55  56  57  58  59  60
                              W   Y   Q   Q   A   P   G   Q   G   P   Q   F   I   F   E   Y   A   N   E   L
X61439    ,TRBV5-3*01         TGG TAC CAA CAG GCC CCG GGT CAG GGG CCC CAG TTT ATC TTT GAA TAT GCT AAT GAG TTA

L36092,U66059,TRBV5-3*01      --- --- --- --- --- --- --- --- --- --- --- --- --- --- --- --- --- --- --- ---

AF009660,TRBV5-3*02           --- --- --- --- --- --- --- --- --- --- --- --- --- --- --- --- --- --- --- ---


                              IMGT________________
                              61  62  63  64  65  66  67  68  69  70  71  72  73  74  75  76  77  78  79  80
                              R                   R   S   E   G   N   F   P       N   R   F   S   G   R   Q
X61439    ,TRBV5-3*01         AGG ... ... ... ... AGA TCA GAA GGA AAC TTC CCT ... AAT CGA TTC TCA GGG CGC CAG

L36092,U66059,TRBV5-3*01      --- ... ... ... ... --- --- --- --- --- --- --- ... --- --- --- --- --- --- ---

AF009660,TRBV5-3*02           --- ... ... ... ... --- --- --- --- --- --- --- ... --- --- --- --- --- --- ---


                              81  82  83  84  85  86  87  88  89  90  91  92  93  94  95  96  97  98  99  100
                              F       H   D   C   C   S   E   M   N   V   S   A   L   E   L   G   D   S   A
X61439    ,TRBV5-3*01         TTC ... CAT GAC TGT TGC TCT GAG ATG AAT GTG AGT GCC TTG GAG CTG GGG GAC TCG GCC

L36092,U66059,TRBV5-3*01      --- ... --- --- --- --- --- --- --- --- --- --- --- --- --- --- --- --- --- ---

AF009660,TRBV5-3*02           --- ... --- --- -A- --- --- --- --- --- --- --- --- --- --- --- --- --- --- ---


                                         ______CDR3-IMGT______
                              101 102 103 104 105 106 107 108 109
                              L   Y   L   C   A   R   S   L
X61439    ,TRBV5-3*01         CTG TAT CTC TGT GCC AGA AGC TTG G

L36092,U66059,TRBV5-3*01      --- --- --- --- --- --- --- --- -

AF009660,TRBV5-3*02           --- --- --- --- --- --- --- --- -
```

Framework and complementarity determining regions

FR1-IMGT: 26	CDR1-IMGT: 5
FR2-IMGT: 17	CDR2-IMGT: 6
FR3-IMGT: 37 (-2 aa: 73, 82)	CDR3-IMGT: 4

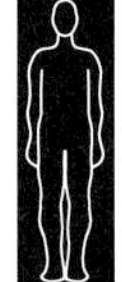

Collier de Perles for human TRBV5-3*01

Accession number: IMGT X61439   EMBL/GenBank/DDBJ: X61439

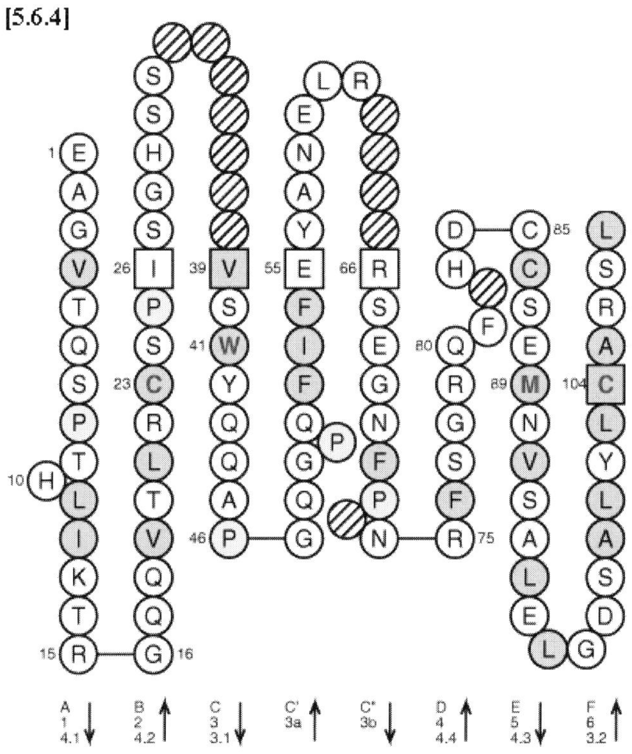

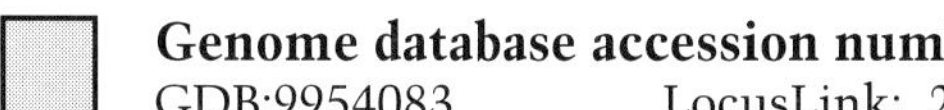

Genome database accession numbers
GDB:9954083   LocusLink: 28612

Nomenclature

TRBV5-4: T cell receptor beta variable 5-4.

Definition and functionality

TRBV5-4 is one of the five functional genes of the TRBV5 subgroup which comprises eight mapped genes in the TRB locus.

Gene location

TRBV5-4 is in the TRB locus on chromosome 7 at 7q34.

Nucleotide and amino acid sequences for human TRBV5-4

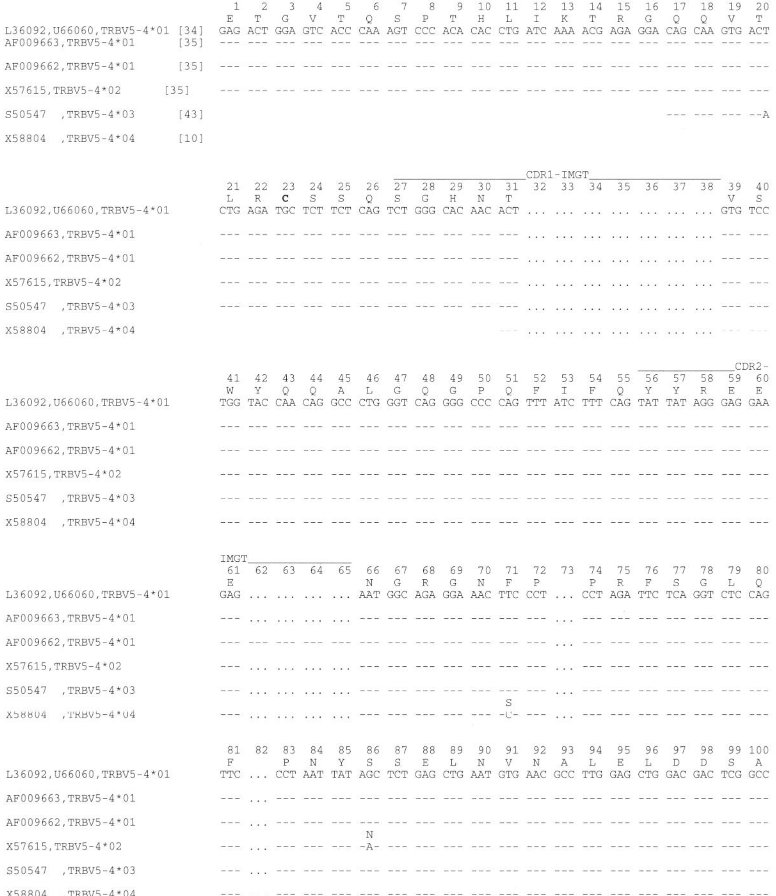

```
                                 1   2   3   4   5   6   7   8   9  10  11  12  13  14  15  16  17  18  19  20
                                 E   T   G   V   T   Q   S   P   T   H   L   I   K   T   R   G   Q   Q   V   T
L36092,U66060,TRBV5-4*01 [34]  GAG ACT GGA GTC ACC CAA AGT CCC ACA CAC CTG ATC AAA ACG AGA GGA CAG CAA GTG ACT
AF009663,TRBV5-4*01      [35]  --- --- --- --- --- --- --- --- --- --- --- --- --- --- --- --- --- --- --- ---
AF009662,TRBV5-4*01      [35]  --- --- --- --- --- --- --- --- --- --- --- --- --- --- --- --- --- --- --- ---
X57615 ,TRBV5-4*02       [35]  --- --- --- --- --- --- --- --- --- --- --- --- --- --- --- --- --- --- --- ---
S50547 ,TRBV5-4*03       [43]                                                          --- --- --- --A
X58804 ,TRBV5-4*04       [10]

                                                            CDR1-IMGT______________________________
                                21  22  23  24  25  26  27  28  29  30  31  32  33  34  35  36  37  38  39  40
                                 L   R   C   S   S   Q   S   G   H   N   T                           V   S
L36092,U66060,TRBV5-4*01       CTG AGA TGC TCT TCT CAG TCT GGG CAC AAC ACT ... ... ... ... ... ... ... GTG TCC
AF009663,TRBV5-4*01            --- --- --- --- --- --- --- --- --- --- --- ... ... ... ... ... ... ... --- ---
AF009662,TRBV5-4*01            --- --- --- --- --- --- --- --- --- --- --- ... ... ... ... ... ... ... --- ---
X57615 ,TRBV5-4*02             --- --- --- --- --- --- --- --- --- --- --- ... ... ... ... ... ... ... --- ---
S50547 ,TRBV5-4*03             --- --- --- --- --- --- --- --- --- --- --- ... ... ... ... ... ... ... --- ---
X58804 ,TRBV5-4*04                                                         ... ... ... ... ... ... ...

                                                                                                    CDR2-
                                41  42  43  44  45  46  47  48  49  50  51  52  53  54  55  56  57  58  59  60
                                 W   Y   Q   Q   A   L   G   Q   G   P   Q   F   I   F   Q   Y   Y   R   E   E
L36092,U66060,TRBV5-4*01       TGG TAC CAA CAG GCC CTG GGT CAG GGG CCC CAG TTT ATC TTT CAG TAT TAT AGG GAG GAA
AF009663,TRBV5-4*01            --- --- --- --- --- --- --- --- --- --- --- --- --- --- --- --- --- --- --- ---
AF009662,TRBV5-4*01            --- --- --- --- --- --- --- --- --- --- --- --- --- --- --- --- --- --- --- ---
X57615 ,TRBV5-4*02             --- --- --- --- --- --- --- --- --- --- --- --- --- --- --- --- --- --- --- ---
S50547 ,TRBV5-4*03             --- --- --- --- --- --- --- --- --- --- --- --- --- --- --- --- --- --- --- ---
X58804 ,TRBV5-4*04             --- --- --- --- --- --- --- --- --- --- --- --- --- --- --- --- --- --- --- ---

                               IMGT_________________
                                61  62  63  64  65  66  67  68  69  70  71  72  73  74  75  76  77  78  79  80
                                 E                   N   G   R   G   N   F   P       P   R   F   S   G   L   Q
L36092,U66060,TRBV5-4*01       GAG ... ... ... ... AAT GGC AGA GGA AAC TTC CCT ... CCT AGA TTC TCA GGT CTC CAG
AF009663,TRBV5-4*01            --- ... ... ... ... --- --- --- --- --- --- --- ... --- --- --- --- --- --- ---
AF009662,TRBV5-4*01            --- ... ... ... ... --- --- --- --- --- --- --- ... --- --- --- --- --- --- ---
X57615 ,TRBV5-4*02             --- ... ... ... ... --- --- --- --- --- --- --- ... --- --- --- --- --- --- ---
S50547 ,TRBV5-4*03             --- ... ... ... ... --- --- --- --- --- --- --- ... --- --- --- --- --- --- ---
                                                                            S
X58804 ,TRBV5-4*04             --- ... ... ... ... --- --- --- --- --- --- -C- ... --- --- --- --- --- --- ---

                                81  82  83  84  85  86  87  88  89  90  91  92  93  94  95  96  97  98  99 100
                                 F       P   N   Y   S   S   E   L   N   V   N   A   L   E   L   D   D   S   A
L36092,U66060,TRBV5-4*01       TTC ... CCT AAT TAT AGC TCT GAG CTG AAT GTG AAC GCC TTG GAG CTG GAC GAC TCG GCC
AF009663,TRBV5-4*01            --- ... --- --- --- --- --- --- --- --- --- --- --- --- --- --- --- --- --- ---
AF009662,TRBV5-4*01            --- ... --- --- --- --- --- --- --- --- --- --- --- --- --- --- --- --- --- ---
                                                    N
X57615 ,TRBV5-4*02             --- ... --- --- --- -A- --- --- --- --- --- --- --- --- --- --- --- --- --- ---
S50547 ,TRBV5-4*03             --- ... --- --- --- --- --- --- --- --- --- --- --- --- --- --- --- --- --- ---
X58804 ,TRBV5-4*04             --- ... --- --- --- --- --- --- --- --- --- --- --- --- --- --- --- --- --- ---
```

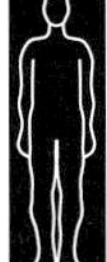

```
                                            _____CDR3-IMGT_____
                      101 102 103 104 105 106 107 108 109
                       L   Y   L   C   A   S   S   L
  L36092,U66060,TRBV5-4*01   CTG TAT CTC TGT GCC AGC AGC TTG G

  AF009663,TRBV5-4*01    --- --- --- --- --- --- --- --- -

  AF009662,TRBV5-4*01    --- --- --- --- --- --- --- --- -

  X57615,TRBV5-4*02      --- --- --- --- --- --- ---        #c

  S50547 ,TRBV5-4*03     --- --- --- --- --- --- ---        #

  X58804 ,TRBV5-4*04     --- --- --- --- --- --- ---        #c


#:  Rearranged
#c: Rearranged cDNA
```

Framework and complementarity determining regions

FR1-IMGT: 26   CDR1-IMGT: 5
FR2-IMGT: 17   CDR2-IMGT: 6
FR3-IMGT: 37 (-2 aa: 73, 82)   CDR3-IMGT: 4

Collier de Perles for human TRBV5-4*01

Accession number: IMGT L36092   EMBL/GenBank/DDBJ: L36092

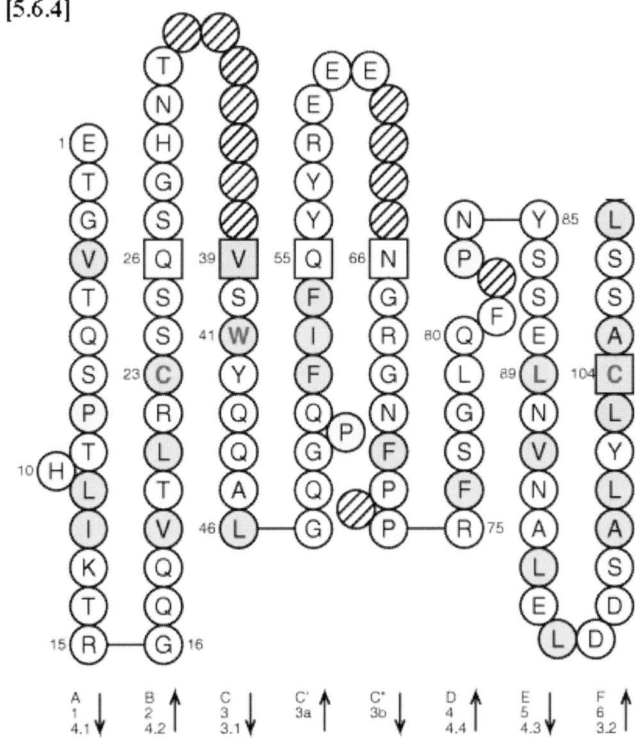

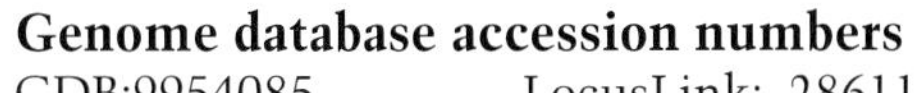

Genome database accession numbers
GDB:9954085   LocusLink: 28611

Nomenclature

TRBV5-5: T cell receptor beta variable 5-5.

Definition and functionality

TRBV5-5 is one of the five functional genes of the TRBV5 subgroup which comprises eight mapped genes in the TRB locus.

Gene location

TRBV5-5 is in the TRB locus on chromosome 7 at 7q34.

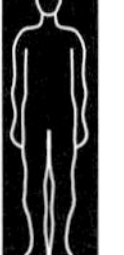

Nucleotide and amino acid sequences for human TRBV5-5

```
                                1   2   3   4   5   6   7   8   9  10  11  12  13  14  15  16  17  18  19  20
                                D   A   G   V   T   Q   S   P   T   H   L   I   K   T   R   G   Q   Q   V   T
L36092,U66060,TRBV5-5*01 [34]  GAC GCT GGA GTC ACC CAA AGT CCC ACA CAC CTG ATC AAA ACG AGA GGA CAG CAA GTG ACT

AF009663,TRBV5-5*01      [35]  --- --- --- --- --- --- --- --- --- --- --- --- --- --- --- --- --- --- --- ---
                                                                                                    H
X57611  ,TRBV5-5*02      [31]  --- --- --- --- --- --- --- --- --- --- --- --- --- --- --- --- --C --- ---

X58801  ,TRBV5-5*03      [10]  --- --- --- --- --- --- --- --- --- --- --- --- --- --- --- --- --- --- --- ---


                                                                          _______________CDR1-IMGT________________
                               21  22  23  24  25  26  27  28  29  30  31  32  33  34  35  36  37  38  39  40
                                L   R   C   S   P   I   S   G   H   K   S                               V   S
L36092,U66060,TRBV5-5*01       CTG AGA TGC TCT CCT ATC TCT GGG CAC AAG AGT ... ... ... ... ... ... ... GTG TCC

AF009663,TRBV5-5*01            --- --- --- --- --- --- --- --- --- --- --- ... ... ... ... ... ... ... --- ---

X57611  ,TRBV5-5*02            --- --- --- --- --- --- --- --- --- --- --- ... ... ... ... ... ... ... --- ---
                                                                E
X58801  ,TRBV5-5*03            --- --- --- --- --- --- --- -A- --- --- --- ... ... ... ... ... ... ... --- ---


                                                                                        ________________CDR2-
                               41  42  43  44  45  46  47  48  49  50  51  52  53  54  55  56  57  58  59  60
                                W   Y   Q   Q   V   L   G   Q   G   P   Q   F   I   F   Q   Y   Y   E   K   E
L36092,U66060,TRBV5-5*01       TGG TAC CAA CAG GTC CTG GGT CAG GGG CCC CAG TTT ATC TTT CAG TAT TAT GAG AAA GAA

AF009663,TRBV5-5*01            --- --- --- --- --- --- --- --- --- --- --- --- --- --- --- --- --- --- --- ---

X57611  ,TRBV5-5*02            --- --- --- --- --- --- --- --- --- --- --- --- --- --- --- --- --- --- --- ---

X58801  ,TRBV5-5*03            --- --- --- --- --- --- --- --- --- --- --- --- --- --- --- --- --- --- --- ---


                               IMGT________________
                               61  62  63  64  65  66  67  68  69  70  71  72  73  74  75  76  77  78  79  80
                                E                   R   G   R   G   N   F   P       D   R   F   S   A   R   Q
L36092,U66060,TRBV5-5*01       GAG ... ... ... ... AGA GGA AGA GGA AAC TTC CCT ... GAT CGA TTC TCA GCT CGC CAG

AF009663,TRBV5-5*01            --- ... ... ... ... --- --- --- --- --- --- --- ... --- --- --- --- --- --- ---

X57611  ,TRBV5-5*02            --- ... ... ... ... --- --- --- --- --- --- --- ... --- --- --- --- --- --- ---

X58801  ,TRBV5-5*03            --- ... ... ... ... --- --- --- --- --- --- --- ... --- --- --- --- --- --- ---


                               81  82  83  84  85  86  87  88  89  90  91  92  93  94  95  96  97  98  99 100
                                F       P   N   Y   S   S   E   L   N   V   N   A   L   L   L   G   D   S   A
L36092,U66060,TRBV5-5*01       TTC ... CCT AAC TAT AGC TCT GAG CTG AAT GTG AAC GCC TTG TTG CTG GGG GAC TCG GCC

AF009663,TRBV5-5*01            --- ... --- --- --- --- --- --- --- --- --- --- --- --- --- --- --- --- --- ---

X57611  ,TRBV5-5*02            --- ... --- --- --- --- --- --- --- --- --- --- --- --- --- --- --- --- --- ---

X58801  ,TRBV5-5*03            --- ... --- --- --- --- --- --- --- --- --- --- --- --- --- --- --- --- --- ---


                                             ______CDR3-IMGT______
                              101 102 103 104 105 106 107 108 109
                                L   Y   L   C   A   S   S   L
L36092,U66060,TRBV5-5*01      CTG TAT CTC TGT GCC AGC AGC TTG G

AF009663,TRBV5-5*01           --- --- --- --- --- --- --- --- -

X57611  ,TRBV5-5*02           --- --- --- --- --- --- ---          #c

X58801  ,TRBV5-5*03           --- --- --- --- --- --- ---          #c
```

#c: Rearranged cDNA

Framework and complementarity determining regions

FR1-IMGT: 26   CDR1-IMGT: 5

FR2-IMGT: 17   CDR2-IMGT: 6

FR3-IMGT: 37 (-2 aa: 73, 82) CDR3-IMGT: 4

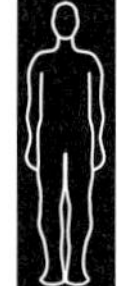

Collier de Perles for human TRBV5-5*01

Accession number: IMGT L36092   EMBL/GenBank/DDBJ: L36092

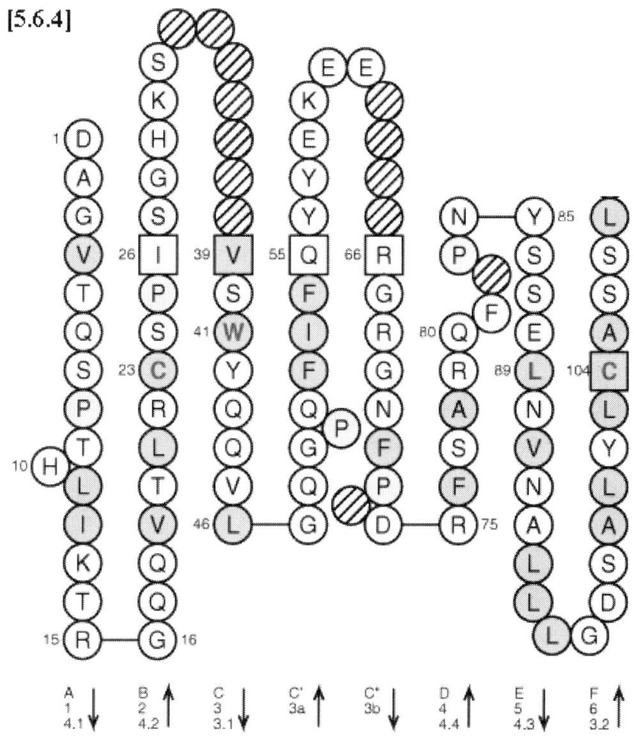

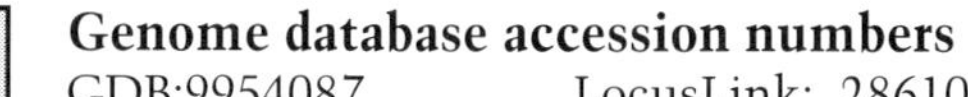

Genome database accession numbers

GDB:9954087   LocusLink: 28610

Nomenclature

TRBV5-6: T cell receptor beta variable 5-6.

Definition and functionality

TRBV5-6 is one of the five functional genes of the TRBV5 subgroup which comprises eight mapped genes in the TRB locus.

Gene location

TRBV5-6 is in the TRB locus on chromosome 7 at 7q34.

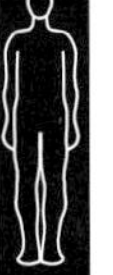

Nucleotide and amino acid sequences for human TRBV5-6

```
                          1    2    3    4    5    6    7    8    9   10   11   12   13   14   15   16   17   18   19   20
                          D    A    G    V    T    Q    S    P    T    H    L    I    K    T    R    G    Q    Q    V    T
L36092,U66060,TRBV5-6*01 [34] GAC GCT GGA GTC ACC CAA AGT CCC ACA CAC CTG ATC AAA ACG AGA GGA CAG CAA GTG ACT

AF009663,TRBV5-6*01      [35] --- --- --- --- --- --- --- --- --- --- --- --- --- --- --- --- --- --- --- ---


                                                                 ______________________CDR1-IMGT__________________
                         21   22   23   24   25   26   27   28   29   30   31   32   33   34   35   36   37   38   39   40
                          L    R    C    S    P    K    S    G    H    D    T                             V    S
L36092,U66060,TRBV5-6*01 CTG AGA TGC TCT CCT AAG TCT GGG CAT GAC ACT ... ... ... ... ... ... ... GTG TCC

AF009663,TRBV5-6*01      --- --- --- --- --- --- --- --- --- --- --- ... ... ... ... ... ... ... --- ---


                                                                                           ________________CDR2-
                         41   42   43   44   45   46   47   48   49   50   51   52   53   54   55   56   57   58   59   60
                          W    Y    Q    Q    A    L    G    Q    G    P    Q    F    I    F    Q    Y    Y    E    E    E
L36092,U66060,TRBV5-6*01 TGG TAC CAA CAG GCC CTG GGT CAG GGG CCC CAG TTT ATC TTT CAG TAT TAT GAG GAG GAA

AF009663,TRBV5-6*01      --- --- --- --- --- --- --- --- --- --- --- --- --- --- --- --- --- --- --- ---


                         IMGT__________________
                         61   62   63   64   65   66   67   68   69   70   71   72   73   74   75   76   77   78   79   80
                          E                             R    Q    R    G    N    F    P         D    R    F    S    G    H    Q
L36092,U66060,TRBV5-6*01 GAG ... ... ... ... AGA CAG AGA GGC AAC TTC CCT ... GAT CGA TTC TCA GGT CAC CAG

AF009663,TRBV5-6*01      --- ... ... ... ... --- --- --- --- --- --- --- ... --- --- --- --- --- --- ---


                         81   82   83   84   85   86   87   88   89   90   91   92   93   94   95   96   97   98   99  100
                          F         P    N    Y    S    S    E    L    N    V    N    A    L    L    L    G    D    S    A
L36092,U66060,TRBV5-6*01 TTC ... CCT AAC TAT AGC TCT GAG CTG AAT GTG AAC GCC TTG TTG CTG GGG GAC TCG GCC

AF009663,TRBV5-6*01      --- ... --- --- --- --- --- --- --- --- --- --- --- --- --- --- --- --- --- ---


                                            ________CDR3-IMGT______
                        101  102  103  104  105  106  107  108  109
                          L    Y    L    C    A    S    S    L
L36092,U66060,TRBV5-6*01 CTC TAT CTC TGT GCC AGC AGC TTG G

AF009663,TRBV5-6*01      --- --- --- --- --- --- --- --- -
```

Framework and complementarity determining regions

FR1-IMGT: 26	CDR1-IMGT: 5
FR2-IMGT: 17	CDR2-IMGT: 6
FR3-IMGT: 37 (-2 aa: 73, 82)	CDR3-IMGT: 4

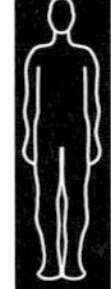

Collier de Perles for human TRBV5-6*01

Accession number: IMGT L36092   EMBL/GenBank/DDBJ: L36092

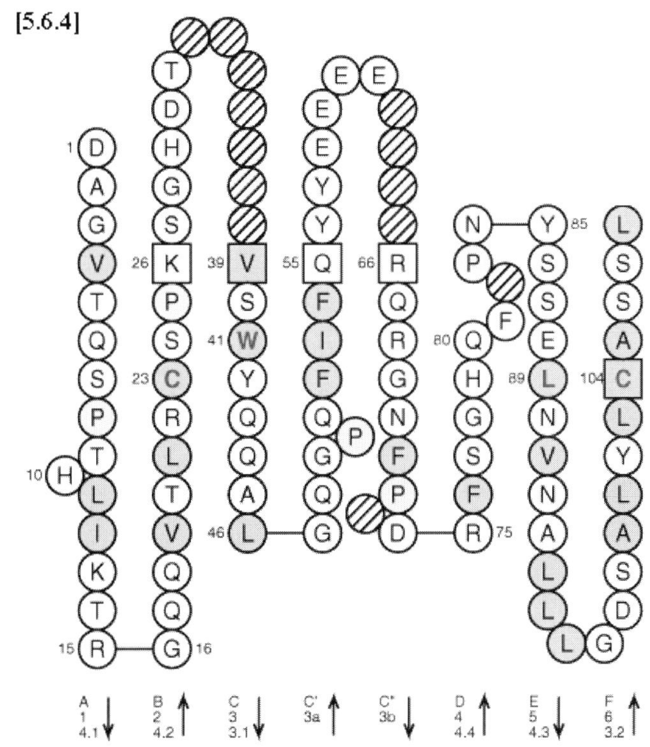

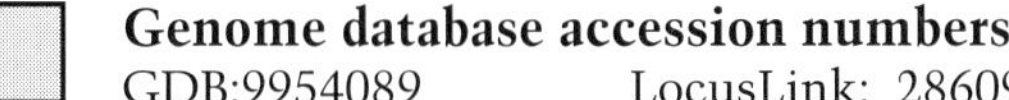

Genome database accession numbers
GDB:9954089   LocusLink: 28609

TRBV5-7

Nomenclature

TRBV5-7: T cell receptor beta variable 5-7.

Definition and functionality

TRBV5-7 is an ORF due to the CONSERVED–TRP (tgg) of the V-EXON, being replaced by a Serine (tcg). TRBV5-7 belongs to the TRBV5 subgroup which comprises eight mapped genes, of which five are functional in the TRB locus.

Gene location

TRBV5-7 is in the TRB locus on chromosome 7 at 7q34.

Nucleotide and amino acid sequences for human TRBV5-7

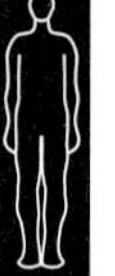

```
                               1   2   3   4   5   6   7   8   9  10  11  12  13  14  15  16  17  18  19  20
                               D   A   G   V   T   Q   S   P   T   H   L   I   K   T   R   G   Q   H   V   T
L36092,U66060,TRBV5-7*01 [34] GAC GCT GGA GTC ACC CAA AGT CCC ACA CAC CTG ATC AAA ACG AGA GGA CAG CAC GTG ACT

AF009663,TRBV5-7*01      [35] --- --- --- --- --- --- --- --- --- --- --- --- --- --- --- --- --- --- --- ---

L26226  ,TRBV5-7*01      [44] --- --- --- --- --- --- --- --- --- --- --- --- --- --- --- --- --- --- --- ---


                                                           ________________________CDR1-IMGT________________________
                              21  22  23  24  25  26  27  28  29  30  31  32  33  34  35  36  37  38  39  40
                               L   R   C   S   P   I   S   G   H   T   S                               V   S
L36092,U66060,TRBV5-7*01      CTG AGA TGC TCT CCT ATC TCT GGG CAC ACC AGT ... ... ... ... ... ... ... GTG TCC

AF009663,TRBV5-7*01           --- --- --- --- --- --- --- --- --- --- --- ... ... ... ... ... ... ... --- ---

L26226  ,TRBV5-7*01           --- --- --- --- --- --- --- --- --- --- --- ... ... ... ... ... ... ... --- ---


                                                                              ____________________________CDR2-
                              41  42  43  44  45  46  47  48  49  50  51  52  53  54  55  56  57  58  59  60
                               S   Y   Q   Q   A   L   G   Q   G   P   Q   F   I   F   Q   Y   Y   E   K   E
L36092,U66060,TRBV5-7*01      TCG TAC CAA CAG GCC CTG GGT CAG GGG CCC CAG TTT ATC TTT CAG TAT TAT GAG AAA GAA

AF009663,TRBV5-7*01           --- --- --- --- --- --- --- --- --- --- --- --- --- --- --- --- --- --- --- ---

L26226  ,TRBV5-7*01           --- --- --- --- --- --- --- --- --- --- --- --- --- --- --- --- --- --- --- ---


                              IMGT________________
                              61  62  63  64  65  66  67  68  69  70  71  72  73  74  75  76  77  78  79  80
                               E                   R   G   R   G   N   F   P       D   Q   F   S   G   H   Q
L36092,U66060,TRBV5-7*01      GAG ... ... ... ... AGA GGA AGA GGA AAC TTC CCT ... GAT CAA TTC TCA GGT CAC CAG

AF009663,TRBV5-7*01           --- ... ... ... ... --- --- --- --- --- --- --- ... --- --- --- --- --- --- ---

L26226  ,TRBV5-7*01           --- ... ... ... ... --- --- --- --- --- --- --- ... --- --- --- --- --- --- ---


                              81  82  83  84  85  86  87  88  89  90  91  92  93  94  95  96  97  98  99 100
                               F       P   N   Y   S   S   E   L   N   V   N   A   L   L   L   G   D   S   A
L36092,U66060,TRBV5-7*01      TTC ... CCT AAC TAT AGC TCT GAG CTG AAT GTG AAC GCC TTG TTG CTA GGG GAC TCG GCC

AF009663,TRBV5-7*01           --- ... --- --- --- --- --- --- --- --- --- --- --- --- --- --- --- --- --- ---

L26226  ,TRBV5-7*01           --- ... --- --- --- --- --- --- --- --- --- --- --- --- --- --- --- --- --- -


                                          ______CDR3-IMGT______
                             101 102 103 104 105 106 107 108 109
                               L   Y   L   C   A   S   S   L
L36092,U66060,TRBV5-7*01      CTC TAT CTC TGT GCC AGC AGC TTG G

AF009663,TRBV5-7*01           --- --- --- --- --- --- --- --- -

L26226  ,TRBV5-7*01                                                          o
```

°: Genomic DNA, but not known as being germline or rearranged

Framework and complementarity determining regions

FR1-IMGT: 26	CDR1-IMGT: 5
FR2-IMGT: 17	CDR2-IMGT: 6
FR3-IMGT: 37 (-2 aa: 73, 82)	CDR3-IMGT: 4

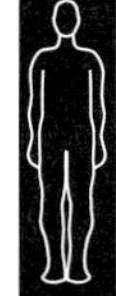

Collier de Perles for human TRBV5-7*01

Accession number: IMGT L36092   EMBL/GenBank/DDBJ: L36092

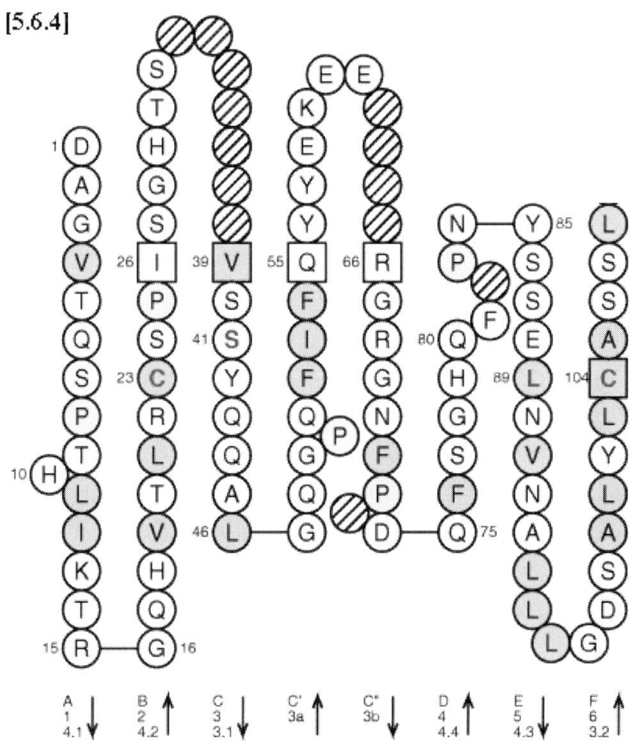

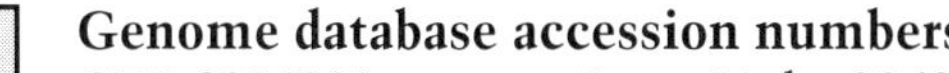

Genome database accession numbers
GDB:9954091   LocusLink: 28608

TRBV5-8

Nomenclature

TRBV5-8: T cell receptor beta variable 5-8.

Definition and functionality

TRBV5-8 is one of the five functional genes of the TRBV5 subgroup which comprises eight mapped genes in the TRB locus.

Gene location

TRBV5-8 is in the TRB locus on chromosome 7 at 7q34.

Nucleotide and amino acid sequences for human TRBV5-8

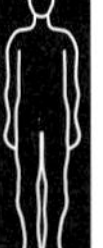

```
                          1   2   3   4   5   6   7   8   9  10  11  12  13  14  15  16  17  18  19  20
                          E   A   G   V   T   Q   S   P   T   H   L   I   K   T   R   G   Q   Q   A   T
L36092,U66060,TRBV5-8*01 [34] GAG GCT GGA GTC ACA CAA AGT CCC ACA CAC CTG ATC AAA ACG AGA GGA CAG CAA GCG ACT
AF009663,TRBV5-8*01      [35] --- --- --- --- --- --- --- --- --- --- --- --- --- --- --- --- --- --- --- ---
X58803   ,TRBV5-8*02     [10]                                                 -  --- --- --- --- ---

                                                                         ____________CDR1-IMGT____________
                         21  22  23  24  25  26  27  28  29  30  31  32  33  34  35  36  37  38  39  40
                          L   R   C   S   P   I   S   G   H   T   S                           V   Y
L36092,U66060,TRBV5-8*01 CTG AGA TGC TCT CCT ATC TCT GGG CAC ACC AGT ... ... ... ... ... ... ... GTG TAC
AF009663,TRBV5-8*01      --- --- --- --- --- --- --- --- --- --- --- ... ... ... ... ... ... ... --- ---
X58803   ,TRBV5-8*02     --- --- --- --- --- --- --- --- --- --- --- ... ... ... ... ... ... ... --- ---

                                                                                     ________________CDR2-
                         41  42  43  44  45  46  47  48  49  50  51  52  53  54  55  56  57  58  59  60
                          W   Y   Q   Q   A   L   G   L   G   L   Q   F   L   L   W   Y   D   E   G   E
L36092,U66060,TRBV5-8*01 TGG TAC CAA CAG GCC CTG GGT CTG GGC CTC CAG TTC CTC CTT TGG TAT GAC GAG GGT GAA
AF009663,TRBV5-8*01      --- --- --- --- --- --- --- --- --- --- --- --- --- --- --- --- --- --- --- ---
                                                                          L
X58803   ,TRBV5-8*02     --- --- --- --- --- --- --- --- --- --- --- C-- --- --- --- --- --- --- --- ---

                         IMGT________
                         61  62  63  64  65  66  67  68  69  70  71  72  73  74  75  76  77  78  79  80
                          E                       R   N   R   G   N   F   P       P   R   F   S   G   R   Q
L36092,U66060,TRBV5-8*01 GAG ... ... ... ... AGA AAC AGA GGA AAC TTC CCT ... CCT AGA TTT TCA GGT CGC CAG
AF009663,TRBV5-8*01      --- ... ... ... ... --- --- --- --- --- --- --- ... --- --- --- --- --- --- ---
X58803   ,TRBV5-8*02     --- ... ... ... ... --- --- --- --- --- --- --- ... --- --- --- --- --- --- ---

                         81  82  83  84  85  86  87  88  89  90  91  92  93  94  95  96  97  98  99 100
                          F       P   N   Y   S   S   E   L   N   V   N   A   L   E   L   E   D   S   A
L36092,U66060,TRBV5-8*01 TTC ... CCT AAT TAT AGC TCT GAG CTG AAT GTG AAC GCC TTG GAG CTG GAG GAC TCG GCC
AF009663,TRBV5-8*01      --- ... --- --- --- --- --- --- --- --- --- --- --- --- --- --- --- --- --- ---
X58803   ,TRBV5-8*02     --- ... --- --- --- --- --- --- --- --- --- --- --- --- --- --- --- --- --- ---

                                          ______CDR3-IMGT______
                        101 102 103 104 105 106 107 108 109
                          L   Y   L   C   A   S   S   L
L36092,U66060,TRBV5-8*01 CTG TAT CTC TGT GCC AGC AGC TTG G
AF009663,TRBV5-8*01      --- --- --- --- --- --- --- --- -
X58803   ,TRBV5-8*02     --- --- --- --- --- --- ---        #c

#c: Rearranged cDNA
```

Framework and complementarity determining regions

FR1-IMGT: 26	CDR1-IMGT: 5
FR2-IMGT: 17	CDR2-IMGT: 6
FR3-IMGT: 37 (-2 aa: 73,82)	CDR3-IMGT: 4

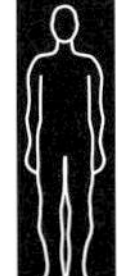

Collier de Perles for human TRBV5-8*01

Accession number: IMGT L36092   EMBL/GenBank/DDBJ: L36092

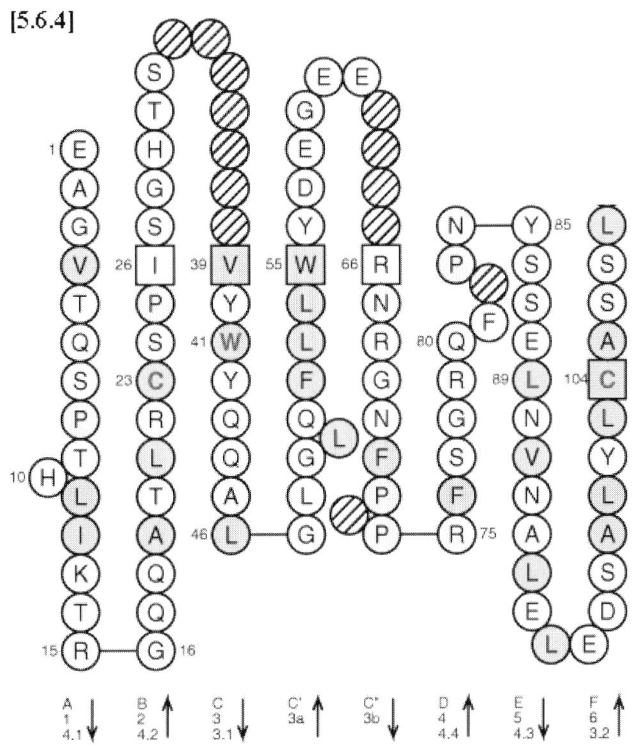

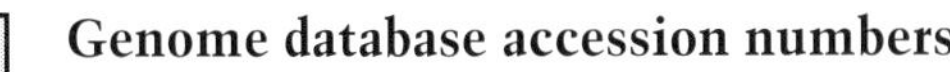

Genome database accession numbers

GDB:9954093   LocusLink: 28607

Nomenclature

TRBV6-1: T cell receptor beta variable 6-1.

Definition and functionality

TRBV6-1 is one of the 5–7 functional genes of the TRBV6 subgroup which comprises 8–9 mapped genes, depending on the haplotypes, in the TRB locus.

Gene location

TRBV6-1 is in the TRB locus on chromosome 7 at 7q34.

Nucleotide and amino acid sequences for human TRBV6-1

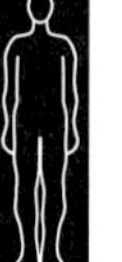

```
                          1   2   3   4   5   6   7   8   9  10  11  12  13  14  15  16  17  18  19  20
                          N   A   G   V   T   Q   T   P   K   F   Q   V   L   K   T   G   Q   S   M   T
X61446    ,TRBV6-1*01  [26] AAT GCT GGT GTC ACT CAG ACC CCA AAA TTC CAG GTC CTG AAG ACA GGA CAG AGC ATG ACA

L36092,U66059,TRBV6-1*01 [34] --- --- --- --- --- --- --- --- --- --- --- --- --- --- --- --- --- --- --- ---


                                                          __________________CDR1-IMGT__________________
                         21  22  23  24  25  26  27  28  29  30  31  32  33  34  35  36  37  38  39  40
                          L   Q   C   A   Q   D   M   N   H   N   S                               M   Y
X61446    ,TRBV6-1*01     CTG CAG TGT GCC CAG GAT ATG AAC CAT AAC TCC ... ... ... ... ... ... ... ATG TAC

L36092,U66059,TRBV6-1*01  --- --- --- --- --- --- --- --- --- --- --- ... ... ... ... ... ... ...


                                                                                          __________CDR2-
                         41  42  43  44  45  46  47  48  49  50  51  52  53  54  55  56  57  58  59  60
                          W   Y   R   Q   D   P   G   M   G   L   R   L   I   Y   Y   S   A   S   E   G
X61446    ,TRBV6-1*01     TGG TAT CGA CAA GAC CCA GGC ATG GGA CTG AGG CTG ATT TAT TAC TCA GCT TCT GAG GGT

L36092,U66059,TRBV6-1*01  --- --- --- --- --- --- --- --- --- --- --- --- --- --- --- --- --- --- --- ---


                         IMGT__________________
                         61  62  63  64  65  66  67  68  69  70  71  72  73  74  75  76  77  78  79  80
                          T                   T   D   K   G   E   V   P       N   G   Y   N   V   S   R
X61446    ,TRBV6-1*01     ACC ... ... ... ... ACT GAC AAA GGA GAA GTC CCC ... AAT GGC TAC AAT GTC TCC AGA

L36092,U66059,TRBV6-1*01  --- ... ... ... ... --- --- --- --- --- --- --- ... --- --- --- --- --- --- ---


                         81  82  83  84  85  86  87  88  89  90  91  92  93  94  95  96  97  98  99 100
                          L       N   K   R   E   F   S   L   R   L   E   S   A   A   P   S   Q   T   S
X61446    ,TRBV6-1*01     TTA ... AAC AAA CGG GAG TTC TCG CTC AGG CTG GAG TCG GCT GCT CCC TCC CAG ACA TCT

L36092,U66059,TRBV6-1*01  --- ... --- --- --- --- --- --- --- --- --- --- --- --- --- --- --- --- --- ---


                                         ______CDR3-IMGT______
                        101 102 103 104 105 106 107 108 109
                          V   Y   F   C   A   S   S   E
X61446    ,TRBV6-1*01     GTG TAC TTC TGT GCC AGC AGT GAA GC

L36092,U66059,TRBV6-1*01  --- --- --- --- --- --- --- --- --
```

Framework and complementarity determining regions

FR1-IMGT: 26   CDR1-IMGT: 5
FR2-IMGT: 17   CDR2-IMGT: 6
FR3-IMGT: 37 (-2 aa: 73, 82)   CDR3-IMGT: 4

Collier de Perles for human TRBV6-1*01

Accession number: IMGT X61446   EMBL/GenBank/DDBJ: X61446

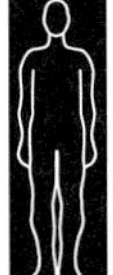

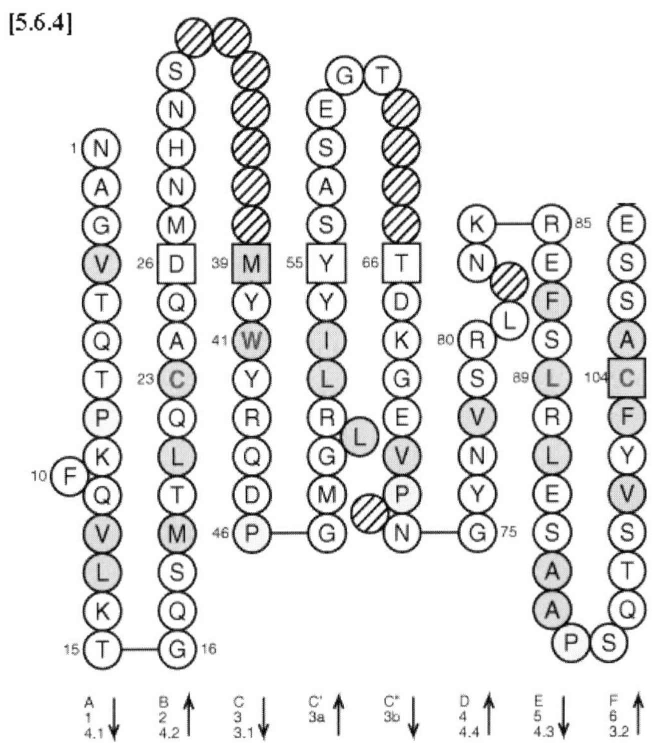

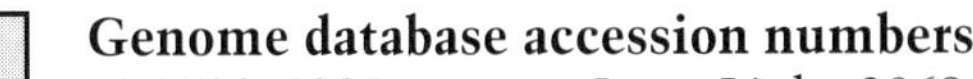

Genome database accession numbers
GDB:9954095   LocusLink: 28606

Nomenclature

TRBV6-2: T cell receptor beta variable 6-2.

Definition and functionality

TRBV6-2 is a functional gene (allele *01) or a pseudogene (alleles *02 and *03). TRBV6-2 belongs to the TRBV6 subgroup which comprises 8–9 mapped genes, of which 5–7 are functional, depending on the haplotypes, in the TRB locus.

TRBV6-2*02 and TRBV6-2*03 are pseudogenes due to a 1 nt DELETION in codon 49, leading to a frameshift.

Gene location

TRBV6-2 is in the TRB locus on chromosome 7 at 7q34.

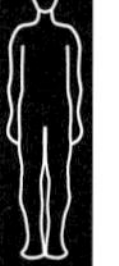

Nucleotide and amino acid sequences for human TRBV6-2

```
                                  1   2   3   4   5   6   7   8   9  10  11  12  13  14  15  16  17  18  19  20
                                  N   A   G   V   T   Q   T   P   K   F   R   V   L   K   T   G   Q   S   M   T
  X61445    ,TRBV6-2*01     [26]  AAT GCT GGT GTC ACT CAG ACC CCA AAA TTC CGG GTC CTG AAG ACA GGA CAG AGC ATG ACA
  U07975    ,TRBV6-2*01     [47]  --- --- --- --- --- --- --- --- --- --- --- --- --- --- --- --- --- --- --- ---
  U07976    ,TRBV6-2*01     [47]  --- --- --- --- --- --- --- --- --- --- --- --- --- --- --- --- --- --- --- ---
  U07978    ,TRBV6-2*01     [47]  --- --- --- --- --- --- --- --- --- --- --- --- --- --- --- --- --- --- --- ---
  L36092,U66059,TRBV6-2*01  [34]  --- --- --- --- --- --- --- --- --- --- --- --- --- --- --- --- --- --- --- ---
  L36190    ,TRBV6-2*01     [34]  --- --- --- --- --- --- --- --- --- --- --- --- --- --- --- --- --- --- --- ---
  AF009660  ,TRBV6-2*01     [35]  --- --- --- --- --- --- --- --- --- --- --- --- --- --- --- --- --- --- --- ---
  X75418    ,TRBV6-2*01     [20]  --- --- --- --- --- --- --- --- --- --- --- --- --- --- --- --- --- --- --- ---
  X75419    ,TRBV6-2*01     [20]  --- --- --- --- --- --- --- --- --- --- --- --- --- --- --- --- --- --- --- ---
  M31347    ,TRBV6-2*02     [17]  --- --- --- --- --- --- --- --- --- --- --- --- --- --- --- --- --- --- --- ---
  [45]      ,TRBV6-2*03           --- --- --- --- --- --- --- --- --- --- --- --- --- --- --- --- --- --- --- ---

                                                                                      ________CDR1-IMGT__________________
                                  21  22  23  24  25  26  27  28  29  30  31  32  33  34  35  36  37  38  39  40
                                  L   L   C   A   Q   D   M   N   H   E   Y                                   M   Y
  X61445    ,TRBV6-2*01           CTG CTG TGT GCC CAG GAT ATG AAC CAT GAA TAC ... ... ... ... ... ... ... ... ATG TAC
  U07975    ,TRBV6-2*01           --- --- --- --- --- --- --- --- --- --- --- ... ... ... ... ... ... ... ... --- ---
  U07976    ,TRBV6-2*01           --- --- --- --- --- --- --- --- --- --- --- ... ... ... ... ... ... ... ... --- ---
  U07978    ,TRBV6-2*01           --- --- --- --- --- --- --- --- --- --- --- ... ... ... ... ... ... ... ... --- ---
  L36092,U66059,TRBV6-2*01        --- --- --- --- --- --- --- --- --- --- --- ... ... ... ... ... ... ... ... --- ---
  L36190    ,TRBV6-2*01           --- --- --- --- --- --- --- --- --- --- --- ... ... ... ... ... ... ... ... --- ---
  AF009660  ,TRBV6-2*01           --- --- --- --- --- --- --- --- --- --- --- ... ... ... ... ... ... ... ... --- ---
  X75418    ,TRBV6-2*01           --- --- --- --- --- --- --- --- --- --- --- ... ... ... ... ... ... ... ... --- ---
  X75419    ,TRBV6-2*01           --- --- --- --- --- --- --- --- --- --- --- ... ... ... ... ... ... ... ... --- ---
  M31347    ,TRBV6-2*02           --- --- --- --- --- --- --- --- --- --- --- ... ... ... ... ... ... ... ... --- ---
                                                                    G                                           C
  [45]      ,TRBV6-2*03           --- --- --- --- --A --- --- --- --- -G- --- ... ... ... ... ... ... ... ... --- -G-

                                                                                          ____________________CDR2-
                                  41  42  43  44  45  46  47  48  49  50  51  52  53  54  55  56  57  58  59  60
                                  W   Y   R   Q   D   P   G   M   G   L   R   L   I   H   Y   S   V   G   E   G
  X61445    ,TRBV6-2*01           TGG TAT CGA CAA GAC CCA GGC ATG GGG CTG AGG CTG ATT CAT TAC TCA GTT GGT GAG GGT
  U07975    ,TRBV6-2*01           --- --- --- --- --- --- --- --- --- --- --- --- --- --- --- --- --- --- --- ---
  U07976    ,TRBV6-2*01           --- --- --- --- --- --- --- --- --- --- --- --- --- --- --- --- --- --- --- ---
  U07978    ,TRBV6-2*01           --- --- --- --- --- --- --- --- --- --- --- --- --- --- --- --- --- --- --- ---
  L36092,U66059,TRBV6-2*01        --- --- --- --- --- --- --- --- --- --- --- --- --- --- --- --- --- --- --- ---
  L36190    ,TRBV6-2*01           --- --- --- --- --- --- --- --- --- --- --- --- --- --- --- --- --- --- --- ---
  AF009660  ,TRBV6-2*01           --- --- --- --- --- --- --- --- --- --- --- --- --- --- --- --- --- --- --- ---
  X75418    ,TRBV6-2*01           --- --- --- --- --- --- --- --- --- --- --- --- --- --- --- --- --- --- --- ---
  X75419    ,TRBV6-2*01           --- --- --- --- --- --- --- --- --- --- --- --- --- --- --- --- --- --- --- ---
                                                              #
  M31347    ,TRBV6-2*02           --- --- --- --- --- --- --- --- --. --- --- --- --- --- --- --- --- --- --- ---
                                                      S       #
  [45]      ,TRBV6-2*03           --- --- --- --- --- --- A-- --- --. --- --- --- --- --- --- --- --- --- --- ---
```

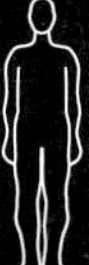

```
                          IMGT____
                           61  62  63  64  65  66  67  68  69  70  71  72  73  74  75  76  77  78  79  80
                           T                        T   A   K   G   E   V   P       D   G   Y   N   V   S   R
X61445      ,TRBV6-2*01   ACA ... ... ... ... ACT GCC AAA GGA GAG GTC CCT ... GAT GGC TAC AAT GTC TCC AGA
U07975      ,TRBV6-2*01   --- ... ... ... ... --- --- --- --- --- --- --- ... --- --- --- --- --- --- ---
U07976      ,TRBV6-2*01   --- ... ... ... ... --- --- --- --- --- --- --- ... --- --- --- --- --- --- ---
U07978      ,TRBV6-2*01   --- ... ... ... ... --- --- --- --- --- --- --- ... --- --- --- --- --- --- ---
L36092,U66059,TRBV6-2*01  --- ... ... ... ... --- --- --- --- --- --- --- ... --- --- --- --- --- --- ---
L36190      ,TRBV6-2*01   --- ... ... ... ... --- --- --- --- --- --- --- ... --- --- --- --- --- --- ---
AF009660    ,TRBV6-2*01   --- ... ... ... ... --- --- --- --- --- --- --- ... --- --- --- --- --- --- ---
X75418      ,TRBV6-2*01   --- ... ... ... ... --- --- --- --- --- --- --- ... --- --- --- --- --- --- ---
X75419      ,TRBV6-2*01   --- ... ... ... ... --- --- --- --- --- --- --- ... --- --- --- --- --- --- ---
M31347      ,TRBV6-2*02   --- ... ... ... ... --- --- --- --- --- --- --- ... --- --- --- --- --- --- ---
[45]        ,TRBV6-2*03   --- ... ... ... ... --- --- --- --- --- --- --- ... --- --- --- --- --- --- ---

                           81  82  83  84  85  86  87  88  89  90  91  92  93  94  95  96  97  98  99 100
                           L       K   K   Q   N   F   L   L   G   L   E   S   A   A   P   S   Q   T   S
X61445      ,TRBV6-2*01   TTA ... AAA AAA CAG AAT TTC CTG CTG GGG TTG GAG TCG GCT GCT CCC TCC CAA ACA TCT
U07975      ,TRBV6-2*01   --- ... --- --- --- --- --- --- --- --- --- --- --- --- --- --- --- --- --- ---
U07976      ,TRBV6-2*01   --- ... --- --- --- --- --- --- --- --- --- --- --- --- --- --- --- --- --- ---
U07978      ,TRBV6-2*01   --- ... --- --- --- --- --- --- --- --- --- --- --- --- --- --- --- --- --- ---
L36092,U66059,TRBV6-2*01  --- ... --- --- --- --- --- --- --- --- --- --- --- --- --- --- --- --- --- ---
L36190      ,TRBV6-2*01   --- ... --- --- --- --- --- --- --- --- --- --- --- --- --- --- --- --- --- ---
AF009660    ,TRBV6-2*01   --- ... --- --- --- --- --- --- --- --- --- --- --- --- --- --- --- --- --- ---
X75418      ,TRBV6-2*01   --- ... --- --- --- --- --- --- --- --- --- --- --- --- -
X75419      ,TRBV6-2*01   --- ... --- --- --- --- --- --- --- --- --- --- --- --- -
M31347      ,TRBV6-2*02   --- ... --- --- --- --- --- --- --- --- --- --- --- --- --- --- --- --- --- ---
[45]        ,TRBV6-2*03   --- ... --- --- --- --- --- --- --- --- --- --- --- --- --- --- --- --- --- ---

                                               ______CDR3-IMGT______
                          101 102 103 104 105 106 107 108 109
                           V   Y   F   C   A   S   S   Y
X61445      ,TRBV6-2*01   GTG TAC TTC TGT GCC AGC AGT TAC TC
U07975      ,TRBV6-2*01   --- --- --- --- --- --- --- --- --
U07976      ,TRBV6-2*01   --- --- --- --- --- --- --- --- --
U07978      ,TRBV6-2*01   --- --- --- --- --- --- --- --- --
L36092,U66059,TRBV6-2*01  --- --- --- --- --- --- --- --- --
L36190      ,TRBV6-2*01   --- --- --- --- --- --- --- --- --
AF009660    ,TRBV6-2*01   --- --- --- --- --- --- --- --- --
X75418      ,TRBV6-2*01
X75419      ,TRBV6-2*01
                                                  P
M31347      ,TRBV6-2*02   --- --- --- --- --- --- --C CCT        #g
[45]        ,TRBV6-2*03   --- --- --- --- --- ---                #
```

```
# (in the sequence): Frameshift
#: Rearranged
#g: Rearranged genomic DNA
```

Framework and complementarity determining regions

FR1-IMGT: 26

FR2-IMGT: 17

FR3-IMGT: 37 (-2 aa: 73, 82)

CDR1-IMGT: 5

CDR2-IMGT: 6

CDR3-IMGT: 4

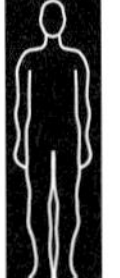

Collier de Perles for human TRBV6-2*01

Accession number: IMGT X61445   EMBL/GenBank/DDBJ: X61445

[5.6.4]

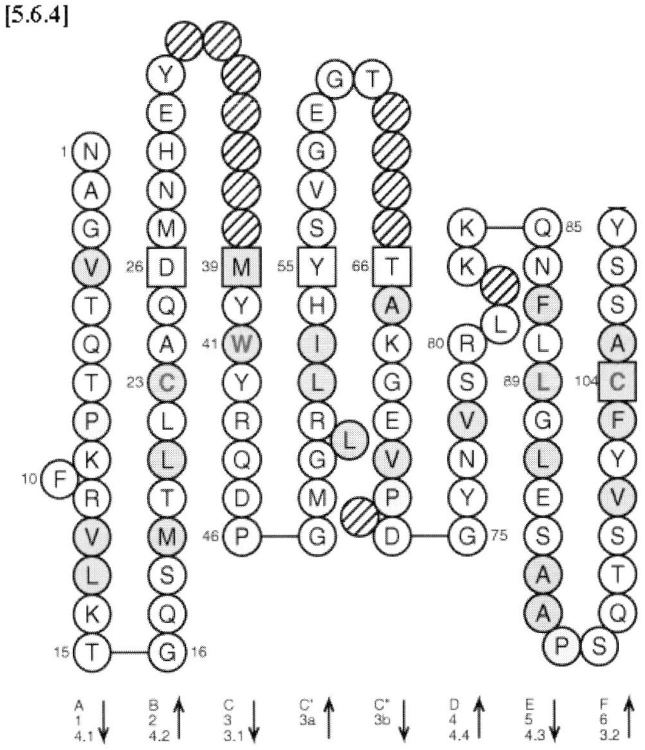

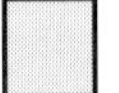

Genome database accession numbers
GDB:9954097   LocusLink: 28605

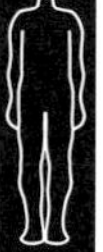

Nomenclature

TRBV6-3: T cell receptor beta variable 6-3.

Definition and functionality

TRBV6-3 is one of the 5–7 functional genes which may or may not be present due to a polymorphism by insertion/deletion. TRBV6-3 belongs to the TRBV6 subgroup which comprises 8–9 mapped genes, depending on the haplotypes, in the TRB locus.

Gene location

TRBV6-3 is in the TRB locus on chromosome 7 at 7q34.

Nucleotide and amino acid sequences for human TRBV6-3

```
                                     1   2   3   4   5   6   7   8   9  10  11  12  13  14  15  16  17  18  19  20
                                     N   A   G   V   T   Q   T   P   K   F   R   V   L   K   T   G   Q   S   M   T
U07978     ,TRBV6-3*01        [47]  AAT GCT GGT GTC ACT CAG ACC CCA AAA TTC CGG GTC CTG AAG ACA GGA CAG AGC ATG ACA

L36092,U66059,TRBV6-3*01      [34]  --- --- --- --- --- --- --- --- --- --- --- --- --- --- --- --- --- --- --- ---

L26229     ,TRBV6-3*01        [44]  --- --- --- --- --- --- --- --- --- --- --- --- --- --- --- --- --- --- --- ---


                                                                          _________________________CDR1-IMGT_________________________
                                    21  22  23  24  25  26  27  28  29  30  31  32  33  34  35  36  37  38  39  40
                                     L   L   C   A   Q   D   M   N   H   E   Y                               M   Y
U07978     ,TRBV6-3*01              CTG CTG TGT GCC CAG GAT ATG AAC CAT GAA TAC ... ... ... ... ... ... ... ATG TAC

L36092,U66059,TRBV6-3*01            --- --- --- --- --- --- --- --- --- --- --- ... ... ... ... ... --- ---

L26229     ,TRBV6-3*01              --- --- --- --- --- --- --- --- --- --- --- ... ... ... ... ... --- ---


                                                                                                      __________CDR2-
                                    41  42  43  44  45  46  47  48  49  50  51  52  53  54  55  56  57  58  59  60
                                     W   Y   R   Q   D   P   G   M   G   L   R   L   I   H   Y   S   V   G   E   G
U07978     ,TRBV6-3*01              TGG TAT CGA CAA GAC CCA GGC ATG GGG CTG AGG CTG ATT CAT TAC TCA GTT GGT GAG GGT

L36092,U66059,TRBV6-3*01            --- --- --- --- --- --- --- --- --- --- --- --- --- --- --- --- --- --- --- ---

L26229     ,TRBV6-3*01              --- --- --- --- --- --- --- --- --- --- --- --- --- --- --- --- --- --- --- ---


                                    IMGT__________________
                                    61  62  63  64  65  66  67  68  69  70  71  72  73  74  75  76  77  78  79  80
                                     T                       T   A   K   G   E   V   P       D   G   Y   N   V   S   R
U07978     ,TRBV6-3*01              ACA ... ... ... ... ACT GCC AAA GGA GAG GTC CCT ... GAT GGC TAC AAT GTC TCC AGA

L36092,U66059,TRBV6-3*01            --- ... ... ... ... --- --- --- --- --- --- --- ... --- --- --- --- --- --- ---

L26229     ,TRBV6-3*01              --- ... ... ... ... --- --- --- --- --- --- --- ... --- --- --- --- --- --- ---


                                    81  82  83  84  85  86  87  88  89  90  91  92  93  94  95  96  97  98  99 100
                                     L       K   K   Q   N   F   L   L   G   L   E   S   A   A   P   S   Q   T   S
U07978     ,TRBV6-3*01              TTA ... AAA AAA CAG AAT TTC CTG CTG GGG TTG GAG TCG GCT GCT CCC TCC CAA ACA TCT

L36092,U66059,TRBV6-3*01            --- ... --- --- --- --- --- --- --- --- --- --- --- --- --- --- --- --- --- ---

L26229     ,TRBV6-3*01              --- ... --- --- --- --- --- --- --- --- --- --- --- --- --- --- --- --- --- ---


                                                    ________CDR3-IMGT________
                                   101 102 103 104 105 106 107 108 109
                                     V   Y   F   C   A   S   S   Y
U07978     ,TRBV6-3*01              GTG TAC TTC TGT GCC AGC AGT TAC TC

L36092,U66059,TRBV6-3*01            --- --- --- --- --- --- --- --- --

L26229     ,TRBV6-3*01                                              o
```

°: Genomic DNA, but not known as being germline or rearranged

Framework and complementarity determining regions

FR1-IMGT: 26   CDR1-IMGT: 5
FR2-IMGT: 17   CDR2-IMGT: 6
FR3-IMGT: 37 (-2 aa: 73, 82) CDR3-IMGT: 4

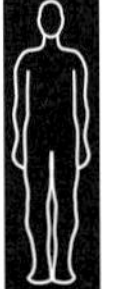

Collier de Perles for human TRBV6-3*01

Accession number: IMGT U07978   EMBL/GenBank/DDBJ: U07978

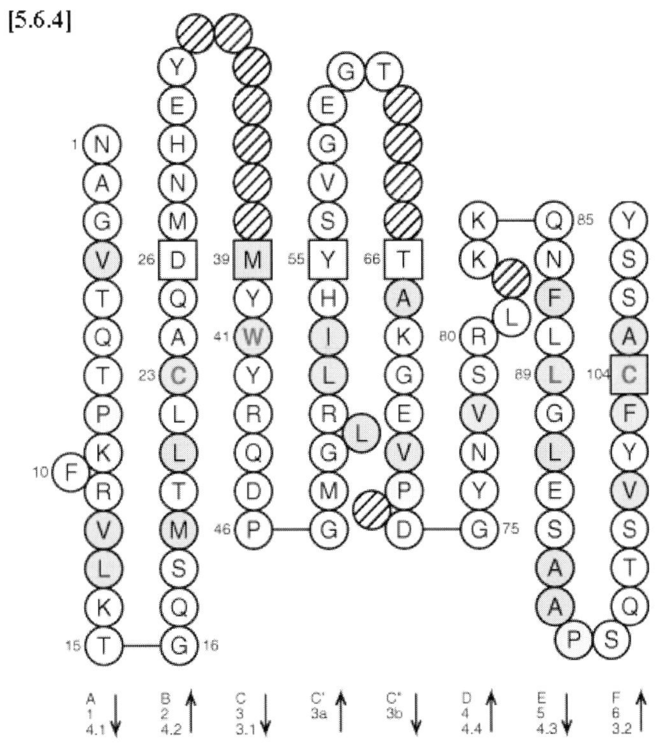

Genome database accession numbers
GDB:9954099   LocusLink: 28604

TRBV6-4

Nomenclature

TRBV6-4: T cell receptor beta variable 6-4.

Definition and functionality

TRBV6-4 is one of the 5–7 functional genes of the TRBV6 subgroup which comprises 8–9 mapped genes, depending on the haplotypes, in the TRB locus.

Gene location

TRBV6-4 is in the TRB locus on chromosome 7 at 7q34.

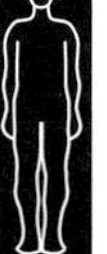

Nucleotide and amino acid sequences for human TRBV6-4

```
                              1   2   3   4   5   6   7   8   9   10  11  12  13  14  15  16  17  18  19  20
                              I   A   G   I   T   Q   A   P   T   S   Q   I   L   A   A   G   R   R   M   T
X61653   ,TRBV6-4*01    [26]  ATT GCT GGG ATC ACC CAG GCA CCA ACA TCT CAG ATC CTG GCA GCA GGA CGG CGC ATG ACA

L36092,U66059,TRBV6-4*01 [34] --- --- --- --- --- --- --- --- --- --- --- --- --- --- --- --- --- --- --- ---
                              T                                                                       S
AF009660,TRBV6-4*02     [35]  -C- --- --- --- --- --- --- --- --- --- --- --- --- --- --- --- A-- --- ---


                                                              ______________CDR1-IMGT____________________
                              21  22  23  24  25  26  27  28  29  30  31  32  33  34  35  36  37  38  39  40
                              L   R   C   T   Q   D   M   R   H   N   A                           M   Y
X61653   ,TRBV6-4*01          CTG AGA TGT ACC CAG GAT ATG AGA CAT AAT GCC ... ... ... ... ... ... ATG TAC

L36092,U66059,TRBV6-4*01      --- --- --- --- --- --- --- --- --- --- --- ... ... ... ... ... ... --- ---

AF009660,TRBV6-4*02           --- --- --- --- --- --- --- --- --- --- --- ... ... ... ... ... ... --- ---


                                                                                          ____________CDR2-
                              41  42  43  44  45  46  47  48  49  50  51  52  53  54  55  56  57  58  59  60
                              W   Y   R   Q   D   L   G   L   G   L   R   L   I   H   Y   S   N   T   A   G
X61653   ,TRBV6-4*01          TGG TAT AGA CAA GAT CTA GGA CTG GGG CTA AGG CTC ATC CAT TAT TCA AAT ACT GCA GGT

L36092,U66059,TRBV6-4*01      --- --- --- --- --- --- --- --- --- --- --- --- --- --- --- --- --- --- --- ---

AF009660,TRBV6-4*02           --- --- --- --- --- --- --- --- --- --- --- --- --- --- --- --- --- --- --- ---


                              IMGT______________________
                              61  62  63  64  65  66  67  68  69  70  71  72  73  74  75  76  77  78  79  80
                              T                   T   G   K   G   E   V   P       D   G   Y   S   V   S   R
X61653   ,TRBV6-4*01          ACC ... ... ... ... ACT GGC AAA GGA GAA GTC CCT ... GAT GGT TAT AGT GTC TCC AGA

L36092,U66059,TRBV6-4*01      --- ... ... ... ... --- --- --- --- --- --- --- ... --- --- --- --- --- --- ---

AF009660,TRBV6-4*02           --- ... ... ... ... --- --- --- --- --- --- --- ... --- --- --- --- --- --- ---


                              81  82  83  84  85  86  87  88  89  90  91  92  93  94  95  96  97  98  99 100
                              A       N   T   D   D   F   P   L   T   L   A   S   A   V   P   S   Q   T   S
X61653   ,TRBV6-4*01          GCA ... AAC ACA GAT GAT TTC CCC CTC ACG TTG GCG TCT GCT GTA CCC TCT CAG ACA TCT

L36092,U66059,TRBV6-4*01      --- ... --- --- --- --- --- --- --- --- --- --- --- --- --- --- --- --- --- ---

AF009660,TRBV6-4*02           --- ... --- --- --- --- --- --- --- --- --- --- --- --- --- --- --- --- --- ---


                                              ______CDR3-IMGT______
                              101 102 103 104 105 106 107 108 109
                              V   Y   F   C   A   S   S   D
X61653   ,TRBV6-4*01          GTG TAC TTC TGT GCC AGC AGT GAC TC

L36092,U66059,TRBV6-4*01      --- --- --- --- --- --- --- --- --

AF009660,TRBV6-4*02           --- --- --- --- --- --- --- --- --
```

Framework and complementarity determining regions

FR1-IMGT: 26	CDR1-IMGT: 5
FR2-IMGT: 17	CDR2-IMGT: 6
FR3-IMGT: 37 (-2 aa: 73, 82)	CDR3-IMGT: 4

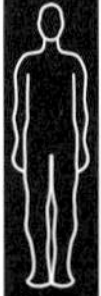

Collier de Perles for human TRBV6-4*01

Accession number: IMGT X61653   EMBL/GenBank/DDBJ: X61653

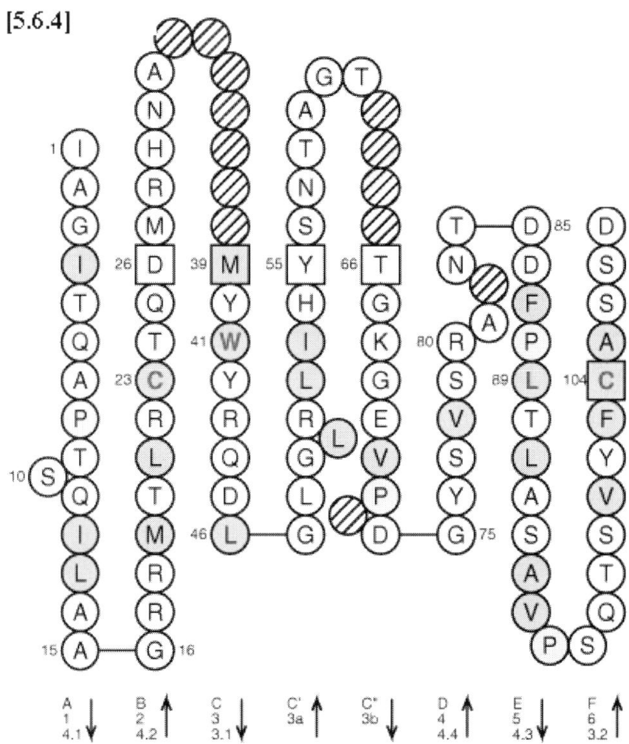

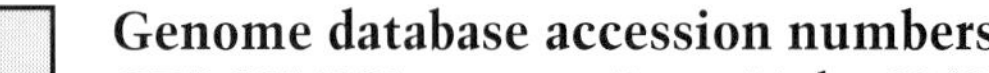

Genome database accession numbers
GDB:9954101   LocusLink: 28603

TRBV6-5

Nomenclature

TRBV6-5: T cell receptor beta variable 6-5.

Definition and functionality

TRBV6-5 is one of the 5–7 functional genes of the TRBV6 subgroup which comprises 8–9 mapped genes, depending on the haplotypes, in the TRB locus.

Gene location

TRBV6-5 is in the TRB locus on chromosome 7 at 7q34.

Nucleotide and amino acid sequences for human TRBV6-5

```
                                       1   2   3   4   5   6   7   8   9  10  11  12  13  14  15  16  17  18  19  20
                                       N   A   G   V   T   Q   T   P   K   F   Q   V   L   K   T   G   Q   S   M   T
L36092,U66059,U66060,TRBV6-5*01 [34]  AAT GCT GGT GTC ACT CAG ACC CCA AAA TTC CAG GTC CTG AAG ACA GGA CAG AGC ATG ACA

AF009662,TRBV6-5*01             [35]  --- --- --- --- --- --- --- --- --- --- --- --- --- --- --- --- --- --- --- ---

AF009663,TRBV6-5*01             [35]  --- --- --- --- --- --- --- --- --- --- --- --- --- --- --- --- --- --- --- ---


                                                                        ____________________CDR1-IMGT____________________
                                      21  22  23  24  25  26  27  28  29  30  31  32  33  34  35  36  37  38  39  40
                                       L   Q   C   A   Q   D   M   N   H   E   Y                               M   S
L36092,U66059,U66060,TRBV6-5*01       CTG CAG TGT GCC CAG GAT ATG AAC CAT GAA TAC ... ... ... ... ... ... ... ATG TCC

AF009662,TRBV6-5*01                   --- --- --- --- --- --- --- --- --- --- --- ... ... ... ... ... ... .. --- ---

AF009663,TRBV6-5*01                   --- --- --- --- --- --- --- --- --- --- --- ... ... ... ... ... ... .. --- ---


                                                                                                          __________CDR2-
                                      41  42  43  44  45  46  47  48  49  50  51  52  53  54  55  56  57  58  59  60
                                       W   Y   R   Q   D   P   G   M   G   L   R   L   I   H   Y   S   V   G   A   G
L36092,U66059,U66060,TRBV6-5*01       TGG TAT CGA CAA GAC CCA GGC ATG GGG CTG AGG CTG ATT CAT TAC TCA GTT GGT GCT GGT

AF009662,TRBV6-5*01                   --- --- --- --- --- --- --- --- --- --- --- --- --- --- --- --- --- --- --- ---

AF009663,TRBV6-5*01                   --- --- --- --- --- --- --- --- --- --- --- --- --- --- --- --- --- --- --- ---


                                      IMGT__________________
                                      61  62  63  64  65  66  67  68  69  70  71  72  73  74  75  76  77  78  79  80
                                       I                       T   D   Q   G   E   V   P       N   G   Y   N   V   S   R
L36092,U66059,U66060,TRBV6-5*01       ATC ... ... ... ... ACT GAC CAA GGA GAA GTC CCC ... AAT GGC TAC AAT GTC TCC AGA

AF009662,TRBV6-5*01                   --- ... ... ... ... --- --- --- --- --- --- --- ... --- --- --- --- --- --- ---

AF009663,TRBV6-5*01                   --- ... ... ... ... --- --- --- --- --- --- --- ... --- --- --- --- --- --- ---


                                      81  82  83  84  85  86  87  88  89  90  91  92  93  94  95  96  97  98  99 100
                                       S       T   T   E   D   F   P   L   R   L   L   S   A   A   P   S   Q   T   S
L36092,U66059,U66060,TRBV6-5*01       TCA ... ACC ACA GAG GAT TTC CCG CTC AGG CTG CTG TCG GCT GCT CCC TCC CAG ACA TCT

AF009662,TRBV6-5*01                   --- ... --- --- --- --- --- --- --- --- --- --- --- --- --- --- --- --- --- ---

AF009663,TRBV6-5*01                   --- ... --- --- --- --- --- --- --- --- --- --- --- --- --- --- --- --- --- ---


                                             ______CDR3-IMGT______
                                     101 102 103 104 105 106 107 108 109
                                       V   Y   F   C   A   S   S   Y
L36092,U66059,U66060,TRBV6-5*01       GTG TAC TTC TGT GCC AGC AGT TAC TC

AF009662,TRBV6-5*01                   --- --- --- --- --- --- --- --- --

AF009663,TRBV6-5*01                   --- --- --- --- --- --- --- --- --
```

Framework and complementarity determining regions

FR1-IMGT: 26	CDR1-IMGT: 5
FR2-IMGT: 17	CDR2-IMGT: 6
FR3-IMGT: 37 (-2 aa: 73, 82)	CDR3-IMGT: 4

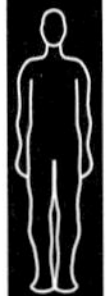

Collier de Perles for human TRBV6-5*01

Accession number: IMGT L36092   EMBL/GenBank/DDBJ: L36092

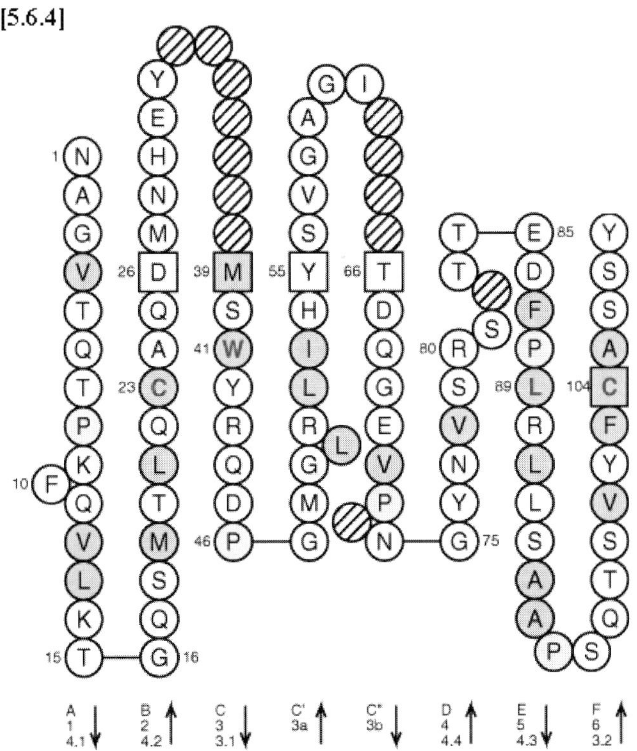

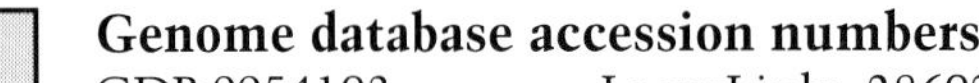

Genome database accession numbers
GDB:9954103   LocusLink: 28602

TRBV6-6

Nomenclature

TRBV6-6: T cell receptor beta variable 6-6.

Definition and functionality

TRBV6-6 is one of the 5–7 functional genes of the TRBV6 subgroup which comprises 8–9 mapped genes, depending on the haplotypes, in the TRB locus.

Gene location

TRBV6-6 is in the TRB locus on chromosome 7 at 7q34.

Nucleotide and amino acid sequences for human TRBV6-6

```
                               1   2   3   4   5   6   7   8   9  10  11  12  13  14  15  16  17  18  19  20
                               N   A   G   V   T   Q   T   P   K   F   R   I   L   K   I   G   Q   S   M   T
L36092,U66060,TRBV6-6*01 [34]  AAT GCT GGT GTC ACT CAG ACC CCA AAA TTC CGC ATC CTG AAG ATA GGA CAG AGC ATG ACA
AF009663,TRBV6-6*01      [35]  --- --- --- --- --- --- --- --- --- --- --- --- --- --- --- --- --- --- --- ---
AF009662,TRBV6-6*02      [35]  --- --- --- --- --- --- --- --- --- --- --- --- --- --- --- --- --- --- --- ---
X58815  ,TRBV6-6*03      [10]  --- --- --- --- --- --- --- --- --- --- --- --- --- --- --- --- --- --- --- ---
X74848  ,TRBV6-6*04      [19]  --- --- --- --- --- --- --- --- --- --- --- --- --- --- --- --- --- --- --- ---
L06892  ,TRBV6-6*05      [36]  --- --- --- --- --- --- --- --- --- --- --- --- --- --- --- --- --- --- --- ---

                                                                   ________________CDR1-IMGT_________________
                              21  22  23  24  25  26  27  28  29  30  31  32  33  34  35  36  37  38  39  40
                               L   Q   C   T   Q   D   M   N   H   N   Y                           M   Y
L36092,U66060,TRBV6-6*01      CTG CAG TGT ACC CAG GAT ATG AAC CAT AAC TAC ... ... ... ... ... ... ... ATG TAC
AF009663,TRBV6-6*01           --- --- --- --- --- --- --- --- --- --- --- ... ... ... ... ... ... ... --- ---
                                           A
AF009662,TRBV6-6*02           --- --- --- G-- --- --- --- --- --- --- --- ... ... ... ... ... ... ... --- ---
                                           A
X58815  ,TRBV6-6*03           --- --- --- G-- --- --- --- --- --- --- --- ... ... ... ... ... ... ... --- ---
                                                                       E
X74848  ,TRBV6-6*04           --- --- --- --- --- --- --- --- --- G-A --- ... ... ... ... ... ... ... --- ---
                                           A
L06892  ,TRBV6-6*05           --- --- --- G-- --- --- --- --- --- --- --- ... ... ... ... ... ... ... --- G--

                                                                                               _________CDR2-
                              41  42  43  44  45  46  47  48  49  50  51  52  53  54  55  56  57  58  59  60
                               W   Y   R   Q   D   P   G   M   G   L   K   L   I   Y   Y   S   V   G   A   G
L36092,U66060,TRBV6-6*01      TGG TAT CGA CAA GAC CCA GGC ATG GGG CTG AAG CTG ATT TAT TAT TCA GTT GGT GCT GGT
AF009663,TRBV6-6*01           --- --- --- --- --- --- --- --- --- --- --- --- --- --- --- --- --- --- --- ---
AF009662,TRBV6-6*02           --- --- --- --- --- --- --- --- --- --- --- --- --- --- --- --- --- --- --- ---
X58815  ,TRBV6-6*03           --- --- --- --- --- --- --- --- --- --- --- --- --- --- --- --- --- --- --- ---
X74848  ,TRBV6-6*04           --- --- --- --- --- --- --- --- --- --- --- --- --- --- --- --- --- --- --- ---
L06892  ,TRBV6-6*05           --- --- --- --- --- --- --- --- --- --- --- --- --- --- --- --- --- --- --- ---

                              IMGT__________________
                              61  62  63  64  65  66  67  68  69  70  71  72  73  74  75  76  77  78  79  80
                               I                       T   D   K   G   E   V   P       N   G   Y   N   V   S   R
L36092,U66060,TRBV6-6*01      ATC ... ... ... ... ACT GAT AAA GGA GAA GTC CCG ... AAT GGC TAC AAC GTC TCC AGA
AF009663,TRBV6-6*01           --- ... ... ... ... --- --- --- --- --- --- --- ... --- --- --- --- --- --- ---
AF009662,TRBV6-6*02           --- ... ... ... ... --- --C --- --- --- --- --- ... --- --- --- --- --- --- ---
X58815  ,TRBV6-6*03           --- ... ... ... ... --- --- --- --- --- --- --- ... --- --- --- --- --- --- ---
X74848  ,TRBV6-6*04           --- ... ... ... ... --- --- --- --- --- --- --- ... --- --- --- --T --- --- ---
L06892  ,TRBV6-6*05           --- ... ... ... ... --- --C --- --- --- --- --- ... --- --- --- --- --- --- ---

                              81  82  83  84  85  86  87  88  89  90  91  92  93  94  95  96  97  98  99 100
                               S       T   T   E   D   F   P   L   R   L   E   L   A   A   P   S   Q   T   S
L36092,U66060,TRBV6-6*01      TCA ... ACC ACA GAG GAT TTC CCG CTC AGG CTG GAG TTG GCT GCT CCC TCC CAG ACA TCT
AF009663,TRBV6-6*01           --- ... --- --- --- --- --- --- --- --- --- --- --- --- --- --- --- --- --- ---
AF009662,TRBV6-6*02           --- ... --- --- --- --- --- --- --- --- --- --- --- --- --- --- --- --- --- ---
X58815  ,TRBV6-6*03           --- ... --- --- --- --- --- --- --- --- --- --- --- --- --- --- --- --- --- ---
X74848  ,TRBV6-6*04           --- ... --- --- --- --- --- --- --- --- --- --- --- --- --- --- --- --- --- ---
                                                                                              A
L06892  ,TRBV6-6*05           --- ... --- --- --- --- --- --- --- --- --- --- --- --- --- G-- --- --- --- ---
```

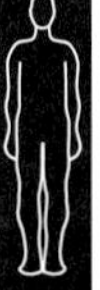

```
                                            ____CDR3-IMGT____
                          101 102 103 104 105 106 107 108 109
                           V   Y   F   C   A   S   S   Y
     L36092,U66060,TRBV6-6*01  GTG TAC TTC TGT GCC AGC AGT TAC TC

     AF009663,TRBV6-6*01       --- --- --- --- --- --- --- --- --

     AF009662,TRBV6-6*02       --- --- --- --- --- --- ---

     X58815  ,TRBV6-6*03       --- --- --- --- --- --- ---              #c
                                                          R
     X74848  ,TRBV6-6*04       --- --- --- --- --- --- --- CGA          #c

     L06892  ,TRBV6-6*05       --- --- --- --- --- --- --C              #c

#c: Rearranged cDNA
```

Framework and complementarity determining regions

FR1-IMGT: 26   CDR1-IMGT: 5
FR2-IMGT: 17   CDR2-IMGT: 6
FR3-IMGT: 37 (-2 aa: 73, 82)   CDR3-IMGT: 4

Collier de Perles for human TRBV6-6*01

Accession number: IMGT L36092   EMBL/GenBank/DDBJ: L36092

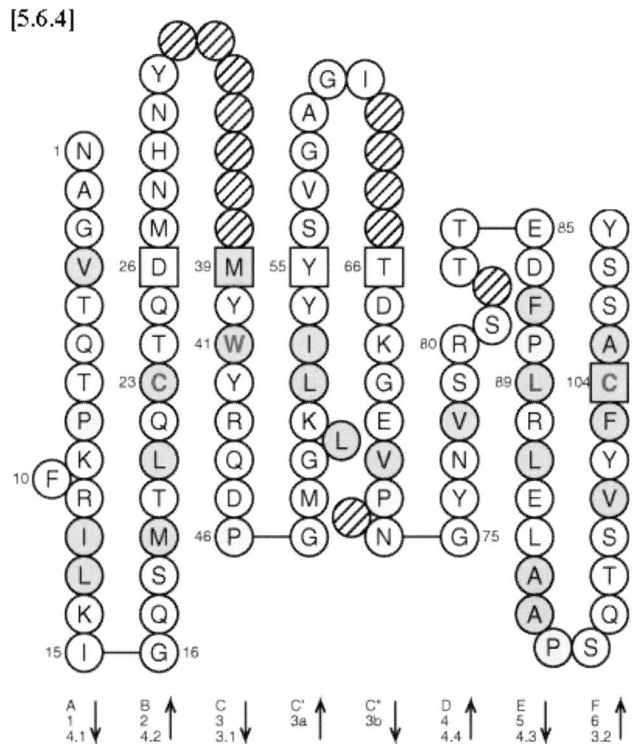

Genome database accession numbers
GDB:9954105   LocusLink: 28601

Nomenclature

TRBV6-7: T cell receptor beta variable 6-7.

Definition and functionality

TRBV6-7 is an ORF due to the CONSERVED–TRP (tgg) of the V-EXON, being replaced by an Arginine (cgg). TRBV6-7 belongs to the TRBV6 subgroup which comprises 8–9 mapped genes, of which 5–7 are functional, depending on the haplotypes, in the TRB locus.

Gene location

TRBV6-7 is in the TRB locus on chromosome 7 at 7q34.

Nucleotide and amino acid sequences for human TRBV6-7

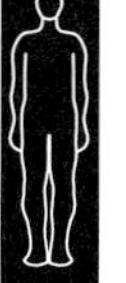

```
                              1   2   3   4   5   6   7   8   9  10  11  12  13  14  15  16  17  18  19  20
                              N   A   G   V   T   Q   T   P   K   F   H   V   L   K   T   G   Q   S   M   T
L36092,U66060,TRBV6-7*01 [34] AAT GCT GGT GTC ACT CAG ACC CCA AAA TTC CAC GTC CTG AAG ACA GGA CAG AGC ATG ACT

AF009663,TRBV6-7*01      [35] --- --- --- --- --- --- --- --- --- --- --- --- --- --- --- --- --- --- --- ---

L26227   ,TRBV6-7*01     [44] --- --- --- --- --- --- --- --- --- --- --- --- --- --- --- --- --- --- --- ---


                                                                          ______________CDR1-IMGT________
                              21  22  23  24  25  26  27  28  29  30  31  32  33  34  35  36  37  38  39  40
                              L   L   C   A   Q   D   M   N   H   E   Y                               M   Y
L36092,U66060,TRBV6-7*01      CTG CTG TGT GCC CAG GAT ATG AAC CAT GAA TAC ... ... ... ... ... ... ... ATG TAT

AF009663,TRBV6-7*01           --- --- --- --- --- --- --- --- --- --- --- ... ... ... ... ... ... ... --- ---

L26227   ,TRBV6-7*01          --- --- --- --- --- --- --- --- --- --- --- ... ... ... ... ... ... ... --- ---


                                                                                      ________________CDR2-
                              41  42  43  44  45  46  47  48  49  50  51  52  53  54  55  56  57  58  59  60
                              R   Y   R   Q   D   P   G   K   G   L   R   L   I   Y   Y   S   V   A   A   A
L36092,U66060,TRBV6-7*01      CGG TAT CGA CAA GAC CCA GGC AAG GGG CTG AGG CTG ATT TAC TAC TCA GTT GCT GCT GCT

AF009663,TRBV6-7*01           --- --- --- --- --- --- --- --- --- --- --- --- --- --- --- --- --- --- --- ---

L26227   ,TRBV6-7*01          --- --- --- --- --- --- --- --- --- --- --- --- --- --- --- --- --- --- --- ---


                              IMGT____
                              61  62  63  64  65  66  67  68  69  70  71  72  73  74  75  76  77  78  79  80
                              L                       T   D   K   G   E   V   P       N   G   Y   N   V   S   R
L36092,U66060,TRBV6-7*01      CTC ... ... ... ... ACT GAC AAA GGA GAA GTT CCC ... AAT GGC TAC AAT GTC TCC AGA

AF009663,TRBV6-7*01           --- ... ... ... ... --- --- --- --- --- --- --- ... --- --- --- --- --- --- ---

L26227   ,TRBV6-7*01          --- ... ... ... ... --- --- --- --- --- --- --- ... --- --- --- --- --- --- ---


                              81  82  83  84  85  86  87  88  89  90  91  92  93  94  95  96  97  98  99 100
                              S       N   T   E   D   F   P   L   K   L   E   S   A   A   P   S   Q   T   S
L36092,U66060,TRBV6-7*01      TCA ... AAC ACA GAG GAT TTC CCC CTC AAG CTG GAG TCA GCT GCT CCC TCT CAG ACT TCT

AF009663,TRBV6-7*01           --- ... --- --- --- --- --- --- --- --- --- --- --- --- --- --- --- --- --- ---

L26227   ,TRBV6-7*01          --- ... --- --- --- --- --- --- --- --- --- --- --- --- --- --- --- --- --- -


                                      _______CDR3-IMGT______
                             101 102 103 104 105 106 107 108 109
                              V   Y   F   C   A   S   S   Y
L36092,U66060,TRBV6-7*01      GTT TAC TTC TGT GCC AGC AGT TAC TC

AF009663,TRBV6-7*01           --- --- --- --- --- --- --- --- --

L26227   ,TRBV6-7*01                                            °
```

°: Genomic DNA, but not known as being germline or rearranged

Framework and complementarity determining regions

FR1-IMGT: 26	CDR1-IMGT: 5
FR2-IMGT: 17	CDR2-IMGT: 6
FR3-IMGT: 37 (-2 aa: 73, 82)	CDR3-IMGT: 4

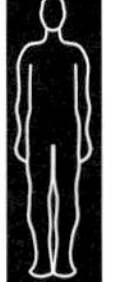

Collier de Perles for human TRBV6-7*01

Accession number: IMGT L36092   EMBL/GenBank/DDBJ: L36092

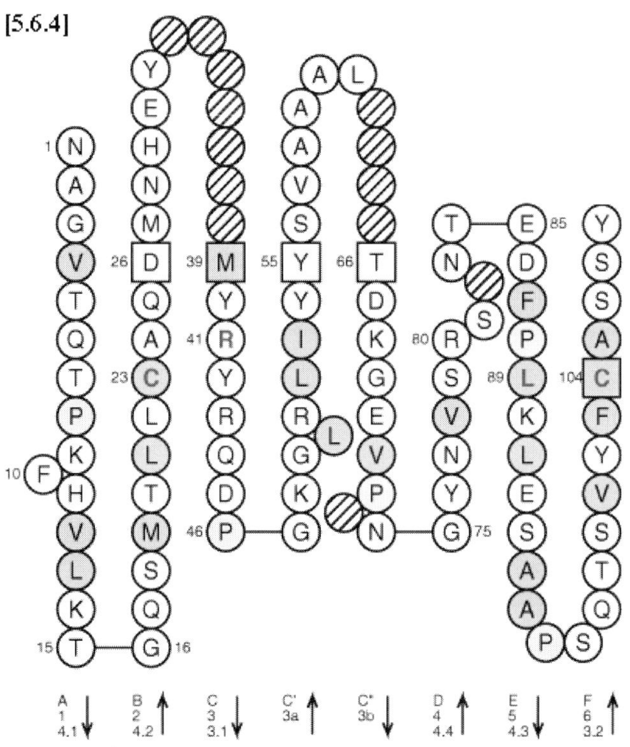

Genome database accession numbers
GDB:9954107   LocusLink: 28600

Nomenclature

TRBV6-8: T cell receptor beta variable 6-8.

Definition and functionality

TRBV6-8 is one of the 5–7 functional genes of the TRBV6 subgroup which comprises 8–9 mapped genes, depending on the haplotypes, in the TRB locus.

Gene location

TRBV6-8 is in the TRB locus on chromosome 7 at 7q34.

Nucleotide and amino acid sequences for human TRBV6-8

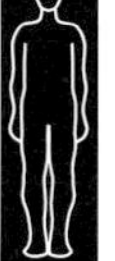

```
                             1   2   3   4   5   6   7   8   9  10  11  12  13  14  15  16  17  18  19  20
                             N   A   G   V   T   Q   T   P   K   F   H   I   L   K   T   G   Q   S   M   T
L36092,U66060,TRBV6-8*01 [34] AAT GCT GGT GTC ACT CAG ACC CCA AAA TTC CAC ATC CTG AAG ACA GGA CAG AGC ATG ACA

AF009663,TRBV6-8*01      [35] --- --- --- --- --- --- --- --- --- --- --- --- --- --- --- --- --- --- --- ---

L26228 ,TRBV6-8*01       [44] --- --- --- --- --- --- --- --- --- --- --- --- --- --- --- --- --- --- --- ---


                                                                          ______________CDR1-IMGT__________________
                             21  22  23  24  25  26  27  28  29  30  31  32  33  34  35  36  37  38  39  40
                             L   Q   C   A   Q   D   M   N   H   G   Y                           M   S
L36092,U66060,TRBV6-8*01     CTG CAG TGT GCC CAG GAT ATG AAC CAT GGA TAC ... ... ... ... ... ... ... ATG TCC

AF009663,TRBV6-8*01          --- --- --- --- --- --- --- --- --- --- --- ... ... ... ... ... ... ... --- ---

L26228 ,TRBV6-8*01           --- --- --- --- --- --- --- --- --- --- --- ... ... ... ... ... ... ... --- ---


                                                                                              ____________CDR2-
                             41  42  43  44  45  46  47  48  49  50  51  52  53  54  55  56  57  58  59  60
                             W   Y   R   Q   D   P   G   M   G   L   R   L   I   Y   Y   S   A   A   A   G
L36092,U66060,TRBV6-8*01     TGG TAT CGA CAA GAC CCA GGC ATG GGG CTG AGA CTG ATT TAC TAC TCA GCT GCT GCT GGT

AF009663,TRBV6-8*01          --- --- --- --- --- --- --- --- --- --- --- --- --- --- --- --- --- --- --- ---

L26228 ,TRBV6-8*01           --- --- --- --- --- --- --- --- --- --- --- --- --- --- --- --- --- --- --- ---


                             IMGT_____________________
                             61  62  63  64  65  66  67  68  69  70  71  72  73  74  75  76  77  78  79  80
                             T                   T   D   K       E   V   P       N   G   Y   N   V   S   R
L36092,U66060,TRBV6-8*01     ACT ... ... ... ... ACT GAC AAA ... GAA GTC CCC ... AAT GGC TAC AAT GTC TCT AGA

AF009663,TRBV6-8*01          --- ... ... ... ... --- --- --- ... --- --- --- ... --- --- --- --- --- --- ---

L26228 ,TRBV6-8*01           --- ... ... ... ... --- --- --- ... --- --- --- ... --- --- --- --- --- --- ---


                             81  82  83  84  85  86  87  88  89  90  91  92  93  94  95  96  97  98  99 100
                             L   N   T   E   D   F   P   L   R   L   V   S   A   A   P   S   Q   T   S
L36092,U66060,TRBV6-8*01     TTA ... AAC ACA GAG GAT TTC CCA CTC AGG CTG GTG TCG GCT GCT CCC TCC CAG ACA TCT

AF009663,TRBV6-8*01          --- ... --- --- --- --- --- --- --- --- --- --- --- --- --- --- --- --- --- ---

L26228 ,TRBV6-8*01           --- ... --- --- --- --- --- --- --- --- --- --- --- --- --- --- --- -- 


                                            ______CDR3-IMGT______
                             101 102 103 104 105 106 107 108 109
                             V   Y   L   C   A   S   S   Y
L36092,U66060,TRBV6-8*01     GTG TAC TTG TGT GCC AGC AGT TAC TC

AF009663,TRBV6-8*01          --- --- --- --- --- --- --- --- ---

L26228 ,TRBV6-8*01                                           o
```

o: Genomic DNA, but not known as being germline or rearranged

Framework and complementarity determining regions

FR1-IMGT: 26	CDR1-IMGT: 5
FR2-IMGT: 17	CDR2-IMGT: 6
FR3-IMGT: 36 (-3 aa: 69, 73, 82)	CDR3-IMGT: 4

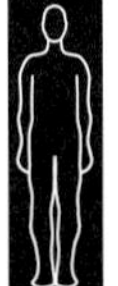

Collier de Perles for human TRBV6-8*01

Accession number: IMGT L36092   EMBL/GenBank/DDBJ: L36092

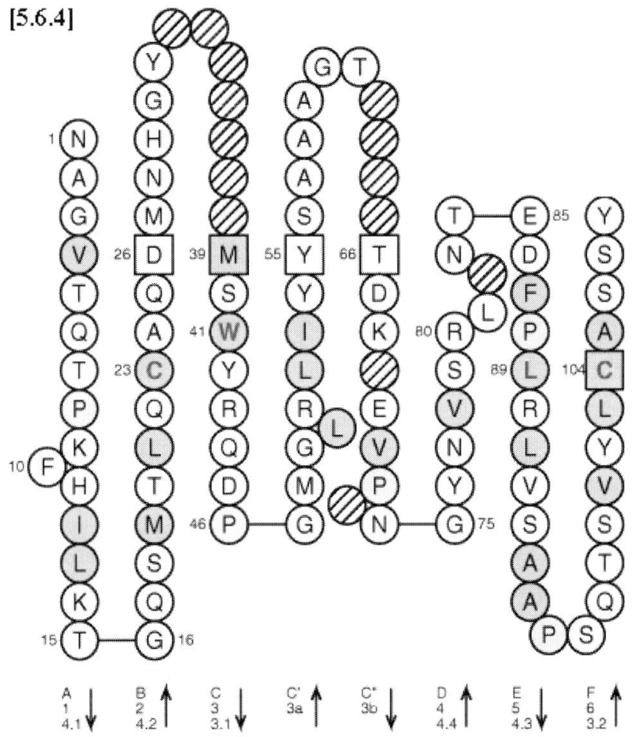

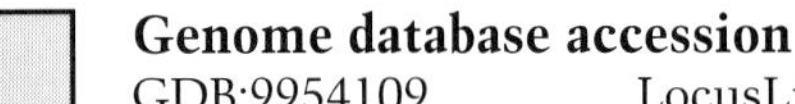

Genome database accession numbers
GDB:9954109   LocusLink: 28599

Nomenclature

TRBV6-9: T cell receptor beta variable 6-9.

Definition and functionality

TRBV6-9 is one of the 5–7 functional genes of the TRBV6 subgroup which comprises 8–9 mapped genes, depending on the haplotypes, in the TRB locus.

Gene location

TRBV6-9 is in the TRB locus on chromosome 7 at 7q34.

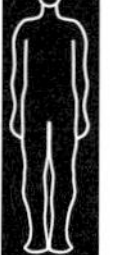

Nucleotide and amino acid sequences for human TRBV6-9

```
                         1    2    3    4    5    6    7    8    9   10   11   12   13   14   15   16   17   18   19   20
                         N    A    G    V    T    Q    T    P    K    F    H    I    L    K    T    G    Q    S    M    T
X61447  ,TRBV6-9*01  [26] AAT  GCT  GGT  GTC  ACT  CAG  ACC  CCA  AAA  TTC  CAC  ATC  CTG  AAG  ACA  GGA  CAG  AGC  ATG  ACA

L36092,U66060,TRBV6-9*01 [34] ---  ---  ---  ---  ---  ---  ---  ---  ---  ---  ---  ---  ---  ---  ---  ---  ---  ---  ---  ---

AF009663,TRBV6-9*01      [35] ---  ---  ---  ---  ---  ---  ---  ---  ---  ---  ---  ---  ---  ---  ---  ---  ---  ---  ---  ---


                                                                      ____________________________CDR1-IMGT________________
                        21   22   23   24   25   26   27   28   29   30   31   32   33   34   35   36   37   38   39   40
                         L    Q    C    A    Q    D    M    N    H    G    Y                                       L    S
X61447  ,TRBV6-9*01      CTG  CAG  TGT  GCC  CAG  GAT  ATG  AAC  CAT  GGA  TAC  ...  ...  ...  ...  ...  ...  ...  TTG  TCC

L36092,U66060,TRBV6-9*01 ---  ---  ---  ---  ---  ---  ---  ---  ---  ---  ---  ...  ...  ...  ...  ...  ...  ...  ---  ---

AF009663,TRBV6-9*01      ---  ---  ---  ---  ---  ---  ---  ---  ---  ---  ---  ...  ...  ...  ...  ...  ...  ...  ---  ---


                                                                                               ________________________CDR2-
                        41   42   43   44   45   46   47   48   49   50   51   52   53   54   55   56   57   58   59   60
                         W    Y    R    Q    D    P    G    M    G    L    R    R    I    H    Y    S    V    A    A    G
X61447  ,TRBV6-9*01      TGG  TAT  CGA  CAA  GAC  CCA  GGC  ATG  GGG  CTG  AGG  CGC  ATT  CAT  TAC  TCA  GTT  GCT  GCT  GGT

L36092,U66060,TRBV6-9*01 ---  ---  ---  ---  ---  ---  ---  ---  ---  ---  ---  ---  ---  ---  ---  ---  ---  ---  ---  ---

AF009663,TRBV6-9*01      ---  ---  ---  ---  ---  ---  ---  ---  ---  ---  ---  ---  ---  ---  ---  ---  ---  ---  ---  ---


                        IMGT_____
                        61   62   63   64   65   66   67   68   69   70   71   72   73   74   75   76   77   78   79   80
                         I                        T    D    K    G    E    V    P         D    G    Y    N    V    S    R
X61447  ,TRBV6-9*01      ATC  ...  ...  ...  ...  ACT  GAC  AAA  GGA  GAA  GTC  CCC  ...  GAT  GGC  TAC  AAT  GTA  TCC  AGA

L36092,U66060,TRBV6-9*01 ---  ...  ...  ...  ...  ---  ---  ---  ---  ---  ---  ---  ...  ---  ---  ---  ---  ---  ---  ---

AF009663,TRBV6-9*01      ---  ...  ...  ...  ...  ---  ---  ---  ---  ---  ---  ---  ...  ---  ---  ---  ---  ---  ---  ---


                        81   82   83   84   85   86   87   88   89   90   91   92   93   94   95   96   97   98   99  100
                         S         N    T    E    D    F    P    L    R    L    E    S    A    A    P    S    Q    T    S
X61447  ,TRBV6-9*01      TCA  ...  AAC  ACA  GAG  GAT  TTC  CCG  CTC  AGG  CTG  GAG  TCA  GCT  GCT  CCC  TCC  CAG  ACA  TCT

L36092,U66060,TRBV6-9*01 ---  ...  ---  ---  ---  ---  ---  ---  ---  ---  ---  ---  ---  ---  ---  ---  ---  ---  ---  ---

AF009663,TRBV6-9*01      ---  ...  ---  ---  ---  ---  ---  ---  ---  ---  ---  ---  ---  ---  ---  ---  ---  ---  ---  ---


                            ______CDR3-IMGT______
                       101  102  103  104  105  106  107  108  109
                         V    Y    F    C    A    S    S    Y
X61447  ,TRBV6-9*01      GTA  TAC  TTC  TGT  GCC  AGC  AGT  TAT  TC

L36092,U66060,TRBV6-9*01 ---  ---  ---  ---  ---  ---  ---  ---  --

AF009663,TRBV6-9*01      ---  ---  ---  ---  ---  ---  ---  ---  --
```

Framework and complementarity determining regions

FR1-IMGT: 26	CDR1-IMGT: 5
FR2-IMGT: 17	CDR2-IMGT: 6
FR3-IMGT: 37 (-2 aa: 73, 82)	CDR3-IMGT: 4

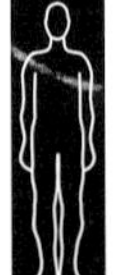

Collier de Perles for human TRBV6-9*01

Accession number: IMGT X61447   EMBL/GenBank/DDBJ: X61447

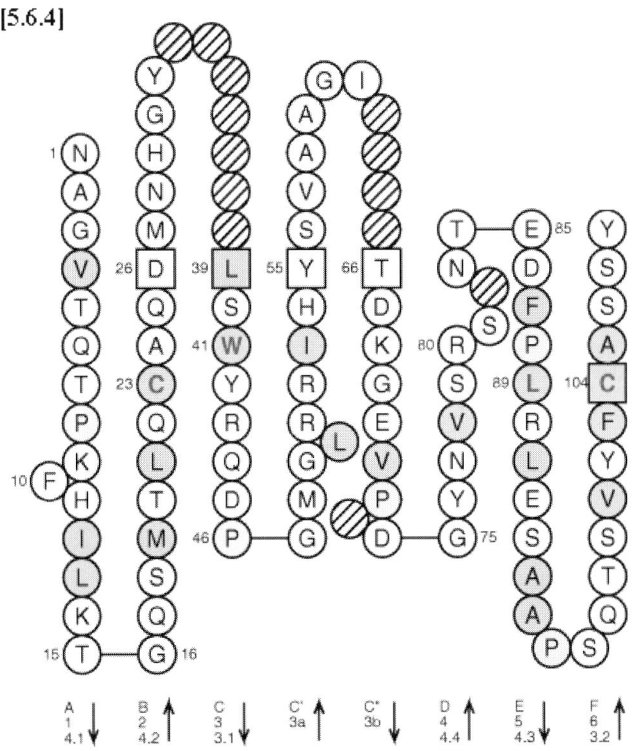

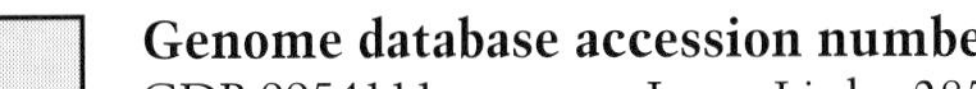

Genome database accession numbers

GDB:9954111   LocusLink: 28598

TRBV7-1

Nomenclature

TRBV7-1: T cell receptor beta variable 7-1.

Definition and functionality

TRBV7-1 is an ORF due to the 1st–CYS of FR1-IMGT, being replaced by a Tyrosine (tat) and, missing V-SPACER and V-NONAMER. TRBV7-1 belongs to the TRBV7 subgroup which comprises nine mapped genes, of which 5–6 are functional in the TRB locus.

Gene location

TRBV7-1 is in the TRB locus on chromosome 7 at 7q34.

Nucleotide and amino acid sequences for human TRBV7-1

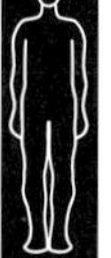

```
                        1    2    3    4    5    6    7    8    9   10   11   12   13   14   15   16   17   18   19   20
                        G    A    G    V    S    Q    S    L    R    H    K    V    A    K    K    G    K    D    V    A
X61444    ,TRBV7-1*01  [26] GGT  GCT  GGA  GTC  TCC  CAG  TCC  CTG  AGA  CAC  AAG  GTA  GCA  AAG  AAG  GGA  AAG  GAT  GTA  GCT

L36092,U66059,TRBV7-1*01 [34]  ---  ---  ---  ---  ---  ---  ---  ---  ---  ---  ---  ---  ---  ---  ---  ---  ---  ---  ---  ---


                                                                        ________________CDR1-IMGT________
                       21   22   23   24   25   26   27   28   29   30   31   32   33   34   35   36   37   38   39   40
                        L    R    Y    D    P    I    S    G    H    N    A                                      L    Y
X61444    ,TRBV7-1*01  CTC  AGA  TAT  GAT  CCA  ATT  TCA  GGT  CAT  AAT  GCC  ...  ...  ...  ...  ...  ...  ...  CTT  TAT

L36092,U66059,TRBV7-1*01  ---  ---  ---  ---  ---  ---  ---  ---  ---  ---  ---  ...  ...  ...  ...  ...  ...  ...  ---  ---


                                                                                                      _________CDR2-
                       41   42   43   44   45   46   47   48   49   50   51   52   53   54   55   56   57   58   59   60
                        W    Y    R    Q    S    L    G    Q    G    L    E    F    P    I    Y    F    Q    G    K    D
X61444    ,TRBV7-1*01  TGG  TAC  CGA  CAG  AGC  CTG  GGG  CAG  GGC  CTG  GAG  TTT  CCA  ATT  TAC  TTC  CAA  GGC  AAG  GAT

L36092,U66059,TRBV7-1*01  ---  ---  ---  ---  ---  ---  ---  ---  ---  ---  ---  ---  ---  ---  ---  ---  ---  ---  ---  ---


                       IMGT________
                       61   62   63   64   65   66   67   68   69   70   71   72   73   74   75   76   77   78   79   80
                        A                       A    D    K    S    G    L    P    R    D    R    F    S    A    Q    R
X61444    ,TRBV7-1*01  GCA  ...  ...  ...  ...  GCA  GAC  AAA  TCG  GGG  CTT  CCC  CGT  GAT  CGG  TTC  TCT  GCA  CAG  AGG

L36092,U66059,TRBV7-1*01  ---  ...  ...  ...  ...  ---  ---  ---  ---  ---  ---  ---  ---  ---  ---  ---  ---  ---  ---  ---


                       81   82   83   84   85   86   87   88   89   90   91   92   93   94   95   96   97   98   99  100
                        S         E    G    S    I    S    T    L    K    F    Q    R    T    Q    Q    G    D    L    A
X61444    ,TRBV7-1*01  TCT  ...  GAG  GGA  TCC  ATC  TCC  ACT  CTG  AAG  TTC  CAG  CGC  ACA  CAG  CAG  GGG  GAC  TTG  GCT

L36092,U66059,TRBV7-1*01  ---  ...  ---  ---  ---  ---  ---  ---  ---  ---  ---  ---  ---  ---  ---  ---  ---  ---  ---  ---


                                    ______CDR3-IMGT______
                      101  102  103  104  105  106  107  108  109
                        V    Y    L    C    A    S    S    S
X61444    ,TRBV7-1*01  GTG  TAT  CTC  TGT  GCC  AGC  AGC  TCA  GC

L36092,U66059,TRBV7-1*01  ---  ---  ---  ---  ---  ---  ---  ---  ---
```

Framework and complementarity determining regions

FR1-IMGT: 26	CDR1-IMGT: 5
FR2-IMGT: 17	CDR2-IMGT: 6
FR3-IMGT: 38 (-1 aa: 82)	CDR3-IMGT: 4

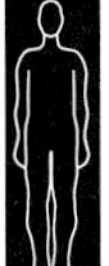

Collier de Perles for human TRBV7-1*01

Accession number: IMGT X61444   EMBL/GenBank/DDBJ: X61444

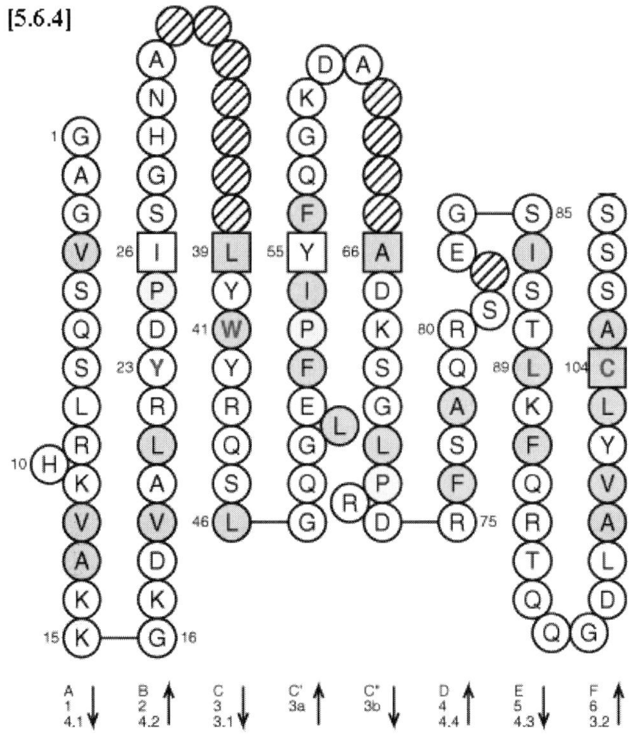

Genome database accession numbers

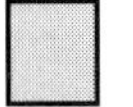

GDB:9954113   LocusLink: 28597

TRBV7-2

Nomenclature

TRBV7-2: T cell receptor beta variable 7-2.

Definition and functionality

TRBV7-2 is one of the 5–6 functional genes of the TRBV7 subgroup which comprises nine mapped genes, in the TRB locus.

Gene location

TRBV7-2 is in the TRB locus on chromosome 7 at 7q34.

Nucleotide and amino acid sequences for human TRBV7-2

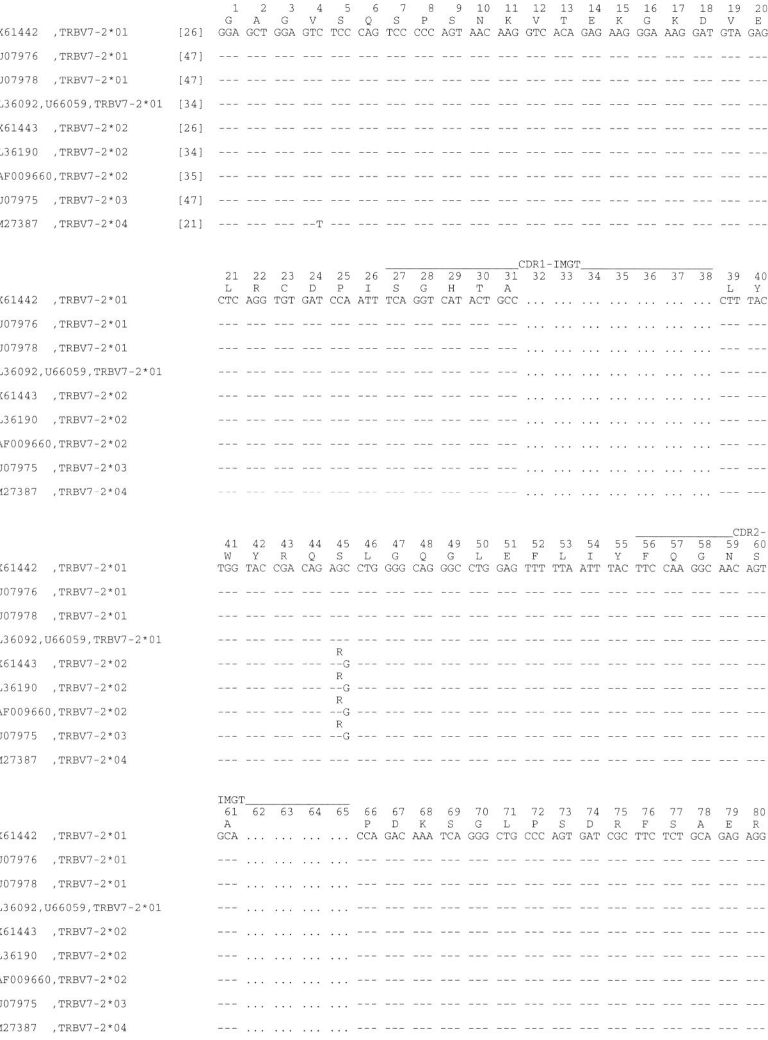

```
                                1   2   3   4   5   6   7   8   9  10  11  12  13  14  15  16  17  18  19  20
                                G   A   G   V   S   Q   S   P   S   N   K   V   T   E   K   G   K   D   V   E
X61442     ,TRBV7-2*01   [26]  GGA GCT GGA GTC TCC CAG TCC CCC AGT AAC AAG GTC ACA GAG AAG GGA AAG GAT GTA GAG
U07976     ,TRBV7-2*01   [47]  --- --- --- --- --- --- --- --- --- --- --- --- --- --- --- --- --- --- --- ---
U07978     ,TRBV7-2*01   [47]  --- --- --- --- --- --- --- --- --- --- --- --- --- --- --- --- --- --- --- ---
L36092,U66059,TRBV7-2*01 [34]  --- --- --- --- --- --- --- --- --- --- --- --- --- --- --- --- --- --- --- ---
X61443     ,TRBV7-2*02   [26]  --- --- --- --- --- --- --- --- --- --- --- --- --- --- --- --- --- --- --- ---
L36190     ,TRBV7-2*02   [34]  --- --- --- --- --- --- --- --- --- --- --- --- --- --- --- --- --- --- --- ---
AF009660,TRBV7-2*02      [35]  --- --- --- --- --- --- --- --- --- --- --- --- --- --- --- --- --- --- --- ---
U07975     ,TRBV7-2*03   [47]  --- --- --- --- --- --- --- --- --- --- --- --- --- --- --- --- --- --- --- ---
M27387     ,TRBV7-2*04   [21]  --- --- --- --T --- --- --- --- --- --- --- --- --- --- --- --- --- --- --- ---

                                                                                      CDR1-IMGT
                               21  22  23  24  25  26  27  28  29  30  31  32  33  34  35  36  37  38  39  40
                                L   R   C   D   P   I   S   G   H   T   A                               L   Y
X61442     ,TRBV7-2*01         CTC AGG TGT GAT CCA ATT TCA GGT CAT ACT GCC ... ... ... ... ... ... ... CTT TAC
U07976     ,TRBV7-2*01         --- --- --- --- --- --- --- --- --- --- --- ... ... ... ... ... ... ... --- ---
U07978     ,TRBV7-2*01         --- --- --- --- --- --- --- --- --- --- --- ... ... ... ... ... ... ... --- ---
L36092,U66059,TRBV7-2*01       --- --- --- --- --- --- --- --- --- --- --- ... ... ... ... ... ... ... --- ---
X61443     ,TRBV7-2*02         --- --- --- --- --- --- --- --- --- --- --- ... ... ... ... ... ... ... --- ---
L36190     ,TRBV7-2*02         --- --- --- --- --- --- --- --- --- --- --- ... ... ... ... ... ... ... --- ---
AF009660,TRBV7-2*02            --- --- --- --- --- --- --- --- --- --- --- ... ... ... ... ... ... ... --- ---
U07975     ,TRBV7-2*03         --- --- --- --- --- --- --- --- --- --- --- ... ... ... ... ... ... ... --- ---
M27387     ,TRBV7-2*04         --- --- --- --- --- --- --- --- --- --- --- ... ... ... ... ... ... ... --- ---

                                                                                                      CDR2-
                               41  42  43  44  45  46  47  48  49  50  51  52  53  54  55  56  57  58  59  60
                                W   Y   R   Q   S   L   G   Q   G   L   E   F   L   I   Y   F   Q   G   N   S
X61442     ,TRBV7-2*01         TGG TAC CGA CAG AGC CTG GGG CAG GGC CTG GAG TTT TTA ATT TAC TTC CAA GGC AAC AGT
U07976     ,TRBV7-2*01         --- --- --- --- --- --- --- --- --- --- --- --- --- --- --- --- --- --- --- ---
U07978     ,TRBV7-2*01         --- --- --- --- --- --- --- --- --- --- --- --- --- --- --- --- --- --- --- ---
L36092,U66059,TRBV7-2*01       --- --- --- --- --- --- --- --- --- --- --- --- --- --- --- --- --- --- --- ---
                                               R
X61443     ,TRBV7-2*02         --- --- --- --- --G --- --- --- --- --- --- --- --- --- --- --- --- --- --- ---
                                               R
L36190     ,TRBV7-2*02         --- --- --- --- --G --- --- --- --- --- --- --- --- --- --- --- --- --- --- ---
                                               R
AF009660,TRBV7-2*02            --- --- --- --- --G --- --- --- --- --- --- --- --- --- --- --- --- --- --- ---
                                               R
U07975     ,TRBV7-2*03         --- --- --- --- --G --- --- --- --- --- --- --- --- --- --- --- --- --- --- ---
M27387     ,TRBV7-2*04         --- --- --- --- --- --- --- --- --- --- --- --- --- --- --- --- --- --- --- ---

                               IMGT
                               61  62  63  64  65  66  67  68  69  70  71  72  73  74  75  76  77  78  79  80
                                A                   P   D   K   S   G   L   P   S   D   R   F   S   A   E   R
X61442     ,TRBV7-2*01         GCA ... ... ... ... CCA GAC AAA TCA GGG CTG CCC AGT GAT CGC TTC TCT GCA GAG AGG
U07976     ,TRBV7-2*01         --- ... ... ... ... --- --- --- --- --- --- --- --- --- --- --- --- --- --- ---
U07978     ,TRBV7-2*01         --- ... ... ... ... --- --- --- --- --- --- --- --- --- --- --- --- --- --- ---
L36092,U66059,TRBV7-2*01       --- ... ... ... ... --- --- --- --- --- --- --- --- --- --- --- --- --- --- ---
X61443     ,TRBV7-2*02         --- ... ... ... ... --- --- --- --- --- --- --- --- --- --- --- --- --- --- ---
L36190     ,TRBV7-2*02         --- ... ... ... ... --- --- --- --- --- --- --- --- --- --- --- --- --- --- ---
AF009660,TRBV7-2*02            --- ... ... ... ... --- --- --- --- --- --- --- --- --- --- --- --- --- --- ---
U07975     ,TRBV7-2*03         --- ... ... ... ... --- --- --- --- --- --- --- --- --- --- --- --- --- --- ---
M27387     ,TRBV7-2*04         --- ... ... ... ... --- --- --- --- --- --- --- --- --- --- --- --- --- --- ---
```

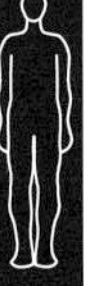

```
                           81  82  83  84  85  86  87  88  89  90  91  92  93  94  95  96  97  98  99 100
                            T       G   G   S   V   S   T   L   T   I   Q   R   T   Q   Q   E   D   S   A
    X61442  ,TRBV7-2*01    ACT ... GGG GGA TCC GTC TCC ACT CTG ACG ATC CAG CGC ACA CAG CAG GAG GAC TCG GCC
    U07976  ,TRBV7-2*01    --- ... --- --- --- --- --- --- --- --- --- --- --- --- --- --- --- --- --- ---
    U07978  ,TRBV7-2*01    --- ... --- --- --- --- --- --- --- --- --- --- --- --- --- --- --- --- --- ---
    L36092,U66059,TRBV7-2*01 --- ... --- --- --- --- --- --- --- --- --- --- --- --- --- --- --- --- --- ---
                                            E
    X61443  ,TRBV7-2*02    --- ... --- -A- --- --- --- --- --- --- --- --- --- --- --- --- --- --- --- ---
                                            E
    L36190  ,TRBV7-2*02    --- ... --- -A- --- --- --- --- --- --- --- --- --- --- --- --- --- --- --- ---
                                            E
    AF009660,TRBV7-2*02    --- ... --- -A- --- --- --- --- --- --- --- --- --- --- --- --- --- --- --- ---
                                            E
    U07975  ,TRBV7-2*03    --- ... --- -A- --- --- --- --- --- --- --- --- --- --- --- --- --- --- --- ---
    M27387  ,TRBV7-2*04        ...


                                         ______CDR3-IMGT______
                           101 102 103 104 105 106 107 108 109
                            V   Y   L   C   A   S   S   L
    X61442  ,TRBV7-2*01    GTG TAT CTC TGT GCC AGC AGC TTA GC
    U07976  ,TRBV7-2*01    --- --- --- --- --- --- --- --- --
    U07978  ,TRBV7-2*01    --- --- --- --- --- --- --- --- --
    L36092,U66059,TRBV7-2*01 --- --- --- --- --- --- --- --- --
    X61443  ,TRBV7-2*02    --- --- --- --- --- --- --- --- --
    L36190  ,TRBV7-2*02    --- --- --- --- --- --- --- --- --
    AF009660,TRBV7-2*02    --- --- --- --- --- --- --- --- --
                                            T
    U07975  ,TRBV7-2*03    --- --- --- --- A-- --- --- --- --
    M27387  ,TRBV7-2*04    --- --- --- --- --- --- --- ---         #c

#c: Rearranged cDNA
```

Framework and complementarity determining regions

FR1-IMGT: 26   CDR1-IMGT: 5
FR2-IMGT: 17   CDR2-IMGT: 6
FR3-IMGT: 38 (-1 aa: 82)   CDR3-IMGT: 4

Collier de Perles for human TRBV7-2*01

Accession number: IMGT X61442   EMBL/GenBank/DDBJ: X61442

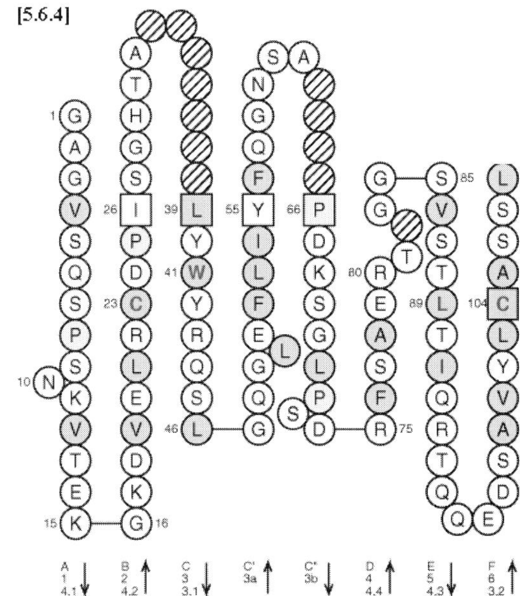

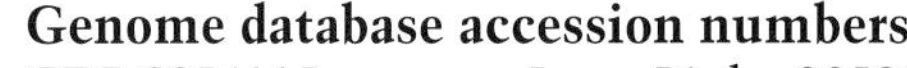

Genome database accession numbers

GDB:9954115   LocusLink: 28596

TRBV7-3

Nomenclature

TRBV7-3: T cell receptor beta variable 7-3.

Definition and functionality

TRBV7-3 is a functional gene (alleles *01, *04 and *05) or an ORF (alleles *02 and *03). TRBV7-3 belongs to TRBV7 subgroup which comprises nine mapped genes, of which 5–6 are functional, in the TRB locus.

TRBV7-3*02 and TRBV7-3*03 are ORF due to the 2nd–CYS (tgt) of FR3-IMGT being replaced by an Arginine (cgt).

Gene location

TRBV7-3 is in the TRB locus on chromosome 7 at 7q34.

Nucleotide and amino acid sequences for human TRBV7-3

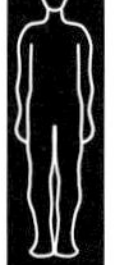

```
                               1   2   3   4   5   6   7   8   9   10  11  12  13  14  15  16  17  18  19  20
                               G   A   G   V   S   Q   T   P   S   N   K   V   T   E   K   G   K   Y   V   E
X61440     ,TRBV7-3*01    [26] GGT GCT GGA GTC TCC CAG ACC CCC AGT AAC AAG GTC ACA GAG AAG GGA AAA TAT GTA GAG
L33104     ,TRBV7-3*01    [1]  --- --- --- --- --- --- --- --- --- --- --- --- --- --- --- --- --- --- --- ---
L36092,U66059,TRBV7-3*01  [34] --- --- --- --- --- --- --- --- --- --- --- --- --- --- --- --- --- --- --- ---
M67511     ,TRBV7-3*01    [28]
M67512     ,TRBV7-3*01    [28]
                                                                                                       D
M97943     ,TRBV7-3*02    [27] --- --- --- --- --- --- --- --- --- --- --- --- --- --- --- --- G-- --- ---
                                                                                                       D
L33103     ,TRBV7-3*02    [1]  --- --- --- --- --- --- --- --- --- --- --- --- --- --- --- --- G-- --- ---
                                                                                                       D
L33105     ,TRBV7-3*03    [1]  --- --- --- --- --- --- --- --- --- --- --- --- --- --- --- --- G-- --- ---
                                                                                                       D
AF009660,TRBV7-3*03       [35] --- --- --- --- --- --- --- --- --- --- --- --- --- --- --- --- G-- --- ---
X74843     ,TRBV7-3*04    [19] --- --- --- --- --- --- --- --- --- --- --- --- --- --- --- --- --- --- ---
                                                                                                   W
M13550     ,TRBV7-3*05    [24]                                                                     TGG ---

                                                                            ____________CDR1-IMGT____________
                               21  22  23  24  25  26  27  28  29  30  31  32  33  34  35  36  37  38  39  40
                               L   R   C   D   P   I   S   G   H   T   A                               L   Y
X61440     ,TRBV7-3*01         CTC AGG TGT GAT CCA ATT TCA GGT CAT ACT GCC ... ... ... ... ... ... ... CTT TAC
L33104     ,TRBV7-3*01         --- --- --- --- --- --- --- --- --- --- --- ... ... ... ... ... ... ... --- ---
L36092,U66059,TRBV7-3*01       --- --- --- --- --- --- --- --- --- --- --- ... ... ... ... ... ... ... --- ---
M67511     ,TRBV7-3*01                         --- --- --- --- --- --- --- ... ... ... ... ... ... ... --- ---
M67512     ,TRBV7-3*01                         --- --- --- --- --- --- --- ... ... ... ... ... ... ... --- ---
M97943     ,TRBV7-3*02         --- --- --- --- --- --- --- --- --- --- --- ... ... ... ... ... ... ... --- ---
L33103     ,TRBV7-3*02         --- --- --- --- --- --- --- --- --- --- --- ... ... ... ... ... ... ... --- ---
L33105     ,TRBV7-3*03         --- --- --- --- --- --- --- --- --- --- --- ... ... ... ... ... ... ... --- ---
AF009660,TRBV7-3*03            --- --- --- --- --- --- --- --- --- --- --- ... ... ... ... ... ... ... --- ---
X74843     ,TRBV7-3*04         --- --- --- --- --- --- --- --- --- --- --- ... ... ... ... ... ... ... --- ---
M13550     ,TRBV7-3*05         --- --- --- --- --- --- --- --- --- --- --- ... ... ... ... ... ... ... --- ---

                                                                                    ________________CDR2-
                               41  42  43  44  45  46  47  48  49  50  51  52  53  54  55  56  57  58  59  60
                               W   Y   R   Q   S   L   G   Q   G   P   E   F   L   I   Y   F   Q   G   T   G
X61440     ,TRBV7-3*01         TGG TAC CGA CAA AGC CTG GGG CAG GGC CCA GAG TTT CTA ATT TAC TTC CAA GGC ACG GGT
L33104     ,TRBV7-3*01         --- --- --- --- --- --- --- --- --- --- --- --- --- --- --- --- --- --- --- ---
L36092,U66059,TRBV7-3*01       --- --- --- --- --- --- --- --- --- --- --- --- --- --- --- --- --- --- --- ---
M67511     ,TRBV7-3*01         --- --- --- --- --- --- --- --- --- --- --- --- --- --- --- --- --- --- --- ---
M67512     ,TRBV7-3*01         --- --- --- --- --- --- --- --- --- --- --- --- --- --- --- --- --- --- --- ---
M97943     ,TRBV7-3*02         --- --- --- --- --- --- --- --- --- --- --- --- --- --- --- --- --- --- --- ---
L33103     ,TRBV7-3*02         --- --- --- --- --- --- --- --- --- --- --- --- --- --- --- --- --- --- --- ---
L33105     ,TRBV7-3*03         --- --- --- --- --- --- --- --- --- --- --- --- --- --- --- --- --- --- --- ---
AF009660,TRBV7-3*03            --- --- --- --- --- --- --- --- --- --- --- --- --- --- --- --- --- --- --- ---
X74843     ,TRBV7-3*04         --- --- --- --- --- --- --- --- --- --- --- --- --- --- --- --- --- --- --- ---
                                                                           L
M13550     ,TRBV7-3*05         --- --- --- --- --- --- --- --- --- --- C-- --- --- --- --- --- --- --- --- ---
```

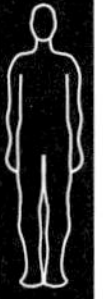

```
                            IMGT_______________
                             61  62  63  64  65  66  67  68  69  70  71  72  73  74  75  76  77  78  79  80
                              A                   A   D   D   S   G   L   P   N   D   R   F   F   A   V   R
X61440     ,TRBV7-3*01       GCG ... ... ... ... GCA GAT GAC TCA GGG CTG CCC AAC GAT CGG TTC TTT GCA GTC AGG

L33104     ,TRBV7-3*01       --- ... ... ... ... --- --- --- --- --- --- --- --- --- --- --- --- --- --- ---

L36092,U66059,TRBV7-3*01     --- ... ... ... ... --- --- --- --- --- --- --- --- --- --- --- --- --- --- ---

M67511     ,TRBV7-3*01       --- ... ... ... ... --- --- --- --- --- --- --- --- --- --- --- --- --- --- ---

M67512     ,TRBV7-3*01       --- ... ... ... ... --- --- --- --- --- --- --- --- --- --- --- --- --- --- ---
                                                                                 K
M97943     ,TRBV7-3*02       --- ... ... ... ... --- --- --- --- --- --- --- --A --- --- --- --- --- --- ---
                                                                                 K
L33103     ,TRBV7-3*02       --- ... ... ... ... --- --- --- --- --- --- --- --A --- --- --- --- --- --- ---
                                                                                 K
L33105     ,TRBV7-3*03       --- ... ... ... ... --- --- --- --- --- --- --- --A --- --- --- --- --- --- ---
                                                                                 K
AF009660,TRBV7-3*03          --- ... ... ... ... --- --- --- --- --- --- --- --A --- --- --- --- --- --- ---

X74843     ,TRBV7-3*04       --- ... ... ... ... --- --- --- --- --- --- --- --- --- --- --- --- --- --- ---

M13550     ,TRBV7-3*05       --- ... ... ... ... --- --- --- --- --- --- --- --- --- --- --- --- --- --- ---


                             81  82  83  84  85  86  87  88  89  90  91  92  93  94  95  96  97  98  99 100
                              P       E   G   S   V   S   T   L   K   I   Q   R   T   E   R   G   D   S   A
X61440     ,TRBV7-3*01       CCT ... GAG GGA TCC GTC TCT ACT CTG AAG ATC CAG CGC ACA GAG CGG GGG GAC TCA GCC

L33104     ,TRBV7-3*01       --- ... --- --- --- --- --- --- --- --- --- --- --- --- --- --- --- --- --- ---

L36092,U66059,TRBV7-3*01     --- ... --- --- --- --- --- --- --- --- --- --- --- --- --- --- --- --- --- ---

M67511     ,TRBV7-3*01       --- ... --- --- --- --- --- --- --- --- --- --- --- --- --- --- --- --- --- ---

M67512     ,TRBV7-3*01       --- ... --- --- --- --- --- --- --- --- --- --- --- --- --- --- --- --- --- ---
                                                                                             Q
M97943     ,TRBV7-3*02       --- ... --- --- --- --- --- --- --- --- --- --- --- --- --- -A- --- --- --- ---
                                                                                             Q
L33103     ,TRBV7-3*02       --- ... --- --- --- --- --- --- --- --- --- --- --- --- --- -A- --- --- --- ---
                                                                                             Q
L33105     ,TRBV7-3*03       --- ... --- --- --- --- --- --- --- --- --- --- --- --- --- -A- --- --- --- ---
                                                                                             Q
AF009660,TRBV7-3*03          --- ... --- --- --- --- --- --- --- --- --- --- --- --- --- -A- --- --- --- ---

X74843     ,TRBV7-3*04       --- ... --- --- --- --- --- --- --- --- --- --- --- --- --- --- --- --- --T ---

M13550     ,TRBV7-3*05       --- ... --- --- --- --- --- --- --- --- --- --- --- --- --- --- --- --- --- ---


                                            ______CDR3-IMGT______
                             101 102 103 104 105 106 107 108 109
                              V   Y   L   C   A   S   S   L
X61440     ,TRBV7-3*01       GTG TAT CTC TGT GCC AGC AGC TTA AC

L33104     ,TRBV7-3*01       --- --- --- --- --- --- --- --- --

L36092,U66059,TRBV7-3*01     --- --- --- --- --- --- --- --- --

M67511     ,TRBV7-3*01       --- --- --- --- ---                    °

M67512     ,TRBV7-3*01       --- --- --- --- ---                    °
                                             R
M97943     ,TRBV7-3*02       --- --- --- C-- --- --- --- --- --
                                             R
L33103     ,TRBV7-3*02       --- --- --- C-- --- --- --- --- --
                              A              R
L33105     ,TRBV7-3*03       -C- --- --- C-- --- --- --- ---
                              A              R
AF009660,TRBV7-3*03          -C- --- --- C-- --- --- --- --- --

X74843     ,TRBV7-3*04       --- --- --- --- --- --- ---           #c

M13550     ,TRBV7-3*05       --- --- --- --- --- --- ---           #c
```

#c: Rearranged cDNA
°: Genomic DNA, but not known as being germline or rearranged

Framework and complementarity determining regions

FR1-IMGT: 26	CDR1-IMGT: 5
FR2-IMGT: 17	CDR2-IMGT: 6
FR3-IMGT: 38 (-1 aa: 82)	CDR3-IMGT: 4

Collier de Perles for human TRBV7-3*01

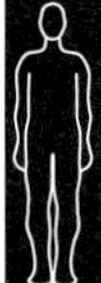

Accession number: IMGT X61440   EMBL/GenBank/DDBJ: X61440

[5.6.4]

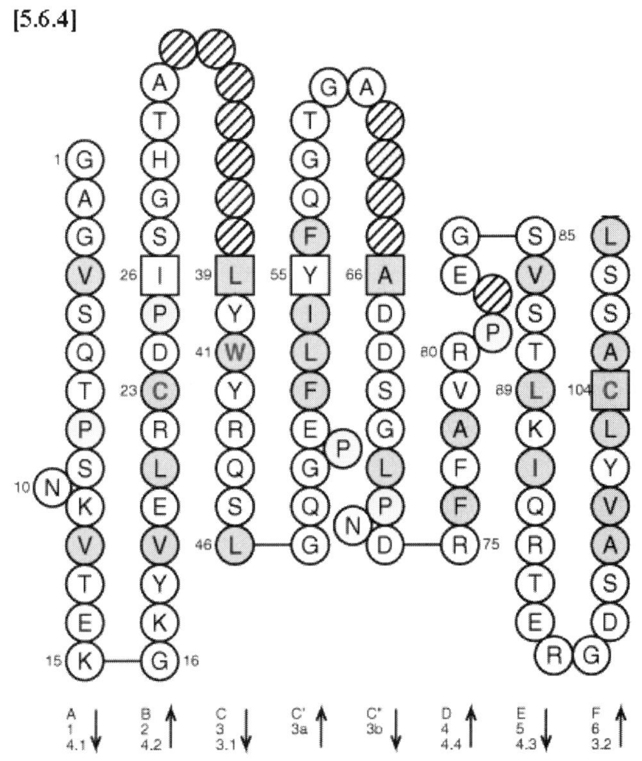

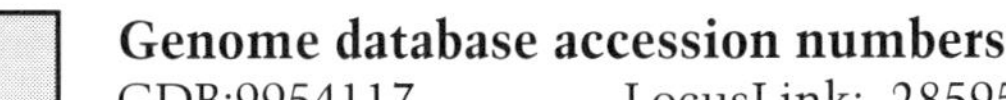

Genome database accession numbers
GDB:9954117   LocusLink: 28595

TRBV7-4

Nomenclature

TRBV7-4: T cell receptor beta variable 7-4.

Definition and functionality

TRBV7-4 is a functional gene (allele *01) or a pseudogene (allele *02). TRBV7-4 belongs to TRBV7 subgroup which comprises nine mapped genes, of which 5–6 are functional, in the TRB locus.

TRBV7-4*02 is a pseudogene due to 1 nt DELETION in codon 85 leading to a frameshift in FR3-IMGT.

Gene location

TRBV7-4 is in the TRB locus on chromosome 7 at 7q34.

Nucleotide and amino acid sequences for human TRBV7-4

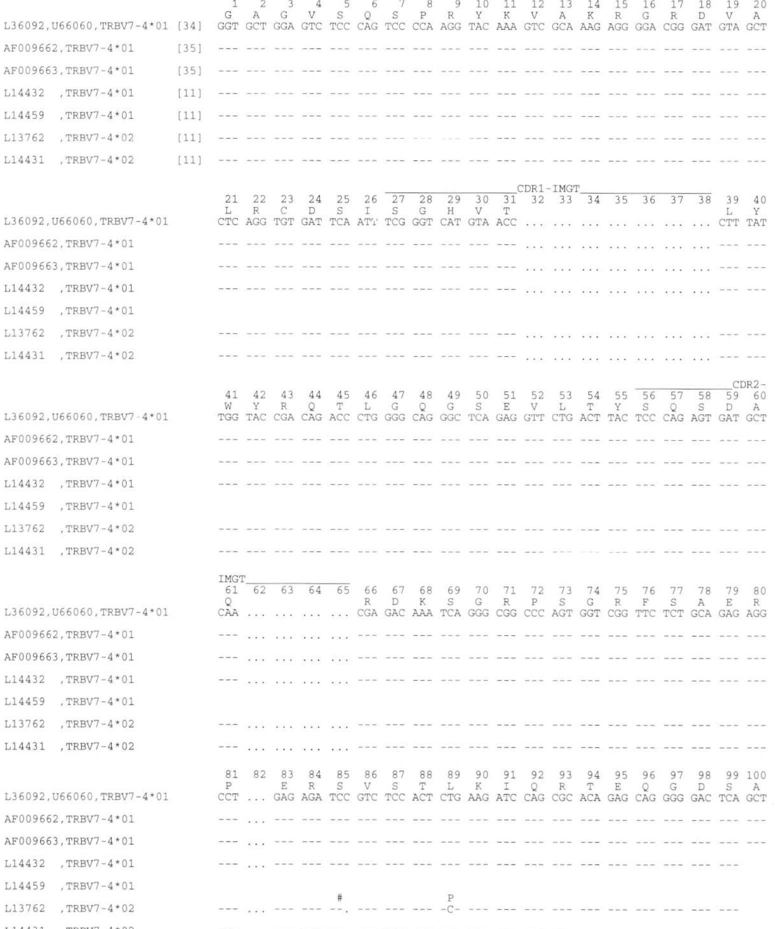

```
                                1   2   3   4   5   6   7   8   9  10  11  12  13  14  15  16  17  18  19  20
                                G   A   G   V   S   Q   S   P   R   Y   K   V   A   K   R   G   R   D   V   A
L36092,U66060,TRBV7-4*01 [34]  GGT GCT GGA GTC TCC CAG TCC CCA AGG TAC AAA GTC GCA AAG AGG GGA CGG GAT GTA GCT
AF009662,TRBV7-4*01      [35]  --- --- --- --- --- --- --- --- --- --- --- --- --- --- --- --- --- --- --- ---
AF009663,TRBV7-4*01      [35]  --- --- --- --- --- --- --- --- --- --- --- --- --- --- --- --- --- --- --- ---
L14432  ,TRBV7-4*01      [11]  --- --- --- --- --- --- --- --- --- --- --- --- --- --- --- --- --- --- --- ---
L14459  ,TRBV7-4*01      [11]  --- --- --- --- --- --- --- --- --- --- --- --- --- --- --- --- --- --- --- ---
L13762  ,TRBV7-4*02      [11]  --- --- --- --- --- --- --- --- --- --- --- --- --- --- --- --- --- --- --- ---
L14431  ,TRBV7-4*02      [11]  --- --- --- --- --- --- --- --- --- --- --- --- --- --- --- --- --- --- --- ---

                                                          ______________CDR1-IMGT_______________
                               21  22  23  24  25  26  27  28  29  30  31  32  33  34  35  36  37  38  39  40
                                L   R   C   D   S   I   S   G   H   V   T                           L   Y
L36092,U66060,TRBV7-4*01       CTC AGG TGT GAT TCA ATT TCG GGT CAT GTA ACC ... ... ... ... ... ... ... CTT TAT
AF009662,TRBV7-4*01            --- --- --- --- --- --- --- --- --- --- --- ... ... ... ... ... ... ... --- ---
AF009663,TRBV7-4*01            --- --- --- --- --- --- --- --- --- --- --- ... ... ... ... ... ... ... --- ---
L14432  ,TRBV7-4*01            --- --- --- --- --- --- --- --- --- --- --- ... ... ... ... ... ... ... --- ---
L14459  ,TRBV7-4*01
L13762  ,TRBV7-4*02            --- --- --- --- --- --- --- --- --- --- --- ... ... ... ... ... ... ... --- ---
L14431  ,TRBV7-4*02            --- --- --- --- --- --- --- --- --- --- --- ... ... ... ... ... ... ... --- ---

                                                                                            ________CDR2-
                               41  42  43  44  45  46  47  48  49  50  51  52  53  54  55  56  57  58  59  60
                                W   Y   R   Q   T   L   G   Q   G   S   E   V   L   T   Y   S   Q   S   D   A
L36092,U66060,TRBV7-4*01       TGG TAC CGA CAG ACC CTG GGG CAG GGC TCA GAG GTT CTG ACT TAC TCC CAG AGT GAT GCT
AF009662,TRBV7-4*01            --- --- --- --- --- --- --- --- --- --- --- --- --- --- --- --- --- --- --- ---
AF009663,TRBV7-4*01            --- --- --- --- --- --- --- --- --- --- --- --- --- --- --- --- --- --- --- ---
L14432  ,TRBV7-4*01            --- --- --- --- --- --- --- --- --- --- --- --- --- --- --- --- --- --- --- ---
L14459  ,TRBV7-4*01
L13762  ,TRBV7-4*02            --- --- --- --- --- --- --- --- --- --- --- --- --- --- --- --- --- --- --- ---
L14431  ,TRBV7-4*02            --- --- --- --- --- --- --- --- --- --- --- --- --- --- --- --- --- --- --- ---

                               IMGT______
                               61  62  63  64  65  66  67  68  69  70  71  72  73  74  75  76  77  78  79  80
                                Q                       R   D   K   S   G   R   P   S   G   R   F   S   A   E   R
L36092,U66060,TRBV7-4*01       CAA ... ... ... ... CGA GAC AAA TCA GGG CGG CCC AGT GGT CGG TTC TCT GCA GAG AGG
AF009662,TRBV7-4*01            --- ... ... ... ... --- --- --- --- --- --- --- --- --- --- --- --- --- --- ---
AF009663,TRBV7-4*01            --- ... ... ... ... --- --- --- --- --- --- --- --- --- --- --- --- --- --- ---
L14432  ,TRBV7-4*01            --- ... ... ... ... --- --- --- --- --- --- --- --- --- --- --- --- --- --- ---
L14459  ,TRBV7-4*01
L13762  ,TRBV7-4*02            --- ... ... ... ... --- --- --- --- --- --- --- --- --- --- --- --- --- --- ---
L14431  ,TRBV7-4*02            --- ... ... ... ... --- --- --- --- --- --- --- --- --- --- --- --- --- --- ---

                               81  82  83  84  85  86  87  88  89  90  91  92  93  94  95  96  97  98  99 100
                                P       E   R   S   V   S   T   L   K   I   Q   R   T   E   Q   G   D   S   A
L36092,U66060,TRBV7-4*01       CCT ... GAG AGA TCC GTC TCC ACT CTG AAG ATC CAG CGC ACA GAG CAG GGG GAC TCA GCT
AF009662,TRBV7-4*01            --- ... --- --- --- --- --- --- --- --- --- --- --- --- --- --- --- --- --- ---
AF009663,TRBV7-4*01            --- ... --- --- --- --- --- --- --- --- --- --- --- --- --- --- --- --- --- ---
L14432  ,TRBV7-4*01            --- ... --- --- --- --- --- --- --- --- --- --- --- --- --- --- --- --- --- ---
L14459  ,TRBV7-4*01
                                                #                       P
L13762  ,TRBV7-4*02            --- ... --- --- --. --- --- --- -C- --- --- --- --- --- --- --- --- --- --- ---
L14431  ,TRBV7-4*02            --- ... --- --- --. --- --- --- --- --- --- --- --- --- --- --- --- --- --- ---
```

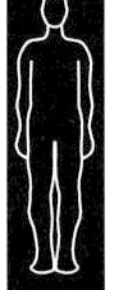

```
                                       ______CDR3-IMGT______
                              101 102 103 104 105 106 107 108 109
                               V   Y   L   C   A   S   S   L
  L36092,U66060,TRBV7-4*01    GTG TAT CTC TGT GCC AGC AGC TTA GC

  AF009662,TRBV7-4*01         --- --- --- --- --- --- --- --- --

  AF009663,TRBV7-4*01         --- --- --- --- --- --- --- --- --

  L14432  ,TRBV7-4*01                                            °

  L14459  ,TRBV7-4*01                                            °

  L13762  ,TRBV7-4*02                                            °

  L14431  ,TRBV7-4*02                                            °

# (in the sequence): Frameshift
°: Genomic DNA, but not known as being germline or rearranged
```

Framework and complementarity determining regions

FR1-IMGT: 26   CDR1-IMGT: 5
FR2-IMGT: 17   CDR2-IMGT: 6
FR3-IMGT: 38 (-1 aa: 82)   CDR3-IMGT: 4

Collier de Perles for human TRBV7-4*01

Accession number: IMGT L36092   EMBL/GenBank/DDBJ: L36092

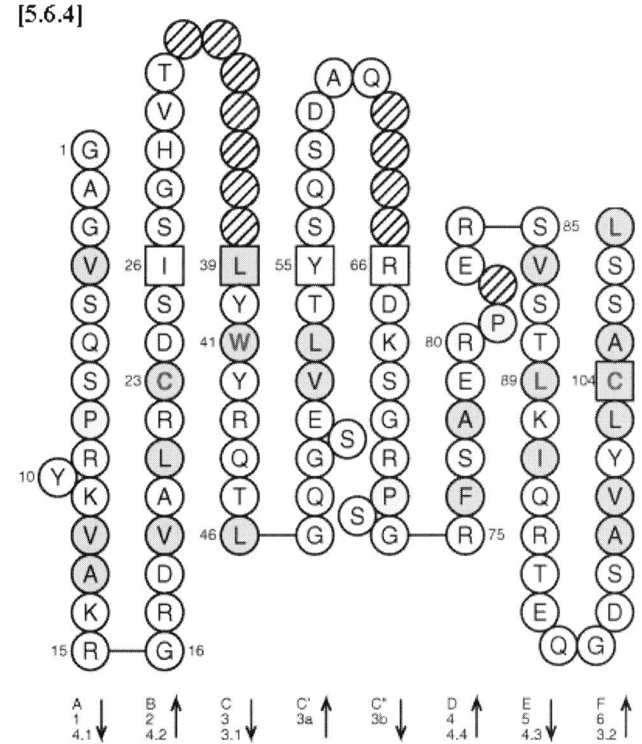

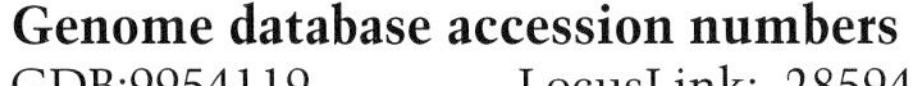

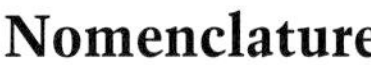

Nomenclature

TRBV7-6: T cell receptor beta variable 7-6.

Definition and functionality

TRBV7-6 is one of the 5–6 functional genes of the TRBV7 subgroup which comprises nine mapped genes, in the TRB locus.

Gene location

TRBV7-6 is in the TRB locus on chromosome 7 at 7q34.

Nucleotide and amino acid sequences for human TRBV7-6

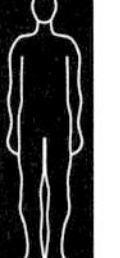

```
                                 1   2   3   4   5   6   7   8   9  10  11  12  13  14  15  16  17  18  19  20
                                 G   A   G   V   S   Q   S   P   R   Y   K   V   T   K   R   G   Q   D   V   A
L36092,U66060,TRBV7-6*01  [34]  GGT GCT GGA GTC TCC CAG TCT CCC AGG TAC AAA GTC ACA AAG AGG GGA CAG GAT GTA GCT
AF009663,TRBV7-6*01       [35]  --- --- --- --- --- --- --- --- --- --- --- --- --- --- --- --- --- --- --- ---
L14480   ,TRBV7-6*01      [11]  --- --- --- --- --- --- --- --- --- --- --- --- --- --- --- --- --- --- --- ---
M97504   ,TRBV7-6*01      [11]  --- --- --- --- --- --- --- --- --- --- --- --- --- --- --- --- --- --- --- ---
X58806   ,TRBV7-6*02      [10]  --- --- --- --- --- --- --- --- --- --- --- --- --- --- --- --- --- --- --- ---

                                                                          ___________________CDR1-IMGT___________________
                                21  22  23  24  25  26  27  28  29  30  31  32  33  34  35  36  37  38  39  40
                                 L   R   C   D   P   I   S   G   H   V   S                               L   Y
L36092,U66060,TRBV7-6*01        CTC AGG TGT GAT CCA ATT TCG GGT CAT GTA TCC ... ... ... ... ... ... ... CTT TAT
AF009663,TRBV7-6*01             --- --- --- --- --- --- --- --- --- --- ---  ... ... ... ... ... ... ... --- ---
L14480   ,TRBV7-6*01            --- --- --- --- --- --- --- --- --- --- ---  ... ... ... ... ... ... ... --- ---
M97504   ,TRBV7-6*01            --- --- --- ---
X58806   ,TRBV7-6*02            --- --- --- --- --- --C --- --- --- --- ---  ... ... ... ... ... ... ... --- ---

                                                                                          _______________CDR2-
                                41  42  43  44  45  46  47  48  49  50  51  52  53  54  55  56  57  58  59  60
                                 W   Y   R   Q   A   L   G   Q   G   P   E   F   L   T   Y   F   N   Y   E   A
L36092,U66060,TRBV7-6*01        TGG TAC CGA CAG GCC CTG GGG CAG GGC CCA GAG TTT CTG ACT TAC TTC AAT TAT GAA GCC
AF009663,TRBV7-6*01             --- --- --- --- --- --- --- --- --- --- --- --- --- --- --- --- --- --- --- ---
L14480   ,TRBV7-6*01            --- --- --- --- --- --- --- --- --- --- --- --- --- --- --- --- --- --- --- ---
M97504   ,TRBV7-6*01
X58806   ,TRBV7-6*02            --- --- --- --- --- --- --- --- --- --- --- --- --- --- --- --- --- --- --- ---

                                IMGT________________
                                61  62  63  64  65  66  67  68  69  70  71  72  73  74  75  76  77  78  79  80
                                 Q                   Q   D   K   S   G   L   P   N   D   R   F   S   A   E   R
L36092,U66060,TRBV7-6*01        CAA ... ... ... ... CAA GAC AAA TCA GGG CTG CCC AAT GAT CGG TTC TCT GCA GAG AGG
AF009663,TRBV7-6*01             --- ... ... ... ... --- --- --- --- --- --- --- --- --- --- --- --- --- --- ---
L14480   ,TRBV7-6*01            --- ... ... ... ... --- --- --- --- --- --- --- --- --- --- --- --- --- --- ---
M97504   ,TRBV7-6*01
X58806   ,TRBV7-6*02            --- ... ... ... ... --- --- --- --- --- --- --- --- --- --- --- --- --- --- ---

                                81  82  83  84  85  86  87  88  89  90  91  92  93  94  95  96  97  98  99 100
                                 P       E   G   S   I   S   T   L   T   I   Q   R   T   E   Q   R   D   S   A
L36092,U66060,TRBV7-6*01        CCT ... GAG GGA TCC ATC TCC ACT CTG ACG ATC CAG CGC ACA GAG CAG CGG GAC TCG GCC
AF009663,TRBV7-6*01             --- ... --- --- --- --- --- --- --- --- --- --- --- --- --- --- --- --- --- ---
L14480   ,TRBV7-6*01            --- ... --- --- --- --- --- --- --- --- --- --- --- --- --- --- --- --- --- ---
M97504   ,TRBV7-6*01
X58806   ,TRBV7-6*02            --- ... --- --- --- --- --- --- --- --- --- --- --- --- --- --- --- --- --- ---

                                          _______CDR3-IMGT_______
                               101 102 103 104 105 106 107 108 109
                                 M   Y   R   C   A   S   S   L
L36092,U66060,TRBV7-6*01        ATG TAT CGC TGT GCC AGC AGC TTA GC
AF009663,TRBV7-6*01             --- --- --- --- --- --- --- --- --
L14480   ,TRBV7-6*01                                                   °
M97504   ,TRBV7-6*01                                                   °
X58806   ,TRBV7-6*02            --- --- --- --- --- --- ---           #c
```

#c: Rearranged cDNA
°: Genomic DNA, but not known as being germline or rearranged

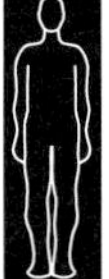

Framework and complementarity determining regions

FR1-IMGT: 26
FR2-IMGT: 17
FR3-IMGT: 38 (-1 aa: 82)

CDR1-IMGT: 5
CDR2-IMGT: 6
CDR3-IMGT: 4

Collier de Perles for human TRBV7-6*01

Accession number: IMGT L36092

EMBL/GenBank/DDBJ: L36092

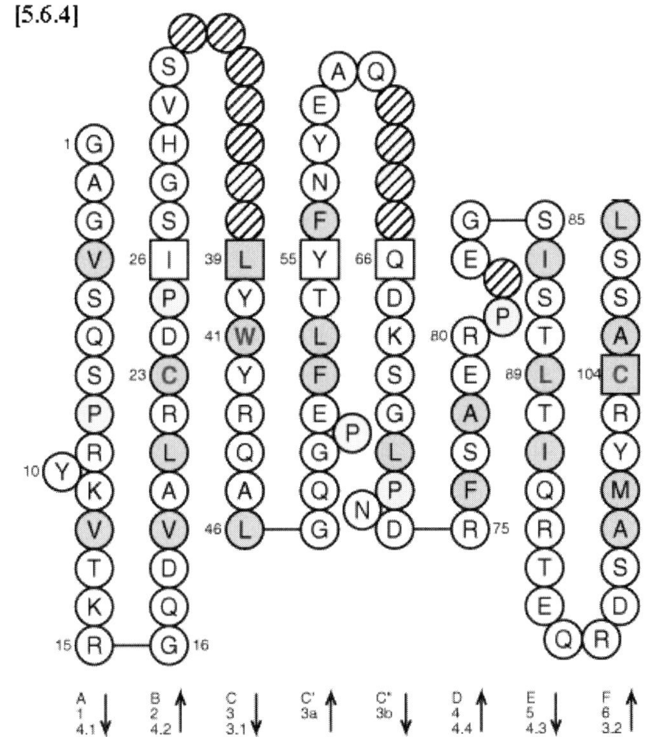

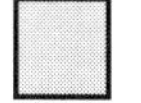

Genome database accession numbers

GDB:9954123   LocusLink: 28592

Nomenclature

TRBV7-7: T cell receptor beta variable 7-7.

Definition and functionality

TRBV7-7 is one of the 5–6 functional genes of the TRBV7 subgroup which comprises nine mapped genes, in the TRB locus.

Gene location

TRBV7-7 is in the TRB locus on chromosome 7 at 7q35.

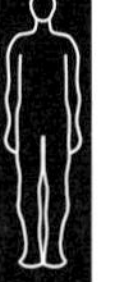

Nucleotide and amino acid sequences for human TRBV7-7

```
                                  1   2   3   4   5   6   7   8   9  10  11  12  13  14  15  16  17  18  19  20
                                  G   A   G   V   S   Q   S   P   R   Y   K   V   T   K   R   G   Q   D   V   T
    L36092,U66060,TRBV7-7*01 [34] GGT GCT GGA GTC TCC CAG TCT CCC AGG TAC AAA GTC ACA AAG AGG GGA CAG GAT GTA ACT
    AF009663,TRBV7-7*01      [35] --- --- --- --- --- --- --- --- --- --- --- --- --- --- --- --- --- --- --- ---
    L14483  ,TRBV7-7*01      [11] --- --- --- --- --- --- --- --- --- --- --- --- --- --- --- --- --- --- --- ---
    M97505  ,TRBV7-7*01      [11] --- --- --- --- --- --- --- --- --- --- --- --- --- --- --- --- --- --- --- ---
    X57607  ,TRBV7-7*02      [31] --- --- --- --- --- --- --- --- --- --- --- --- --- --- --- --- --- --- --- ---

                                                                      ________________________CDR1-IMGT________________________
                                 21  22  23  24  25  26  27  28  29  30  31  32  33  34  35  36  37  38  39  40
                                  L   R   C   D   P   I   S   S   H   A   T                               L   Y
    L36092,U66060,TRBV7 7*01     CTC AGG TGT GAT CCA ATT TCG AGT CAT GCA ACC ... ... ... ... ... ... ... CTT TAT
    AF009663,TRBV7-7*01          --- --- --- --- --- --- --- --- --- --- ---                     ... ... --- ---
    L14483  ,TRBV7-7*01          --- --- --- --- --- --- --- --- --- --- ---                         ... --- ---
    M97505  ,TRBV7-7*01          --- --- ---
                                                                      V
    X57607  ,TRBV7-7*02          --- --- --- --- --- --- --- --- --- -T- ---             ... ... ... --- ---

                                                                                      ________________CDR2-
                                 41  42  43  44  45  46  47  48  49  50  51  52  53  54  55  56  57  58  59  60
                                  W   Y   Q   Q   A   L   G   Q   G   P   E   F   L   T   Y   F   N   Y   E   A
    L36092,U66060,TRBV7-7*01     TGG TAT CAA CAG GCC CTG GGG CAG GGC CCA GAG TTT CTG ACT TAC TTC AAT TAT GAA GCT
    AF009663,TRBV7-7*01          --- --- --- --- --- --- --- --- --- --- --- --- --- --- --- --- --- --- --- ---
    L14483  ,TRBV7-7*01          --- --- --- --- --- --- --- --- --- --- --- --- --- --- --- --- --- --- --- ---
    M97505  ,TRBV7-7*01
    X57607  ,TRBV7-7*02          --- --- --- --- --- --- --- --- --- --- --- --- --- --- --- --- --- --- --- ---

    IMGT________________
                                 61  62  63  64  65  66  67  68  69  70  71  72  73  74  75  76  77  78  79  80
                                  Q                   P   D   K   S   G   L   P   S   D   R   F   S   A   E   R
    L36092,U66060,TRBV7-7*01     CAA ... ... ... ... CCA GAC AAA TCA GGG CTG CCC AGT GAT CGG TTC TCT GCA GAG AGG
    AF009663,TRBV7-7*01          --- ... ... ... ... --- --- --- --- --- --- --- --- --- --- --- --- --- --- ---
    L14483  ,TRBV7-7*01          --- ... ... --- --- --- --- --- --- --- --- --- --- --- --- --- --- --- --- ---
    M97505  ,TRBV7-7*01
    X57607  ,TRBV7-7*02          --- ... ... ... ... --- --- --- --- --- --- --- --- --- --- --- --- --- --- ---

                                 81  82  83  84  85  86  87  88  89  90  91  92  93  94  95  96  97  98  99 100
                                  P       E   G   S   I   S   T   L   T   I   Q   R   T   E   Q   R   D   S   A
    L36092,U66060,TRBV7-7*01     CCT ... GAG GGA TCC ATC TCC ACT CTG ACG ATT CAG CGC ACA GAG CAG CGG GAC TCA GCC
    AF009663,TRBV7-7*01          --- ... --- --- --- --- --- --- --- --- --- --- --- --- --- --- --- --- --- ---
    L14483  ,TRBV7-7*01          --- ... --- --- --- --- --- --- --- --- --- --- --- --- --- --- --- --- --- ---
    M97505  ,TRBV7-7*01
    X57607  ,TRBV7-7*02          --- ... --- --- --- --- --- --- --- --- --- --- --- --- --- --- --- --- --- ---

                                         ________CDR3-IMGT________
                                101 102 103 104 105 106 107 108 109
                                  M   Y   R   C   A   S   S   L
    L36092,U66060,TRBV7-7*01     ATG TAT CGC TGT GCC AGC AGC TTA GC
    AF009663,TRBV7-7*01          --- --- --- --- --- --- --- --- --
    L14483  ,TRBV7-7*01                                                         o
    M97505  ,TRBV7-7*01                                                         o
    X57607  ,TRBV7-7*02          --- --- --- --- --- --- ---                    #c
```

#c: Rearranged cDNA
o: Genomic DNA, but not known as being germline or rearranged

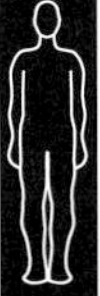

Framework and complementarity determining regions

FR1-IMGT: 26
FR2-IMGT: 17
FR3-IMGT: 38 (-1 aa: 82)

CDR1-IMGT: 5
CDR2-IMGT: 6
CDR3-IMGT: 4

Collier de Perles for human TRBV7-7*01

Accession number: IMGT L36092

EMBL/GenBank/DDBJ: L36092

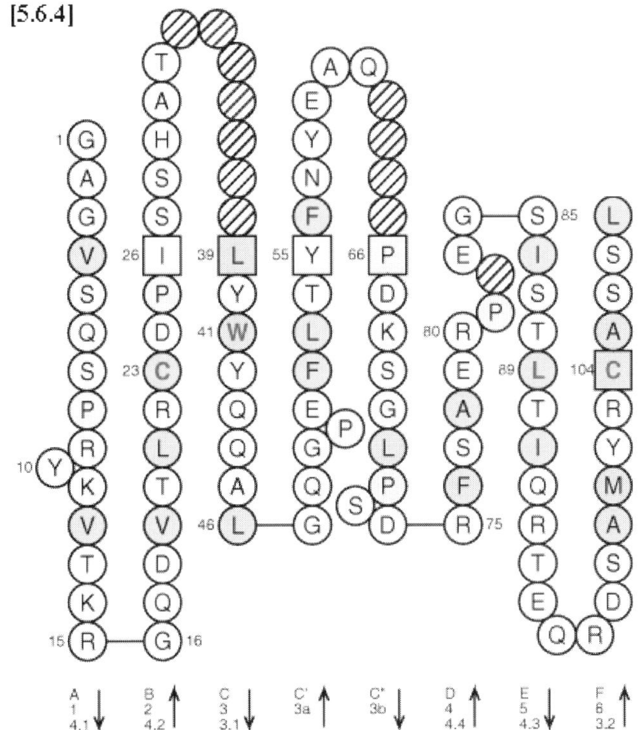

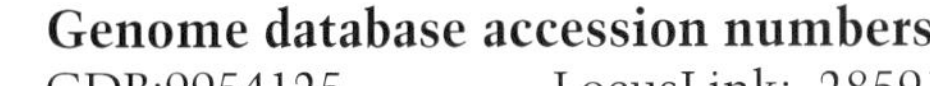

Genome database accession numbers
GDB:9954125   LocusLink: 28591

Nomenclature

TRBV7-8: T cell receptor beta variable 7-8.

Definition and functionality

TRBV7-8 is one of the 5–6 functional genes of the TRBV7 subgroup which comprises nine mapped genes, in the TRB locus.

Gene location

TRBV7-8 is in the TRB locus on chromosome 7 at 7q34.

Nucleotide and amino acid sequences for human TRBV7-8

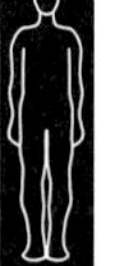

```
                            1    2    3    4    5    6    7    8    9   10   11   12   13   14   15   16   17   18   19   20
                            G    A    G    V    S    Q    S    P    R    Y    K    V    A    K    R    G    Q    D    V    A
M11953     ,TRBV7-8*01 [18] GGT  GCT  GGA  GTC  TCC  CAG  TCC  CCT  AGG  TAC  AAA  GTC  GCA  AAG  AGA  GGA  CAG  GAT  GTA  GCT

L36092,U66060,TRBV7-8*01 [34] ---  ---  ---  ---  ---  ---  ---  ---  ---  ---  ---  ---  ---  ---  ---  ---  ---  ---  ---  ---

AF009663,TRBV7-8*01    [35] ---  ---  ---  ---  ---  ---  ---  ---  ---  ---  ---  ---  ---  ---  ---  ---  ---  ---  ---  ---

X61441     ,TRBV7-8*02 [13] ---  ---  ---  ---  ---  ---  ---  ---  ---  ---  ---  ---  ---  ---  ---  ---  ---  ---  ---  ---

M27384     ,TRBV7-8*03 [21] ---  ---  ---  ---  ---  ---  ---  ---  ---  ---  ---  ---  ---  ---  ---  ---  ---  ---  ---  ---


                                                             ______________CDR1-IMGT______
                            21   22   23   24   25   26   27   28   29   30   31   32   33   34   35   36   37   38   39   40
                            L    R    C    D    P    I    S    G    H    V    S                                       L    F
M11953     ,TRBV7-8*01      CTC  AGG  TGT  GAT  CCA  ATT  TCG  GGT  CAT  GTA  TCC  ...  ...  ...  ...  ...  ...  ...  CTT  TTT

L36092,U66060,TRBV7-8*01    ---  ---  ---  ---  ---  ---  ---  ---  ---  ---  ---                                 ---  ---

AF009663,TRBV7-8*01         ---  ---  ---  ---  ---  ---  ---  ---  ---  ---  ---                                 ---  ---

X61441     ,TRBV7-8*02      ---  ---  ---  ---  ---  ---  ---  ---  ---  ---  ---                                 ---  ---

M27384     ,TRBV7-8*03      ---  ---  ---  ---  ---  ---  ---  ---  ---  ---  ---                                 ---  ---


                                                                                                 ______________CDR2-
                            41   42   43   44   45   46   47   48   49   50   51   52   53   54   55   56   57   58   59   60
                            W    Y    Q    Q    A    L    G    Q    G    P    E    F    L    T    Y    F    Q    N    E    A
M11953     ,TRBV7-8*01      TGG  TAC  CAA  CAG  GCC  CTG  GGG  CAG  GGG  CCA  GAG  TTT  CTG  ACT  TAT  TTC  CAG  AAT  GAA  GCT

L36092,U66060,TRBV7-8*01    ---  ---  ---  ---  ---  ---  ---  ---  ---  ---  ---  ---  ---  ---  ---  ---  ---  ---  ---  ---

AF009663,TRBV7-8*01         ---  ---  ---  ---  ---  ---  ---  ---  ---  ---  ---  ---  ---  ---  ---  ---  ---  ---  ---  ---

X61441     ,TRBV7-8*02      ---  ---  ---  ---  ---  ---  ---  ---  ---  ---  ---  ---  ---  ---  ---  ---  ---  ---  ---  ---

M27384     ,TRBV7-8*03      ---  ---  ---  ---  ---  --C  ---  ---  ---  ---  ---  ---  ---  ---  ---  ---  ---  ---  ---  ---


                            IMGT________________
                            61   62   63   64   65   66   67   68   69   70   71   72   73   74   75   76   77   78   79   80
                            Q                        L    D    K    S    G    L    P    S    D    R    F    F    A    E    R
M11953     ,TRBV7-8*01      CAA  ...  ...  ...  ...  CTA  GAC  AAA  TCG  GGG  CTG  CCC  AGT  GAT  CGC  TTC  TTT  GCA  GAA  AGG

L36092,U66060,TRBV7-8*01    ---  ...  ...  ...  ...  ---  ---  ---  ---  ---  ---  ---  ---  ---  ---  ---  ---  ---  ---  ---

AF009663,TRBV7-8*01         ---  ...  ...  ...  ...  ---  ---  ---  ---  ---  ---  ---  ---  ---  ---  ---  ---  ---  ---  ---

X61441     ,TRBV7-8*02      ---  ...  ...  ...  ...  ---  ---  ---  ---  ---  ---  ---  ---  ---  ---  ---  ---  ---  ---  ---

M27384     ,TRBV7-8*03      ---  ...  ...  ...  ...  ---  ---  ---  ---  ---  ---  ---  ---  ---  ---  ---  ---  ---  ---  ---


                            81   82   83   84   85   86   87   88   89   90   91   92   93   94   95   96   97   98   99  100
                            P         E    G    S    V    S    T    L    K    I    Q    R    T    Q    Q    E    D    S    A
M11953     ,TRBV7-8*01      CCT  ...  GAG  GGA  TCC  GTC  TCC  ACT  CTG  AAG  ATC  CAG  CGC  ACA  CAG  CAG  GAG  GAC  TCC  GCC

L36092,U66060,TRBV7-8*01    ---  ...  ---  ---  ---  ---  ---  ---  ---  ---  ---  ---  ---  ---  ---  ---  ---  ---  ---  ---

AF009663,TRBV7-8*01         ---  ...  ---  ---  ---  ---  ---  ---  ---  ---  ---  ---  ---  ---  ---  ---  ---  ---  ---  ---

                                                                                                           K
X61441     ,TRBV7-8*02      ---  ...  ---  ---  ---  ---  ---  ---  ---  ---  ---  ---  ---  ---  ---  A--  ---  ---  ---  ---

M27384     ,TRBV7-8*03      ---  ...  ---  ---  ---  ---  ---  ---  ---  ---  ---  ---  ---  ---  ---  ---  ---  ---  ---  ---


                                             ______CDR3-IMGT______
                           101  102  103  104  105  106  107  108  109
                            V    Y    L    C    A    S    S    L
M11953     ,TRBV7-8*01      GTG  TAT  CTC  TGT  GCC  AGC  AGC  TTA  GC

L36092,U66060,TRBV7-8*01    ---  ---  ---  ---  ---  ---  ---  ---  --

AF009663,TRBV7-8*01         ---  ---  ---  ---  ---  ---  ---  ---  --

X61441     ,TRBV7-8*02      ---  ---  ---  ---  ---  ---  ---  ---  --

                                                                 R
M27384     ,TRBV7-8*03      ---  ---  ---  ---  ---  ---  ---  CG-       #c
```

#c: Rearranged cDNA

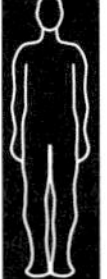

Framework and complementarity determining regions

FR1-IMGT: 26
FR2-IMGT: 17
FR3-IMGT: 38 (-1 aa: 82)

CDR1-IMGT: 5
CDR2-IMGT: 6
CDR3-IMGT: 4

Collier de Perles for human TRBV7-8*01

Accession number: IMGT M11953   EMBL/GenBank/DDBJ: M11953

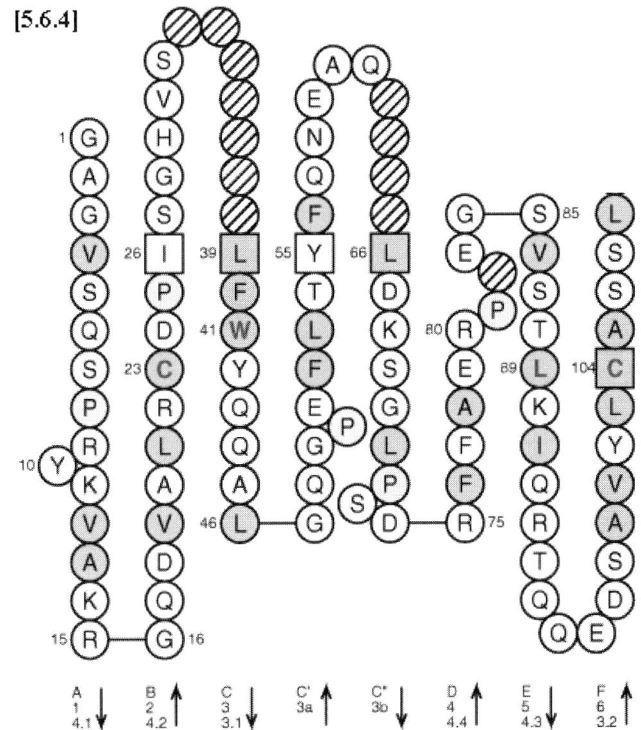

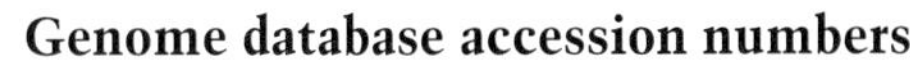

Genome database accession numbers

GDB:9954127   LocusLink: 28590

Nomenclature

TRBV7-9: T cell receptor beta variable 7-9.

Definition and functionality

TRBV7-9 is one of the 5–6 functional genes of the TRBV7 subgroup which comprises nine mapped genes, in the TRB locus.

Gene location

TRBV7-9 is in the TRB locus on chromosome 7 at 7q34.

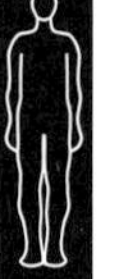

Nucleotide and amino acid sequences for human TRBV7-9

```
                            1   2   3   4   5   6   7   8   9  10  11  12  13  14  15  16  17  18  19  20
                            D   T   G   V   S   Q   N   P   R   H   K   I   T   K   R   G   Q   N   V   T
L36092,U66060,TRBV7-9*01 [34] GAT ACT GGA GTC TCC CAG AAC CCC AGA CAC AAG ATC ACA AAG AGG GGA CAG AAT GTA ACT
AF009661,TRBV7-9*01      [35] --- --- --- --- --- --- --- --- --- --- --- --- --- --- --- --- --- --- --- ---
U03115  ,TRBV7-9*01      [39]                                             - --- --- --- --- --- --- --- --- ---
X64741  ,TRBV7-9*01      [13] --- --- --- --- --- --- --- --- --- --- --- --- --- --- --- --- --- --- --- ---
                                                                             N
M15564  ,TRBV7-9*02      [23] --- --- --- --- --- --- --- --- --- --- --C --- --- --- --- --- --- --- --- ---
                                                          D
AF009663,TRBV7-9*03      [35] --- --- --- --- --- --- G-- --- --- --- --- --- --- --- --- --- --- --- --- ---
                              I   S               H
M14261  ,TRBV7-9*04      [41] ATA T-- --- --- --- --C --- --- --- --- --- --- --- --- --- --- --- --- --- ---
M27385  ,TRBV7-9*05      [21] --- --- --- --- --- --- --- --- --- --- --- --- --- --- --- --- --- --- --- ---
X74844  ,TRBV7-9*06      [19] --- --- --- --- --- --- --- --- --- --- --- --- --- --- --- --- --- --- --- ---
L14854  ,TRBV7-9*07      [15]
```

```
                                                         ________________CDR1-IMGT________________
                           21  22  23  24  25  26  27  28  29  30  31  32  33  34  35  36  37  38  39  40
                            F   R   C   D   P   I   S   E   H   N   R                               L   Y
L36092,U66060,TRBV7-9*01    TTC AGG TGT GAT CCA ATT TCT GAA CAC AAC CGC ... ... ... ... ... ... ... CTT TAT
AF009661,TRBV7-9*01         --- --- --- --- --- --- --- --- --- --- --- ... ... ... ... ... ... ... --- ---
U03115  ,TRBV7-9*01         --- --- --- --- --- --- --- --- --- --- --- ... ... ... ... ... ... ... --- ---
X64741  ,TRBV7-9*01         --- --- --- --- --- --- --- --- --- --- --- ... ... ... ... ... ... ... --- ---
M15564  ,TRBV7-9*02         --- --- --- --- --- --- --- --- --- --- --- ... ... ... ... ... ... ... --- ---
AF009663,TRBV7-9*03         --- --- --- --- --- --- --- --- --- --- --- ... ... ... ... ... ... ... --- ---
M14261  ,TRBV7-9*04         --- --- --- --- --- --- --- --- --- --- --- ... ... ... ... ... ... ... --- ---
M27385  ,TRBV7-9*05         --- --- --- --- --- --- --- --- --- --- --- ... ... ... ... ... ... ... --- ---
X74844  ,TRBV7-9*06         --- --- --- --- --- --- --- --- --- --- --- ... ... ... ... ... ... ... --- ---
L14854  ,TRBV7-9*07                                 --- --- --- --- --- ... ... ... ... ... ... ... --- ---
```

```
                                                                                         ____________CDR2-
                           41  42  43  44  45  46  47  48  49  50  51  52  53  54  55  56  57  58  59  60
                            W   Y   R   Q   T   L   G   Q   G   P   E   F   L   T   Y   F   Q   N   E   A
L36092,U66060,TRBV7-9*01    TGG TAC CGA CAG ACC CTG GGG CAG GGC CCA GAG TTT CTG ACT TAC TTC CAG AAT GAA GCT
AF009661,TRBV7-9*01         --- --- --- --- --- --- --- --- --- --- --- --- --- --- --- --- --- --- --- ---
U03115  ,TRBV7-9*01         --- --- --- --- --- --- --- --- --- --- --- --- --- --- --- --- --- --- --- ---
X64741  ,TRBV7-9*01         --- --- --- --- --- --- --- --- --- --- --- --- --- --- --- --- --- --- --- ---
M15564  ,TRBV7-9*02         --- --- --- --- --- --- --- --- --- --- --- --- --- --- --- --- --- --- --- ---
AF009663,TRBV7-9*03         --- --- --- --- --- --- --- --- --- --- --- --- --- --- --- --- --- --- --- ---
                                            N   P
M14261  ,TRBV7-9*04         --- --- --- --- -A- -CT --- --- --- --- --- --- --- --- --- --- --- --- --- ---
M27385  ,TRBV7-9*05         --- --- --- --- --- --- --- --- --- --- --- --- --- --- --- --- --- --- --- ---
X74844  ,TRBV7-9*06         --- --- --- --- --- --- --- --- --- --- --- --- --- --- --- --- --- --- --- ---
L14854  ,TRBV7-9*07         --- --- --- --- --- --- --- --- --- --- --- --- --- --- --- --- --- --- --- ---
```

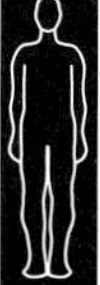

```
                    IMGT_______________
                    61  62  63  64  65  66  67  68  69  70  71  72  73  74  75  76  77  78  79  80
                    Q                   L   E   K   S   R   L   L   S   D   R   F   S   A   E   R
L36092,U66060,TRBV7-9*01  CAA ... ... ... ... CTA GAA AAA TCA AGG CTG CTC AGT GAT CGG TTC TCT GCA GAG AGG

AF009661,TRBV7-9*01  --- ... .. .. ... --- --- --- --- --- --- --- --- --- --- --- --- --- --- ---

U03115 ,TRBV7-9*01   --- ... .. .. ... --- --- --- --- --- --- --- --- --- --- --- --- --- --- ---

X64741 ,TRBV7-9*01   --- ... .. .. ... --- --- --- --- --- --- --- --- --- --- --- --- ---

M15564 ,TRBV7-9*02   --- ... .. .. ... --- --- --- --- --- --- --- --- --- --- --- --- --- --- ---

AF009663,TRBV7-9*03  --- ... .. .. ... --- --- --- --- --- --- --- --- --- --- --- --- --- --- ---
                                                                G                           I
M14261 ,TRBV7-9*04   --- ... .. .. ... --G --- --- --- G-- --- --- --- --- --- A-- --- --- --- ---

M27385 ,TRBV7-9*05   --- ... .. .. ... --- --- --- --- --- --- --- --- --- --- --- --- --- --- ---

X74844 ,TRBV7-9*06   --- ... .. .. ... --- --- --- --- --- --- --- --- --- --- --- --- --- --- ---

L14854 ,TRBV7-9*07   --- ... .. .. ... --- --- --- --- --- --- --- --- --- --- --- --- --- --- ---


                    81  82  83  84  85  86  87  88  89  90  91  92  93  94  95  96  97  98  99 100
                    P       K   G   S   F   S   T   L   E   I   Q   R   T   E   Q   G   D   S   A
L36092,U66060,TRBV7-9*01  CCT ... AAG GGA TCT TTC TCC ACC TTG GAG ATC CAG CGC ACA GAG CAG GGG GAC TCG GCC

AF009661,TRBV7-9*01  --- ... --- --- --- --- --- --- --- --- --- --- --- --- --- --- --- --- --- ---

U03115 ,TRBV7-9*01   --- ... --- --- --- --- --- --- --- --- --- --- --- --- --- --- --- --- --- ---

X64741 ,TRBV7-9*01

M15564 ,TRBV7-9*02   --- ... --- --- --- --- --- --- --- --- --- --- --- --- --- --- --- --- --- ---

AF009663,TRBV7-9*03  --- ... --- --- --- --- --- --- --- --- --- --- --- --- --- --- --- --- --- ---

M14261 ,TRBV7-9*04   --- ... --- --- --- --- --- --- --- --- --- --- --- --- --- --- --- --- --- ---
                                            L
M27385 ,TRBV7-9*05   --- ... --- --- --- C-- --- --- --- --- --- --- --- --- --- --- --- --- --- ---
                                            L
X74844 ,TRBV7-9*06   --- ... --- --- --- C-T --- --- --- --- --- --- --- --- --- --- --- --- --- ---
                                                                                    E
L14854 ,TRBV7-9*07   --- ... --- --- --- --- --- --- --- --- --- --- --- --- --- G-- --- --- --- ---


                              _____CDR3-IMGT______
                    101 102 103 104 105 106 107 108 109
                    M   Y   L   C   A   S   S   L
L36092,U66060,TRBV7-9*01  ATG TAT CTC TGT GCC AGC AGC TTA GC
AF009661,TRBV7-9*01  --- --- --- --- --- --- --- --- --

U03115 ,TRBV7-9*01   --- --- --- --- --- --- --- --- --

X64741 ,TRBV7-9*01   --- --- --- --- --- --- --- --- --      °

M15564 ,TRBV7-9*02   --- --- --- --- --- --- --- ---        #c

AF009663,TRBV7-9*03  --- --- --- --- --- --- ---             #c
                                                    S
M14261 ,TRBV7-9*04   --- --- --- --- --- --- --- -CT         #c
                                                T   K
M27385 ,TRBV7-9*05   --- --- --- --- --- --- -C- AA-         #c
                                                T   L
X74844 ,TRBV7-9*06   --- --- --- --- --- --- -CG --G         #c
                                                    S
L14854 ,TRBV7-9*07   --- --- --- --- --- --- --- AGT         #c
```

#c: Rearranged cDNA
°: Genomic DNA, but not known as being germline or rearranged

Framework and complementarity determining regions

FR1-IMGT: 26
FR2-IMGT: 17
FR3-IMGT: 38 (-1 aa: 82)

CDR1-IMGT: 5
CDR2-IMGT: 6
CDR3-IMGT: 4

Collier de Perles for human TRBV7-9*01

Accession number: IMGT L36092   EMBL/GenBank/DDBJ: L36092

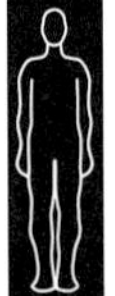

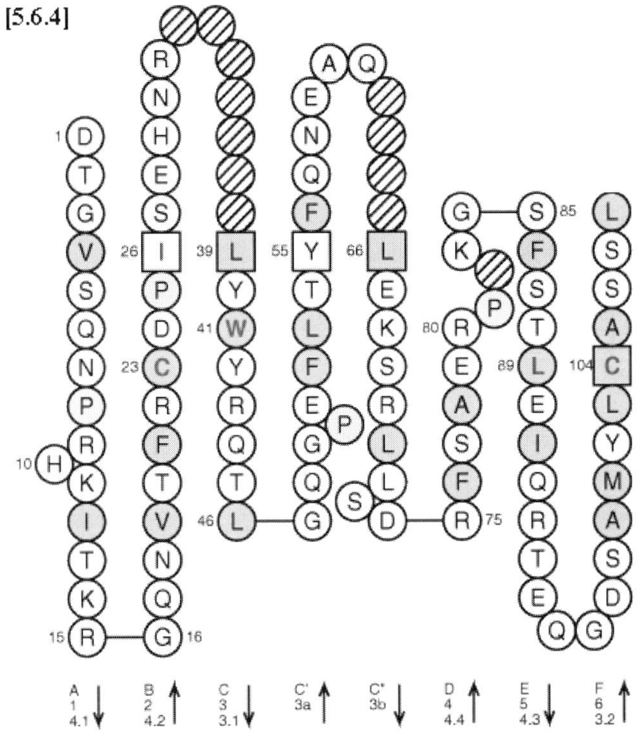

Genome database accession numbers
GDB:9954129   LocusLink: 28589

Nomenclature

TRBV9: T cell receptor beta variable 9.

Definition and functionality

TRBV9 is the unique functional gene of the TRBV9 subgroup which only comprises this mapped gene, in the TRB locus.

Gene location

TRBV9 is in the TRB locus on chromosome 7 at 7q34.

Nucleotide and amino acid sequences for human TRBV9

```
                          1   2   3   4   5   6   7   8   9   10  11  12  13  14  15  16  17  18  19  20
                          D   S   G   V   T   Q   T   P   K   H   L   I   T   A   T   G   Q   R   V   T
L36092,U66059,TRBV9*01 [34] GAT TCT GGA GTC ACA CAA ACC CCA AAG CAC CTG ATC ACA GCA ACT GGA CAG CGA GTG ACG

AF009660,TRBV9*02      [35] --- --- --- --- --- --- --- --- --- --- --- --- --- --- --- --- --- --- --- ---

M27380  ,TRBV9*03      [21] --- --- --- --- --- --- --- --- --- --- --- --- --- --- --- --- --- --- --- ---


                                                              ________________CDR1-IMGT________________
                          21  22  23  24  25  26  27  28  29  30  31  32  33  34  35  36  37  38  39  40
                          L   R   C   S   P   R   S   G   D   L   S                               V   Y
L36092,U66059,TRBV9*01    CTG AGA TGC TCC CCT AGG TCT GGA GAC CTC TCT ... ... ... ... ... ... ... GTG TAC

AF009660,TRBV9*02         --- --- --- --- --- --- --- --- --- --- --- ... ... ... ... --- ---

M27380  ,TRBV9*03         --- --- --- --- --- --- --- --- --- --- --- ... ... ... ... --- ---


                                                                              ______________CDR2-
                          41  42  43  44  45  46  47  48  49  50  51  52  53  54  55  56  57  58  59  60
                          W   Y   Q   Q   S   L   D   Q   G   L   Q   F   L   I   Q   Y   Y   N   G   E
L36092,U66059,TRBV9*01    TGG TAC CAA CAG AGC CTG GAC CAG GGC CTC CAG TTC CTC ATT CAG TAT TAT AAT GGA GAA
                                                                          H
AF009660,TRBV9*02         --- --- --- --- --- --- --- --- --- --- --- --- --- --- --C --- --- --- ---

M27380  ,TRBV9*03         --- --- --- --- --- --- --- --- --- --- --- --- --- --- --A --- --- --- --- ---


                          IMGT________________
                          61  62  63  64  65  66  67  68  69  70  71  72  73  74  75  76  77  78  79  80
                          E                       R   A   K   G   N   I   L       E   R   F   S   A   Q   Q
L36092,U66059,TRBV9*01    GAG ... ... ... ... AGA GCA AAA GGA AAC ATT CTT ... GAA CGA TTC TCC GCA CAA CAG

AF009660,TRBV9*02         --- ... ... ... ... --- --- --- --- --- --- --- ... --- --- --- --- --- ---

M27380  ,TRBV9*03         --- ... ... ... ... --- --- --- --- --- --- --- ... --- --- --- --- --- ---


                          81  82  83  84  85  86  87  88  89  90  91  92  93  94  95  96  97  98  99 100
                          F       P   D   L   H   S   E   L   N   L   S   S   L   E   L   G   D   S   A
L36092,U66059,TRBV9*01    TTC ... CCT GAC TTG CAC TCT GAA CTA AAC CTG AGC TCT CTG GAG CTG GGG GAC TCA GCT

AF009660,TRBV9*02         --- ... --- --- --- --- --- --- --- --- --- --- --- --- --- --- --- --- --- ---

M27380  ,TRBV9*03         --- ... --- --- --- --- --- --- --- --- --- --- --- --- --- --- --- --- --- ---


                              ______CDR3-IMGT______
                          101 102 103 104 105 106 107 108 109
                          L   Y   F   C   A   S   S   V
L36092,U66059,TRBV9*01    TTG TAT TTC TGT GCC AGC AGC GTA G
                                                  R       L
AF009660,TRBV9*02         --- --- --- --- --- --A --- T-G

M27380  ,TRBV9*03         --- --- --- --- --- --- ---                  #c

#c: Rearranged cDNA
```

Framework and complementarity determining regions

FR1-IMGT: 26   CDR1-IMGT: 5
FR2-IMGT: 17   CDR2-IMGT: 6
FR3-IMGT: 37 (-2 aa: 73, 82)   CDR3-IMGT: 4

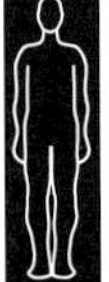

Collier de Perles for human TRBV9*01

Accession number: IMGT L36092   EMBL/GenBank/DDBJ: L36092

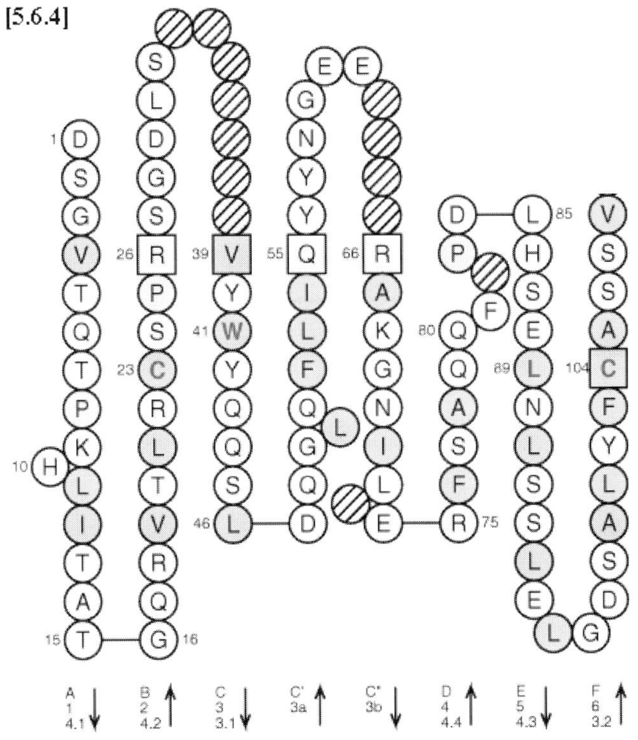

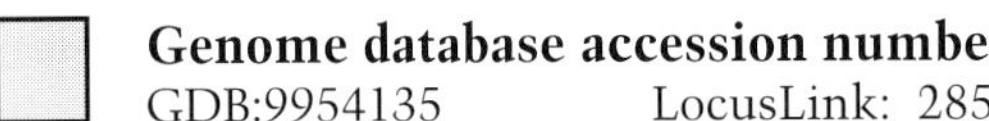

Genome database accession numbers
GDB:9954135   LocusLink: 28586

Nomenclature

TRBV10-1: T cell receptor beta variable 10-1.

Definition and functionality

TRBV10-1 is a functional gene (alleles *01 and *02) or a pseudogene (allele *03). TRBV10-1 belongs to TRBV10 subgroup which comprises three mapped genes, of which 2–3 are functional, in the TRB locus.

TRBV10-1*03 is a pseudogene due to Glutamic acid (gag) 92 replaced by a STOP-CODON (tag), in the FR3-IMGT.

Gene location

TRBV10-1 is in the TRB locus on chromosome 7 at 7q34.

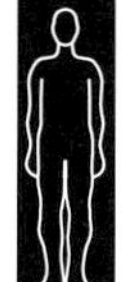

Nucleotide and amino acid sequences for human TRBV10-1

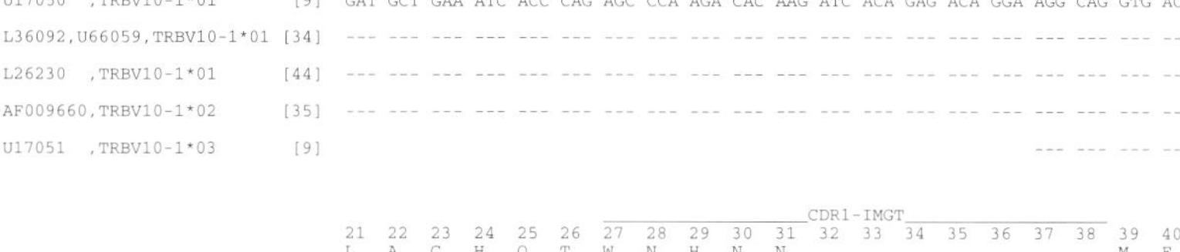

```
                                 1   2   3   4   5   6   7   8   9  10  11  12  13  14  15  16  17  18  19  20
                                 D   A   E   I   T   Q   S   P   R   H   K   I   T   E   T   G   R   Q   V   T
U17050     ,TRBV10-1*01    [9]  GAT GCT GAA ATC ACC CAG AGC CCA AGA CAC AAG ATC ACA GAG ACA GGA AGG CAG GTG ACC
L36092,U66059,TRBV10-1*01 [34]  --- --- --- --- --- --- --- --- --- --- --- --- --- --- --- --- --- --- --- ---
L26230     ,TRBV10-1*01   [44]  --- --- --- --- --- --- --- --- --- --- --- --- --- --- --- --- --- --- --- ---
AF009660,TRBV10-1*02      [35]  --- --- --- --- --- --- --- --- --- --- --- --- --- --- --- --- --- --- --- ---
U17051     ,TRBV10-1*03    [9]                                                                  --- --- --- ---

                                                                             CDR1-IMGT
                                21  22  23  24  25  26  27  28  29  30  31  32  33  34  35  36  37  38  39  40
                                 L   A   C   H   Q   T   W   N   H   N   N                                   M   F
U17050     ,TRBV10-1*01        TTG GCG TGT CAC CAG ACT TGG AAC CAC AAC AAT ... ... ... ... ... ... ... ATG TTC
L36092,U66059,TRBV10-1*01      --- --- --- --- --- --- --- --- --- --- ---  ... ... ... ... ...  ... ... --- ---
L26230     ,TRBV10-1*01        --- --- --- --- --- --- --- --- --- --- ---  ... ... ... ... ...  ... ... --- ---
AF009660,TRBV10-1*02           --- --- --- --- --- --- --- --- --- --- ---  ... ... ... ... ...  ... ... --- ---
U17051     ,TRBV10-1*03        --- --- --- --- --- --- --- --- --- --- ---  ... ... ... ... ...  ... ... --- ---

                                                                                             ____________CDR2-
                                41  42  43  44  45  46  47  48  49  50  51  52  53  54  55  56  57  58  59  60
                                 W   Y   R   Q   D   L   G   H   G   L   R   L   I   H   Y   S   Y   G   V   Q
U17050     ,TRBV10-1*01        TGG TAT CGA CAA GAC CTG GGA CAT GGG CTG AGG CTG ATC CAT TAC TCA TAT GGT GTT CAA
L36092,U66059,TRBV10-1*01      --- --- --- --- --- --- --- --- --- --- --- --- --- --- --- --- --- --- --- ---
L26230     ,TRBV10-1*01        --- --- --- --- --- --- --- --- --- --- --- --- --- --- --- --- --- --- --- ---
AF009660,TRBV10-1*02           --- --- --- --- --- --- --- --- --- --- --- --- --- --- --- --- --- --- --- --C  (H)
U17051     ,TRBV10-1*03        --- --- --- --- --- --- --- --- --- --- --- --- --- --- --- --- --- --- --- --C  (H)

                                IMGT________
                                61  62  63  64  65  66  67  68  69  70  71  72  73  74  75  76  77  78  79  80
                                 D                   T   N   K   G   E   V   S       D   G   Y   S   V   S   R
U17050     ,TRBV10-1*01        GAC ... ... ... ... ACT AAC AAA GGA GAA GTC TCA ... GAT GGC TAC AGT GTC TCT AGA
L36092,U66059,TRBV10-1*01      --- ... ... ... ... --- --- --- --- --- --- --- ... --- --- --- --- --- --- ---
L26230     ,TRBV10-1*01        --- ... ... ... ... --- --- --- --- --- --- --- ... --- --- --- --- --- --- ---
AF009660,TRBV10-1*02           --- ... ... ... ... --- --- --- --- --- --- --- ... --- --- --- --- --- --- ---
U17051     ,TRBV10-1*03        --- ... ... ... ... --- --- --- --- --- --- --- ... --- --- --- --- --- --- ---

                                81  82  83  84  85  86  87  88  89  90  91  92  93  94  95  96  97  98  99 100
                                 S       N   T   E   D   L   P   L   T   L   E   S   A   A   S   S   Q   T   S
U17050     ,TRBV10-1*01        TCA ... AAC ACA GAG GAC CTC CCC CTC ACT CTG GAG TCT GCT GCC TCC TCC CAG ACA TCT
L36092,U66059,TRBV10-1*01      --- ... --- --- --- --- --- --- --- --- --- --- --- --- --- --- --- --- --- ---
L26230     ,TRBV10-1*01        --- ... --- --- --- --- --- --- --- --- --- --- --- --- --- --- --- --- --- ---
AF009660,TRBV10-1*02           --- ... --- --- --- --- --- --- --- --- --- --- --- --- --- --- --- --- --- ---
U17051     ,TRBV10-1*03        --- ... --- --- --- --- --- --- --- --- --- T-- --- --- --- --- --- --- --- ---
                                                                             *
```

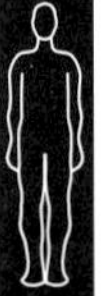

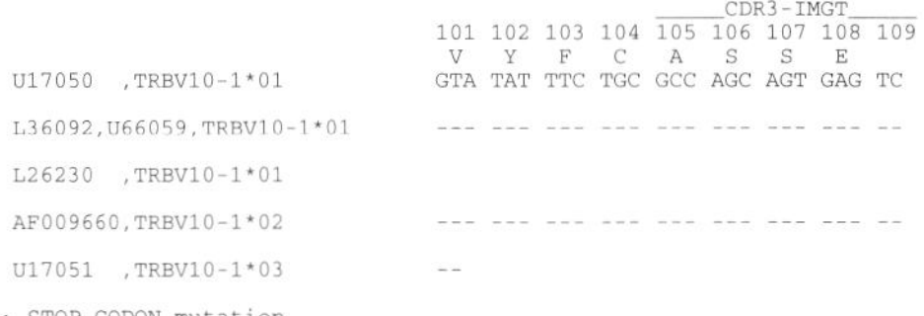

```
                                         ____CDR3-IMGT____
                                101 102 103 104 105 106 107 108 109
                                 V   Y   F   C   A   S   S   E
    U17050   ,TRBV10-1*01       GTA TAT TTC TGC GCC AGC AGT GAG TC

    L36092,U66059,TRBV10-1*01   --- --- --- --- --- --- --- --- --

    L26230   ,TRBV10-1*01                                          o

    AF009660,TRBV10-1*02        --- --- --- --- --- --- --- --- --

    U17051   ,TRBV10-1*03       --                                 o

*: STOP-CODON mutation
o: Genomic DNA, but not known as being germline or rearranged
```

Framework and complementarity determining regions

FR1-IMGT: 26   CDR1-IMGT: 5
FR2-IMGT: 17   CDR2-IMGT: 6
FR3-IMGT: 37 (-2 aa: 73, 82)   CDR3-IMGT: 4

Collier de Perles for human TRBV10-1*01

Accession number: IMGT U17050   EMBL/GenBank/DDBJ: U17050

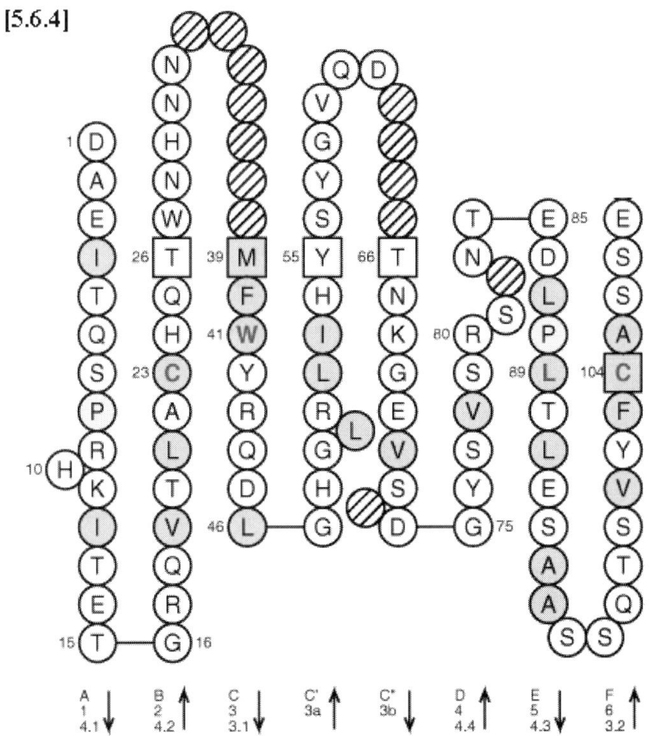

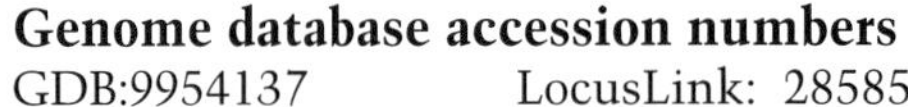

Genome database accession numbers
GDB:9954137   LocusLink: 28585

TRBV10-2

Nomenclature

TRBV10-2: T cell receptor beta variable 10-2.

Definition and functionality

TRBV10-2 is one of the 2–3 functional genes of the TRBV10 subgroup which comprises three mapped genes, in the TRB locus.

Gene location

TRBV10-2 is in the TRB locus on chromosome 7 at 7q34.

Nucleotide and amino acid sequences for human TRBV10-2

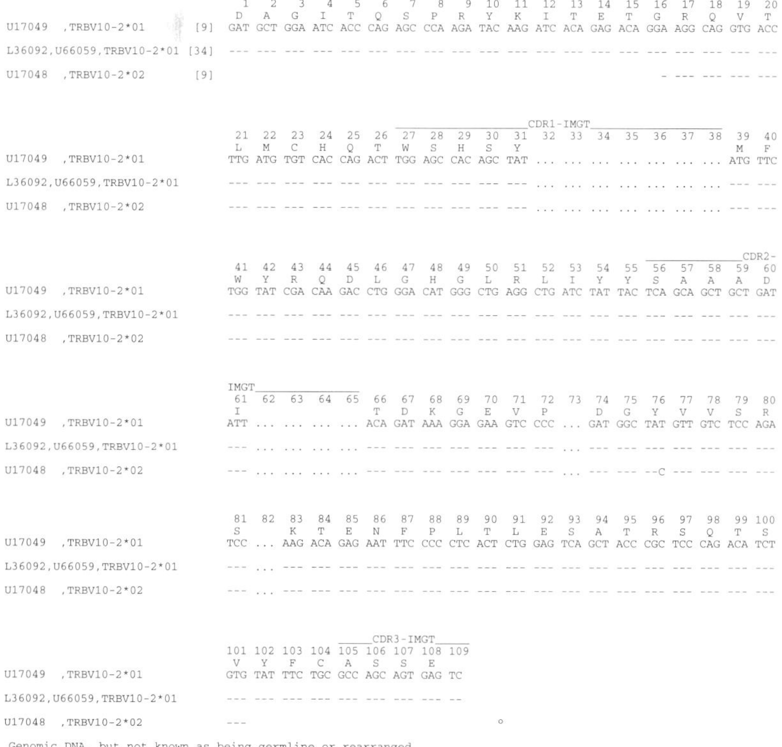

```
                          1   2   3   4   5   6   7   8   9  10  11  12  13  14  15  16  17  18  19  20
                          D   A   G   I   T   Q   S   P   R   Y   K   I   T   E   T   G   R   Q   V   T
U17049    ,TRBV10-2*01  [9] GAT GCT GGA ATC ACC CAG AGC CCA AGA TAC AAG ATC ACA GAG ACA GGA AGG CAG GTG ACC

L36092,U66059,TRBV10-2*01 [34] --- --- --- --- --- --- --- --- --- --- --- --- --- --- --- --- --- --- --- ---

U17048    ,TRBV10-2*02  [9]                                                          -   --- --- --- ---


                                                                      ____________CDR1-IMGT____________
                         21  22  23  24  25  26  27  28  29  30  31  32  33  34  35  36  37  38  39  40
                          L   M   C   H   Q   T   W   S   H   S   Y                               M   F
U17049    ,TRBV10-2*01   TTG ATG TGT CAC CAG ACT TGG AGC CAC AGC TAT ... ... ... ... ... ... ... ATG TTC

L36092,U66059,TRBV10-2*01 --- --- --- --- --- --- --- --- --- --- --- ... ... ... ... ... ... --- ---

U17048    ,TRBV10-2*02   --- --- --- --- --- --- --- --- --- --- --- ... ... ... ... ... ... --- ---


                                                                                      ____________CDR2-
                         41  42  43  44  45  46  47  48  49  50  51  52  53  54  55  56  57  58  59  60
                          W   Y   R   Q   D   L   G   H   G   L   R   L   I   Y   Y   S   A   A   A   D
U17049    ,TRBV10-2*01   TGG TAT CGA CAA GAC CTG GGA CAT GGG CTG AGG CTG ATC TAT TAC TCA GCA GCT GCT GAT

L36092,U66059,TRBV10-2*01 --- --- --- --- --- --- --- --- --- --- --- --- --- --- --- --- --- --- --- ---

U17048    ,TRBV10-2*02   --- --- --- --- --- --- --- --- --- --- --- --- --- --- --- --- --- --- --- ---


                         IMGT____________
                         61  62  63  64  65  66  67  68  69  70  71  72  73  74  75  76  77  78  79  80
                          I                   T   D   K   G   E   V   P       D   G   Y   V   V   S   R
U17049    ,TRBV10-2*01   ATT ... ... ... ... ACA GAT AAA GGA GAA GTC CCC ... GAT GGC TAT GTT GTC TCC AGA

L36092,U66059,TRBV10-2*01 --- ... ... ... ... --- --- --- --- --- --- --- ... --- --- --- --- --- --- ---

U17048    ,TRBV10-2*02   --- ... ... ... ... --- --- --- --- --- --- --- ... --- --- --C --- --- --- ---


                         81  82  83  84  85  86  87  88  89  90  91  92  93  94  95  96  97  98  99 100
                          S       K   T   E   N   F   P   L   T   L   E   S   A   T   R   S   Q   T   S
U17049    ,TRBV10-2*01   TCC ... AAG ACA GAG AAT TTC CCC CTC ACT CTG GAG TCA GCT ACC CGC TCC CAG ACA TCT

L36092,U66059,TRBV10-2*01 --- ... --- --- --- --- --- --- --- --- --- --- --- --- --- --- --- --- --- ---

U17048    ,TRBV10-2*02   --- ... --- --- --- --- --- --- --- --- --- --- --- --- --- --- --- --- --- ---


                                         ______CDR3-IMGT______
                        101 102 103 104 105 106 107 108 109
                          V   Y   F   C   A   S   S   E
U17049    ,TRBV10-2*01   GTG TAT TTC TGC GCC AGC AGT GAG TC

L36092,U66059,TRBV10-2*01 --- --- --- --- --- --- --- --- --

U17048    ,TRBV10-2*02   ---                                   °
```

°: Genomic DNA, but not known as being germline or rearranged

Framework and complementarity determining regions

FR1-IMGT: 26	CDR1-IMGT: 5
FR2-IMGT: 17	CDR2-IMGT: 6
FR3-IMGT: 37 (-2 aa: 73, 82)	CDR3-IMGT: 4

Collier de Perles for human TRBV10-2*01

Accession number: IMGT U17049   EMBL/GenBank/DDBJ: U17049

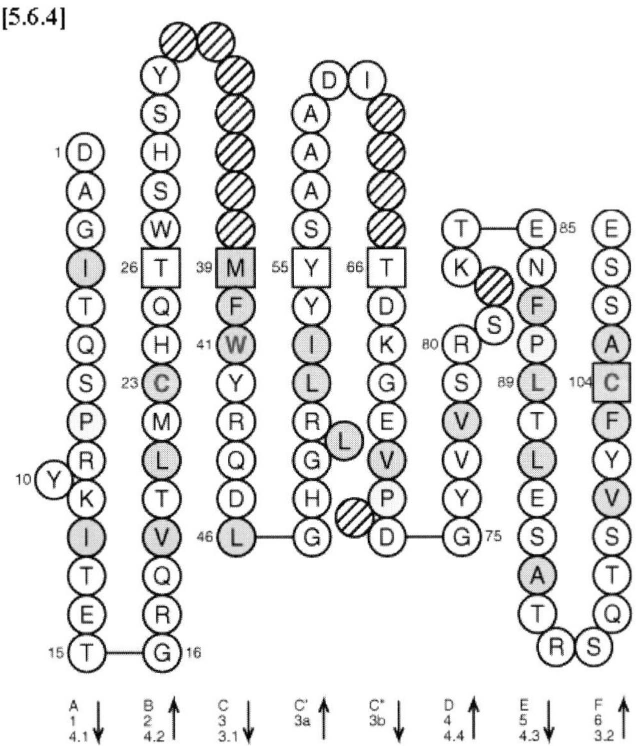

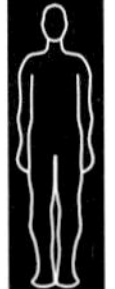

Genome database accession numbers
GDB:9954139   LocusLink: 28584

TRBV10-3

Nomenclature

TRBV10-3: T cell receptor beta variable 10-3.

Definition and functionality

TRBV10-3 is one of the 2–3 functional genes of the TRBV10 subgroup which comprises three mapped genes, in the TRB locus.

Gene location

TRBV10-3 is in the TRB locus on chromosome 7 at 7q34.

Nucleotide and amino acid sequences for human TRBV10-3

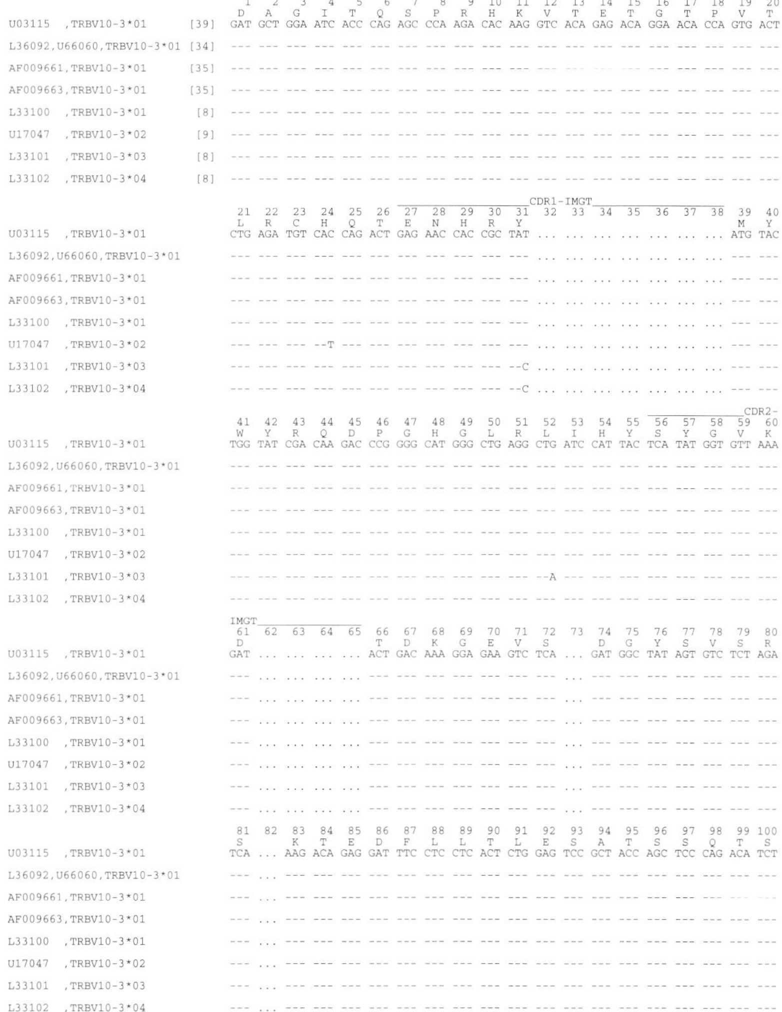

```
                             1   2   3   4   5   6   7   8   9  10  11  12  13  14  15  16  17  18  19  20
                             D   A   G   I   T   Q   S   P   R   H   K   V   T   E   T   G   T   P   V   T
U03115    ,TRBV10-3*01 [39] GAT GCT GGA ATC ACC CAG AGC CCA AGA CAC AAG GTC ACA GAG ACA GGA ACA CCA GTG ACT
L36092,U66060,TRBV10-3*01 [34] --- --- --- --- --- --- --- --- --- --- --- --- --- --- --- --- --- --- --- ---
AF009661,TRBV10-3*01 [35] --- --- --- --- --- --- --- --- --- --- --- --- --- --- --- --- --- --- --- ---
AF009663,TRBV10-3*01 [35] --- --- --- --- --- --- --- --- --- --- --- --- --- --- --- --- --- --- --- ---
L33100    ,TRBV10-3*01  [8] --- --- --- --- --- --- --- --- --- --- --- --- --- --- --- --- --- --- --- ---
U17047    ,TRBV10-3*02  [9] --- --- --- --- --- --- --- --- --- --- --- --- --- --- --- --- --- --- --- ---
L33101    ,TRBV10-3*03  [8] --- --- --- --- --- --- --- --- --- --- --- --- --- --- --- --- --- --- --- ---
L33102    ,TRBV10-3*04  [8] --- --- --- --- --- --- --- --- --- --- --- --- --- --- --- --- --- --- --- ---

                                                             CDR1-IMGT________________________
                            21  22  23  24  25  26  27  28  29  30  31  32  33  34  35  36  37  38  39  40
                             L   R   C   H   Q   T   E   N   H   R   Y                           M   Y
U03115    ,TRBV10-3*01      CTG AGA TGT CAC CAG ACT GAG AAC CAC CGC TAT ... ... ... ... ... ... ... ATG TAC
L36092,U66060,TRBV10-3*01   --- --- --- --- --- --- --- --- --- --- --- ... ... ... ... ... ... ... --- ---
AF009661,TRBV10-3*01        --- --- --- --- --- --- --- --- --- --- --- ... ... ... ... ... ... ... --- ---
AF009663,TRBV10-3*01        --- --- --- --- --- --- --- --- --- --- --- ... ... ... ... ... ... ... --- ---
L33100    ,TRBV10-3*01      --- --- --- --- --- --- --- --- --- --- --- ... ... ... ... ... ... ... --- ---
U17047    ,TRBV10-3*02      --- --- --- --T --- --- --- --- --- --- --- ... ... ... ... ... ... ... --- ---
L33101    ,TRBV10-3*03      --- --- --- --- --- --- --- --- --- --- --C ... ... ... ... ... ... ... --- ---
L33102    ,TRBV10-3*04      --- --- --- --- --- --- --- --- --- --- --C ... ... ... ... ... ... ... --- ---

                                                                                         CDR2-
                            41  42  43  44  45  46  47  48  49  50  51  52  53  54  55  56  57  58  59  60
                             W   Y   R   Q   D   P   G   H   G   L   R   L   I   H   Y   S   Y   G   V   K
U03115    ,TRBV10-3*01      TGG TAT CGA CAA GAC CCG GGG CAT GGG CTG AGG CTG ATC CAT TAC TCA TAT GGT GTT AAA
L36092,U66060,TRBV10-3*01   --- --- --- --- --- --- --- --- --- --- --- --- --- --- --- --- --- --- --- ---
AF009661,TRBV10-3*01        --- --- --- --- --- --- --- --- --- --- --- --- --- --- --- --- --- --- --- ---
AF009663,TRBV10-3*01        --- --- --- --- --- --- --- --- --- --- --- --- --- --- --- --- --- --- --- ---
L33100    ,TRBV10-3*01      --- --- --- --- --- --- --- --- --- --- --- --- --- --- --- --- --- --- --- ---
U17047    ,TRBV10-3*02      --- --- --- --- --- --- --- --- --- --- --- --- --- --- --- --- --- --- --- ---
L33101    ,TRBV10-3*03      --- --- --- --- --- --- --- --- --- --- --- --A --- --- --- --- --- --- --- ---
L33102    ,TRBV10-3*04      --- --- --- --- --- --- --- --- --- --- --- --- --- --- --- --- --- --- --- ---

                            IMGT________________________
                            61  62  63  64  65  66  67  68  69  70  71  72  73  74  75  76  77  78  79  80
                             D                   T   D   K   G   E   V   S       D   G   Y   S   V   S   R
U03115    ,TRBV10-3*01      GAT ... ... ... ... ACT GAC AAA GGA GAA GTC TCA ... GAT GGC TAT AGT GTC TCT AGA
L36092,U66060,TRBV10-3*01   --- ... ... ... ... --- --- --- --- --- --- --- ... --- --- --- --- --- --- ---
AF009661,TRBV10-3*01        --- ... ... ... ... --- --- --- --- --- --- --- ... --- --- --- --- --- --- ---
AF009663,TRBV10-3*01        --- ... ... ... ... --- --- --- --- --- --- --- ... --- --- --- --- --- --- ---
L33100    ,TRBV10-3*01      --- ... ... ... ... --- --- --- --- --- --- --- ... --- --- --- --- --- --- ---
U17047    ,TRBV10-3*02      --- ... ... ... ... --- --- --- --- --- --- --- ... --- --- --- --- --- --- ---
L33101    ,TRBV10-3*03      --- ... ... ... ... --- --- --- --- --- --- --- ... --- --- --- --- --- --- ---
L33102    ,TRBV10-3*04      --- ... ... ... ... --- --- --- --- --- --- --- ... --- --- --- --- --- --- ---

                            81  82  83  84  85  86  87  88  89  90  91  92  93  94  95  96  97  98  99 100
                             S       K   T   E   D   F   L   L   T   L   E   S   A   T   S   S   Q   T   S
U03115    ,TRBV10-3*01      TCA ... AAG ACA GAG GAT TTC CTC CTC ACT CTG GAG TCC GCT ACC AGC TCC CAG ACA TCT
L36092,U66060,TRBV10-3*01   --- ... --- --- --- --- --- --- --- --- --- --- --- --- --- --- --- --- --- ---
AF009661,TRBV10-3*01        --- ... --- --- --- --- --- --- --- --- --- --- --- --- --- --- --- --- --- ---
AF009663,TRBV10-3*01        --- ... --- --- --- --- --- --- --- --- --- --- --- --- --- --- --- --- --- ---
L33100    ,TRBV10-3*01      --- ... --- --- --- --- --- --- --- --- --- --- --- --- --- --- --- --- --- ---
U17047    ,TRBV10-3*02      --- ... --- --- --- --- --- --- --- --- --- --- --- --- --- --- --- --- --- ---
L33101    ,TRBV10-3*03      --- ... --- --- --- --- --- --- --- --- --- --- --- --- --- --- --- --- --- ---
L33102    ,TRBV10-3*04      --- ... --- --- --- --- --- --- --- --- --- --- --- --- --- --- --- --- --- ---
```

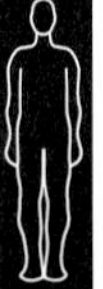

```
                                        ________CDR3-IMGT________
                              101 102 103 104 105 106 107 108 109
                               V   Y   F   C   A   I   S   E
   U03115    ,TRBV10-3*01     GTG TAC TTC TGT GCC ATC AGT GAG TC

   L36092,U66060,TRBV10-3*01  --- --- --- --- --- --- --- --- --

   AF009661,TRBV10-3*01       --- --- --- --- --- --- --- --- --

   AF009663,TRBV10-3*01       --- --- --- --- --- --- --- --- --

   L33100    ,TRBV10-3*01     --- --- --- ---                        °

   U17047    ,TRBV10-3*02     --- --- --- --- --- --- --- --- --

   L33101    ,TRBV10-3*03     --- --- --- ---                        °

   L33102    ,TRBV10-3*04     --- --- --- ---                        °
```

°: Genomic DNA, but not known as being germline or rearranged

Framework and complementarity determining regions

FR1-IMGT: 26   CDR1-IMGT: 5
FR2-IMGT: 17   CDR2-IMGT: 6
FR3-IMGT: 37 (-2 aa: 73, 82)   CDR3-IMGT: 4

Collier de Perles for human TRBV10-3*01

Accession number: IMGT U03115   EMBL/GenBank/DDBJ: U03115

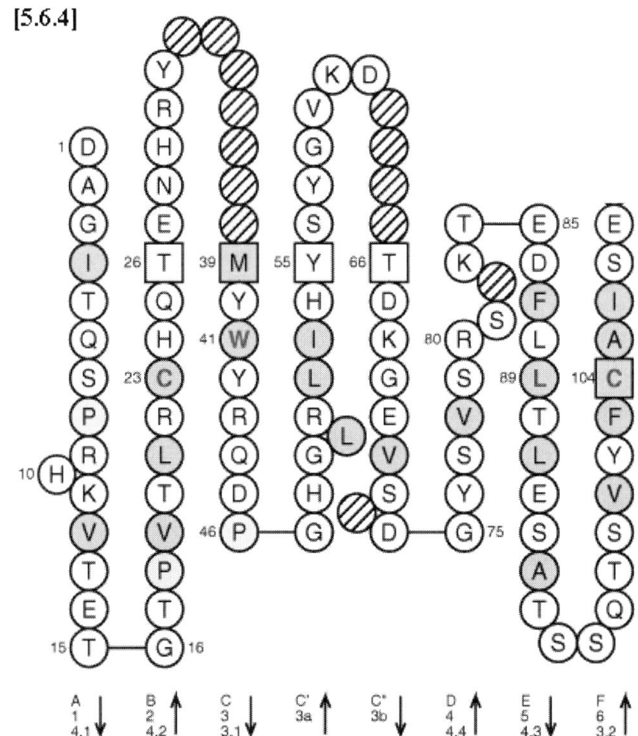

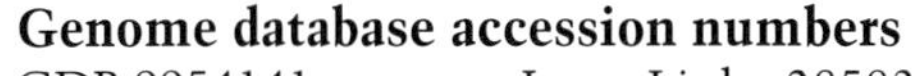

Genome database accession numbers
GDB:9954141   LocusLink: 28583

TRBV11-1

Nomenclature

TRBV11-1: T cell receptor beta variable 11-1.

Definition and functionality

TRBV11-1 is one of the three functional genes of the TRBV11 subgroup which comprises three mapped genes, in the TRB locus.

Gene location

TRBV11-1 is in the TRB locus on chromosome 7 at 7q34.

Nucleotide and amino acid sequences for human TRBV11-1

```
                            1   2   3   4   5   6   7   8   9  10  11  12  13  14  15  16  17  18  19  20
                            E   A   E   V   A   Q   S   P   R   Y   K   I   T   E   K   S   Q   A   V   A
M33233    ,TRBV11-1*01 [46] GAA GCT GAA GTT GCC CAG TCC CCC AGA TAT AAG ATT ACA GAG AAA AGC CAG GCT GTG GCT

L36092,U66059,TRBV11-1*01 [34] --- --- --- --- --- --- --- --- --- --- --- --- --- --- --- --- --- --- --- ---


                                                                   ___________CDR1-IMGT___________
                           21  22  23  24  25  26  27  28  29  30  31  32  33  34  35  36  37  38  39  40
                            F   W   C   D   P   I   S   G   H   A   T                               L   Y
M33233    ,TRBV11-1*01     TTT TGG TGT GAT CCT ATT TCT GGC CAT GCT ACC ... ... ... ... ... ... ... CTT TAC

L36092,U66059,TRBV11-1*01  --- --- --- --- --- --- --- --- --- --- --- ... ... ... ... ... ... ... --- ---


                                                                               _______________CDR2-
                           41  42  43  44  45  46  47  48  49  50  51  52  53  54  55  56  57  58  59  60
                            W   Y   R   Q   I   L   G   Q   G   P   E   L   L   V   Q   F   Q   D   E   S
M33233    ,TRBV11-1*01     TGG TAC CGG CAG ATC CTG GGA CAG GGC CCG GAG CTT CTG GTT CAA TTT CAG GAT GAG AGT

L36092,U66059,TRBV11-1*01  --- --- --- --- --- --- --- --- --- --- --- --- --- --- --- --- --- --- --- ---


                           IMGT________________
                           61  62  63  64  65  66  67  68  69  70  71  72  73  74  75  76  77  78  79  80
                            V                   V   D   D   S   Q   L   P   K   D   R   F   S   A   E   R
M33233    ,TRBV11-1*01     GTA ... ... ... ... GTA GAT GAT TCA CAG TTG CCT AAG GAT CGA TTT TCT GCA GAG AGG

L36092,U66059,TRBV11-1*01  --- ... ... ... ... --- --- --- --- --- --- --- --- --- --- --- --- --- --- ---


                           81  82  83  84  85  86  87  88  89  90  91  92  93  94  95  96  97  98  99 100
                            L       K   G   V   D   S   T   L   K   I   Q   P   A   E   L   G   D   S   A
M33233    ,TRBV11-1*01     CTC ... AAA GGA GTA GAC TCC ACT CTC AAG ATC CAG CCT GCA GAG CTT GGG GAC TCG GCC

L36092,U66059,TRBV11-1*01  --- ... --- --- --- --- --- --- --- --- --- --- --- --- --- --- --- --- --- ---


                                           ______CDR3-IMGT______
                          101 102 103 104 105 106 107 108 109
                            M   Y   L   C   A   S   S   L
M33233    ,TRBV11-1*01     ATG TAT CTC TGT GCC AGC AGC TTA GC

L36092,U66059,TRBV11-1*01  --- --- --- --- --- --- --- --- --
```

Framework and complementarity determining regions

FR1-IMGT: 26

FR2-IMGT: 17

FR3-IMGT: 38 (-1 aa: 82)

CDR1-IMGT: 5

CDR2-IMGT: 6

CDR3-IMGT: 4

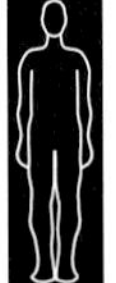

Collier de Perles for human TRBV11-1*01

Accession number: IMGT M33233   EMBL/GenBank/DDBJ: M33233

[5.6.4]

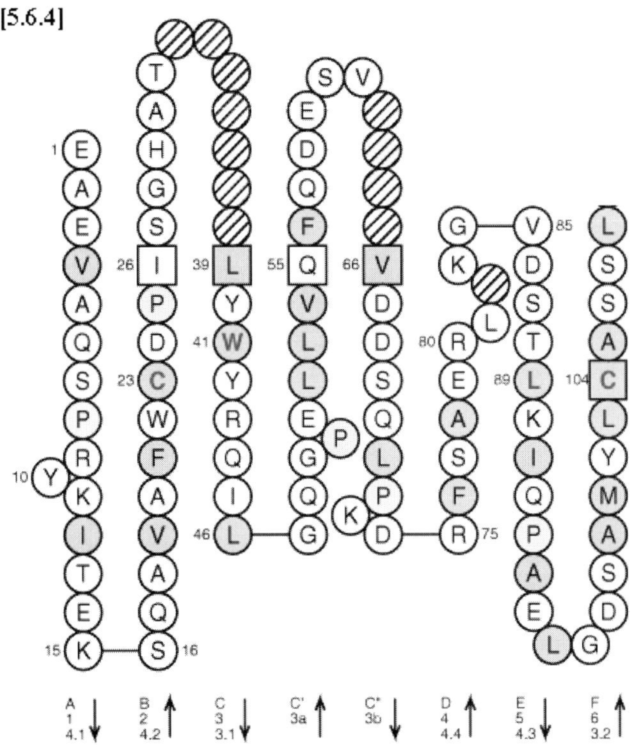

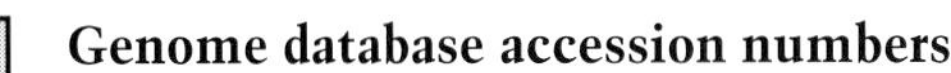

Genome database accession numbers
GDB:9954143   LocusLink: 28582

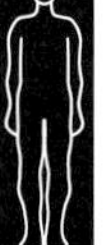

Nomenclature

TRBV11-2: T cell receptor beta variable 11-2.

Definition and functionality

TRBV11-2 is one of the three functional genes of the TRBV11 subgroup which comprises three mapped genes, in the TRB locus.

Gene location

TRBV11-2 is in the TRB locus on chromosome 7 at 7q34.

Nucleotide and amino acid sequences for human TRBV11-2

```
                                1    2    3    4    5    6    7    8    9   10   11   12   13   14   15   16   17   18   19   20
                                E    A    G    V    A    Q    S    P    R    Y    K    I    I    E    K    R    Q    S    V    A
L36092,U66059,TRBV11-2*01 [34] GAA  GCT  GGA  GTT  GCC  CAG  TCT  CCC  AGA  TAT  AAG  ATT  ATA  GAG  AAA  AGG  CAG  AGT  GTG  GCT

M33235   ,TRBV11-2*02    [46]  ---  ---  ---  ---  ---  ---  ---  ---  ---  ---  ---  ---  ---  ---  ---  ---  ---  ---  ---  ---

X58796   ,TRBV11-2*03    [10]  ---  ---  ---  ---  ---  ---  ---  ---  ---  ---  ---  ---  ---  ---  ---  ---  ---  ---  ---  ---


                                                                           ________________CDR1-IMGT________________
                               21   22   23   24   25   26   27   28   29   30   31   32   33   34   35   36   37   38   39   40
                                F    W    C    N    P    I    S    G    H    A    T                                  L    Y
L36092,U66059,TRBV11-2*01      TTT  TGG  TGC  AAT  CCT  ATA  TCT  GGC  CAT  GCT  ACC  ...  ...  ...  ...  ...  ...  ...  CTT  TAC

M33235   ,TRBV11-2*02          ---  ---  ---  ---  ---  ---  ---  ---  ---  ---  ---  ...  ...  ...  ...  ...  ...  ...  ---  ---

X58796   ,TRBV11-2*03          ---  ---  ---  ---  ---  ---  ---  ---  ---  ---  ---  ...  ...  ...  ...  ...  ...  ...  ---  ---


                                                                                                    ____________________CDR2-
                               41   42   43   44   45   46   47   48   49   50   51   52   53   54   55   56   57   58   59   60
                                W    Y    Q    Q    I    L    G    Q    G    P    K    L    L    I    Q    F    Q    N    N    G
L36092,U66059,TRBV11-2*01      TGG  TAC  CAG  CAG  ATC  CTG  GGA  CAG  GGC  CCA  AAG  CTT  CTG  ATT  CAG  TTT  CAG  AAT  AAC  GGT

M33235   ,TRBV11-2*02          ---  ---  ---  ---  ---  ---  ---  ---  ---  ---  ---  ---  ---  ---  ---  ---  ---  ---  ---  ---

X58796   ,TRBV11-2*03          ---  ---  ---  ---  ---  ---  ---  ---  ---  ---  ---  ---  ---  ---  ---  ---  ---  ---  ---  ---


                               IMGT_________________
                               61   62   63   64   65   66   67   68   69   70   71   72   73   74   75   76   77   78   79   80
                                V                        V    D    D    S    Q    L    P    K    D    R    F    S    A    E    R
L36092,U66059,TRBV11-2*01      GTA  ...  ...  ...  ...  GTG  GAT  GAT  TCA  CAG  TTG  CCT  AAG  GAT  CGA  TTT  TCT  GCA  GAG  AGG

M33235   ,TRBV11-2*02          ---  ...  ...  ...  ...  ---  ---  ---  ---  ---  ---  ---  ---  ---  ---  ---  ---  ---  ---  ---

X58796   ,TRBV11-2*03          ---  ...  ...  ...  ...  ---  ---  ---  ---  ---  ---  ---  ---  ---  ---  ---  ---  ---  ---  ---


                               81   82   83   84   85   86   87   88   89   90   91   92   93   94   95   96   97   98   99  100
                                L         K    G    V    D    S    T    L    K    I    Q    P    A    K    L    E    D    S    A
L36092,U66059,TRBV11-2*01      CTC  ...  AAA  GGA  GTA  GAC  TCC  ACT  CTC  AAG  ATC  CAG  CCT  GCA  AAG  CTT  GAG  GAC  TCG  GCC
                                                                                                          N
M33235   ,TRBV11-2*02          ---  ...  ---  ---  ---  ---  ---  ---  ---  ---  ---  ---  ---  ---  ---  ---  ---  A--  ---  ---

X58796   ,TRBV11-2*03          ---  ...  ---  ---  ---  ---  ---  ---  ---  ---  ---  --A  ---  ---  ---  ---  ---  ---  ---  ---


                                              ______CDR3-IMGT______
                              101  102  103  104  105  106  107  108  109
                                V    Y    L    C    A    S    S    L
L36092,U66059,TRBV11-2*01     GTG  TAT  CTC  TGT  GCC  AGC  AGC  TTA  GA

M33235   ,TRBV11-2*02         ---  ---  ---  ---  ---  ---  ---  --T            °

X58796   ,TRBV11-2*03         ---  ---  ---  ---  ---  ---  ---                 #c
```

#c: Rearranged cDNA
°: Genomic DNA, but not known as being germline or rearranged

Framework and complementarity determining regions

FR1-IMGT: 26   CDR1-IMGT: 5
FR2-IMGT: 17   CDR2-IMGT: 6
FR3-IMGT: 38 (-1 aa: 82)   CDR3-IMGT: 4

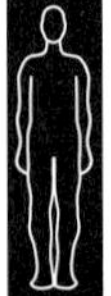

Collier de Perles for human TRBV11-2*01

Accession number: IMGT L36092   EMBL/GenBank/DDBJ: L36092

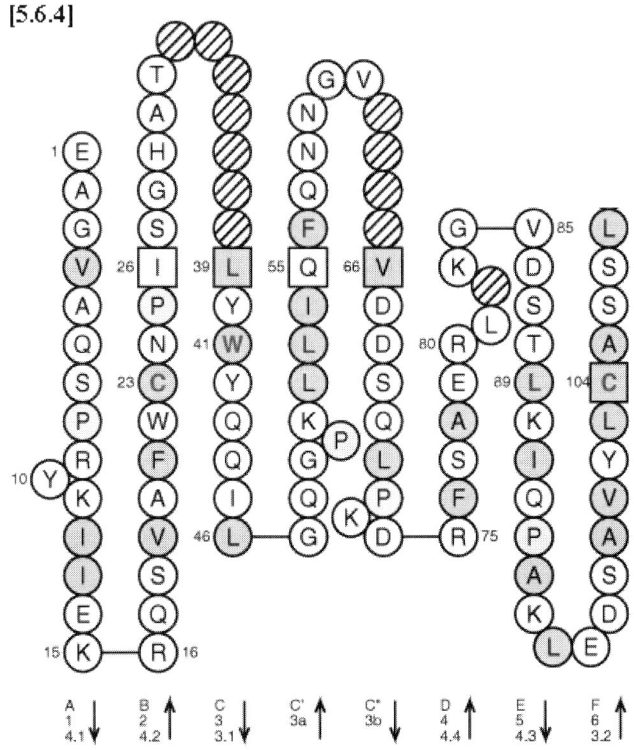

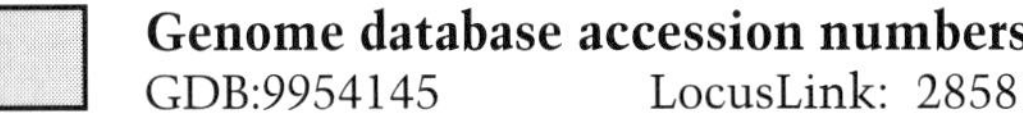

Genome database accession numbers

GDB:9954145   LocusLink: 28581

TRBV11-3

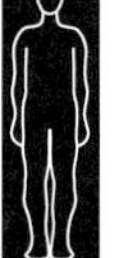

Nomenclature

TRBV11-3: T cell receptor beta variable 11-3.

Definition and functionality

TRBV11-3 is one of the three functional genes of the TRBV11 subgroup which comprises three mapped genes, in the TRB locus.

Gene location

TRBV11-3 is in the TRB locus on chromosome 7 at 7q34.

Nucleotide and amino acid sequences for human TRBV11-3

```
                              1   2   3   4   5   6   7   8   9  10  11  12  13  14  15  16  17  18  19  20
                              E   A   G   V   V   Q   S   P   R   Y   K   I   I   E   K   K   Q   P   V   A
M33234      ,TRBV11-3*01 [46] GAA GCT GGA GTG GTT CAG TCT CCC AGA TAT AAG ATT ATA GAG AAA AAA CAG CCT GTG GCT
U03115      ,TRBV11-3*01 [39] --- --- --- --- --- --- --- --- --- --- --- --- --- --- --- --- --- --- --- ---
L36092,U66060,TRBV11-3*01 [34] --- --- --- --- --- --- --- --- --- --- --- --- --- --- --- --- --- --- --- ---
AF009661    ,TRBV11-3*01 [35] --- --- --- --- --- --- --- --- --- --- --- --- --- --- --- --- --- --- --- ---
AF009663    ,TRBV11-3*01 [35] --- --- --- --- --- --- --- --- --- --- --- --- --- --- --- --- --- --- --- ---
X58797      ,TRBV11-3*02 [10] --- --- --- --- --- --- --- --- --- --- --- --- --- --- --- --- --G --- --- ---
M62377      ,TRBV11-3*03 [33] --- --- --- --- --- --- G-  --- --- --- --- --- --- --- --- --- --G --- --- ---
[13]        ,TRBV11-3*04      --- --- --- --- --- --- --- --- --- --- --- --- --- --- --- --- --- --- --- ---

                                                      ________________CDR1-IMGT_______________
                             21  22  23  24  25  26  27  28  29  30  31  32  33  34  35  36  37  38  39  40
                              F   W   C   N   P   I   S   G   H   N   T                           L   Y
M33234      ,TRBV11-3*01      TTT TGG TGC AAT CCT ATT TCT GGC CAC AAT ACC ... ... ... ... ... ... ... CTT TAC
U03115      ,TRBV11-3*01      --- --- --- --- --- --- --- --- --- --- --- ... ... ... ... ... ... ... --- ---
L36092,U66060,TRBV11-3*01    --- --- --- --- --- --- --- --- --- --- --- ... ... ... ... ... ... ... --- ---
AF009661    ,TRBV11-3*01      --- --- --- --- --- --- --- --- --- --- --- ... ... ... ... ... ... ... --- ---
AF009663    ,TRBV11-3*01      --- --- --- --- --- --- --- --- --- --- --- ... ... ... ... ... ... ... --- ---
X58797      ,TRBV11-3*02      --- --- --- --- --- --- --- --- --- --- --- ... ... ... ... ... ... ... --- ---
M62377      ,TRBV11-3*03      --- --- --- --- --A --- --- --- --- --- --- ... ... ... ... ... ... ... --- ---
[13]        ,TRBV11-3*04      --- --- --- --- --- --- --- --- --- --- --- ... ... ... ... ... ... ... --- ---

                                                                                          ___________CDR2-
                             41  42  43  44  45  46  47  48  49  50  51  52  53  54  55  56  57  58  59  60
                              W   Y   L   Q   N   L   G   Q   G   P   E   L   L   I   R   Y   E   N   E   E
M33234      ,TRBV11-3*01      TGG TAC CTG CAG AAC TTG GGA CAG GGC CCG GAG CTT CTG ATT CGA TAT GAG AAT GAG GAA
U03115      ,TRBV11-3*01      --- --- --- --- --- --- --- --- --- --- --- --- --- --- --- --- --- --- --- ---
L36092,U66060,TRBV11-3*01    --- --- --- --- --- --- --- --- --- --- --- --- --- --- --- --- --- --- --- ---
AF009661    ,TRBV11-3*01      --- --- --- --- --- --- --- --- --- --- --- --- --- --- --- --- --- --- --- ---
AF009663    ,TRBV11-3*01      --- --- --- --- --- --- --- --- --- --- --- --- --- --- --- --- --- --- --- ---
                                      R
X58797      ,TRBV11-3*02      --- --- -G- --- --- --- --- --- --- --- --- --- --- --- --- --- --- --- --- ---
M62377      ,TRBV11-3*03      --- --- --- --- --- --- --- --- --- --- --- --- --- --- --- --- --- --- --- ---
                                      R
[13]        ,TRBV11-3*04      --- --- -G- --- --- --- --- --- --- --- --- --- --- --- --- --- --- --- --- ---

                             IMGT_______________
                             61  62  63  64  65  66  67  68  69  70  71  72  73  74  75  76  77  78  79  80
                              A                   V   D   D   S   Q   L   P   K   D   R   F   S   A   E   R
M33234      ,TRBV11-3*01      GCA ... ... ... ... GTA GAC GAT TCA CAG TTG CCT AAG GAT CGA TTT TCT GCA GAG AGG
U03115      ,TRBV11-3*01      --- ... ... ... ... --- --- --- --- --- --- --- --- --- --- --- --- --- --- ---
L36092,U66060,TRBV11-3*01    --- ... ... ... ... --- --- --- --- --- --- --- --- --- --- --- --- --- --- ---
AF009661    ,TRBV11-3*01      --- ... ... ... ... --- --- --- --- --- --- --- --- --- --- --- --- --- --- ---
AF009663    ,TRBV11-3*01      --- ... ... ... ... --- --- --- --- --- --- --- --- --- --- --- --- --- --- ---
X58797      ,TRBV11-3*02      --- ... ... ... ... --- --- --- --- --- --- --- --- --- --- --- --- --- --- ---
M62377      ,TRBV11-3*03      --- ... ... ... ... --- --- --- --- --- --- --- --- --- --- --- --- --- --- ---
[13]        ,TRBV11-3*04      --- ... ... ... ... --- --- --- --- --- --- --- --- --- --- --- --- --- --- ---

                             81  82  83  84  85  86  87  88  89  90  91  92  93  94  95  96  97  98  99 100
                              L       K   G   V   D   S   T   L   K   I   Q   P   A   E   L   G   D   S   A
M33234      ,TRBV11-3*01      CTC ... AAA GGA GTA GAC TCC ACT CTC AAG ATC CAG CCT GCA GAG CTT GGG GAC TCG GCC
U03115      ,TRBV11-3*01      --- ... --- --- --- --- --- --- --- --- --- --- --- --- --- --- --- --- --- ---
L36092,U66060,TRBV11-3*01    --- ... --- --- --- --- --- --- --- --- --- --- --- --- --- --- --- --- --- ---
AF009661    ,TRBV11-3*01      --- ... --- --- --- --- --- --- --- --- --- --- --- --- --- --- --- --- --- ---
AF009663    ,TRBV11-3*01      --- ... --- --- --- --- --- --- --- --- --- --- --- --- --- --- --- --- --- ---
X58797      ,TRBV11-3*02      --- ... --- --- --- --- --- --- --- --- --- --- --- --- --- --- --- --- --- ---
M62377      ,TRBV11-3*03      --- ... --- --- --- --- --- --- --- --- --- --- --A --- --- --- --- --- --- ---
[13]        ,TRBV11-3*04      --- ... --- --- --- --- --- --- --- --- --- --- --- --- --- --- --- --- --- ---
```

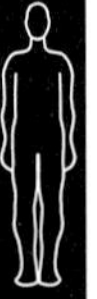

```
                                          ______CDR3-IMGT______
                        101 102 103 104 105 106 107 108 109
                         V   Y   L   C   A   S   S   L
      M33234   ,TRBV11-3*01   GTG TAT CTC TGT GCC AGC AGC TTA GA

      U03115   ,TRBV11-3*01   --- --- --- --- --- --- --- --- --

      L36092,U66060,TRBV11-3*01   --- --- --- --- --- --- --- --- --

      AF009661,TRBV11-3*01   --- --- --- --- --- --- --- --- --

      AF009663,TRBV11-3*01   --- --- --- --- --- --- --- --- --

      X58797   ,TRBV11-3*02   --- --- --- --- --- --- ---            #c
                               M
      M62377   ,TRBV11-3*03   A-- --- --- --- --- --- ---            #c

      [13]     ,TRBV11-3*04   --- --- --- --- --- --- ---            #
```

#: Rearranged
#c: Rearranged cDNA

Framework and complementarity determining regions

FR1-IMGT: 26   CDR1-IMGT: 5
FR2-IMGT: 17   CDR2-IMGT: 6
FR3-IMGT: 38 (-1 aa: 82)   CDR3-IMGT: 4

Collier de Perles for human TRBV11-3*01

Accession number: IMGT M33234   EMBL/GenBank/DDBJ: M33234

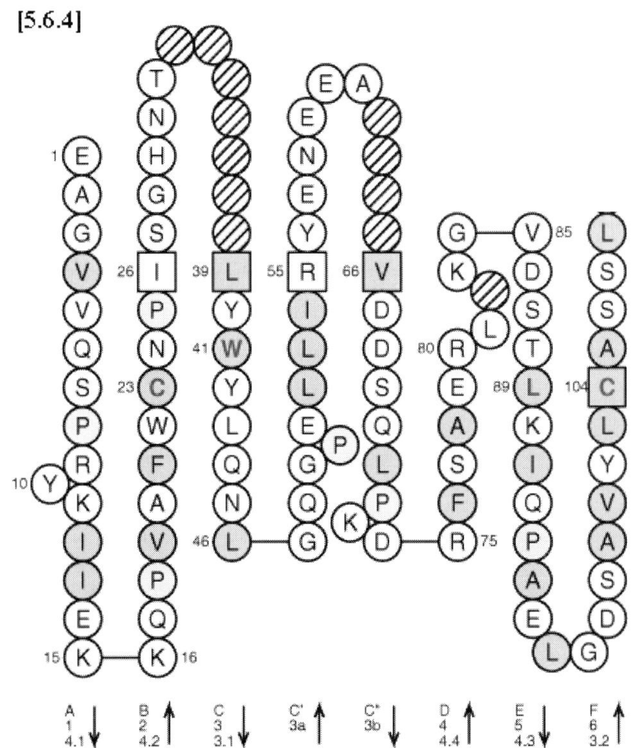

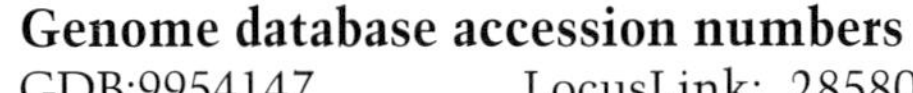

Genome database accession numbers
GDB:9954147   LocusLink: 28580

TRBV12-3

Nomenclature

TRBV12-3: T cell receptor beta variable 12-3.

Definition and functionality

TRBV12-3 is one of the three functional genes of the TRBV12 subgroup which comprises five mapped genes, in the TRB locus.

Gene location

TRBV12-3 is in the TRB locus on chromosome 7 at 7q34.

Nucleotide and amino acid sequences for human TRBV12-3

```
                              1   2   3   4   5   6   7   8   9  10  11  12  13  14  15  16  17  18  19  20
                              D   A   G   V   I   Q   S   P   R   H   E   V   T   E   M   G   Q   E   V   T
X07192   ,TRBV12-3*01   [38] GAT GCT GGA GTT ATC CAG TCA CCC CGC CAT GAG GTG ACA GAG ATG GGA CAA GAA GTG ACT

U03115   ,TRBV12-3*01   (39] --- --- --- --- --- --- --- --- --- --- --- --- --- --- --- --- --- --- --- ---

L36092,U66060,TRBV12-3*01 [34] --- --- --- --- --- --- --- --- --- --- --- --- --- --- --- --- --- --- --- ---

AF009661,TRBV12-3*01   [35] --- --- --- --- --- --- --- --- --- --- --- --- --- --- --- --- --- --- --- ---


                                                                        ________________CDR1-IMGT________________
                             21  22  23  24  25  26  27  28  29  30  31  32  33  34  35  36  37  38  39  40
                              L   R   C   K   P   I   S   G   H   N   S                               L   F
X07192   ,TRBV12-3*01        CTG AGA TGT AAA CCA ATT TCA GGC CAC AAC TCC ... ... ... ... ... ... ... CTT TTC

U03115   ,TRBV12-3*01        --- --- --- --- --- --- --- --- --- --- --- ... ... ... ... ... ... ... --- ---

L36092,U66060,TRBV12-3*01    --- --- --- --- --- --- --- --- --- --- --- ... ... ... ... ... ... ... --- ---

AF009661,TRBV12-3*01         --- --- --- --- --- --- --- --- --- --- --- ... ... ... ... ... ... ... --- ---


                                                                                            ___________________CDR2-
                             41  42  43  44  45  46  47  48  49  50  51  52  53  54  55  56  57  58  59  60
                              W   Y   R   Q   T   M   M   R   G   L   E   L   L   I   Y   F   N   N   N   V
X07192   ,TRBV12-3*01        TGG TAC AGA CAG ACC ATG ATG CGG GGA CTG GAG TTG CTC ATT TAC TTT AAC AAC AAC GTT

U03115   ,TRBV12-3*01        --- --- --- --- --- --- --- --- --- --- --- --- --- --- --- --- --- --- --- ---

L36092,U66060,TRBV12-3*01    --- --- --- --- --- --- --- --- --- --- --- --- --- --- --- --- --- --- --- ---

AF009661,TRBV12-3*01         --- --- --- --- --- --- --- --- --- --- --- --- --- --- --- --- --- --- --- ---


                             IMGT_______
                             61  62  63  64  65  66  67  68  69  70  71  72  73  74  75  76  77  78  79  80
                              P                   I   D   D   S   G   M   P   E   D   R   F   S   A   K   M
X07192   ,TRBV12-3*01        CCG ... ... ... ... ATA GAT GAT TCA GGG ATG CCC GAG GAT CGA TTC TCA GCT AAG ATG

U03115   ,TRBV12-3*01        --- ... ... ... ... --- --- --- --- --- --- --- --- --- --- --- --- --- --- ---

L36092,U66060,TRBV12-3*01    --- ... ... ... ... --- --- --- --- --- --- --- --- --- --- --- --- --- --- ---

AF009661,TRBV12-3*01         --- ... ... ... ... --- --- --- --- --- --- --- --- --- --- --- --- --- --- ---


                             81  82  83  84  85  86  87  88  89  90  91  92  93  94  95  96  97  98  99 100
                              P       N   A   S   F   S   T   L   K   I   Q   P   S   E   P   R   D   S   A
X07192   ,TRBV12-3*01        CCT ... AAT GCA TCA TTC TCC ACT CTG AAG ATC CAG CCC TCA GAA CCC AGG GAC TCA GCT

U03115   ,TRBV12-3*01        --- ...

L36092,U66060,TRBV12-3*01    --- ... --- --- --- --- --- --- --- --- --- --- --- --- --- --- --- --- --- ---

AF009661,TRBV12-3*01         --- ... --- --- --- --- --- --- --- --- --- --- --- --- --- --- --- --- --- ---


                                         ________CDR3-IMGT________
                            101 102 103 104 105 106 107 108 109
                              V   Y   F   C   A   S   S   L
X07192   ,TRBV12-3*01        GTG TAC TTC TGT GCC AGC AGT TTA GC

U03115   ,TRBV12-3*01        --- --- --- --- --- --- --- --- --

L36092,U66060,TRBV12-3*01    --- --- --- --- --- --- --- --- --

AF009661,TRBV12-3*01         --- --- --- --- --- --- --- --- --
```

Framework and complementarity determining regions

FR1-IMGT: 26   CDR1-IMGT: 5
FR2-IMGT: 17   CDR2-IMGT: 6
FR3-IMGT: 38 (-1 aa: 82)   CDR3-IMGT: 4

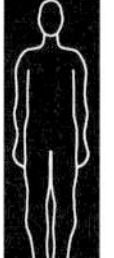

Collier de Perles for human TRBV12-3*01

Accession number: IMGT X07192   EMBL/GenBank/DDBJ: X07192

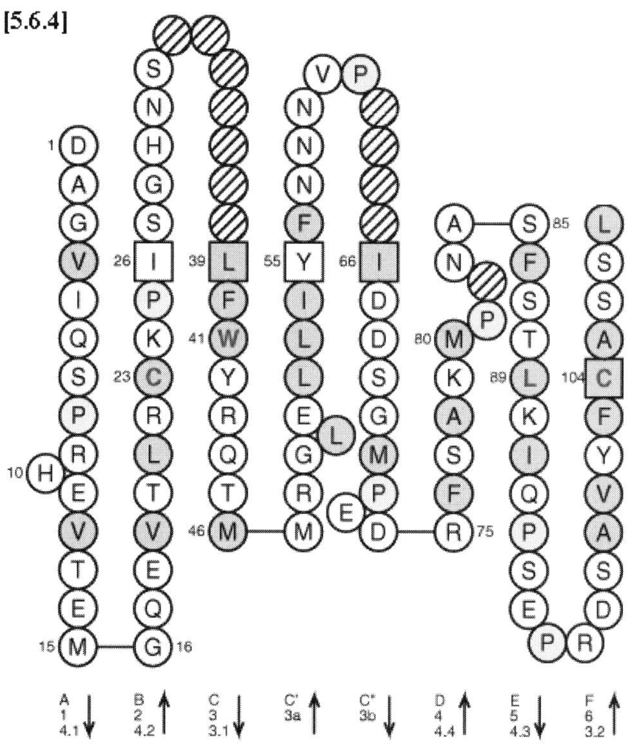

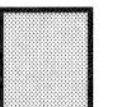

Genome database accession numbers
GDB:9954153   LocusLink: 28577

Nomenclature

TRBV12-4: T cell receptor beta variable 12-4.

Definition and functionality

TRBV12-4 is one of the three functional genes of the TRBV12 subgroup which comprises five mapped genes, in the TRB locus.

Gene location

TRBV12-4 is in the TRB locus on chromosome 7 at 7q34.

Nucleotide and amino acid sequences for human TRBV12-4

```
                                 1   2   3   4   5   6   7   8   9   10  11  12  13  14  15  16  17  18  19  20
                                 D   A   G   V   I   Q   S   P   R   H   E   V   T   E   M   G   Q   E   V   T
K02546     ,TRBV12-4*01     [37] GAT GCT GGA GTT ATC CAG TCA CCC CGG CAC GAG GTG ACA GAG ATG GGA CAA GAA GTG ACT
X07222     ,TRBV12-4*01     [38] --- --- --- --- --- --- --- --- --- --- --- --- --- --- --- --- --- --- --- ---
U03115     ,TRBV12-4*01     [39] --- --- --- --- --- --- --- --- --- --- --- --- --- --- --- --- --- --- --- ---
L36092,U66060,TRBV12-4*01   [34] --- --- --- --- --- --- --- --- --- --- --- --- --- --- --- --- --- --- --- ---
M14264     ,TRBV12-4*02     [41] --- --- --- --- --- --- --- --- --- --- --- --- --- --- --- --- --- --- --- ---

                                                                         CDR1-IMGT
                                 21  22  23  24  25  26  27  28  29  30  31  32  33  34  35  36  37  38  39  40
                                 L   R   C   K   P   I   S   G   H   D   Y                           L   F
K02546     ,TRBV12-4*01          CTG AGA TGT AAA CCA ATT TCA GGA CAC GAC TAC ... ... ... ... ... ... ... CTT TTC
X07222     ,TRBV12-4*01          --- --- --- --- --- --- --- --- --- --- --- ... ... ... ... ... ... ... --- ---
U03115     ,TRBV12-4*01          --- --- --- --- --- --- --- --- --- --- --- ... ... ... ... ... ... ... --- ---
L36092,U66060,TRBV12-4*01        --- --- --- --- --- --- --- --- --- --- --- ... ... ... ... ... ... ... --- ---
M14264     ,TRBV12-4*02          --- --- --- --- --- --- --- --- --- --T --- --- ... ... ... ... ... ... --- ---

                                                                                                     CDR2-
                                 41  42  43  44  45  46  47  48  49  50  51  52  53  54  55  56  57  58  59  60
                                 W   Y   R   Q   T   M   M   R   G   L   E   L   L   I   Y   F   N   N   N   V
K02546     ,TRBV12-4*01          TGG TAC AGA CAG ACC ATG ATG CGG GGA CTG GAG TTG CTC ATT TAC TTT AAC AAC AAC GTT
X07222     ,TRBV12-4*01          --- --- --- --- --- --- --- --- --- --- --- --- --- --- --- --- --- --- --- ---
U03115     ,TRBV12-4*01          --- --- --- --- --- --- --- --- --- --- --- --- --- --- --- --- --- --- --- ---
L36092,U66060,TRBV12-4*01        --- --- --- --- --- --- --- --- --- --- --- --- --- --- --- --- --- --- --- ---
M14264     ,TRBV12-4*02          --- --- --- --- --- --- --- --- --- --- --- --- --- --- --- --- --- --- --- ---

                                 IMGT
                                 61  62  63  64  65  66  67  68  69  70  71  72  73  74  75  76  77  78  79  80
                                 P                       I   D   D   S   G   M   P   E   D   R   F   S   A   K   M
K02546     ,TRBV12-4*01          CCG ... ... ... ... ... ATA GAT GAT TCA GGG ATG CCC GAG GAT CGA TTC TCA GCT AAG ATG
X07222     ,TRBV12-4*01          --- ... ... ... ... ... --- --- --- --- --- --- --- --- --- --- --- --- --- --- ---
U03115     ,TRBV12-4*01          --- ... ... ... ... ... --- --- --- --- --- --- --- --- --- --- --- --- --- --- ---
L36092,U66060,TRBV12-4*01        --- ... ... ... ... ... --- --- --- --- --- --- --- --- --- --- --- --- --- --- ---
M14264     ,TRBV12-4*02          --- ... ... ... ... ... --- --- --- --- --- --- --- --- --- --- --- --- --- --- ---

                                 81  82  83  84  85  86  87  88  89  90  91  92  93  94  95  96  97  98  99  100
                                 P       N   A   S   F   S   T   L   K   I   Q   P   S   E   P   R   D   S   A
K02546     ,TRBV12-4*01          CCT ... AAT GCA TCA TTC TCC ACT CTG AAG ATC CAG CCC TCA GAA CCC AGG GAC TCA GCT
X07222     ,TRBV12-4*01          --- ... --- --- --- --- --- --- --- --- --- --- --- --- --- --- --- --- --- ---
U03115     ,TRBV12-4*01          --- ... --- --- --- --- --- --- --- --- --- --- --- --- --- --- --- --- --- ---
L36092,U66060,TRBV12-4*01        --- ... --- --- --- --- --- --- --- --- --- --- --- --- --- --- --- --- --- ---
                                                                         R
M14264     ,TRBV12-4*02          --- ... --- --- --- --- --- --- --- -G- --- --- --- --- --- --- --- --- --- ---

                                             CDR3-IMGT
                                 101 102 103 104 105 106 107 108 109
                                 V   Y   F   C   A   S   S   L
K02546     ,TRBV12-4*01          GTG TAC TTC TGT GCC AGC AGT TTA GC
X07222     ,TRBV12-4*01          --- --- --- --- --- --- --- --- --
U03115     ,TRBV12-4*01          --- --- --- --- --- --- --- --- --
L36092,U66060,TRBV12-4*01        --- --- --- --- --- --- --- --- --
M14264     ,TRBV12-4*02          --- --- --- --- --- --- --- ---       #c
```

#c: Rearranged cDNA

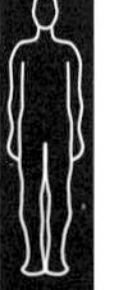

Framework and complementarity determining regions

FR1-IMGT: 26
FR2-IMGT: 17
FR3-IMGT: 38 (-1 aa: 82)

CDR1-IMGT: 5
CDR2-IMGT: 6
CDR3-IMGT: 4

Collier de Perles for human TRBV12-4*01

Accession number: IMGT K02546   EMBL/GenBank/DDBJ: K02546

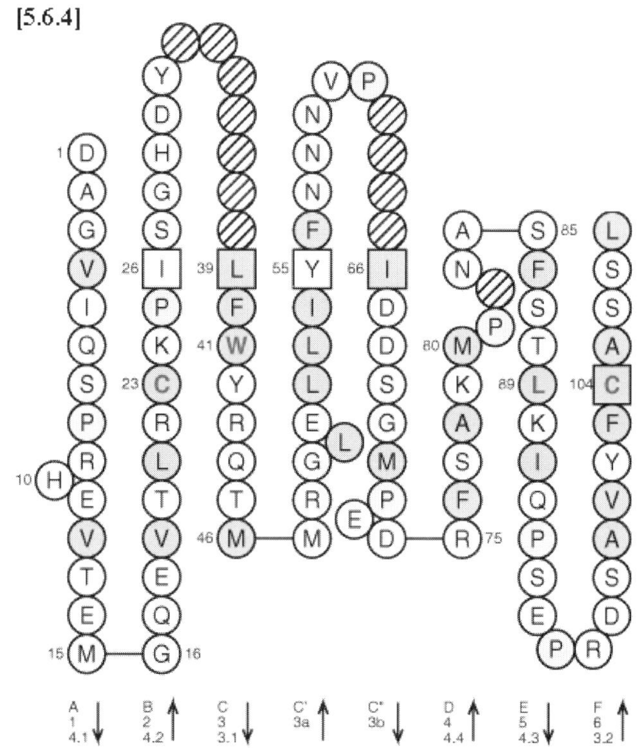

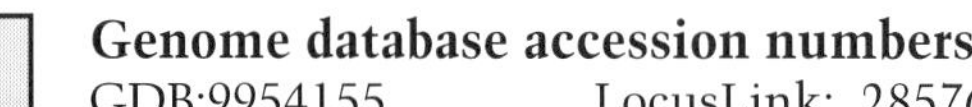

Genome database accession numbers

GDB:9954155   LocusLink: 28576

TRBV12-5

Nomenclature

TRBV12-5: T cell receptor beta variable 12-5.

Definition and functionality

TRBV12-5 is one of the three functional genes of the TRBV12 subgroup which comprises five mapped genes, in the TRB locus.

Gene location

TRBV12-5 is in the TRB locus on chromosome 7 at 7q34.

Nucleotide and amino acid sequences for human TRBV12-5

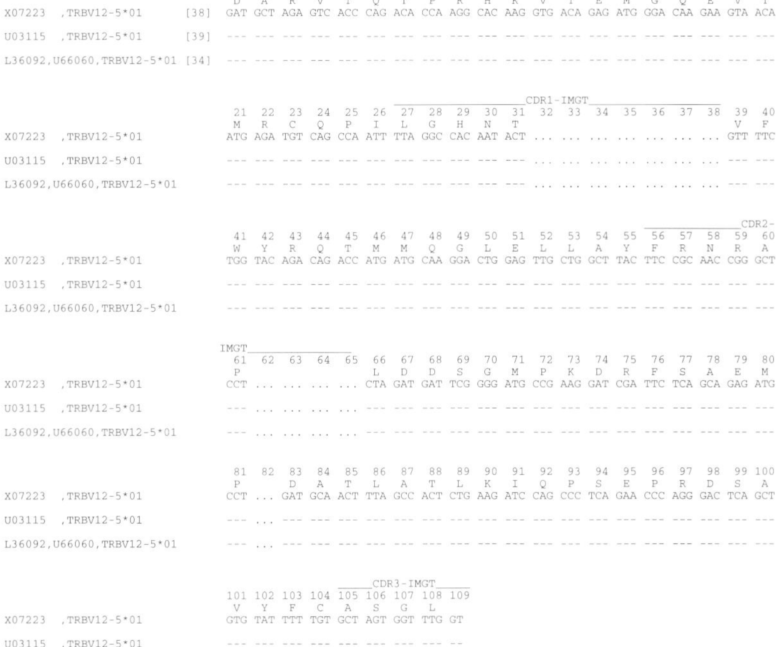

```
                          1   2   3   4   5   6   7   8   9  10  11  12  13  14  15  16  17  18  19  20
                          D   A   R   V   T   Q   T   P   R   H   K   V   T   E   M   G   Q   E   V   T
X07223    ,TRBV12-5*01  [38] GAT GCT AGA GTC ACC CAG ACA CCA AGG CAC AAG GTG ACA GAG ATG GGA CAA GAA GTA ACA

U03115    ,TRBV12-5*01  [39] --- --- --- --- --- --- --- --- --- --- --- --- --- --- --- --- --- --- --- ---

L36092,U66060,TRBV12-5*01 [34] --- --- --- --- --- --- --- --- --- --- --- --- --- --- --- --- --- --- --- ---


                                                                        ________________CDR1-IMGT________________
                         21  22  23  24  25  26  27  28  29  30  31  32  33  34  35  36  37  38  39  40
                          M   R   C   Q   P   I   L   G   H   N   T                                   V   F
X07223    ,TRBV12-5*01       ATG AGA TGT CAG CCA ATT TTA GGC CAC AAT ACT ... ... ... ... ... ... ... GTT TTC

U03115    ,TRBV12-5*01       --- --- --- --- --- --- --- --- --- --- --- ... ... ... ... ... ... ... --- ---

L36092,U66060,TRBV12-5*01    --- --- --- --- --- --- --- --- --- --- --- ... ... ... ... ... ... ... --- ---


                                                                                        ________________CDR2-
                         41  42  43  44  45  46  47  48  49  50  51  52  53  54  55  56  57  58  59  60
                          W   Y   R   Q   T   M   M   Q   G   L   E   L   L   A   Y   F   R   N   R   A
X07223    ,TRBV12-5*01       TGG TAC AGA CAG ACC ATG ATG CAA GGA CTG GAG TTG CTG GCT TAC TTC CGC AAC CGG GCT

U03115    ,TRBV12-5*01       --- --- --- --- --- --- --- --- --- --- --- --- --- --- --- --- --- --- --- ---

L36092,U66060,TRBV12-5*01    --- --- --- --- --- --- --- --- --- --- --- --- --- --- --- --- --- --- --- ---


                         IMGT________________
                         61  62  63  64  65  66  67  68  69  70  71  72  73  74  75  76  77  78  79  80
                          P                   L   D   D   S   G   M   P   K   D   R   F   S   A   E   M
X07223    ,TRBV12-5*01       CCT ... ... ... ... CTA GAT GAT TCG GGG ATG CCG AAG GAT CGA TTC TCA GCA GAG ATG

U03115    ,TRBV12-5*01       --- ... ... ... ... --- --- --- --- --- --- --- --- --- --- --- --- --- --- ---

L36092,U66060,TRBV12-5*01    --- ... ... ... ... --- --- --- --- --- --- --- --- --- --- --- --- --- --- ---


                         81  82  83  84  85  86  87  88  89  90  91  92  93  94  95  96  97  98  99 100
                          P       D   A   T   L   A   T   L   K   I   Q   P   S   E   P   R   D   S   A
X07223    ,TRBV12-5*01       CCT ... GAT GCA ACT TTA GCC ACT CTG AAG ATC CAG CCC TCA GAA CCC AGG GAC TCA GCT

U03115    ,TRBV12-5*01       --- ... --- --- --- --- --- --- --- --- --- --- --- --- --- --- --- --- --- ---

L36092,U66060,TRBV12-5*01    --- ... --- --- --- --- --- --- --- --- --- --- --- --- --- --- --- --- --- ---


                                            ______CDR3-IMGT______
                        101 102 103 104 105 106 107 108 109
                          V   Y   F   C   A   S   G   L
X07223    ,TRBV12-5*01       GTG TAT TTT TGT GCT AGT GGT TTG GT

U03115    ,TRBV12-5*01       --- --- --- --- --- --- --- --- --

L36092,U66060,TRBV12-5*01    --- --- --- --- --- --- --- --- --
```

Framework and complementarity determining regions

FR1-IMGT: 26	CDR1-IMGT: 5
FR2-IMGT: 17	CDR2-IMGT: 6
FR3-IMGT: 38 (-1 aa: 82)	CDR3-IMGT: 4

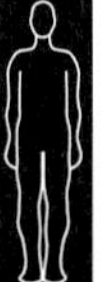

Collier de Perles for human TRBV12-5*01

Accession number: IMGT X07223   EMBL/GenBank/DDBJ: X07223

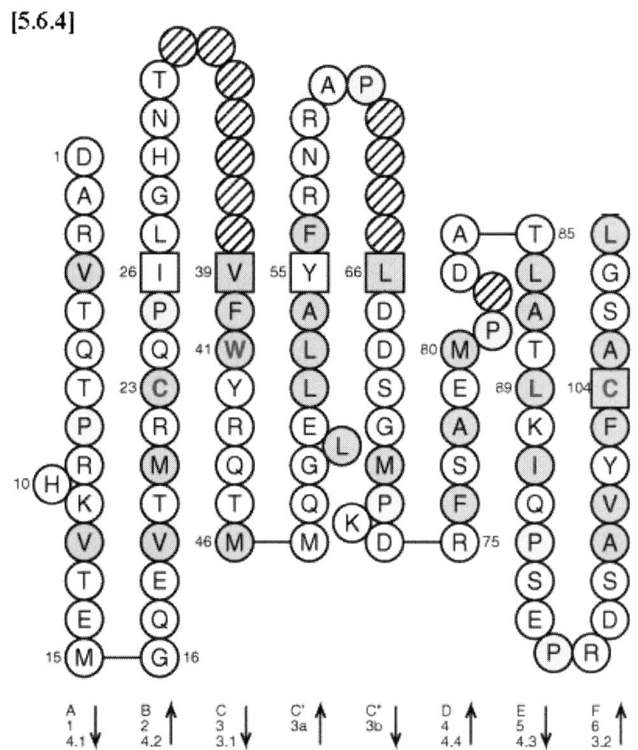

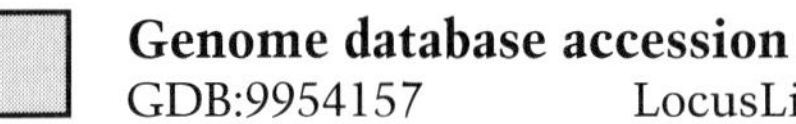

Genome database accession numbers
GDB:9954157   LocusLink: 28575

Nomenclature

TRBV13: T cell receptor beta variable 13.

Definition and functionality

TRBV13 is the unique functional gene of the TRBV13 subgroup which only comprises this mapped gene, in the TRB locus.

Gene location

TRBV13 is in the TRB locus on chromosome 7 at 7q34.

Nucleotide and amino acid sequences for human TRBV13

```
                             1   2   3   4   5   6   7   8   9   10  11  12  13  14  15  16  17  18  19  20
                             A   A   G   V   I   Q   S   P   R   H   L   I   K   E   K   R   E   T   A   T
U03115    ,TRBV13*01  [39]   GCT GCT GGA GTC ATC CAG TCC CCA AGA CAT CTG ATC AAA GAA AAG AGG GAA ACA GCC ACT

L36092,U66060,TRBV13*01 [34] --- --- --- --- --- --- --- --- --- --- --- --- --- --- --- --- --- --- --- ---

AF009661,TRBV13*01   [35]    --- --- --- --- --- --- --- --- --- --- --- --- --- --- --- --- --- --- --- ---

AF009663,TRBV13*01   [35]    --- --- --- --- --- --- --- --- --- --- --- --- --- --- --- --- --- --- --- ---

U96844    ,TRBV13*01 [29]    --- --- --- --- --- --- --- --- --- --- --- --- --- --- --- --- --- --- --- ---
                                                                                 R
M62378    ,TRBV13*02 [33]    --- --- --- --- --- --- --- --- --- --- --- --- -G- --- --- --- --- --- --- ---


                                                               __________CDR1-IMGT__________________________
                             21  22  23  24  25  26  27  28  29  30  31  32  33  34  35  36  37  38  39  40
                             L   K   C   Y   P   I   P   R   H   D   T                               V   Y
U03115    ,TRBV13*01         CTG AAA TGC TAT CCT ATC CCT AGA CAC GAC ACT ... ... ... ... ... ... ... GTC TAC

L36092,U66060,TRBV13*01      --- --- --- --- --- --- --- --- --- --- --- ... ... ... ... ... ... ... --- ---

AF009661,TRBV13*01           --- --- --- --- --- --- --- --- --- --- --- ... ... ... ... ... ... ... --- ---

AF009663,TRBV13*01           --- --- --- --- --- --- --- --- --- --- --- ... ... ... ... ... ... ... --- ---

U96844    ,TRBV13*01         --- --- --- --- --- --- --- --- --- --- --- ... ... ... ... ... ... ... --- ---

M62378    ,TRBV13*02         --- --- --- --- --- --- --- --- --- --- --- ... ... ... ... ... ... ... --- ---


                                                                                         ________________CDR2-
                             41  42  43  44  45  46  47  48  49  50  51  52  53  54  55  56  57  58  59  60
                             W   Y   Q   Q   G   P   G   Q   D   P   Q   F   L   I   S   F   Y   E   K   M
U03115    ,TRBV13*01         TGG TAC CAG CAG GGT CCA GGT CAG GAC CCC CAG TTC CTC ATT TCG TTT TAT GAA AAG ATG

L36092,U66060,TRBV13*01      --- --- --- --- --- --- --- --- --- --- --- --- --- --- --- --- --- --- --- ---

AF009661,TRBV13*01           --- --- --- --- --- --- --- --- --- --- --- --- --- --- --- --- --- --- --- ---

AF009663,TRBV13*01           --- --- --- --- --- --- --- --- --- --- --- --- --- --- --- --- --- --- --- ---

U96844    ,TRBV13*01         --- --- --- --- --- --- --- --- --- --- --- --- --- --- --- --- --- --- --- ---
                                                                                     F
M62378    ,TRBV13*02         --- --- --- --C --- --- --- --- --- --- --- T-- --- --- --- --- --- --- --- ---


                             IMGT________________
                             61  62  63  64  65  66  67  68  69  70  71  72  73  74  75  76  77  78  79  80
                             Q                   S   D   K   G   S   I   P       D   R   F   S   A   Q   Q
U03115    ,TRBV13*01         CAG ... ... ... ... AGC GAT AAA GGA AGC ATC CCT ... GAT CGA TTC TCA GCT CAA CAG

L36092,U66060,TRBV13*01      --- ... ... ... ... --- --- --- --- --- --- --- ... --- --- --- --- --- --- ---

AF009661,TRBV13*01           --- ... ... ... ... --- --- --- --- --- --- --- ... --- --- --- --- --- --- ---

AF009663,TRBV13*01           --- ... ... ... ... --- --- --- --- --- --- --- ... --- --- --- --- --- --- ---

U96844    ,TRBV13*01         --- ... ... ... ... --- --- --- --- --- --- --- ... --- --- --- --- --- --- ---

M62378    ,TRBV13*02         --- ... ... ... ... --- --- --- --- --- --- --- ... --- --- --- --- --- --- ---


                             81  82  83  84  85  86  87  88  89  90  91  92  93  94  95  96  97  98  99  100
                             F       S   D   Y   H   S   E   L   N   M   S   S   L   E   L   G   D   S   A
U03115    ,TRBV13*01         TTC ... AGT GAC TAT CAT TCT GAA CTG AAC ATG AGC TCC TTG GAG CTG GGG GAC TCA GCC

L36092,U66060,TRBV13*01      --- ... --- --- --- --- --- --- --- --- --- --- --- --- --- --- --- --- --- ---

AF009661,TRBV13*01           --- ... --- --- --- --- --- --- --- --- --- --- --- --- --- --- --- --- --- ---

AF009663,TRBV13*01           --- ... --- --- --- --- --- --- --- --- --- --- --- --- --- --- --- --- --- ---

U96844    ,TRBV13*01         --- ... --- --- --- --- --- --- --- --- --- --- --- --- --- --- --- --- --- ---

M62378    ,TRBV13*02         --- ... --- --- --- --- --- --- --- --- --- --- --- --- --- --- --- --- --- ---
```

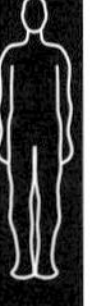

```
                                           ____CDR3-IMGT____
                              101 102 103 104 105 106 107 108 109
                               L   Y   F   C   A   S   S   L
   U03115    ,TRBV13*01        CTG TAC TTC TGT GCC AGC AGC TTA GG

   L36092,U66060,TRBV13*01     --- --- --- --- --- --- --- --- --

   AF009661,TRBV13*01          --- --- --- --- --- --- --- --- --

   AF009663,TRBV13*01          --- --- --- --- --- --- --- --- --

   U96844    ,TRBV13*01        --- --- --- --- --- --- --- --- --

   M62378    ,TRBV13*02        --- --- --- --- --- --- ---              #c

#c: Rearranged cDNA
```

Framework and complementarity determining regions

FR1-IMGT: 26   CDR1-IMGT: 5
FR2-IMGT: 17   CDR2-IMGT: 6
FR3-IMGT: 37 (-2 aa: 73, 82)   CDR3-IMGT: 4

Collier de Perles for human TRBV13*01

Accession number: IMGT U03115   EMBL/GenBank/DDBJ: U03115

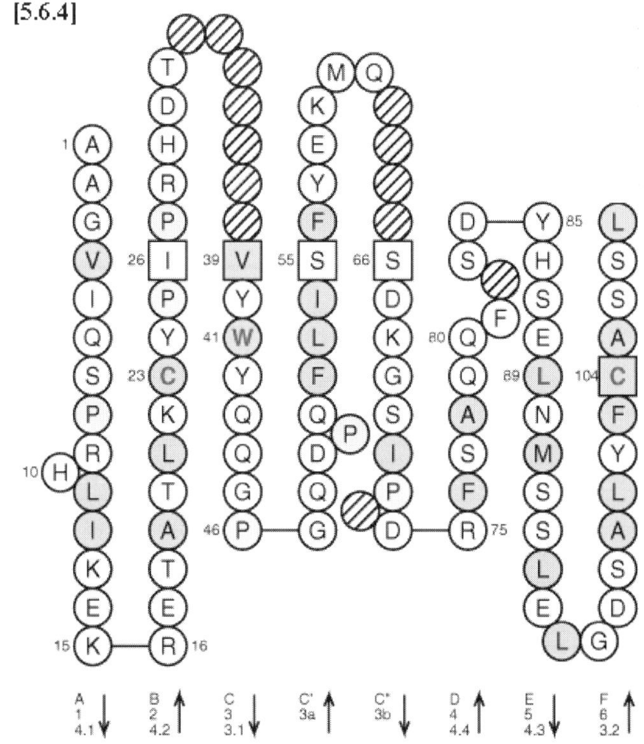

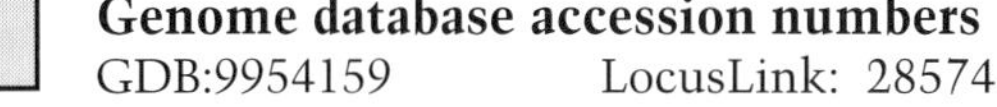

Genome database accession numbers

GDB:9954159   LocusLink: 28574

TRBV14

Nomenclature

TRBV14: T cell receptor beta variable 14.

Definition and functionality

TRBV14 is the unique functional gene of the TRBV14 subgroup which only comprises this mapped gene, in the TRB locus.

Gene location

TRBV14 is in the TRB locus on chromosome 7 at 7q34.

Nucleotide and amino acid sequences for human TRBV14

```
                                1    2    3    4    5    6    7    8    9   10   11   12   13   14   15   16   17   18   19   20
                                E    A    G    V    T    Q    F    P    S    H    S    V    I    E    K    G    Q    T    V    T
X06154     ,TRBV14*01    [40]  GAA  GCT  GGA  GTT  ACT  CAG  TTC  CCC  AGC  CAC  AGC  GTA  ATA  GAG  AAG  GGC  CAG  ACT  GTG  ACT

U03115     ,TRBV14*01    [39]  ---  ---  ---  ---  ---  ---  ---  ---  ---  ---  ---  ---  ---  ---  ---  ---  ---  ---  ---  ---

L36092,U66060,TRBV14*01  [34]  ---  ---  ---  ---  ---  ---  ---  ---  ---  ---  ---  ---  ---  ---  ---  ---  ---  ---  ---  ---

X57722     ,TRBV14*02    [31]  ---  ---  ---  ---  ---  ---  ---  ---  ---  ---  ---  ---  ---  ---  ---  ---  ---  ---  ---  ---


                                                                        ________________CDR1-IMGT________________
                               21   22   23   24   25   26   27   28   29   30   31   32   33   34   35   36   37   38   39   40
                                L    R    C    D    P    I    S    G    H    D    N                                  L    Y
X06154     ,TRBV14*01          CTG  AGA  TGT  GAC  CCA  ATT  TCT  GGA  CAT  GAT  AAT  ...  ...  ...  ...  ...  ...  ...  CTT  TAT

U03115     ,TRBV14*01          ---  ---  ---  ---  ---  ---  ---  ---  ---  ---  ---  ...  ...  ...  ...  ...  ...  ...  ---  ---

L36092,U66060,TRBV14*01        ---  ---  ---  ---  ---  ---  ---  ---  ---  ---  ---  ...  ...  ...  ...  ...  ...  ...  ---  ---

X57722     ,TRBV14*02          ---  ---  ---  ---  ---  ---  ---  ---  ---  ---  ---  ...  ...  ...  ...  ...  ...  ...  ---  ---


                                                                                               ________________CDR2-
                               41   42   43   44   45   46   47   48   49   50   51   52   53   54   55   56   57   58   59   60
                                W    Y    R    R    V    M    G    K    E    I    K    F    L    L    H    F    V    K    E    S
X06154     ,TRBV14*01          TGG  TAT  CGA  CGT  GTT  ATG  GGA  AAA  GAA  ATA  AAA  TTT  CTG  TTA  CAT  TTT  GTG  AAA  GAG  TCT

U03115     ,TRBV14*01          ---  ---  ---  ---  ---  ---  ---  ---  ---  ---  ---  ---  ---  ---  ---  ---  ---  ---  ---  ---

L36092,U66060,TRBV14*01        ---  ---  ---  ---  ---  ---  ---  ---  ---  ---  ---  ---  ---  ---  ---  ---  ---  ---  ---  ---

X57722     ,TRBV14*02          ---  ---  ---  ---  ---  ---  ---  ---  ---  ---  ---  ...  ...  ...  ...  ...  ...  ...  ---  ---


                               IMGT________________
                               61   62   63   64   65   66   67   68   69   70   71   72   73   74   75   76   77   78   79   80
                                K                        Q    D    E    S    G    M    P    N    N    R    F    L    A    E    R
X06154     ,TRBV14*01          AAA  ...  ...  ...  ...  CAG  GAT  GAG  TCC  GGT  ATG  CCC  AAC  AAT  CGA  TTC  TTA  GCT  GAA  AGG

U03115     ,TRBV14*01          ---  ...  ...  ...  ...  ---  ---  ---  ---  ---  ---  ---  ---  ---  ---  ---  ---  ---  ---  ---

L36092,U66060,TRBV14*01        ---  ...  ...  ...  ...  ---  ---  ---  ---  ---  ---  ---  ---  ---  ---  ---  ---  ---  ---  ---

X57722     ,TRBV14*02          ---  ...  ...  ...  ...  ---  ---  --A  ---  ---  ---  ---  ---  ---  ---  ---  ---  ---  ---  ---


                               81   82   83   84   85   86   87   88   89   90   91   92   93   94   95   96   97   98   99  100
                                T         G    G    T    Y    S    T    L    K    V    Q    P    A    E    L    E    D    S    G
X06154     ,TRBV14*01          ACT  ...  GGA  GGG  ACG  TAT  TCT  ACT  CTG  AAG  GTG  CAG  CCT  GCA  GAA  CTG  GAG  GAT  TCT  GGA

U03115     ,TRBV14*01          ---  ...  ---  ---  ---  ---  ---  ---  ---  ---  ---  ---  ---  ---  ---  ---  ---  ---  ---  ---

L36092,U66060,TRBV14*01        ---  ...  ---  ---  ---  ---  ---  ---  ---  ---  ---  ---  ---  ---  ---  ---  ---  ---  ---  ---

X57722     ,TRBV14*02          ---  ...  ---  ---  ---  ---  ---  ---  ---  ---  ---  ---  ---  ---  ---  ---  ---  ---  ---  ---


                                                    ________CDR3-IMGT________
                              101  102  103  104  105  106  107  108  109
                                V    Y    F    C    A    S    S    Q
X06154     ,TRBV14*01         GTT  TAT  TTC  TGT  GCC  AGC  AGC  CAA  GA

U03115     ,TRBV14*01         ---  ---  ---  ---  ---  ---  ---  ---  --

L36092,U66060,TRBV14*01       ---  ---  ---  ---  ---  ---  ---  ---  --

X57722     ,TRBV14*02         ---  ---  ---  ---  ---  ---  ---                  #g
```

#g: Rearranged genomic DNA

Framework and complementarity determining regions

FR1-IMGT: 26
FR2-IMGT: 17
FR3-IMGT: 38 (-1 aa: 82)

CDR1-IMGT: 5
CDR2-IMGT: 6
CDR3-IMGT: 4

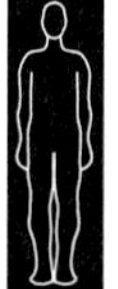

Collier de Perles for human TRBV14*01

Accession number: IMGT X06154   EMBL/GenBank/DDBJ: X06154

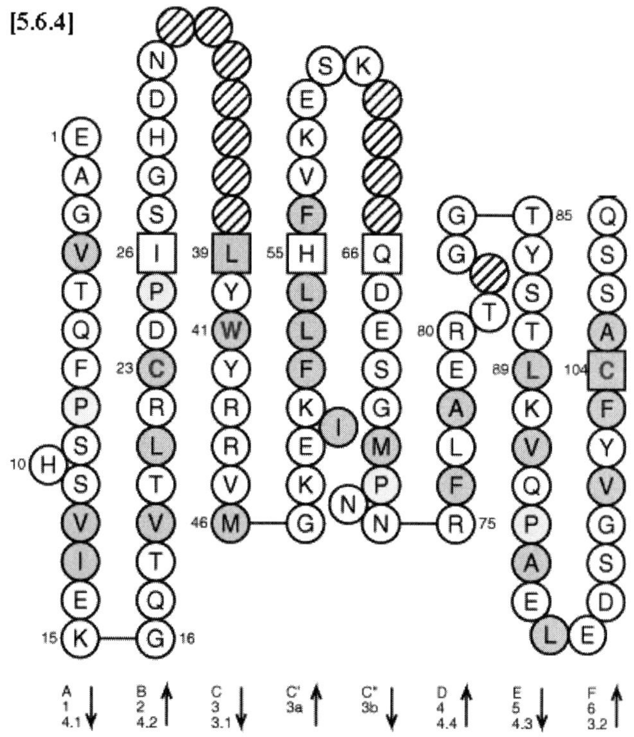

Genome database accession numbers
GDB:9954161   LocusLink: 28573

TRBV15

Nomenclature

TRBV15: T cell receptor beta variable 15.

Definition and functionality

TRBV15 is the unique functional gene of the TRBV15 subgroup which only comprises this mapped gene, in the TRB locus.

Gene location

TRBV15 is in the TRB locus on chromosome 7 at 7q34.

Nucleotide and amino acid sequences for human TRBV15

```
                          1   2   3   4   5   6   7   8   9  10  11  12  13  14  15  16  17  18  19  20
                          D   A   M   V   I   Q   N   P   R   Y   Q   V   T   Q   F   G   K   P   V   T
U03115   ,TRBV15*01 [39] GAT GCC ATG GTC ATC CAG AAC CCA AGA TAC CAG GTT ACC CAG TTT GGA AAG CCA GTG ACC

L36092,U66060,TRBV15*01 [34] --- --- --- --- --- --- --- --- --- --- --- --- --- --- --- --- --- --- --- ---

X58800   ,TRBV15*02 [10] --- --- --- --- --- --- --- --- --- --- --- --- --- --- --- --- --- --- --- ---
                                                                      R
M62376   ,TRBV15*03 [33] --- --- --- --- --- --- --- --- --- --- -G- --- --- --- --- --- --- --- --- ---


                                                                    ________CDR1-IMGT________
                         21  22  23  24  25  26  27  28  29  30  31  32  33  34  35  36  37  38  39  40
                          L   S   C   S   Q   T   L   N   H   N   V                           M   Y
U03115   ,TRBV15*01      CTG AGT TGT TCT CAG ACT TTG AAC CAT AAC GTC ... ... ... ... ... ... ATG TAC

L36092,U66060,TRBV15*01 --- --- --- --- --- --- --- --- --- --- --- ... ... ... ... ... ... --- ---

X58800   ,TRBV15*02     --- --- --- --- --- --- --- --- --- --- --- ... ... ... ... ... ... --- ---

M62376   ,TRBV15*03     --- --- --- --- --- --- --- --- --- --- --- ... ... ... ... ... ... --- ---


                                                                            ________________CDR2-
                         41  42  43  44  45  46  47  48  49  50  51  52  53  54  55  56  57  58  59  60
                          W   Y   Q   Q   K   S   S   Q   A   P   K   L   L   F   H   Y   Y   D   K   D
U03115   ,TRBV15*01     TGG TAC CAG CAG AAG TCA AGT CAG GCC CCA AAG CTG CTG TTC CAC TAC TAT GAC AAA GAT

L36092,U66060,TRBV15*01 --- --- --- --- --- --- --- --- --- --- --- --- --- --- --- --- --- --- --- ---

X58800   ,TRBV15*02     --- --- --- --- --- --- --- --- --- --- --- --- --- --- --- --- --- --- --- ---
                                                                                    N
M62376   ,TRBV15*03     --- --- --- --- --- --- --- --- --- --- --- --- --- --- --- A-- --- ---


                         IMGT________________
                         61  62  63  64  65  66  67  68  69  70  71  72  73  74  75  76  77  78  79  80
                          F                   N   N   E   A   D   T   P       D   N   F   Q   S   R   R
U03115   ,TRBV15*01     TTT ... ... ... ... AAC AAT GAA GCA GAC ACC CCT ... GAT AAC TTC CAA TCC AGG AGG

L36092,U66060,TRBV15*01 --- ... ... ... ... --- --- --- --- --- --- --- ... --- --- --- --- --- ---

X58800   ,TRBV15*02     --- ... ... ... ... --- --- --- --- --- --- --- ... --- --- --- --- --- ---

M62376   ,TRBV15*03     --- ... ... ... ... --- --- --- --- --- --- --- ... --- --- --- --- --- ---


                         81  82  83  84  85  86  87  88  89  90  91  92  93  94  95  96  97  98  99 100
                          P       N   T   S   F   C   F   L   D   I   R   S   P   G   L   G   D   T   A
U03115   ,TRBV15*01     CCG ... AAC ACT TCT TTC TGC TTT CTT GAC ATC CGC TCA CCA GGC CTG GGG GAC ACA GCC

L36092,U66060,TRBV15*01 --- ... --- --- --- --- --- --- --- --- --- --- --- --- --- --- --- --- ---
                                                                                                    A
X58800   ,TRBV15*02     --- ... --- --- --- --- --- --- --- --- --- --- --- --- --- --- --- G-- ---
                                                                                                    A
M62376   ,TRBV15*03     --- ... --- --- --- --- --- --- --A --- --- --- --- --- --- --- --- G-- ---


                                         ________CDR3-IMGT________
                        101 102 103 104 105 106 107 108 109
                          M   Y   L   C   A   T   S   R
U03115   ,TRBV15*01     ATG TAC CTG TGT GCC ACC AGC AGA GA

L36092,U66060,TRBV15*01 --- --- --- --- --- --- --- --- --

X58800   ,TRBV15*02     --- --- --- --- --- --- ---            #c
                                         Q
M62376   ,TRBV15*03     --- --- -A- --- --- --- ---            #c
```

#c: Rearranged cDNA

Framework and complementarity determining regions

FR1-IMGT: 26

FR2-IMGT: 17

FR3-IMGT: 37 (-2 aa: 73, 82)

CDR1-IMGT: 5

CDR2-IMGT: 6

CDR3-IMGT: 4

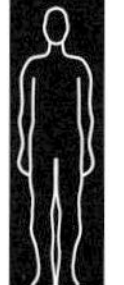

Collier de Perles for human TRBV15*01

Accession number: IMGT U03115   EMBL/GenBank/DDBJ: U03115

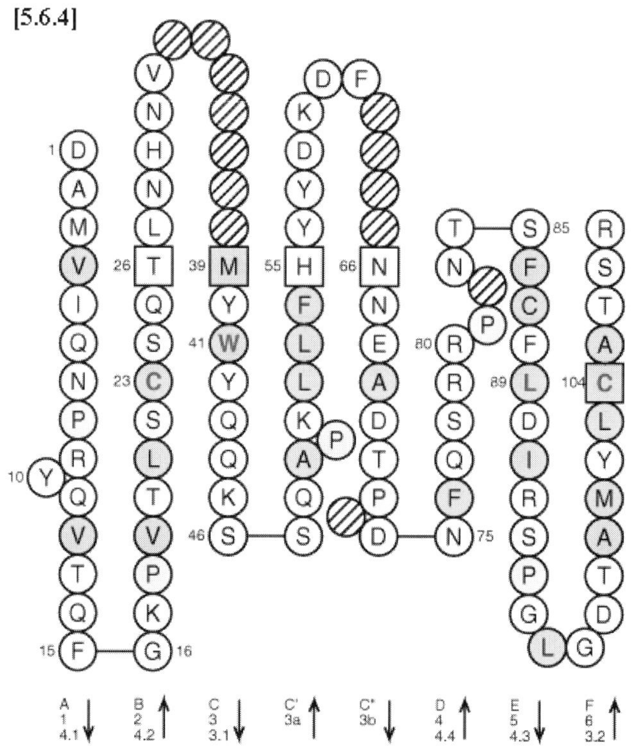

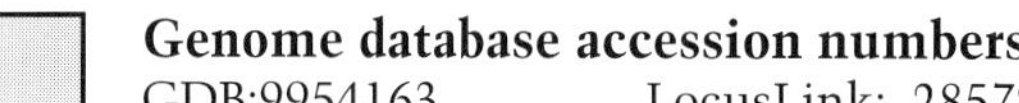

Genome database accession numbers
GDB:9954163   LocusLink: 28572

Nomenclature

TRBV16: T cell receptor beta variable 16.

Definition and functionality

TRBV16 is a functional gene (alleles *01 and *03) or a pseudogene (allele *02). TRBV16 belongs to the TRBV16 subgroup which only comprises this mapped gene, in the TRB locus.

TRBV16*02 is a pseudogene due to Tyrosine (tat) 31 being replaced by a STOP-CODON (tag), in the FR1-IMGT.

Gene location

TRBV16 is in the TRB locus on chromosome 7 at 7q34.

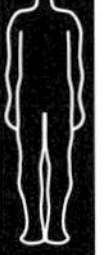

Nucleotide and amino acid sequences for human TRBV16

```
                                1    2    3    4    5    6    7    8    9   10   11   12   13   14   15   16   17   18   19   20
                                G    E    E    V    A    Q    T    P    K    H    L    V    R    G    E    G    Q    K    A    K
  L26231    ,TRBV16*01     [44] GGT  GAA  GAA  GTC  GCC  CAG  ACT  CCA  AAA  CAT  CTT  GTC  AGA  GGG  GAA  GGA  CAG  AAA  GCA  AAA

  U03115    ,TRBV16*02     [39] ---  ---  ---  ---  ---  ---  ---  ---  ---  ---  ---  ---  ---  ---  ---  ---  ---  ---  ---  ---

  L36092,U66060,TRBV16*02  [34] ---  ---  ---  ---  ---  ---  ---  ---  ---  ---  ---  ---  ---  ---  ---  ---  ---  ---  ---  ---

  L26054    ,TRBV16*03     [12] ---  ---  ---  ---  ---  ---  ---  ---  ---  ---  ---  ---  ---  ---  ---  ---  ---  ---  ---  ---


                                                                              ______________________CDR1-IMGT__________________
                                21   22   23   24   25   26   27   28   29   30   31   32   33   34   35   36   37   38   39   40
                                L    Y    C    A    P    I    K    G    H    S    Y                                      V    F
  L26231    ,TRBV16*01          TTA  TAT  TGT  GCC  CCA  ATA  AAA  GGA  CAC  AGT  TAT  ...  ...  ...  ...  ...  ...  ...  GTT  TTT
                                                                              *
  U03115    ,TRBV16*02          ---  ---  ---  ---  ---  ---  ---  ---  ---  ---  --G  ...  ...  ...  ...  ...  ...  ...  ---  ---
                                                                              *
  L36092,U66060,TRBV16*02       ---  ---  ---  ---  ---  ---  ---  ---  ---  ---  --G  ...  ...  ...  ...  ...  ...  ...  ---  ---

  L26054    ,TRBV16*03          ---  ---  ---  ---  ---  ---  ---  ---  ---  ---  ---  ...  ...  ...  ...  ...  ...  ...  ---  ---


                                                                                        ___________________________CDR2-
                                41   42   43   44   45   46   47   48   49   50   51   52   53   54   55   56   57   58   59   60
                                W    Y    Q    Q    V    L    K    N    E    F    K    F    L    I    S    F    Q    N    E    N
  L26231    ,TRBV16*01          TGG  TAC  CAA  CAG  GTC  CTG  AAA  AAC  GAG  TTC  AAG  TTC  TTG  ATT  TCC  TTC  CAG  AAT  GAA  AAT

  U03115    ,TRBV16*02          ---  ---  ---  ---  ---  ---  ---  ---  ---  ---  ---  ---  ---  ---  ---  ---  ---  ---  ---  ---

  L36092,U66060,TRBV16*02       ---  ---  ---  ---  ---  ---  ---  ---  ---  ---  ---  ---  ---  ---  ---  ---  ---  ---  ---  ---
                                                                                             V
  L26054    ,TRBV16*03          ---  ---  ---  ---  ---  ---  ---  ---  ---  ---  ---  G--  ---  ---  ---  ---  ---  ---  ---  ---


                                IMGT________________
                                61   62   63   64   65   66   67   68   69   70   71   72   73   74   75   76   77   78   79   80
                                V                        F    D    E    T    G    M    P    K    E    R    F    S    A    K    C
  L26231    ,TRBV16*01          GTC  ...  ...  ...  ...  TTT  GAT  GAA  ACA  GGT  ATG  CCC  AAG  GAA  AGA  TTT  TCA  GCT  AAG  TGC

  U03115    ,TRBV16*02          ---  ...  ...  ...  ...  ---  ---  ---  ---  ---  ---  ---  ---  ---  ---  ---  ---  ---  ---  ---

  L36092,U66060,TRBV16*02       ---  ...  ...  ...  ...  ---  ---  ---  ---  ---  ---  ---  ---  ---  ---  ---  ---  ---  ---  ---

  L26054    ,TRBV16*03          ---  ...  ...  ...  ...  ---  ---  ---  ---  ---  ---  ---  ---  ---  ---  ---  ---  ---  ---  ---


                                81   82   83   84   85   86   87   88   89   90   91   92   93   94   95   96   97   98   99  100
                                L         P    N    S    P    C    S    L    E    I    Q    A    T    K    L    E    D    S    A
  L26231    ,TRBV16*01          CTC  ...  CCA  AAT  TCA  CCC  TGT  AGC  CTT  GAG  ATC  CAG  GCT  ACG  AAG  CTT  GAG  GAT  TCA  GCA

  U03115    ,TRBV16*02          ---  ...  ---  ---  ---  ---  ---  ---  ---  ---  ---  ---  ---  ---  ---  ---  ---  ---  ---  ---

  L36092,U66060,TRBV16*02       ---  ...  ---  ---  ---  ---  ---  ---  ---  ---  ---  ---  ---  ---  ---  ---  ---  ---  ---  ---

  L26054    ,TRBV16*03          ---  ...  ---  ---  ---  ---  ---  ---  ---  ---  ---  ---  ---  ---  ---  ---  ---  ---  ---  ---


                                           ______CDR3-IMGT______
                               101  102  103  104  105  106  107  108  109
                                V    Y    F    C    A    S    S    Q
  L26231    ,TRBV16*01          GTG  TAT  TTT  TGT  GCC  AGC  AGC  CAA  TC

  U03115    ,TRBV16*02          ---  ---  ---  ---  ---  ---  ---  ---  --

  L36092,U66060,TRBV16*02       ---  ---  ---  ---  ---  ---  ---  ---  --

  L26054    ,TRBV16*03          ---  ---  ---  ---  ---  ---  ---            #c

*: STOP-CODON mutation
#c: Rearranged cDNA
```

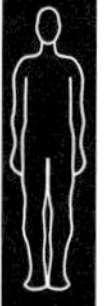

Framework and complementarity determining regions

FR1-IMGT: 26
FR2-IMGT: 17
FR3-IMGT: 38 (-1 aa: 82)

CDR1-IMGT: 5
CDR2-IMGT: 6
CDR3-IMGT: 4

Collier de Perles for human TRBV16*01

Accession number: IMGT L26231

EMBL/GenBank/DDBJ: L26231

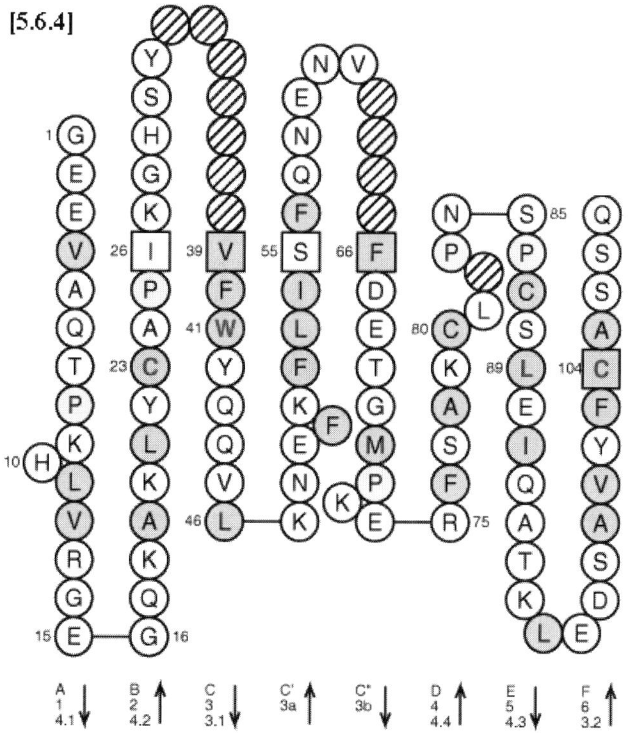

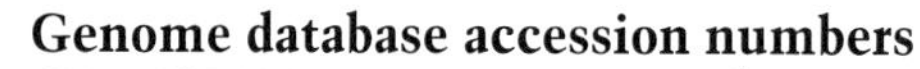

Genome database accession numbers

GDB:9954165   LocusLink: 28571

TRBV17

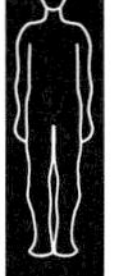

Nomenclature

TRBV17: T cell receptor beta variable 17.

Definition and functionality

TRBV17 is an ORF of the TRBV17 subgroup which only comprises this mapped gene, in the TRB locus.

TRBV17 is an ORF due to 2nd–CYS of FR3-IMGT being replaced by Tyrosine (tac).

Gene location

TRBV17 is in the TRB locus on chromosome 7 at 7q34.

Nucleotide and amino acid sequences for human TRBV17

```
                            1   2   3   4   5   6   7   8   9   10  11  12  13  14  15  16  17  18  19  20
                            E   P   G   V   S   Q   T   P   R   H   K   V   T   N   M   G   Q   E   V   I
U03115    ,TRBV17*01   [39] GAG CCT GGA GTC AGC CAG ACC CCC AGA CAC AAG GTC ACC AAC ATG GGA CAG GAG GTG ATT

L36092,U66060,TRBV17*01 [34] --- --- --- --- --- --- --- --- --- --- --- --- --- --- --- --- --- --- --- ---


                                                            ____________________CDR1-IMGT________________
                            21  22  23  24  25  26  27  28  29  30  31  32  33  34  35  36  37  38  39  40
                            L   R   C   D   P   S   S   G   H   M   F                           V   H
U03115    ,TRBV17*01        CTG AGG TGC GAT CCA TCT TCT GGT CAC ATG TTT ... ... ... ... ... ... ... GTT CAC

L36092,U66060,TRBV17*01     --- --- --- --- --- --- --- --- --- --- --- ... ... ... ... ... ... ... --- ---


                                                                                    ________________CDR2-
                            41  42  43  44  45  46  47  48  49  50  51  52  53  54  55  56  57  58  59  60
                            W   Y   R   Q   N   L   R   Q   E   M   K   L   L   I   S   F   Q   Y   Q   N
U03115    ,TRBV17*01        TGG TAC CGA CAG AAT CTG AGG CAA GAA ATG AAG TTG CTG ATT TCC TTC CAG TAC CAA AAC

L36092,U66060,TRBV17*01     --- --- --- --- --- --- --- --- --- --- --- --- --- --- --- --- --- --- --- ---


                            IMGT________________
                            61  62  63  64  65  66  67  68  69  70  71  72  73  74  75  76  77  78  79  80
                            I                   A   V   D   S   G   M   P   K   E   R   F   T   A   E   R
U03115    ,TRBV17*01        ATT ... ... ... ... GCA GTT GAT TCA GGG ATG CCC AAG GAA CGA TTC ACA GCT GAA AGA

L36092,U66060,TRBV17*01     --- ... ... ... ... --- --- --- --- --- --- --- --- --- --- --- --- --- --- ---


                            81  82  83  84  85  86  87  88  89  90  91  92  93  94  95  96  97  98  99  100
                            P       N   G   T   S   S   T   L   K   I   H   P   A   E   P   R   D   S   A
U03115    ,TRBV17*01        CCT ... AAC GGA ACG TCT TCC ACG CTG AAG ATC CAT CCC GCA GAG CCG AGG GAC TCA GCC

L36092,U66060,TRBV17*01     --- ... --- --- --- --- --- --- --- --- --- --- --- --- --- --- --- --- --- ---


                                            ____CDR3-IMGT____
                            101 102 103 104 105 106 107 108
                            V   Y   L   Y   S   S   G
U03115    ,TRBV17*01        GTG TAT CTC TAC AGT AGC GGT GG

L36092,U66060,TRBV17*01     --- --- --- --- --- --- --- --
```

Framework and complementarity determining regions

FR1-IMGT: 26

FR2-IMGT: 17

FR3-IMGT: 38 (-1 aa: 82)

CDR1-IMGT: 5

CDR2-IMGT: 6

CDR3-IMGT: 3

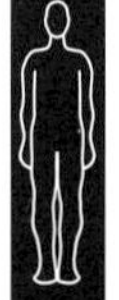

Collier de Perles for human TRBV17*01

Accession number: IMGT U03115   EMBL/GenBank/DDBJ: U03115

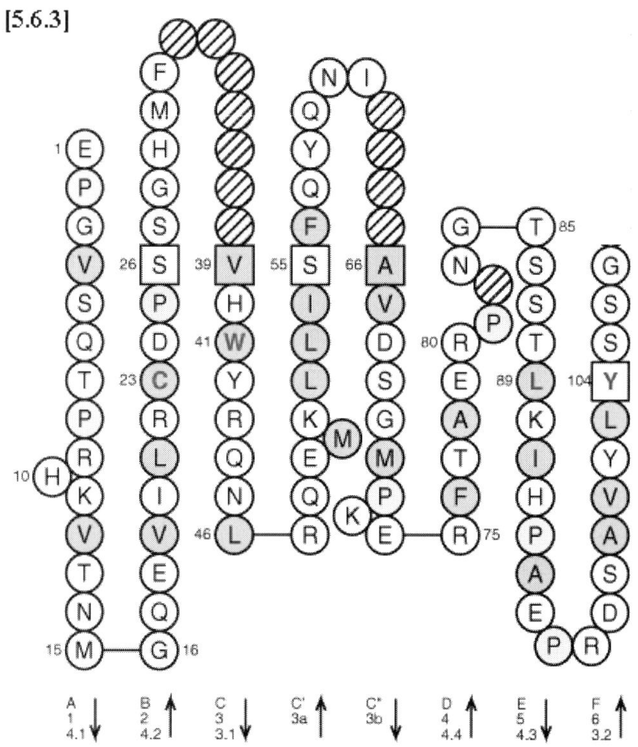

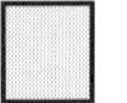

Genome database accession numbers
GDB:9954167   LocusLink: 28570

Nomenclature

TRBV18: T cell receptor beta variable 18.

Definition and functionality

TRBV18 is the unique functional gene of the TRBV18 subgroup which only comprises this mapped gene, in the TRB locus.

Gene location

TRBV18 is in the TRB locus on chromosome 7 at 7q34.

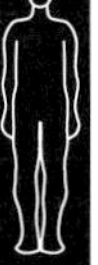

Nucleotide and amino acid sequences for human TRBV18

```
                          1   2   3   4   5   6   7   8   9  10  11  12  13  14  15  16  17  18  19  20
                          N   A   G   V   M   Q   N   P   R   H   L   V   R   R   R   G   Q   E   A   R
L36092,U66060,TRBV18*01 [34] AAT GCC GGC GTC ATG CAG AAC CCA AGA CAC CTG GTC AGG AGG AGG GGA CAG GAG GCA AGA

                                                           ____________________CDR1-IMGT____________________
                         21  22  23  24  25  26  27  28  29  30  31  32  33  34  35  36  37  38  39  40
                          L   R   C   S   P   M   K   G   H   S   H                                   V   Y
L36092,U66060,TRBV18*01  CTG AGA TGC AGC CCA ATG AAA GGA CAC AGT CAT ... ... ... ... ... ... ... GTT TAC

                                                                                 ____________________CDR2-
                         41  42  43  44  45  46  47  48  49  50  51  52  53  54  55  56  57  58  59  60
                          W   Y   R   Q   L   P   E   E   G   L   K   F   M   V   Y   L   Q   K   E   N
L36092,U66060,TRBV18*01  TGG TAT CGG CAG CTC CCA GAG GAA GGT CTG AAA TTC ATG GTT TAT CTC CAG AAA GAA AAT

                         IMGT____________________
                         61  62  63  64  65  66  67  68  69  70  71  72  73  74  75  76  77  78  79  80
                          I                       I   D   E   S   G   M   P   K   E   R   F   S   A   E   F
L36092,U66060,TRBV18*01  ATC ... ... ... ... ATA GAT GAG TCA GGA ATG CCA AAG GAA CGA TTT TCT GCT GAA TTT

                         81  82  83  84  85  86  87  88  89  90  91  92  93  94  95  96  97  98  99 100
                          P       K   E   G   P   S   I   L   R   I   Q   Q   V   V   R   G   D   S   A
L36092,U66060,TRBV18*01  CCC ... AAA GAG GGC CCC AGC ATC CTG AGG ATC CAG CAG GTA GTG CGA GGA GAT TCG GCA

                                                 ______CDR3-IMGT______
                        101 102 103 104 105 106 107 108 109
                          A   Y   F   C   A   S   S   P
L36092,U66060,TRBV18*01  GCT TAT TTC TGT GCC AGC TCA CCA CC
```

Framework and complementarity determining regions

FR1-IMGT: 26   CDR1-IMGT: 5
FR2-IMGT: 17   CDR2-IMGT: 6
FR3-IMGT: 38 (-1 aa: 82)   CDR3-IMGT: 4

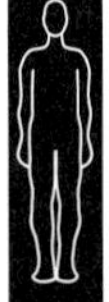

Collier de Perles for human TRBV18*01

Accession number: IMGT L36092 EMBL/GenBank/DDBJ: L36092

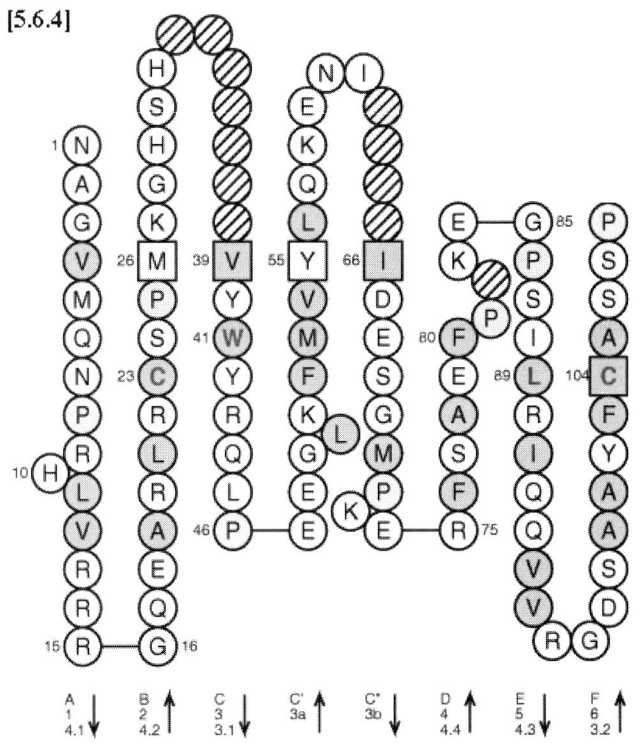

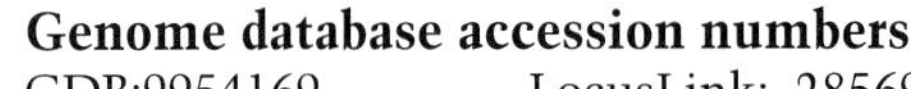

Genome database accession numbers
GDB:9954169 LocusLink: 28569

TRBV19

Nomenclature
TRBV19: T cell receptor beta variable 19.

Definition and functionality

TRBV19 is the unique functional gene of the TRBV19 subgroup which only comprises this mapped gene, in the TRB locus.

Gene location

TRBV19 is in the TRB locus on chromosome 7 at 7q34.

Nucleotide and amino acid sequences for human TRBV19

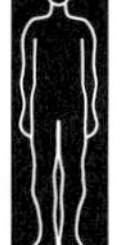

```
                                    1   2   3   4   5   6   7   8   9  10  11  12  13  14  15  16  17  18  19  20
                                    D   G   G   I   T   Q   S   P   K   Y   L   F   R   K   E   G   Q   N   V   T
U48260     ,TRBV19*01         [25] GAT GGT GGA ATC ACT CAG TCC CCA AAG TAC CTG TTC AGA AAG GAA GGA CAG AAT GTG ACC
L36092,U66060,U66061,TRBV19*01 [34] --- --- --- --- --- --- --- --- --- --- --- --- --- --- --- --- --- --- --- ---
U48259     ,TRBV19*02         [25] --- --- --- --- --- --- --- --- --- --- --- --- --- --- --- --- --- --- --- ---
M97725     ,TRBV19*03         [16] --- --- --- --- --- --- --- --- --- --- --- --- --- --- --- --- --- --- --- ---


                                                                        _________CDR1-IMGT_________
                                   21  22  23  24  25  26  27  28  29  30  31  32  33  34  35  36  37  38  39  40
                                    L   S   C   E   Q   N   L   N   H   D   A                           M   Y
U48260     ,TRBV19*01              CTG AGT TGT GAA CAG AAT TTG AAC CAC GAT GCC ... ... ... ... ... ... ... ATG TAC
L36092,U66060,U66061,TRBV19*01     --- --- --- --- --- --- --- --- --- --- --- ... ... ... ... ... ... --- ---
U48259     ,TRBV19*02              --- --- --- --- --- --- --- --- --- --- --- ... ... ... ... ... ... --- ---
M97725     ,TRBV19*03              --- --- --- --- --- --- --- --- --- --- --- ... ... ... ... ... ... --- ---


                                                                                        ___________CDR2-
                                   41  42  43  44  45  46  47  48  49  50  51  52  53  54  55  56  57  58  59  60
                                    W   Y   R   Q   D   P   G   Q   G   L   R   L   I   Y   Y   S   Q   I   V   N
U48260     ,TRBV19*01              TGG TAC CGA CAG GAC CCA GGG CAA GGG CTG AGA TTG ATC TAC TAC TCA CAG ATA GTA AAT
L36092,U66060,U66061,TRBV19*01     --- --- --- --- --- --- --- --- --- --- --- --- --- --- --- --- --- --- --- ---
                                                       V                               H
U48259     ,TRBV19*02              --- --- --- --- -T- --- --- --- --- --- --- --- --- --- --- --C --- --- ---
                                                                                       H
M97725     ,TRBV19*03              --- --- --- --- --- --- --- --- --- --- --- --- --- --- --- --C --- --- ---


                                   IMGT_______________
                                   61  62  63  64  65  66  67  68  69  70  71  72  73  74  75  76  77  78  79  80
                                    D                       F   Q   K   G   D   I   A       E   G   Y   S   V   S   R
U48260     ,TRBV19*01              GAC ... ... ... ... TTT CAG AAA GGA GAT ATA GCT ... GAA GGG TAC AGC GTC TCT CGG
L36092,U66060,U66061,TRBV19*01     --- ... ... ... ... --- --- --- --- --- --- --- ... --- --- --- --- --- ---
U48259     ,TRBV19*02              --- ... ... ... ... --- --- --- --- --- --- --- ... --- --- --- --- --- ---
M97725     ,TRBV19*03              --- ... ... ... ... --- --- --- --- --- --- --- ... --- --- --- --- --- ---


                                   81  82  83  84  85  86  87  88  89  90  91  92  93  94  95  96  97  98  99 100
                                    E       K   K   E   S   F   P   L   T   V   T   S   A   Q   K   N   P   T   A
U48260     ,TRBV19*01              GAG ... AAG AAG GAA TCC TTT CCT CTC ACT GTG ACA TCG GCC CAA AAG AAC CCG ACA GCT
L36092,U66060,U66061,TRBV19*01     --- ... --- --- --- --- --- --- --- --- --- --- --- --- --- --- --- --- --- ---
U48259     ,TRBV19*02              --- ... --- --- --- --- --- --- --- --- --- --- --- --- --- --- --- --- --- ---
M97725     ,TRBV19*03              --- ... --- --- --- --- --- --- --- --- --- --- --- --- --- --- --- --- --- ---


                                               ______CDR3-IMGT______
                                  101 102 103 104 105 106 107 108 109
                                    F   Y   L   C   A   S   S   I
U48260     ,TRBV19*01             TTC TAT CTC TGT GCC AGT AGT ATA GA
L36092,U66060,U66061,TRBV19*01    --- --- --- --- --- --- --- --- --
U48259     ,TRBV19*02             --- --- --- --- --- --- --- --- --
M97725     ,TRBV19*03             --- --- --- --- --- --- --C           #c

#c: Rearranged cDNA
```

Framework and complementarity determining regions

FR1-IMGT: 26	CDR1-IMGT: 5
FR2-IMGT: 17	CDR2-IMGT: 6
FR3-IMGT: 37 (-2 aa: 73, 82)	CDR3-IMGT: 4

Collier de Perles for human TRBV19*01

Accession number: IMGT U48260   EMBL/GenBank/DDBJ: U48260

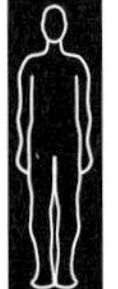

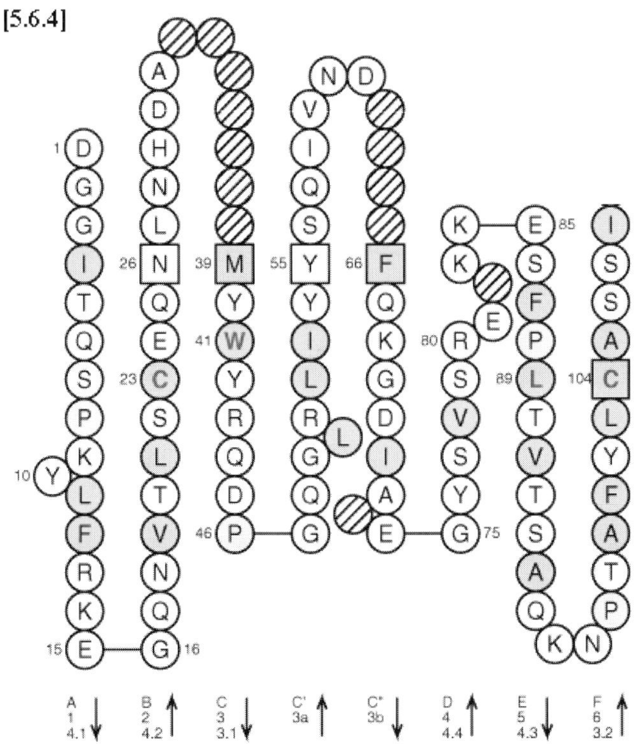

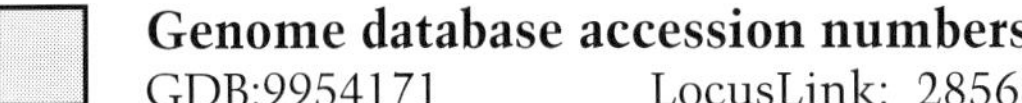

Genome database accession numbers
GDB:9954171   LocusLink: 28568

TRBV20-1

Nomenclature

TRBV20-1: T cell receptor beta variable 20-1.

Definition and functionality

TRBV20-1 is the unique functional gene of the TRBV20-1 subgroup which only comprises this mapped gene, in the TRB locus.

Gene location

TRBV20-1 is in the TRB locus on chromosome 7 at 7q34.

Nucleotide and amino acid sequences for human TRBV20-1

```
                                        1   2   3   4   5   6   7   8   9   10  11  12  13  14  15  16  17  18  19  20
                                        G   A   V   V   S   Q   H   P   S   W   V   I   C   K   S   G   T   S   V   K
M11955     ,TRBV20-1*01          [18]  GGT GCT GTC GTC TCT CAA CAT CCG AGC TGG GTT ATC TGT AAG AGT GGA ACC TCT GTG AAG
L36092,U66060,U66061,TRBV20-1*01 [34]  --- --- --- --- --- --- --- --- --- --- --- --- --- --- --- --- --- --- --- ---
                                                                            R
X72719     ,TRBV20-1*02          [6]   --- --- --- --- --- --- --- --- --- A-- --- --- --- --- --- --- --- --- --- ---
M11954     ,TRBV20-1*03          [18]  --- --- --- --- --- --- --- --- --- --- --- --- --- --- --- --- --- --- --- ---
                                                                            R
M14263     ,TRBV20-1*04          [41]  --- --- --- --- --- --- --- --- --- A-- --- --- --- --- --- --- --- --- --- ---
                                                                            R
X57604     ,TRBV20-1*05          [31]  --- --- --- --- --- --- --- --- --- A-- --- --- --- --- --- --- --- --- --- ---
                                                                            R
D13088     ,TRBV20-1*06          [30]  --- --- --- --- --- --- --- --- --T A-- --- --- --- --- --- --- --- --- --- ---
                                                                            R
X74852     ,TRBV20-1*07          [19]  --- --- --- --- --- --- --- --- --- A-- --- --- --- --- --- --- --- --- --- ---

                                                               CDR1-IMGT
                                        21  22  23  24  25  26  27  28  29  30  31  32  33  34  35  36  37  38  39  40
                                        I   E   C   R   S   L   D   F   Q   A   T   T                       M   F
M11955     ,TRBV20-1*01                ATC GAG TGC CGT TCC CTG GAC TTT CAG GCC ACA ACT ... ... ... ... ... ... ATG TTT
L36092,U66060,U66061,TRBV20-1*01       --- --- --- --- --- --- --- --- --- --- --- --- ... ... ... ... ... ... --- ---
X72719     ,TRBV20-1*02                --- --- --- --- --- --- --- --- --- --- --- --- ... ... ... ... ... ... --- ---
M11954     ,TRBV20-1*03                --- --- --- --- --- --- --- --- --- --- --- --- ... ... ... ... ... ... --- ---
M14263     ,TRBV20-1*04                --- --- --- --- --- T-- --- --- --- --- --- --- ... ... ... ... ... ... --- ---
X57604     ,TRBV20-1*05                --- --- --- --- --- --- --- --- --- --- --- --- ... ... ... ... ... ... --- ---
D13088     ,TRBV20-1*06                --- --- --- --- --- --- --- --- --- --- --- --- ... ... ... ... ... ... --- ---
X74852     ,TRBV20-1*07                --- --- --- --- --- --- --- --- --- --- --- --- ... ... ... ... ... ... --- ---

                                                                                                        CDR2-
                                        41  42  43  44  45  46  47  48  49  50  51  52  53  54  55  56  57  58  59  60
                                        W   Y   R   Q   F   P   K   Q   S   L   M   L   M   A   T   S   N   E   G   S
M11955     ,TRBV20-1*01                TGG TAT CGT CAG TTC CCG AAA CAG AGT CTC ATG CTG ATG GCA ACT TCC AAT GAG GGC TCC
L36092,U66060,U66061,TRBV20-1*01       --- --- --- --- --- --- --- --- --- --- --- --- --- --- --- --- --- --- --- ---
X72719     ,TRBV20-1*02                --- --- --- --- --- --- --- --- --- --- --- --- --- --- --- --- --- --- --- ---
                                                                                                                    C
M11954     ,TRBV20-1*03                --- --- --- --- --- --- --- --- --- --- --- --- --- --- --- --- --- --- --- -G-
                                                                K
M14263     ,TRBV20-1*04                --- --- --- --- --- --- --- A-- --- --- --- --- --- --- --- --- --- --- --- ---
                                                                K
X57604     ,TRBV20-1*05                --- --- --- --- --- --- --- A-- --- --- --- --- --- --- --- --- --- --- --- ---
                                                                K
D13088     ,TRBV20-1*06                --- --- --- --- --- --- --- A-- --- --- --- --- --- --- --- --- --- --- --- ---
                                                                K               Q   I
X74852     ,TRBV20-1*07                --- --- --- --- --- --- --- A-- --- --- -A- --C --- --- --- --- --- --- --- ---

IMGT
                                        61  62  63  64  65  66  67  68  69  70  71  72  73  74  75  76  77  78  79  80
                                        K   A               T   Y   E   Q   G   V   E   K   D   K   F   L   I   N   H
M11955     ,TRBV20-1*01                AAG GCC ... ... ... ACA TAC GAG CAA GGC GTC GAG AAG GAC AAG TTT CTC ATC AAC CAT
L36092,U66060,U66061,TRBV20-1*01       --- --- ... ... ... --- --- --- --- --- --- --- --- --- --- --- --- --- --- ---
X72719     ,TRBV20-1*02                --- --- ... ... ... --- --- --- --- --- --- --- --- --- --- --- --- --- --- ---
M11954     ,TRBV20-1*03                --- --- ... ... ... --- --- --- --- --- --- --- --- --- --- --- --- --- --- ---
M14263     ,TRBV20-1*04                --- --- ... ... ... --- --- --- --- --- --- --- --- --- --- --- --- --- --- ---
X57604     ,TRBV20-1*05                --- --- ... ... ... --- --- --- --- --- --- --- --- --- --- --- --- --- --- ---
D13088     ,TRBV20-1*06                --- --- ... ... ... --- --- --- --- --- --- --- --- --- --- --- --- --- --- ---
X74852     ,TRBV20-1*07                --- --- ... ... ... --- --- --- --- --- --- --- --- --- --- --- --- --- --- ---

                                        81  82  83  84  85  86  87  88  89  90  91  92  93  94  95  96  97  98  99 100
                                        A       S   L   T   L   S   T   L   T   V   T   S   A   H   P   E   D   S   S
M11955     ,TRBV20-1*01                GCA ... AGC CTG ACC TTG TCC ACT CTG ACA GTG ACC AGT GCC CAT CCT GAA GAC AGC AGC
L36092,U66060,U66061,TRBV20-1*01       --- ... --- --- --- --- --- --- --- --- --- --- --- --- --- --- --- --- --- ---
X72719     ,TRBV20-1*02                --- ... --- --- --- --- --- --- --- --- --- --- --- --- --- --- --- --- --- ---
M11954     ,TRBV20-1*03                --- ... --- --- --- --- --- --- --- --- --- --- --- --- --- --- --- --- --- ---
M14263     ,TRBV20-1*04                --- ... --- --- --- --- --- --- --- --- --- --- --- --- --- --- --- --- --- ---
X57604     ,TRBV20-1*05                --- ... --- --- --- --- --- --- --- --- --- --- --- --- --- --- --- --- --- ---
D13088     ,TRBV20-1*06                --- ... --- --- --- --- --- --- --- --- --- --- --- --- --- --- --- --- --- ---
X74852     ,TRBV20-1*07                --- ... --- --- --- --- --- --- --- --- --- --- --- --- --- --- --- --- --- ---
```

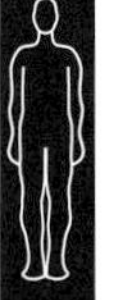

```
                                             ___CDR3-IMGT___
                                  101 102 103 104 105 106 107 108
                                   F   Y   I   C   S   A   R
M11955    ,TRBV20-1*01            TTC TAC ATC TGC AGT GCT AGA GA

L36092,U66060,U66061,TRBV20-1*01  --- --- --- --- --- --- --- --

X72719    ,TRBV20-1*02            --- --- --- --- --- ---

M11954    ,TRBV20-1*03            --- --- --- --- --- ---         #g
                                                          S
M14263    ,TRBV20-1*04            --- --- --- --- --- --- --T     #c

X57604    ,TRBV20-1*05            --- --- --- --- --- ---         #g

D13088    ,TRBV20-1*06            --- --- --- --- --- ---         #c

X74852    ,TRBV20-1*07            --- --- --- --- --- ---         #c

#c: Rearranged cDNA
#g: Rearranged genomic DNA
```

Framework and complementarity determining regions

FR1-IMGT: 26   CDR1-IMGT: 6
FR2-IMGT: 17   CDR2-IMGT: 7
FR3-IMGT: 38 (-1 aa: 82)   CDR3-IMGT: 3

Collier de Perles for human TRBV20-1*01

Accession number: IMGT M11955   EMBL/GenBank/DDBJ: M11955

[6.7.3]

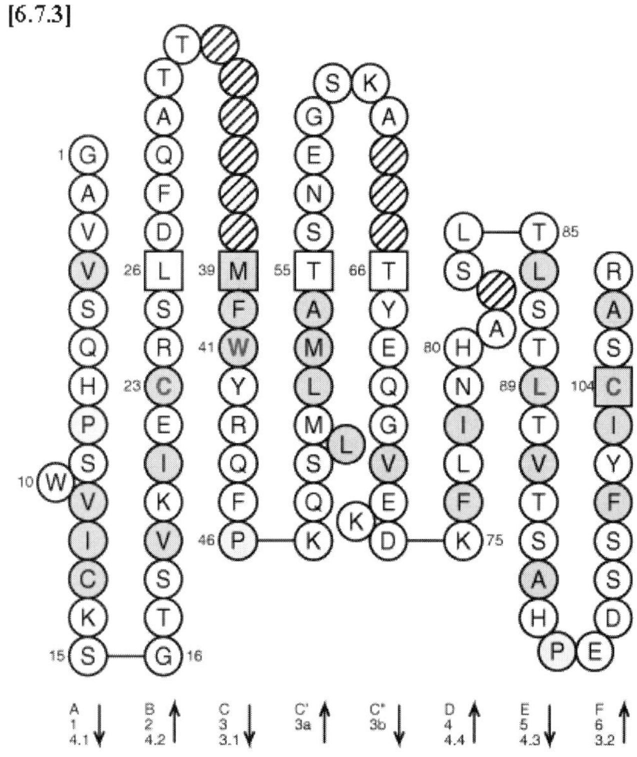

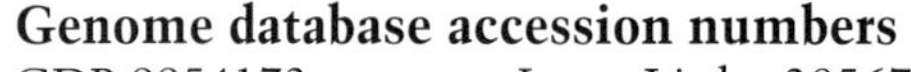

Genome database accession numbers
GDB:9954173   LocusLink: 28567

TRBV23-1

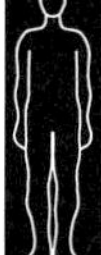

Nomenclature

TRBV23-1: T cell receptor beta variable 23-1.

Definition and functionality

TRBV23-1 is an ORF of the TRBV23 subgroup which only comprises this mapped gene, in the TRB locus.

TRBV23-1 is an ORF due to a mutation in the DONOR–SPLICE (ngt being replaced by nat).

Gene location

TRBV23-1 is in the TRB locus on chromosome 7 at 7q34.

Nucleotide and amino acid sequences for human TRBV23-1

```
                              1   2   3   4   5   6   7   8   9  10  11  12  13  14  15  16  17  18  19  20
                              H   A   K   V   T   Q   T   P   G   H   L   V   K   G   K   G   Q   K   T   K
L36092,U66061,TRBV23-1*01 [34] CAT GCC AAA GTC ACA CAG ACT CCA GGA CAT TTG GTC AAA GGA AAA GGA CAG AAA ACA AAG

L48730   ,TRBV23-1*01    [7]  --- --- --- --- --- --- --- --- --- --- --- --- --- --- --- --- --- --- --- ---

L27614   ,TRBV23-1*01    [3]  --- --- --- --- --- --- --- --- --- --- --- --- --- --- --- --- --- --- --- ---


                                                                      ______________CDR1-IMGT________________
                             21  22  23  24  25  26  27  28  29  30  31  32  33  34  35  36  37  38  39  40
                              M   D   C   T   P   E   K   G   H   T   F                               V   Y
L36092,U66061,TRBV23-1*01    ATG GAT TGT ACC CCC GAA AAA GGA CAT ACT TTT ... ... ... ... ... ... ... GTT TAT

L48730   ,TRBV23-1*01        --- --- --- --- --- --- --- --- --- --- --- ... ... ... ... ... ... ... --- ---

L27614   ,TRBV23-1*01        --- --- --- --- --- --- --- --- --- --- --- ... ... ... ... ... ... ... --- ---


                                                                                          ________________CDR2-
                             41  42  43  44  45  46  47  48  49  50  51  52  53  54  55  56  57  58  59  60
                              W   Y   Q   Q   N   Q   N   K   E   F   M   L   L   I   S   F   Q   N   E   Q
L36092,U66061,TRBV23-1*01    TGG TAT CAA CAG AAT CAG AAT AAA GAG TTT ATG CTT TTG ATT TCC TTT CAG AAT GAA CAA

L48730   ,TRBV23-1*01        --- --- --- --- --- --- --- --- --- --- --- --- --- --- --- --- --- --- --- ---

L27614   ,TRBV23-1*01        --- --- --- --- --- --- --- --- --- --- --- --- --- --- --- --- --- --- --- ---


                             IMGT________________
                             61  62  63  64  65  66  67  68  69  70  71  72  73  74  75  76  77  78  79  80
                              V                   L   Q   E   T   E   M   H   K   K   R   F   S   S   Q   C
L36092,U66061,TRBV23-1*01    GTT ... ... ... ... CTT CAA GAA ACG GAG ATG CAC AAG AAG CGA TTC TCA TCT CAA TGC

L48730   ,TRBV23-1*01        --- ... ... ... ... --- --- --- --- --- --- --- --- --- --- --- --- --- --- ---

L27614   ,TRBV23-1*01        --- ... ... ... ... --- --- --- --- --- --- --- --- --- --- --- --- --- --- ---


                             81  82  83  84  85  86  87  88  89  90  91  92  93  94  95  96  97  98  99 100
                              P       K   N   A   P   C   S   L   A   I   L   S   S   E   P   G   D   T   A
L36092,U66061,TRBV23-1*01    CCC ... AAG AAC GCA CCC TGC AGC CTG GCA ATC CTG TCC TCA GAA CCG GGA GAC ACG GCA

L48730   ,TRBV23-1*01        --- ... --- --- --- --- --- --- --- --- --- --- --- --- --- --- --- --- --- ---

L27614   ,TRBV23-1*01        --- ... --- --- --- --- --- --- --- ---


                                      ______CDR3-IMGT______
                            101 102 103 104 105 106 107 108 109
                              L   Y   L   C   A   S   S   Q
L36092,U66061,TRBV23-1*01    CTG TAT CTC TGC GCC AGC AGT CAA TC

L48730   ,TRBV23-1*01        --- --- --- --- --- --- --- --- --

L27614   ,TRBV23-1*01                                                  o
```

°: Genomic DNA, but not known as being germline or rearranged

Framework and complementarity determining regions

FR1-IMGT: 26

FR2-IMGT: 17

FR3-IMGT: 38 (-1 aa: 82)

CDR1-IMGT: 5

CDR2-IMGT: 6

CDR3-IMGT: 4

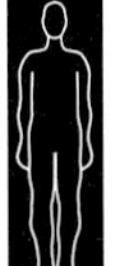

Collier de Perles for human TRBV23-1*01

Accession number: IMGT L36092   EMBL/GenBank/DDBJ: L36092

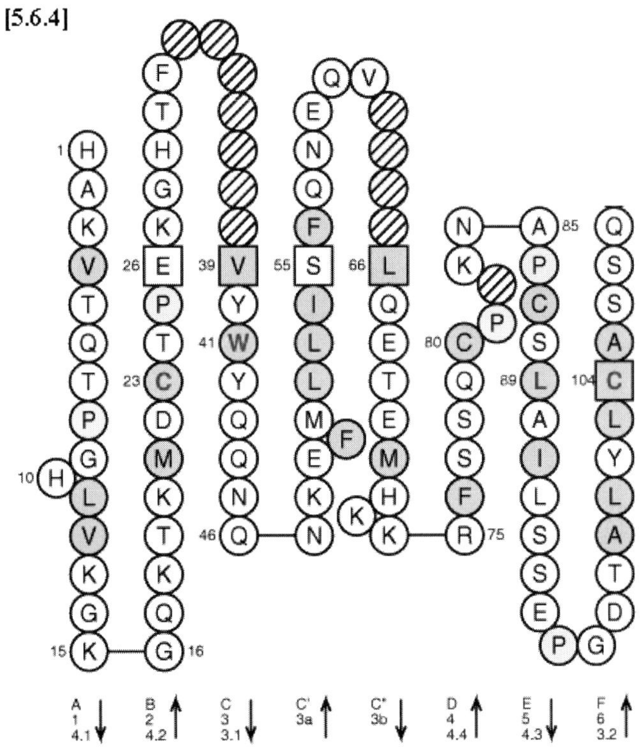

Genome database accession numbers
GDB:9954179   LocusLink: 28564

TRBV24-1

Nomenclature

TRBV24-1: T cell receptor beta variable 24-1.

Definition and functionality

TRBV24-1 is the unique functional gene of the TRBV24-1 subgroup which only comprises this mapped gene, in the TRB locus.

Gene location

TRBV24-1 is in the TRB locus on chromosome 7 at 7q34.

Nucleotide and amino acid sequences for human TRBV24-1

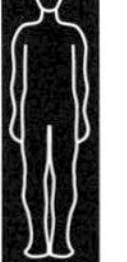

```
                             1   2   3   4   5   6   7   8   9   10  11  12  13  14  15  16  17  18  19  20
                             D   A   D   V   T   Q   T   P   R   N   R   I   T   K   T   G   K   R   I   M
M11951   ,TRBV24-1*01   [18] GAT GCT GAT GTT ACC CAG ACC CCA AGG AAT AGG ATC ACA AAG ACA GGA AAG AGG ATT ATG

L27612   ,TRBV24-1*01    [3] --- --- --- --- --- --- --- --- --- --- --- --- --- --- --- --- --- --- --- ---

L36092,U66061,TRBV24-1*01 [34] --- --- --- --- --- --- --- --- --- --- --- --- --- --- --- --- --- --- --- ---


                                                                     ____________________CDR1-IMGT____________________
                             21  22  23  24  25  26  27  28  29  30  31  32  33  34  35  36  37  38  39  40
                             L   E   C   S   Q   T   K   G   H   D   R                               M   Y
M11951   ,TRBV24-1*01        CTG GAA TGT TCT CAG ACT AAG GGT CAT GAT AGA ... ... ... ... ... ... ... ATG TAC

L27612   ,TRBV24-1*01        --- --- --- --- --- --- --- --- --- --- --- ... ... ... ... ... ... ... --- ---

L36092,U66061,TRBV24-1*01    --- --- --- --- --- --- --- --- --- --- --- ... ... ... ... ... ... ... --- ---


                                                                                         __________________CDR2-
                             41  42  43  44  45  46  47  48  49  50  51  52  53  54  55  56  57  58  59  60
                             W   Y   R   Q   D   P   G   L   G   L   R   L   I   Y   Y   S   F   D   V   K
M11951   ,TRBV24-1*01        TGG TAT CGA CAA GAC CCA GGA CTG GGC CTA CGG TTG ATC TAT TAC TCC TTT GAT GTC AAA

L27612   ,TRBV24-1*01        --- --- --- --- --- --- --- --- --- --- --- --- --- --- --- --- --- --- --- ---

L36092,U66061,TRBV24-1*01    --- --- --- --- --- --- --- --- --- --- --- --- --- --- --- --- --- --- --- ---


                             IMGT________________
                             61  62  63  64  65  66  67  68  69  70  71  72  73  74  75  76  77  78  79  80
                             D                   I   N   K   G   E   I   S       D   G   Y   S   V   S   R
M11951   ,TRBV24-1*01        GAT ... ... ... ... ATA AAC AAA GGA GAG ATC TCT ... GAT GGA TAC AGT GTC TCT CGA

L27612   ,TRBV24-1*01        --- ... ... ... ... --- --- --- --- --- --- --- ... --- --- --- --- --- --- ---

L36092,U66061,TRBV24-1*01    --- ... ... ... ... --- --- --- --- --- --- --- ... --- --- --- --- --- --- ---


                             81  82  83  84  85  86  87  88  89  90  91  92  93  94  95  96  97  98  99 100
                             Q       A   Q   A   K   F   S   L   S   L   E   S   A   I   P   N   Q   T   A
M11951   ,TRBV24-1*01        CAG ... GCA CAG GCT AAA TTC TCC CTG TCC CTA GAG TCT GCC ATC CCC AAC CAG ACA GCT

L27612   ,TRBV24-1*01        --- ... --- --- --- --- --- --- --- --- --- --- --- --- --- --- --- --- --- ---

L36092,U66061,TRBV24-1*01    --- ... --- --- --- --- --- --- --- --- --- --- --- --- --- --- --- --- --- ---


                                         ______CDR3-IMGT______
                            101 102 103 104 105 106 107 108 109
                             L   Y   F   C   A   T   S   D   L
M11951   ,TRBV24-1*01        CTT TAC TTC TGT GCC ACC AGT GAT TTG

L27612   ,TRBV24-1*01        --- --- --- --- --- --- --- --- ---

L36092,U66061,TRBV24-1*01    --- --- --- --- --- --- --- --- ---
```

Framework and complementarity determining regions

FR1-IMGT: 26   CDR1-IMGT: 5
FR2-IMGT: 17   CDR2-IMGT: 6
FR3-IMGT: 37 (-2 aa: 73, 82)   CDR3-IMGT: 5

Collier de Perles for human TRBV24-1*01

Accession number: IMGT M11951   EMBL/GenBank/DDBJ: M11951

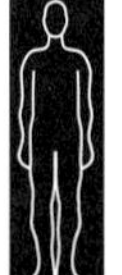

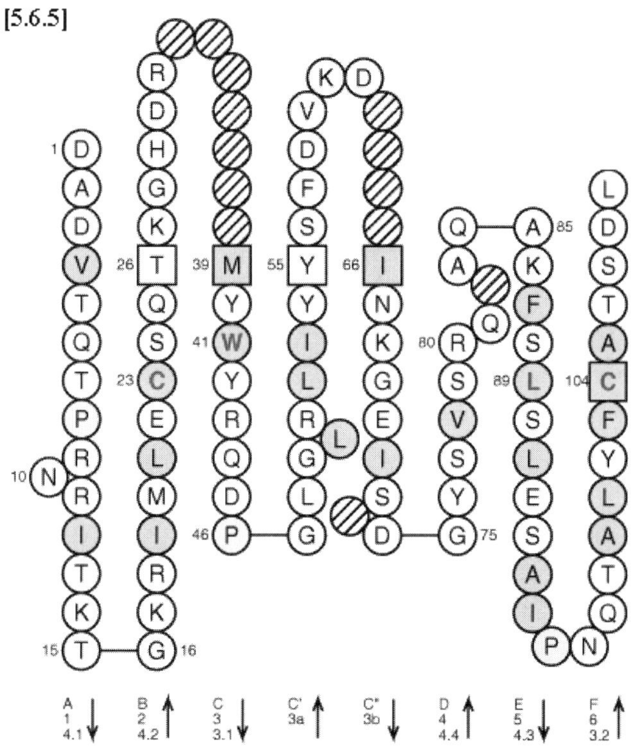

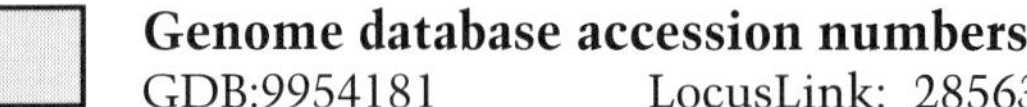

Genome database accession numbers
GDB:9954181   LocusLink: 28563

TRBV25-1

Nomenclature

TRBV25-1: T cell receptor beta variable 25-1.

Definition and functionality

TRBV25-1 is the unique functional gene of the TRBV25-1 subgroup which only comprises this mapped gene, in the TRB locus.

Gene location

TRBV25-1 is in the TRB locus on chromosome 7 at 7q34.

Nucleotide and amino acid sequences for human TRBV25-1

```
                               1   2   3   4   5   6   7   8   9  10  11  12  13  14  15  16  17  18  19  20
                               E   A   D   I   Y   Q   T   P   R   Y   L   V   I   G   T   G   K   K   I   T
L36092,U66061,TRBV25-1*01 [34] GAA GCT GAC ATC TAC CAG ACC CCA AGA TAC CTT GTT ATA GGG ACA GGA AAG AAG ATC ACT

L27610    ,TRBV25-1*01    [3]  --- --- --- --- --- --- --- --- --- --- --- --- --- --- --- --- --- --- --- ---


                                                                   ________________CDR1-IMGT________________
                               21  22  23  24  25  26  27  28  29  30  31  32  33  34  35  36  37  38  39  40
                               L   E   C   S   Q   T   M   G   H   D   K                           M   Y
L36092,U66061,TRBV25-1*01      CTG GAA TGT TCT CAA ACC ATG GGC CAT GAC AAA ... ... ... ... ... ... ... ATG TAC

L27610    ,TRBV25-1*01         --- --- --- --- --- --- --- --- --- --- --- ... ... ... ... ... ... ... --- ---


                                                                                           ____________CDR2-
                               41  42  43  44  45  46  47  48  49  50  51  52  53  54  55  56  57  58  59  60
                               W   Y   Q   Q   D   P   G   M   E   L   H   L   I   H   Y   S   Y   G   V   N
L36092,U66061,TRBV25-1*01      TGG TAT CAA CAA GAT CCA GGA ATG GAA CTA CAC CTC ATC CAC TAT TCC TAT GGA GTT AAT

L27610    ,TRBV25-1*01         --- --- --- --- --- --- --- --- --- --- --- --- --- --- --- --- --- --- --- ---


                               IMGT________________
                               61  62  63  64  65  66  67  68  69  70  71  72  73  74  75  76  77  78  79  80
                               S                   T   E   K   G   D   L   S       S   E   S   T   V   S   R
L36092,U66061,TRBV25-1*01      TCC ... ... ... ... ACA GAG AAG GGA GAT CTT TCC ... TCT GAG TCA ACA GTC TCC AGA

L27610    ,TRBV25-1*01         --- ... ... ... ... --- --- --- --- --- --- --- ... --- --- --- --- --- --- ---


                               81  82  83  84  85  86  87  88  89  90  91  92  93  94  95  96  97  98  99 100
                               I       R   T   E   H   F   P   L   T   L   E   S   A   R   P   S   H   T   S
L36092,U66061,TRBV25-1*01      ATA ... AGG ACG GAG CAT TTT CCC CTG ACC CTG GAG TCT GCC AGG CCC TCA CAT ACC TCT

L27610    ,TRBV25-1*01         --- ... --- --- --- --- --- --- --- --- --- --- --- --- --- --- --- --- --- --


                                           ______CDR3-IMGT______
                              101 102 103 104 105 106 107 108 109
                               Q   Y   L   C   A   S   S   E
L36092,U66061,TRBV25-1*01      CAG TAC CTC TGT GCC AGC AGT GAA TA

L27610    ,TRBV25-1*01
```

Framework and complementarity determining regions

FR1-IMGT: 26

FR2-IMGT: 17

FR3-IMGT: 37 (-2 aa: 73, 82)

CDR1-IMGT: 5

CDR2-IMGT: 6

CDR3-IMGT: 4

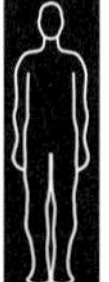

Collier de Perles for human TRBV25-1*01

Accession number: IMGT L36092   EMBL/GenBank/DDBJ: L36092

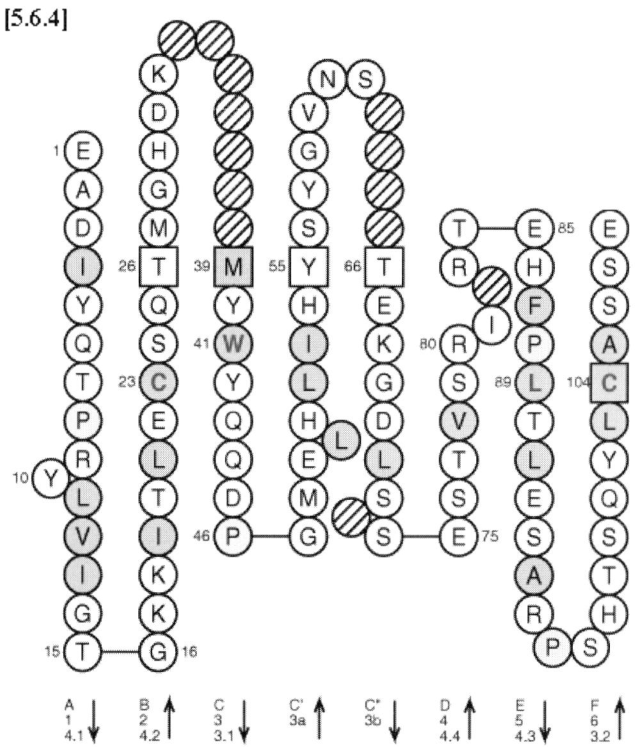

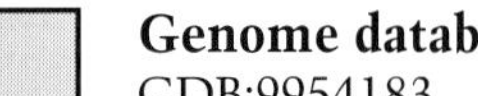

Genome database accession numbers
GDB:9954183   LocusLink: 28562

Nomenclature

TRBV27: T cell receptor beta variable 27.

Definition and functionality

TRBV27 is the unique functional gene of the TRBV27 subgroup which only comprises this mapped gene, in the TRB locus.

Gene location

TRBV27 is in the TRB locus on chromosome 7 at 7q34.

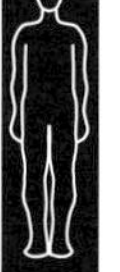

Nucleotide and amino acid sequences for human TRBV27

```
                                1    2    3    4    5    6    7    8    9   10   11   12   13   14   15   16   17   18   19   20
                                E    A    Q    V    T    Q    N    P    R    Y    L    I    T    V    T    G    K    K    L    T
L36092,U66061,TRBV27*01 [34]   GAA  GCC  CAA  GTG  ACC  CAG  AAC  CCA  AGA  TAC  CTC  ATC  ACA  GTG  ACT  GGA  AAG  AAG  TTA  ACA


                                                                   ________________________CDR1-IMGT________________________
                               21   22   23   24   25   26   27   28   29   30   31   32   33   34   35   36   37   38   39   40
                                V    T    C    S    Q    N    M    N    H    E    Y                                      M    S
L36092,U66061,TRBV27*01        GTG  ACT  TGT  TCT  CAG  AAT  ATG  AAC  CAT  GAG  TAT  ...  ...  ...  ...  ...  ...  ...  ATG  TCC


                                                                                               ________________________CDR2-
                               41   42   43   44   45   46   47   48   49   50   51   52   53   54   55   56   57   58   59   60
                                W    Y    R    Q    D    P    G    L    G    L    R    Q    I    Y    Y    S    M    N    V    E
L36092,U66061,TRBV27*01        TGG  TAT  CGA  CAA  GAC  CCA  GGG  CTG  GGC  TTA  AGG  CAG  ATC  TAC  TAT  TCA  ATG  AAT  GTT  GAG


                               IMGT________________________
                               61   62   63   64   65   66   67   68   69   70   71   72   73   74   75   76   77   78   79   80
                                V                             T    D    K    G    D    V    P         E    G    Y    K    V    S    R
L36092,U66061,TRBV27*01        GTG  ...  ...  ...  ...  ACT  GAT  AAG  GGA  GAT  GTT  CCT  ...  GAA  GGG  TAC  AAA  GTC  TCT  CGA


                               81   82   83   84   85   86   87   88   89   90   91   92   93   94   95   96   97   98   99  100
                                K         E    K    R    N    F    P    L    I    L    E    S    P    S    P    N    Q    T    S
L36092,U66061,TRBV27*01        AAA  ...  GAG  AAG  AGG  AAT  TTC  CCC  CTG  ATC  CTG  GAG  TCG  CCC  AGC  CCC  AAC  CAG  ACC  TCT


                                              ________CDR3-IMGT________
                              101  102  103  104  105  106  107  108  109
                                L    Y    F    C    A    S    S    L
L36092,U66061,TRBV27*01        CTG  TAC  TTC  TGT  GCC  AGC  AGT  TTA  TC
```

Framework and complementarity determining regions

FR1-IMGT: 26	CDR1-IMGT: 5
FR2-IMGT: 17	CDR2-IMGT: 6
FR3-IMGT: 37 (-2 aa: 73, 82)	CDR3-IMGT: 4

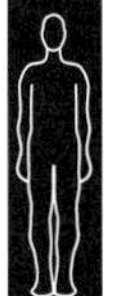

Collier de Perles for human TRBV27*01

Accession number: IMGT L36092   EMBL/GenBank/DDBJ: L36092

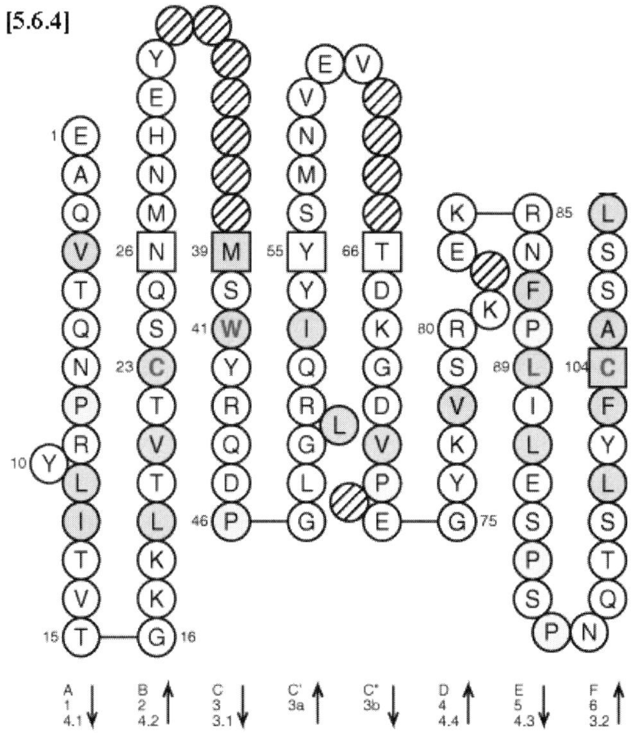

Genome database accession numbers
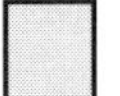
GDB:9954187   LocusLink: 28560

TRBV28

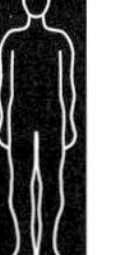

Nomenclature

TRBV28: T cell receptor beta variable 28.

Definition and functionality

TRBV28 is the unique functional gene of the TRBV28 subgroup which only comprises this mapped gene, in the TRB locus.

Gene location

TRBV28 is in the TRB locus on chromosome 7 at 7q34.

Nucleotide and amino acid sequences for human TRBV28

```
                          1    2    3    4    5    6    7    8    9   10   11   12   13   14   15   16   17   18   19   20
                          D    V    K    V    T    Q    S    S    R    Y    L    V    K    R    T    G    E    K    V    F
U08314   ,TRBV28*01  [32] GAT  GTG  AAA  GTA  ACC  CAG  AGC  TCG  AGA  TAT  CTA  GTC  AAA  AGG  ACG  GGA  GAG  AAA  GTT  TTT

L36092,U66061,TRBV28*01 [34] ---  ---  ---  ---  ---  ---  ---  ---  ---  ---  ---  ---  ---  ---  ---  ---  ---  ---  ---  ---

M18464   ,TRBV28*01  [42] ---  ---  ---  ---  ---  ---  ---  ---


                                                                        __________________CDR1-IMGT__________________
                         21   22   23   24   25   26   27   28   29   30   31   32   33   34   35   36   37   38   39   40
                          L    E    C    V    Q    D    M    D    H    E    N                                  M    F
U08314   ,TRBV28*01      CTG  GAA  TGT  GTC  CAG  GAT  ATG  GAC  CAT  GAA  AAT  ...  ...  ...  ...  ...  ...  ...  ATG  TTC

L36092,U66061,TRBV28*01  ---  ---  ---  ---  ---  ---  ---  ---  ---  ---  ---  ...  ...  ...  ...  ...  ...  ...  ---  ---

M18464   ,TRBV28*01


                                                                                                      ________CDR2-
                         41   42   43   44   45   46   47   48   49   50   51   52   53   54   55   56   57   58   59   60
                          W    Y    R    Q    D    P    G    L    G    L    R    L    I    Y    F    S    Y    D    V    K
U08314   ,TRBV28*01      TGG  TAT  CGA  CAA  GAC  CCA  GGT  CTG  GGG  CTA  CGG  CTG  ATC  TAT  TTC  TCA  TAT  GAT  GTT  AAA

L36092,U66061,TRBV28*01  ---  ---  ---  ---  ---  ---  ---  ---  ---  ---  ---  ---  ---  ---  ---  ---  ---  ---  ---  ---

M18464   ,TRBV28*01


                         IMGT_________________
                         61   62   63   64   65   66   67   68   69   70   71   72   73   74   75   76   77   78   79   80
                          M                        K    E    K    G    D    I    P         E    G    Y    S    V    S    R
U08314   ,TRBV28*01      ATG  ...  ...  ...  ...  AAA  GAA  AAA  GGA  GAT  ATT  CCT  ...  GAG  GGG  TAC  AGT  GTC  TCT  AGA

L36092,U66061,TRBV28*01  ---  ...  ...  ...  ...  ---  ---  ---  ---  ---  ---  ---  ...  ---  ---  ---  ---  ---  ---  ---

M18464   ,TRBV28*01


                         81   82   83   84   85   86   87   88   89   90   91   92   93   94   95   96   97   98   99  100
                          E         K    K    E    R    F    S    L    I    L    E    S    A    S    T    N    Q    T    S
U08314   ,TRBV28*01      GAG  ...  AAG  AAG  GAG  CGC  TTC  TCC  CTG  ATT  CTG  GAG  TCC  GCC  AGC  ACC  AAC  CAG  ACA  TCT

L36092,U66061,TRBV28*01  ---  ...  ---  ---  ---  ---  ---  ---  ---  ---  ---  ---  ---  ---  ---  ---  ---  ---  ---  ---

M18464   ,TRBV28*01


                                              ________CDR3-IMGT______
                        101  102  103  104  105  106  107  108  109
                          M    Y    L    C    A    S    S    L
U08314   ,TRBV28*01      ATG  TAC  CTC  TGT  GCC  AGC  AGT  TTA  TG

L36092,U66061,TRBV28*01  ---  ---  ---  ---  ---  ---  ---  ---  ---

M18464   ,TRBV28*01                                           o
```

°: Genomic DNA, but not known as being germline or rearranged

Framework and complementarity determining regions

FR1-IMGT: 26	CDR1-IMGT: 5
FR2-IMGT: 17	CDR2-IMGT: 6
FR3-IMGT: 37 (-2 aa: 73, 82)	CDR3-IMGT: 4

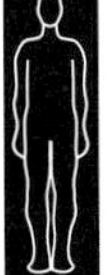

Collier de Perles for human TRBV28*01

Accession number: IMGT U08314   EMBL/GenBank/DDBJ: U08314

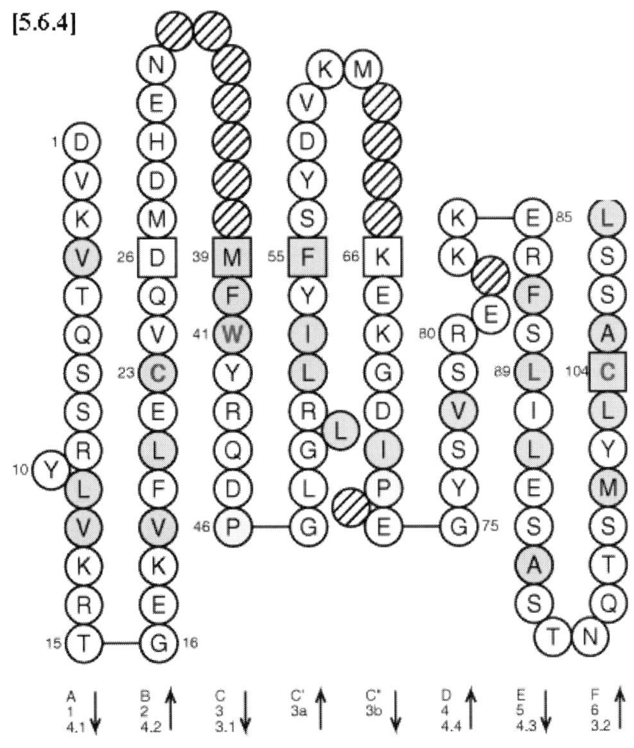

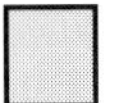

Genome database accession numbers
GDB:9954189   LocusLink: 28559

Nomenclature

TRBV29-1: T cell receptor beta variable 29-1.

Definition and functionality

TRBV29-1 is the unique functional gene of the TRBV29-1 subgroup which only comprises this mapped gene, in the TRB locus.

Gene location

TRBV29-1 is in the TRB locus on chromosome 7 at 7q34.

Nucleotide and amino acid sequences for human TRBV29-1

```
                              1   2   3   4   5   6   7   8   9   10  11  12  13  14  15  16  17  18  19  20
                              S   A   V   I   S   Q   K   P   S   R   D   I   C   Q   R   G   T   S   L   T
L36092,U66061,TRBV29-1*01 [34] AGT GCT GTC ATC TCT CAA AAG CCA AGC AGG GAT ATC TGT CAA CGT GGA ACC TCC CTG ACG

L27623    ,TRBV29-1*01     [3] --- --- --- --- --- --- --- --- --- --- --- --- --- --- --- --- --- --- --- ---

M13847    ,TRBV29-1*02     [5] --- --- --- --- --- --- --- --- --- --- --- --- --- --- --- --- --- --- --- ---

X04926    ,TRBV29-1*03    [22]                                                                             ---


                                                               ________________CDR1-IMGT________________
                              21  22  23  24  25  26  27  28  29  30  31  32  33  34  35  36  37  38  39  40
                              I   Q   C   Q   V   D   S   Q   V   T   M                               M   F
L36092,U66061,TRBV29-1*01     ATC CAG TGT CAA GTC GAT AGC CAA GTC ACC ATG ... ... ... ... ... ... ... ATG TTC

L27623    ,TRBV29-1*01       --- --- --- --- --- --- --- --- --- --- --- ... ... ... ... ... ... ... --- ---

M13847    ,TRBV29-1*02       --- --- --- --- --- --- --- --- --- --- --- ... ... ... ... ... ... ... --- ---
                                                                                                      I
X04926    ,TRBV29-1*03       --- --- --- --- --- --- --- --- --- --- --- ... ... ... ... ... ... ... --A ---


                                                                                      __________________CDR2-
                              41  42  43  44  45  46  47  48  49  50  51  52  53  54  55  56  57  58  59  60
                              W   Y   R   Q   Q   P   G   Q   S   L   T   L   I   A   T   A   N   Q   G   S
L36092,U66061,TRBV29-1*01     TGG TAC CGT CAG CAA CCT GGA CAG AGC CTG ACA CTG ATC GCA ACT GCA AAT CAG GGC TCT

L27623    ,TRBV29-1*01       --- --- --- --- --- --- --- --- --- --- --- --- --- --- --- --- --- --- --- ---

M13847    ,TRBV29-1*02       --- --- --- --- --- --- --- --- --- --- --- --- --- --- --- --- --- --- --- ---

X04926    ,TRBV29-1*03       --- --- --- --- --- --- --- --- --- --- --- --- --- --- --- --- --- --- --- ---


                              IMGT_______________
                              61  62  63  64  65  66  67  68  69  70  71  72  73  74  75  76  77  78  79  80
                              E   A           T   Y   E   S   G   F   V   I   D   K   F   P   I   S   R
L36092,U66061,TRBV29-1*01     GAG GCC ... ... ... ACA TAT GAG AGT GGA TTT GTC ATT GAC AAG TTT CCC ATC AGC CGC

L27623    ,TRBV29-1*01       --- --- ... ... ... --- --- --- --- --- --- --- --- --- --- --- --- --- --- ---

M13847    ,TRBV29-1*02       --- --- ... ... ... --- --- --- --- --- --- --- --- --- --- --- --- --- --- ---

X04926    ,TRBV29-1*03       --- --- ... ... ... --- --- --- --- --- --- --- --- --- --- --- --- --- --- ---


                              81  82  83  84  85  86  87  88  89  90  91  92  93  94  95  96  97  98  99 100
                              P       N   L   T   F   S   T   L   T   V   S   N   M   S   P   E   D   S   S
L36092,U66061,TRBV29-1*01     CCA ... AAC CTA ACA TTC TCA ACT CTG ACT GTG AGC AAC ATG AGC CCT GAA GAC AGC AGC

L27623    ,TRBV29-1*01       --- ... --- --- --- --- --- --- --- --- --- --- --- --- --- --- --- --- --- ---
                                                          S
M13847    ,TRBV29-1*02       --- ... --- --- --- --- --- -G- --- --- --- --- --- --- --- --- --- --- --- ---

X04926    ,TRBV29-1*03       --- ... --- --- --- --- --- --- --- --- --- --- --- --- --- --- --- --- --- ---


                                              ____CDR3-IMGT____
                              101 102 103 104 105 106 107 108
                              I   Y   L   C   S   V   E
L36092,U66061,TRBV29-1*01     ATA TAT CTC TGC AGC GTT GAA GA

L27623    ,TRBV29-1*01

M13847    ,TRBV29-1*02       --- --- --- --- --- --- ---             #c
                                                  A   G
X04926    ,TRBV29-1*03       --- --- --- --- --- -CG -GC             #c

#c: Rearranged cDNA
```

Framework and complementarity determining regions

FR1-IMGT: 26	CDR1-IMGT: 5
FR2-IMGT: 17	CDR2-IMGT: 7
FR3-IMGT: 38 (-1 aa: 82)	CDR3-IMGT: 3

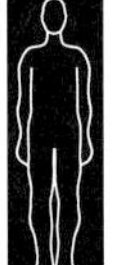

Collier de Perles for human TRBV29-1*01

Accession number: IMGT L36092   EMBL/GenBank/DDBJ: L36092

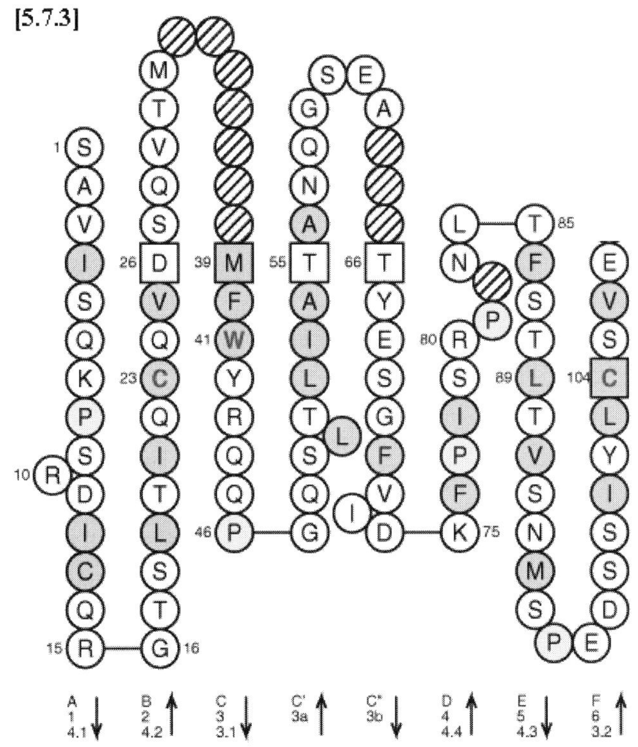

Genome database accession numbers
GDB:9954191   LocusLink: 28558

TRBV30

Nomenclature

TRBV30: T cell receptor beta variable 30.

Definition and functionality

TRBV30 is a functional gene (alleles *01, *02, *04, *05) or a pseudogene (allele *03). TRBV30 belongs to the TRBV30 subgroup which only comprises this mapped gene, in the TRB locus.

TRBV30*03 is a pseudogene due to Arginine (cga) 43 being replaced by a STOP-CODON (tga) in the FR2-IMGT.

Gene location

TRBV30 is in the TRB locus on chromosome 7 at 7q34.

Nucleotide and amino acid sequences for human TRBV30

```
                           1   2   3   4   5   6   7   8   9  10  11  12  13  14  15  16  17  18  19  20
                           S   Q   T   I   H   Q   W   P   A   T   L   V   Q   P   V   G   S   P   L   S
L36092,U66061,TRBV30*01 [34] TCT CAG ACT ATT CAT CAA TGG CCA GCG ACC CTG GTG CAG CCT GTG GGC AGC CCG CTC TCT
Z13967    ,TRBV30*02    [4]  --- --- --- --- --- --- --- --- --- --- --- --- --- --- --- --- --- --- --- ---
[4]       ,TRBV30*03         --- --- --- --- --- --- --- --- --- --- --- --- --- --- --- --- --- --- --- ---
M13554    ,TRBV30*04   [24]      --- --- --- --- --- --- --- --- --- --- --- --- --- --- --- --- --- --- ---
L06893    ,TRBV30*05   [36] --- --- --- --- --- --- --- --- --- --- --- --- --- --- --- --- --- --- --- --C

                                                            ________CDR1-IMGT________
                           21  22  23  24  25  26  27  28  29  30  31  32  33  34  35  36  37  38  39  40
                           L   E   C   T   V   E   G   T   S   N   P   N                           L   Y
L36092,U66061,TRBV30*01    CTG GAG TGC ACT GTG GAG GGA ACA TCA AAC CCC AAC ... ... ... ... ... ... CTA TAC
Z13967    ,TRBV30*02       --- --- --- --- --- --- --- --- --- --- --- --- ... ... ... ... ... ... --- ---
[4]       ,TRBV30*03       --- --- --- --- --- --- --- --- --- --- --- --- ... ... ... ... ... ... --- ---
M13554    ,TRBV30*04       --- --- --- --- --- --- --- --- --- --- --- --- ... ... ... ... ... ... --- ---
L06893    ,TRBV30*05       --- --- --- --- --- --- --- --- --- --- --- --- ... ... ... ... ... ... --- ---

                                                                                   ________CDR2-
                           41  42  43  44  45  46  47  48  49  50  51  52  53  54  55  56  57  58  59  60
                           W   Y   R   Q   A   A   G   R   G   L   Q   L   L   F   Y   S   V   G   I   G
L36092,U66061,TRBV30*01    TGG TAC CGA CAG GCT GCA GGC AGG GGC CTC CAG CTG CTC TTC TAC TCC GTT GGT ATT GGC
Z13967    ,TRBV30*02       --- --- --- --- --- --- --- --- --- --- --- --- --- --- --- --- --- --- --- ---
                                       *
[4]       ,TRBV30*03       --- --- T-- --- --- --- --- --- --- --- --- --- --- --- --- --- --- --- --- ---
                                                                                       I               D
M13554    ,TRBV30*04       --- --- --- --- --- --- --- --- --- --- --- --- --- --- --- --- A-- --- --- -A-
L06893    ,TRBV30*05       --- --- --- --- --- --- --A C-- --- --- --- --- --- --- --- --- --- --- --- ---

                           IMGT________
                           61  62  63  64  65  66  67  68  69  70  71  72  73  74  75  76  77  78  79  80
                                                  Q   I   S   S   E   V   P       Q   N   L   S   A   S   R
L36092,U66061,TRBV30*01    ... ... ... ... ... CAG ATC AGC TCT GAG GTG CCC ... CAG AAT CTC TCA GCC TCC AGA
Z13967    ,TRBV30*02       ... ... ... ... ... --- --- --- --- --- --- --- ... --- --- --- --- --- --- ---
[4]       ,TRBV30*03       ... ... ... ... ... --- --- --- --- --- --- --- ... --- --- --- --- --- --- ---
M13554    ,TRBV30*04       ... ... ... ... ... --- --- --- --- --- --- --- ... --- --- --- --- --- --- ---
L06893    ,TRBV30*05       ... ... ... ... ... --- --- --- --- --- --- --- ... --- --- --- --- --- --- ---

                           81  82  83  84  85  86  87  88  89  90  91  92  93  94  95  96  97  98  99 100
                           P       Q   D   R   Q   F   I   L   S   S   K   K   L   L   L   S   D   S   G
L36092,U66061,TRBV30*01    CCC ... CAG GAC CGG CAG TTC ATC CTG AGT TCT AAG AAG CTC CTT CTC AGT GAC TCT GGC
Z13967    ,TRBV30*02       --- ... --- --- --- --- --- --- --- --- --- --- --- --- --C --- --- --- --- ---
                           S
[4]       ,TRBV30*03       T-- ... --- --- --- --- --- --- --- --- --- --- --- --- --- --- --- --- --- ---
M13554    ,TRBV30*04       --- ... --- --- --- --- --- --T --- --- --- --- --- --- --C --- --- --- --- ---
L06893    ,TRBV30*05       --- ... --- --- --- --- --- --- --- --- --- --- --- --- --- --- --- --- --- ---
```

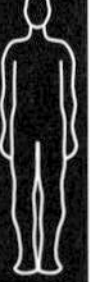

```
                                    ___CDR3-IMGT___
                         101 102 103 104 105 106 107 108
                          F   Y   L   C   A   W   S
    L36092,U66061,TRBV30*01 TTC TAT CTC TGT GCC TGG AGT GT

    Z13967   ,TRBV30*02    --- --- --- --- --- --- --- --

    [4]      ,TRBV30*03    --- --- --- --- --- --- --- --

    M13554   ,TRBV30*04    --- --- --- --- --- --- ---      #c
                                                     G
    L06893   ,TRBV30*05    --- --- --- --- --- --- G-A      #c

    *: STOP-CODON mutation
    #c: Rearranged cDNA
```

Framework and complementarity determining regions

FR1-IMGT: 26   CDR1-IMGT: 6
FR2-IMGT: 17   CDR2-IMGT: 5
FR3-IMGT: 37 (-2 aa: 73, 82)   CDR3-IMGT: 3

Collier de Perles for human TRBV30*01

Accession number: IMGT L36092   EMBL/GenBank/DDBJ: L36092

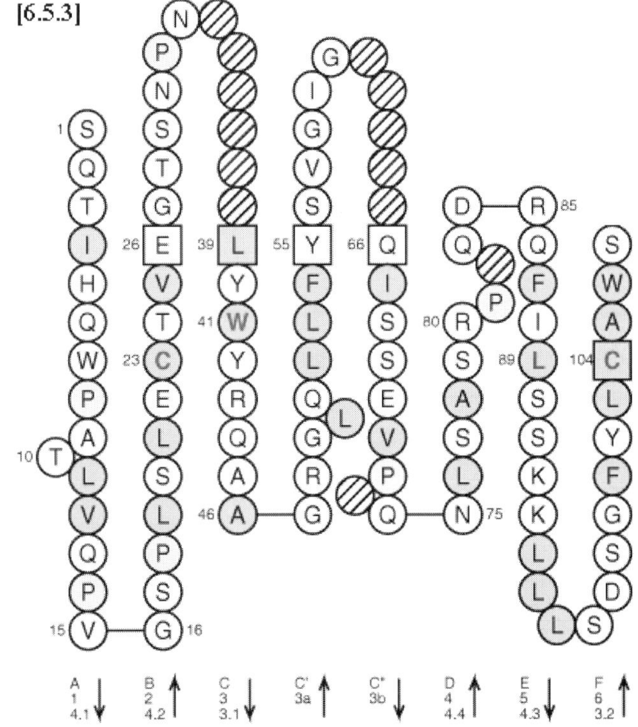

Genome database accession numbers
GDB:9954193   LocusLink: 28557

Protein display of the human TRB V-REGIONs

*Only the *01 allele of each functional or ORF V-REGION is shown. TRBV genes are listed, for each subgroup, according to their position from 5′ to 3′ in the locus. N-glycosylation sites (NXS/T, where X is different from P) are underlined.*

TRBV gene	FR1-IMGT (1–26)	CDR1-IMGT (27–38)	FR2-IMGT (39–55)	CDR2-IMGT (56–65)	FR3-IMGT (66–104)	CDR3-IMGT (105–115)
L36092 , TRBV2	EPEVTQTPSHQVTQMGQEVILRCVPI	SNHLY.......	FYWYRQILGQKVEFLVS	FYNNEI....	SEKSEIFDDQFSVERP.DGSNFTLKIRSTKLEDSAMYFC	ASSE.......
U07977 , TRBV3-1	DTAVSQTPKYLVTQMGNDKSIKCEQN	LGHDT.......	MYWYKQDSKKFLKIMFS	YNNKEL....	IINETVP.NRFSPKSP.DKAHLNLHINSLELGDSAVYFC	ASSQ.......
U07977 , TRBV4-1	DTEVTQTPKHLVMGMTNKKSLKCEQH	MGHRA.......	MYWYKQKAKKPPELMFV	YSYEKL....	SINESVP.SRFSPECP.NSSLLNLHLHALQPEDSALYLC	ASSQ.......
U07975 , TRBV4-2	ETGVTQTPRHLVMGMTNKKSLKCEQH	LGHNA.......	MYWYKQSAKKPLELMFV	YNFKEQ....	TENNSVP.SRFSPECP.NSSHLFLHLHTLQPEDSALYLC	ASSQ.......
U07978 , TRBV4-3	ETGVTQTPRHLVMGMTNKKSLKCEQH	LGHNA.......	MYWYKQSAKKPLELMFV	YSLEER....	VENNSVP.SRFSPECP.NSSHLFLHLHTLQPEDSALYLC	ASSQ.......
L36092 , TRBV5-1	KAGVTQTPRYLIKTRGQQVTLSCSPI	SGHRS.......	VSWYQQTPGQGLQFLFE	YFSETQ....	RNKGNFP.GRFSGRQF.SNSRSEMNVSTLELGDSALYLC	ASSL.......
X61439 , TRBV5-3	EAGVTQSPTHLIKTRGQQVTLRCSPI	SGHSS.......	VSWYQQAPGQGPQFIFE	YANELR....	RSEGNFP.NRFSGRQF.HDCCSEMNVSALELGDSALYLC	ARSL.......
L36092 , TRBV5-4	ETGVTQSPTHLIKTRGQQVTLRCSSQ	SGHNT.......	VSWYQQALGQGPQFIFQ	YYREEE....	NGRGNFP.PRFSGLQF.PNYSSELNVNALELDDSALYLC	ASSL.......
L36092 , TRBV5-5	DAGVTQSPTHLIKTRGQQVTLRCSPI	SGHKS.......	VSWYQQVLGQGPQFIFQ	YYEKEE....	RGRGNFP.DRFSARQF.PNYSSELNVNALLLGDSALYLC	ASSL.......
L36092 , TRBV5-6	DAGVTQSPTHLIKTRGQQVTLRCSPK	SGHDT.......	VSWYQQALGQGPQFIFQ	YYEEEE....	RQRGNFP.DRFSGHQF.PNYSSELNVNALLLGDSALYLC	ASSL.......
L36092 , TRBV5-7	DAGVTQSPTHLIKTRGQHVTLRCSPI	SGHTS.......	VSSYQQALGQGPQFIFQ	YYEKEE....	RGRGNFP.DQFSGHQF.PNYSSELNVNALLLGDSALYLC	ASSL.......
L36092 , TRBV5-8	EAGVTQSPTHLIKTRGQQATLRCSPI	SGHTS.......	VYWYQQALGLGLQFLLW	YDEGEE....	RNRGNFP.PRFSGRQF.PNYSSELNVNALELEDSALYLC	ASSL.......
X61446 , TRBV6-1	NAGVTQTPKFQVLKTGQSMTLQCAQD	MNHNS.......	MYWYRQDPGMGLRLIYY	SASEGT....	TDKGEVP.NGYNVSRL.NKREFSLRLESAAPSQTSVYFC	ASSE.......
X61445 , TRBV6-2	NAGVTQTPKFRVLKTGQSMTLLCAQD	MNHEY.......	MYWYRQDPGMGLRLIHY	SVGEGT....	TAKGEVP.DGYNVSRL.KKQNFLLGLESAAPSQTSVYFC	ASSY.......
U07978 , TRBV6-3	NAGVTQTPKFRVLKTGQSMTLLCAQD	MNHEY.......	MYWYRQDPGMGLRLIHY	SVGEGT....	TAKGEVP.DGYNVSRL.KKQNFLLGLESAAPSQTSVYFC	ASSY.......
X61653 , TRBV6-4	IAGITQAPTSQILAAGRRMTLRCTQD	MRHNA.......	MYWYRQDLGLGLRLIHY	SNTAGT....	TGKGEVP.DGYSVSRA.NTDDFPLTLASAVPSQTSVYFC	ASSD.......
L36092 , TRBV6-5	NAGVTQTPKFQVLKTGQSMTLQCAQD	MNHEY.......	MSWYRQDPGMGLRLIHY	SVGAGI....	TDQGEVP.NGYNVSRS.TTEDFPLRLLSAAPSQTSVYFC	ASSY.......
L36092 , TRBV6-6	NAGVTQTPKFRILKIGQSMTLQCTQD	MNHNY.......	MYWYRQDPGMGLKLIYY	SVGAGI....	TDKGEVP.NGYNVSRS.TTEDFPLRLELAAPSQTSVYFC	ASSY.......
L36092 , TRBV6-7	NAGVTQTPKFHVLKTGQSMTLLCAQD	MNHEY.......	MYRYRQDPGKGLRLIYY	SVAAAL....	TDKGEVP.NGYNVSRS.NTEDFPLKLESAAPSQTSVYFC	ASSY.......
L36092 , TRBV6-8	NAGVTQTPKFHILKTGQSMTLQCAQD	MNHGY.......	MSWYRQDPGMGLRLIYY	SAAAGT....	TDK.EVP.NGYNVSRL.NTEDFPLRLVSAAPSQTSVYFC	ASSY.......
X61447 , TRBV6-9	NAGVTQTPKFHILKTGQSMTLQCAQD	MNHGY.......	LSWYRQDPGMGLRRIHY	SVAAGI....	TDKGEVP.DGYNVSRS.NTEDFPLRLESAAPSQTSVYFC	ASSY.......
X61444 , TRBV7-1	GAGVSQSLRHKVAKKGKDVALRYDPI	SGHNA.......	LYWYRQSLGQGLEFPIY	FQGKDA....	ADKSGLPRDRFSAQRS.EGSISTLKFQRTQQGDLAVYLC	ASSS.......
X61442 , TRBV7-2	GAGVSQSPSNKVTEKGKDVELRCDPI	SGHTA.......	LYWYRQSLGQGLEFLIY	FQGNSA....	PDKSGLPSDRFSAERT.GGSVSTLTIQRTQQEDSAVYLC	ASSL.......
X61440 , TRBV7-3	GAGVSQTPSNKVTEKGKYVELRCDPI	SGHTA.......	LYWYRQSLGQGPEFLIY	FQGTGA....	ADDSGLPNDRFFAVRP.EGSVSTLKIQRTERGDSAVYLC	ASSL.......
L36092 , TRBV7-4	GAGVSQSPRYKVAKRGRDVALRCDSI	SGHVT.......	LYWYRQTLGQGSEVLTY	SQSDAQ....	RDKSGRPSGRFSAERP.ERSVSTLKIQRTEQGDSAVYLC	ASSL.......
L36092 , TRBV7-6	GAGVSQSPRYKVTKRGQDVALRCDPI	SGHVS.......	LYWYRQALGQGPEFLTY	FNYEAQ....	QDKSGLPNDRFSAERP.EGSISTLTIQRTEQRDSAMYRC	ASSL.......
L36092 , TRBV7-7	GAGVSQSPRYKVTKRGQDVTLRCDPI	SSHAT.......	LYWYQQALGQGPEFLTY	FNYEAQ....	PDKSGLPSDRFSAERP.EGSISTLTIQRTEQRDSAMYRC	ASSL.......
M11953 , TRBV7-8	GAGVSQSPRYKVAKRGQDVALRCDPI	SGHVS.......	LFWYQQALGQGPEFLTY	FQNEAQ....	LDKSGLPSDRFFAERP.EGSVSTLKIQRTQQEDSAVYLC	ASSL.......
L36092 , TRBV7-9	DTGVSQNPRHKITKRGQNVTFRCDPI	SEHNR.......	LYWYRQTLGQGPEFLTY	FQNEAQ....	LEKSRLLSDRFSAERP.KGSFSTLEIQRTEQGDSAMYLC	ASSL.......

Continued

Continued

TRBV gene		FR1-IMGT (1-26)	CDR1-IMGT (27-38)	FR2-IMGT (39-55)	CDR2-IMGT (56-65)	FR3-IMGT (66-104)	CDR3-IMGT (105-115)
L36092	,TRBV9	DSGVTQTPKHLITATGQRVTLRCSPR	SGDLS.......	VYWYQQSLDQGLQFLIQ	YYNGEE....	RAKGNIL.ERFSAQQF.PDLHSELNLSSLELGDSALYFC	ASSV.......
U17050	,TRBV10-1	DAEITQSPRHKITETGRQVTLACHQT	WNHNN.......	MFWYRQDLGHGLRLIHY	SYGVQD....	TNKGEVS.DGYSVSRS.NTEDLPLTLESAASSQTSVYFC	ASSE.......
U17049	,TRBV10-2	DAGITQSPRYKITETGRQVTLMCHQT	WSHSY.......	MFWYRQDLGHGLRLIYY	SAAADI....	TDKGEVP.DGYVVSRS.KTENFPLTLESATRSQTSVYFC	ASSE.......
U03115	,TRBV10-3	DAGITQSPRHKVTETGTPVTLRCHQT	ENHRY.......	MYWYRQDPGHGLRLIHY	SYGVKD....	TDKGEVS.DGYSVSRS.KTEDFLLTLESATSSQTSVYFC	AISE.......
M33233	,TRBV11-1	EAEVAQSPRYKITEKSQAVAFWCDPI	SGHAT.......	LYWYRQILGQGPELLVQ	FQDESV....	VDDSQLPKDRFSAERL.KGVDSTLKIQPAELGDSAMYLC	ASSL.......
L36092	,TRBV11-2	EAGVAQSPRYKIIEKRQSVAFWCNPI	SGHAT.......	LYWYQQILGQGPKLLIQ	FQNNGV....	VDDSQLPKDRFSAERL.KGVDSTLKIQPAKLEDSAVYLC	ASSL.......
M33234	,TRBV11-3	EAGVVQSPRYKIIEKKQPVAFWCNPI	SGHNT.......	LYWYLQNLGQGPELLIR	YENEEA....	VDDSQLPKDRFSAERL.KGVDSTLKIQPAELGDSAVYLC	ASSL.......
X07192	,TRBV12-3	DAGVIQSPRHEVTEMGQEVTLRCKPI	SGHNS.......	LFWYRQTMMRGLELLIY	FNNNVP....	IDDSGMPEDRFSAKMP.NASFSTLKIQPSEPRDSAVYFC	ASSL.......
K02546	,TRBV12-4	DAGVIQSPRHEVTEMGQEVTLRCKPI	SGHDY.......	LFWYRQTMMRGLELLIY	FNNNVP....	IDDSGMPEDRFSAKMP.NASFSTLKIQPSEPRDSAVYFC	ASSL.......
X07223	,TRBV12-5	DARVTQTPRHKVTEMGQEVTMRCQPI	LGHNT.......	VFWYRQTMMQGLELLAY	FRNRAP....	LDDSGMPKDRFSAEMP.DATLATLKIQPSEPRDSAVYFC	ASGL.......
U03115	,TRBV13	AAGVIQSPRHLIKEKRETATLKCYPI	PRHDT.......	VYWYQQGPGQDPQFLIS	FYEKMQ....	SDKGSIP.DRFSAQQF.SDYHSELNMSSLELGDSALYFC	ASSL.......
X06154	,TRBV14	EAGVTQFPSHSVIEKGQTVTLRCDPI	SGHDN.......	LYWYRRVMGKEIKFLLH	FVKESK....	QDESGMPNNRFLAERT.GGTYSTLKVQPAELEDSGVYFC	ASSQ.......
U03115	,TRBV15	DAMVIQNPRYQVTQFGKPVTLSCSQT	LNHNV.......	MYWYQQKSSQAPKLLFH	YYDKDF....	NNEADTP.DNFQSRRP.NTSFCFLDIRSPGLGDTAMYLC	ATSR.......
L26231	,TRBV16	GEEVAQTPKHLVRGEGQKAKLYCAPI	KGHSY.......	VFWYQQVLKNEFKFLIS	FQNENV....	FDETGMPKERFSAKCL.PNSPCSLEIQATKLEDSAVYFC	ASSQ.......
U03115	,TRBV17	EPGVSQTPRHKVTNMGQEVILRCDPS	SGHMF.......	VHWYRQNLRQEMKLLIS	FQYQNI....	AVDSGMPKERFTAERP.NGTSSTLKIHPAEPRDSAVYLY	SSG.......
L36092	,TRBV18	NAGVMQNPRHLVRRRGQEARLRCSPM	KGHSH.......	VYWYRQLPEEGLKFMVY	LQKENI....	IDESGMPKERFSAEFP.KEGPSILRIQQVVRGDSAAYFC	ASSP.......
U48260	,TRBV19	DGGITQSPKYLFRKEGQNVTLSCEQN	LNHDA.......	MYWYRQDPGQGLRLIYY	SQIVND....	FQKGDIA.EGYSVSRE.KKESFPLTVTSAQKNPTAFYLC	ASSI.......
M11955	,TRBV20-1	GAVVSQHPSWVICKSGTSVKIECRSL	DFQATT......	MFWYRQFPKQSLMLMAT	SNEGSKA...	TYEQGVEKDKFLINHA.SLTLSTLTVTSAHPEDSSFYIC	SAR.......
L36092	,TRBV23-1	HAKVTQTPGHLVKGKGQKTKMDCTPE	KGHTF.......	VYWYQQNQNKEFMLLIS	FQNEQV....	LQETEMHKKRFSSQCP.KNAPCSLAILSSEPGDTALYLC	ASSQ.......
M11951	,TRBV24-1	DADVTQTPRNRITKTGKRIMLECSQT	KGHDR.......	MYWYRQDPGLGLRLIYY	SFDVKD....	INKGEIS.DGYSVSRQ.AQAKFSLSLESAIPNQTALYFC	ATSDL.......
L36092	,TRBV25-1	EADIYQTPRYLVIGTGKKITLECSQT	MGHDK.......	MYWYQQDPGMELHLIHY	SYGVNS....	TEKGDLS.SESTVSRI.RTEHFPLTLESARPSHTSQYLC	ASSE.......
L36092	,TRBV27	EAQVTQNPRYLITVTGKKLTVTCSQN	MNHEY.......	MSWYRQDPGLGLRQIYY	SMNVEV....	TDKGDVP.EGYKVSRK.EKRNFPLILESPSPNQTSLYFC	ASSL.......
U08314	,TRBV28	DVKVTQSSRYLVKRTGEKVFLECVQD	MDHEN.......	MFWYRQDPGLGLRLIYF	SYDVKM....	KEKGDIP.EGYSVSRE.KKERFSLILESASTNQTSMYLC	ASSL.......
L36092	,TRBV29-1	SAVISQKPSRDICQRGTSLTIQCQVD	SQVTM.......	MFWYRQQPGQSLTLIAT	ANQGSEA...	TYESGFVIDKFPISRP.NLTFSTLTVSNMSPEDSSIYLC	SVE.......
L36092	,TRBV30	SQTIHQWPATLVQPVGSPLSLECTVE	GTSNPN......	LYWYRQAAGRGLQLLFY	SVGIG.....	QISSEVP.QNLSASRP.QDRQFILSSKKLLLSDSGFYLC	AWS.......

Recombination signals

Only the recombination signal of the *01 allele of each functional or ORF TRB V-REGION is shown. Non-conserved nucleotides taken into account for the ORF functionality definition are shown in bold and italic.

TRAV	V Recombination Signal (V-RS)		
gene name	V-HEPTAMER	(bp)	V-NONAMER
TRBV2*01	CACAGCC	23	GCAAAATCC
TRBV3-1*01	CACAGCC	23	GCACAAACC
TRBV4-1*01	CACAGCC	23	GCAGAAACC
TRBV4-2*01	CACAGCC	23	GCAGAAACC
TRBV4-3*01	CACAGCC	23	GCAGAAACC
TRBV5-1*01	CACAGCC	23	GCACAAACC
TRBV5-3*01 (ORF)	CACAGCC	23	GCACTAATC
TRBV5-4*01	CACAGCC	23	ACATAAACT
TRBV5-5*01	CACAGCC	23	ATATAAACT
TRBV5-6*01	CACAGCC	23	ATATAAACT
TRBV5-7*01 (ORF)	CACAGCC	23	ATATAAACT
TRBV5-8*01	CACAGCC	23	ATATAAACT
TRBV6-1*01	CACAGCG	23	ACATAAAGG
TRBV6-2*01	CACAGTG	23	ACAGAAAGG
TRBV6-3*01	CACAGTG	23	ACAGAAAGG
TRBV6-4*01	CACAGTG	23	ACATAAATG
TRBV6-5*01	CACAGCG	23	ACATAAAGG
TRBV6-6*01	CACAGCG	23	ACATAAAGG
TRBV6-7*01 (ORF)	CACAGCG	23	ACATAAAGG
TRBV6-8*01	CACAGCG	23	ACATAAAGG
TRBV6-9*01	CACAGCG	23	ACATAAAGG
TRBV7-1*01 (ORF)	CACAGCA	del	del
TRBV7-2*01	CACAGCA	23	TCATAAACC
TRBV7-3*01	CACAGCA	23	TCATAAACC
TRBV7-4*01	CACAGCG	23	TCACAAACC
TRBV7-6*01	CACAGTG	23	TCACAAACC
TRBV7-7*01	CACAGCA	23	TCACAAACC
TRBV7-8*01	CACAGCA	23	TCACAAACC
TRBV7-9*01	CACAGCA	23	TCACAAACC
TRBV9*01	CACAGCC	23	GCAATAACA
TRBV10-1*01	CACAGTG	23	ACATAAAGG
TRBV10-2*01	CACAGTG	23	ACGGAAATG
TRBV10-3*01	CACAGTG	23	ACGTAAACA
TRBV11-1*01	CACAGCG	22	GCACAAAAC
TRBV11-2*01	CACAGTG	23	GCAGAAAAC
TRBV11-3*01	CACAGTG	23	GCAGAAAAC
TRBV12-3*01	CACAGCG	23	GCAGAAAAC
TRBV12-4*01	CACAGCG	23	GCAGAAACC
TRBV12-5*01	CACAGCG	23	GCAGAAACC
TRBV13*01	CACAGAC	23	ACCCAAACC
TRBV14*01	CACAGTG	23	GCAAAACCA
TRBV15*01	CACAGAG	23	TCATAAACC
TRBV16*01	CACAGTG	23	CACAGACTC
TRBV17*01 (ORF)	CACAGCA	23	GTGCAAACC
TRBV18*01	CACATTG	23	CCACAAACA
TRBV19*01	CACAGTG	23	GCATAAATG
TRBV20-1*01	CACAGCG	23	GCAAGAACC
TRBV23-1*01 (ORF)	CACAGCA	23	ACACAAACT
TRBV24-1*01	CACAGTG	23	ACAGAAAGA
TRBV25-1*01	CACAGTG	23	ACAGAAAGG
TRBV27*01	CACAGTG	23	ACAAAAACA
TRBV28*01	CACAGCG	23	ACAAAAAGA
TRBV29-1*01	CACAGTG	23	GCAAGAACC
TRBV30*01	CACACTG	23	GCAAAAACC

del: deleted

References

1 Barron, K.S. et al., unpublished.
2 Boitel, B. et al. (1992) J. Exp. Med. 175, 765–777.
3 Charmley, P. et al. (1995) Genomics 25, 150–156.
4 Charmley, P. et al. (1993) J. Exp. Med. 177, 135–143.
5 Concannon, P. et al. (1986) Proc. Natl Acad. Sci. USA 83, 6598–6602.
6 Cornélis, F. et al. (1993) Eur. J. Immunol. 23, 1277–1283.
7 Currier, J.R. et al. unpublished.
8 Day, C.E. et al. (1992) Hum. Immunol. 34, 196–202.
9 Deulofeut, H. et al. (1995) Hum. Immunol. 43, 227–230.
10 Ferradini, L. et al. (1991) Eur. J. Immunol. 21, 935–942.
11 Gomolka, M. et al. (1993) Immunogenetics 37, 257–265.
12 Hall, M.A. et al. (1994) Eur. J. Immunol. 24, 641–645.
13 Hansen, T. et al. (1992) Scand. J. Immunol. 36, 285–290.
14 Hansen, T. et al. (1991) Tissue Antigens 38, 99–103.
15 Hoffman, R.W. et al. (1993) J. Immunol. 151, 6460–6469.
16 Hurley, C.K. et al. (1993) J. Immunol. 150, 1314–1324.
17 Ikuta, K. et al. (1986) Nucleic Acids Res. 14, 4899–4909.
18 Ikuta, K. et al. (1985) Proc. Natl Acad. Sci. USA 82, 7701–7705.
19 Jores, R. et al. (1993) J. Immunol. 151, 6110–6122.
20 Kay, R.A. et al. (1994) Eur. J. Immunol. 24, 2863–2867.
21 Kimura, N. et al. (1987) Eur. J. Immunol. 17, 375–383.
22 Kimura, N. et al. (1986) J. Exp. Med. 164, 739–750.
23 Leiden, J.M. et al. (1986) Immunogenetics 24, 17–23.
24 Leiden, J.N. et al. (1986) Proc. Natl Acad. Sci. USA 83, 4456–4460.
25 Li, Y. et al. (1996) Hum. Immunol. 49, 85–95.
26 Li, Y. et al. (1991) J. Exp. Med. 174, 1537–1547.
27 Luyrink, L. et al. (1993) Proc. Natl Acad. Sci. USA 90, 4369–4373.
28 Maksymowych, W.P. et al. (1992) Immunogenetics 35, 257–262.
29 Nickerson, D.A. et al., unpublished.
30 Obata, F. et al. (1993) Immunogenetics. 38 67–70.
31 Plaza, A. et al. (1992) J. Immunol. 147, 4360–4365.
32 Posnett, D.N. et al. (1994) J. Exp. Med. 179, 1707–1711.
33 Robinson, M.A. et al. (1991) J. Immunol. 146, 4392–4397.
34 Rowen, L. et al. (1996) Science 272, 1755–1762. (see Note)
35 Rowen, L. et al., unpublished.
36 Santamaria, P. et al. (1993) Immunogenetics 38, 163–163.
37 Siu, G. et al. (1984) Cell 37, 393–401.
38 Siu, G. et al. (1986) J. Exp. Med. 164, 1600–1614.
39 Slightom, J.L. et al. (1994) Genomics 20, 146–168.
40 Smith, W.J. et al. (1987) Nucleic Acids Res. 15, 4991–4991.
41 Tillinghast, J.P. et al. (1986) Science 233, 879–883.
42 Triebel, F. et al. (1988) J. Immunol. 140, 300–304.
43 Van Schooten, W.C. et al. (1992) Proc. Natl Acad. Sci. USA 89, 11244–11248.
44 Wei, S. et al. (1994) Immunogenetics. 40, 27–36.
45 Weiss, S. et al., unpublished.
46 Wilson, R.K. et al. (1990) Immunogenetics 32, 406–412.

[47] Zhao, T.M. et al. (1994) J. Exp. Med. 180, 1405–1414.

Note:
The original L36092 sequence (684 973 bp) has been split in EMBL into three sequences of 267 156 bp (U66059), 215 422 bp (U66060), and 232 650 bp (U66061); L36092 has become secondary accession number of U66059, U66060, and U66061. In IMGT, the original sequence L36092, which is fully annotated, has also been kept as primary accession number, in addition to U66059, U66060, and U66061.

THE HUMAN
T CELL RECEPTOR
TRG GENES

Part 1

TRGC

TRGC1

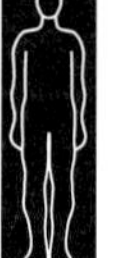

Nomenclature

TRGC1: T cell receptor gamma constant 1.

Definition and functionality

TRGC1 is one of the two functional genes of the TRGC group which comprises two mapped genes, TRGC1 and TRGC2. TRGC1 and TRGC2 result from a recent duplication.

Gene location

TRGC1 is in the TRG locus on chromosome 7 at 7p14. TRGC1 is preceded by three functional joining genes TRGJP1, TRGJP, and TRGJ1.

Nucleotide and amino acid sequences for human TRGC1

The nucleotide in parentheses at the beginning of exons comes from a DONOR–SPLICE (n from ngt).

The Cysteines involved in the intrachain disulfide bridges are shown with their number and letter **C** in bold.

N-glycosylation sites (NXS/T, where X is different from P) are underlined.

```
                                     1   2   3   4   5   6   7   8   9  10  11  12  13  14  15  16  17  18  19  20
                                     D   K   Q   L   D   A   D   V   S   P   K   P   T   I   F   L   P   S   I   A
M14996  ,TRGC1*01,lambdaD19 (EX1)[2] (G)AT AAA CAA CTT GAT GCA GAT GTT TCC CCC AAG CCC ACT ATT TTT CTT CCT TCA ATT GCT
M13915  ,TRGC1*01              [1] (-)-- --- --- --- --- --- --- --- --- --- --- --- --- --- --- --- --- --- --- ---
M17325  ,TRGC1*01,Tgamma5 (cDNA)[3] (-)-- --- --- --- --- --- --- --- --- --- --- --- --- --- --- --- --- --- --- ---
AF159056,TRGC1*01              [4] (-)-- --- --- --- --- --- --- --- --- --- --- --- --- --- --- --- --- --- --- ---
M14999  ,TRGC1*02,lambdaRgamma [2] (-)-- --- --- --- --- --- --- --- --- --- --- --- --- --- --- --- --- --G --- ---
M13914  ,TRGC1*02              [1] (-)-- --- --- --- --- --- --- --- --- --- --- --- --- --- --- --- --- --G --- ---

                                    21  22  23  24  25  26  27  28  29  30  31  32  33  34  35  36  37  38  39  40
                                     E   T   K   L   Q   K   A   G   T   Y   L   C   L   L   E   K   F   F   P   D
M14996  ,TRGC1*01,lambdaD19 (EX1)   GAA ACA AAG CTC CAG AAG GCT GGA ACA TAC CTT TGT CTT CTT GAG AAA TTT TTC CCT GAT
M13915  ,TRGC1*01                   --- --- --- --- --- --- --- --- --- --- --- --- --- --- --- --- --- --- --- ---
M17325  ,TRGC1*01,Tgamma5 (cDNA)    --- --- --- --- --- --- --- --- --- --- --- --- --- --- --- --- --- --- --- ---
AF159056,TRGC1*01                   --- --- --- --- --- --- --- --- --- --- --- --- --- --- --- --- --- --- --- ---
M14999  ,TRGC1*02,lambdaRgamma      --- --- --A --- --- --- --- --- --- --- --- --- --- --- --- --- --- --- --A ---
M13914  ,TRGC1*02                   --- --- --A --- --- --- --- --- --- --- --- --- --- --- --- --- --- --- --A ---

                                    41  42  43  44  45  46  47  48  49  50  51  52  53  54  55  56  57  58  59  60
                                     V   I   K   I   H   W   Q   E   K   K   S   N   T   I   L   G   S   Q   E   G
M14996  ,TRGC1*01,lambdaD19 (EX1)   GTT ATT AAG ATA CAT TGG CAA GAA AAG AAG AGC AAC ACG ATT CTG GGA TCC CAG GAG GGG
M13915  ,TRGC1*01                   --- --- --- --- --- --- --- --- --- --- --- --- -
M17325  ,TRGC1*01,Tgamma5 (cDNA)    --- --- --- --- --- --- --- --- --- --- --- --- --- --- --- --- --- --- --- ---
AF159056,TRGC1*01                   --- --- --- --- --- --- --- --- --- --- --- --- --- --- --- --- --- --- --- ---
                                     I
M14999  ,TRGC1*02,lambdaRgamma      A-- --- --- --- --- --- --- --- --- --- --- --- --- --- --- --- --- --- --- ---
                                     I
M13914  ,TRGC1*02                   A-- --- --- --- --- --- --- --- --- --- --- --- --- --- --- -

                                    61  62  63  64  65  66  67  68  69  70  71  72  73  74  75  76  77  78  79  80
                                     N   T   M   K   T   N   D   T   Y   M   K   F   S   W   L   T   V   P   E   K
M14996  ,TRGC1*01,lambdaD19 (EX1)   AAC ACC ATG AAG ACT AAC GAC ACA TAC ATG AAA TTT AGC TGG TTA ACG GTG CCA GAA AAG
M17325  ,TRGC1*01,Tgamma5 (cDNA)    --- --- --- --- --- --- --- --- --- --- --- --- --- --- --- --- --- --- --- ---
AF159056,TRGC1*01                   --- --- --- --- --- --- --- --- --- --- --- --- --- --- --- --- --- --- --- ---
                                                                                                                  E
M14999  ,TRGC1*02,lambdaRgamma      --- --- --- --- --- --- --- --- --- --- --- --- --- --- --- --- --- --- --- G--

                                    81  82  83  84  85  86  87  88  89  90  91  92  93  94  95  96  97  98  99 100
                                     S   L   D   K   E   H   R   C   I   V   R   H   E   N   N   K   N   G   V   D
M14996  ,TRGC1*01,lambdaD19 (EX1)   TCA CTG GAC AAA GAA CAC AGA TGT ATC GTC AGA CAT GAG AAT AAT AAA AAC GGA GTT GAT
M17325  ,TRGC1*01,Tgamma5 (cDNA)    --- --- --- --- --- --- --- --- --- --- --- --- --- --- --- --- --- --- --- ---
AF159056,TRGC1*01                   --- --- --- --- --- --- --- --- --- --- --- --- --- --- --- --- --- --- --- ---
                                                                                                              I
M14999  ,TRGC1*02,lambdaRgamma      --- --- --- --- --- --- --- --- --- --- --- --- --- --- --- --- --- --- A-- ---
```

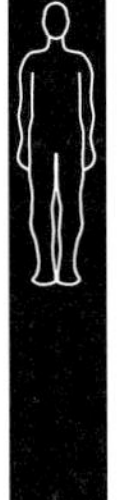

```
                                   101 102 103 104 105 106 107 108 109 110
                                    Q   E   I   I   F   P   P   I   K   T
M14991   ,TRGC1*01,lambdaD19 (EX1)  CAA GAA ATT ATC TTT CCT CCA ATA AAG ACA G
M17325   ,TRGC1*01,Tgamma5 (cDNA)   --- --- --- --- --- --- --- --- --- --- -
AF159056,TRGC1*01                   --- --- --- --- --- --- --- --- --- --- -
M14999   ,TRGC1*02,lambdaRgamma     -


                                     1   2   3   4   5   6   7   8   9   10  11  12  13  14  15  16
                                     D   V   I   T   M   D   P   K   D   N   C   S   K   D   A   N
M14997   ,TRGC1*01,lambdaD19 (EX2) [2] AT GTC ATC ACA ATG GAT CCC AAA GAC AAT TGT TCA AAA GAT GCA AAT G
M17325   ,TRGC1*01,Tgamma5 (cDNA)   -- --- --- --- --- --- --- --- --- --- --- --- --- --- --- --- -
AF159056,TRGC1*01                   -- --- --- --- --- --- --- --- --- --- --- --- --- --- --- --- -


                                     1   2   3   4   5   6   7   8   9   10  11  12  13  14  15  16  17  18  19  20
                                     D   T   L   L   L   Q   L   T   N   M   Y   L   L   L   L   T   S   A   Y   Y
M14998   ,TRGC1*01,lambdaD19 (EX3)  AT ACA CTA CTG CTG CAG CTC ACA AAC ACC TCT GCA TAT TAC ATG TAC CTC CTC CTG CTC
M17325   ,TRGC1*01,Tgamma5 (cDNA)   -- --- --- --- --- --- --- --- --- --- --- --- --- --- --- --- --- --- --- ---
AF159056,TRGC1*01                   -- --- --- --- --- --- --- --- --- --- --- --- --- --- --- --- --- --- --- ---


                                    21  22  23  24  25  26  27  28  29  30  31  32  33  34  35  36  37  38  39  40
                                     L   K   S   V   V   Y   F   A   I   I   T   C   C   L   L   R   R   T   A   F
M14998   ,TRGC1*01,lambdaD19 (EX3)  CTC AAG AGT GTG GTC TAT TTT GCC ATC ATC ACC TGC TGT CTG CTT AGA AGA ACG GCT TTC
M17325   ,TRGC1*01,Tgamma5 (cDNA)   --- --- --- --- --- --- --- --- --- --- --- --- --- --- --- --- --- --- --- ---
AF159056,TRGC1*01                   --- --- --- --- --- --- --- --- --- --- --- --- --- --- --- --- --- --- --- ---


                                    41  42  43  44  45  46  47
                                     C   C   N   G   E   K   S   *
M14998   ,TRGC1*01,lambdaD19 (EX3)  TGC TGC AAT GGA GAG AAA TCA
M17325   ,TRGC1*01,Tgamma5 (cDNA)   --- --- --- --- --- --- ---
AF159056,TRGC1*01                   --- --- --- --- --- --- ---
```

Genome database accession numbers

GDB:120408   LocusLink: 6966

References

[1] Lefranc, M.-P. and Rabbitts T.H. (1985) Nature 316, 464–466.
[2] Lefranc, M.-P. et al. (1986) Proc. Natl Acad. Sci. USA 83, 9596–9600.
[3] Pelicci, P.G. et al. (1987) Science 237, 1051–1055.
[4] Zhan, M. et al., unpublished.

Protein display

Protein display of the TRGC1 gene is shown on page 372.

Nomenclature

TRGC2(2x): T cell receptor gamma constant 2 (2x).

Definition and functionality

TRGC2 is one of the two functional genes of the TRGC group which comprises two mapped genes. TRGC1 and TRGC2 result from a recent duplication. The TRGC2 gene has four or five exons due to the duplication or triplication of exon 2. These polymorphic TRGC2 genes are designated as TRGC2(2x) and TRGC2(3x) respectively.

Based on sequence similarity with the TRGC2(3x) exons, and taking into account the evolution of the TRGC2 polymorphism as a result of unequal crossings-over[4], the duplicated exon 2 of TRGC2(2x) is designated as EX2T or EX2R.

EX2R, but not EX2T, has one N-glycosylation site.

Gene location

TRGC2 is in the TRG locus on chromosome 7 at 7p14. TRGC2 is preceded by two functional joining genes TRGJP2 and TRGJ2.

Nucleotide and amino acid sequences for human TRGC2(2x)

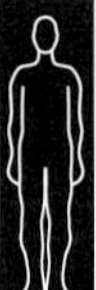

The nucleotide between parentheses at the beginning of exons comes from a DONOR–SPLICE (n from ngt).
The Cysteines involved in the intrachain disulfide bridges are shown with their number and letter **C** in bold.
N-glycosylation sites (NXS/T, where X is different from P) are underlined.

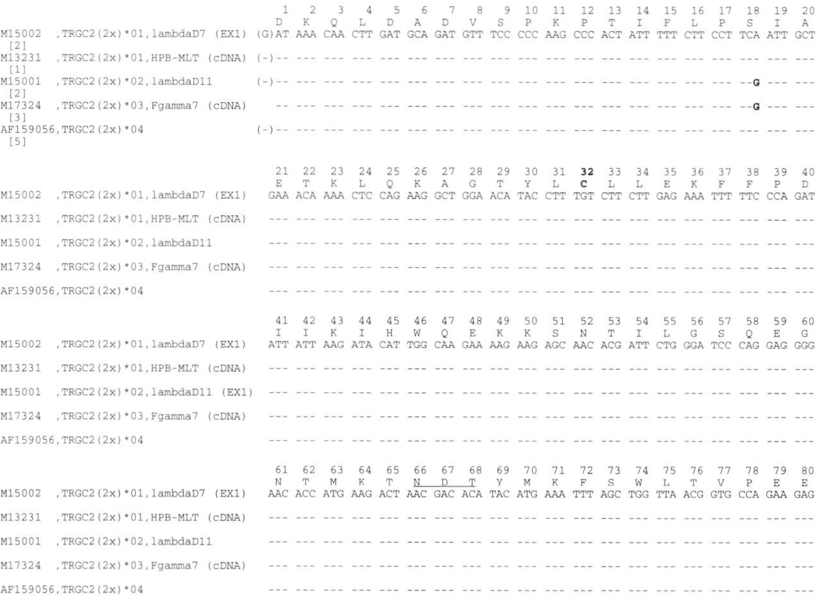

```
                                       1    2    3    4    5    6    7    8    9   10   11   12   13   14   15   16   17   18   19   20
                                       D    K    Q    L    D    A    D    V    S    P    K    P    T    I    F    L    P    S    I    A
M15002   ,TRGC2(2x)*01,lambdaD7  (EX1) (G)AT AAA  CAA  CTT  GAT  GCA  GAT  GTT  TCC  CCC  AAG  CCC  ACT  ATT  TTT  CTT  CCT  TCA  ATT  GCT
  [2]
M13231   ,TRGC2(2x)*01,HPB-MLT  (cDNA) (-)--  ---  ---  ---  ---  ---  ---  ---  ---  ---  ---  ---  ---  ---  ---  ---  ---  ---  ---  ---
  [1]
M15001   ,TRGC2(2x)*02,lambdaD11       (-)--  --G  ---  ---  ---  ---  ---  ---  ---  ---  ---  ---  ---  ---  ---  ---  --G  ---  ---
  [2]
M17324   ,TRGC2(2x)*03,Fgamma7  (cDNA)   --  --G  ---  ---  ---  ---  ---  ---  ---  ---  ---  ---  ---  ---  ---  ---  --G  ---  ---
  [3]
AF159056,TRGC2(2x)*04                  (-)--  ---  ---  ---  ---  ---  ---  ---  ---  ---  ---  ---  ---  ---  ---  ---  ---  ---  ---  ---
  [5]

                                      21   22   23   24   25   26   27   28   29   30   31   32   33   34   35   36   37   38   39   40
                                       E    T    K    L    Q    K    A    G    T    Y    L    C    L    L    E    K    F    F    P    D
M15002   ,TRGC2(2x)*01,lambdaD7  (EX1) GAA  ACA  AAA  CTC  CAG  AAG  GCT  GGA  ACA  TAC  CTT  TGT  CTT  CTT  GAG  AAA  TTT  TTC  CCA  GAT

M13231   ,TRGC2(2x)*01,HPB-MLT  (cDNA) ---  ---  ---  ---  ---  ---  ---  ---  ---  ---  ---  ---  ---  ---  ---  ---  ---  ---  ---  ---

M15001   ,TRGC2(2x)*02,lambdaD11       ---  ---  ---  ---  ---  ---  ---  ---  ---  ---  ---  ---  ---  ---  ---  ---  ---  ---  ---  ---

M17324   ,TRGC2(2x)*03,Fgamma7  (cDNA) ---  ---  ---  ---  ---  ---  ---  ---  ---  ---  ---  ---  ---  ---  ---  ---  ---  ---  ---  ---

AF159056,TRGC2(2x)*04                  ---  ---  ---  ---  ---  ---  ---  ---  ---  ---  ---  ---  ---  ---  ---  ---  ---  ---  ---  ---

                                      41   42   43   44   45   46   47   48   49   50   51   52   53   54   55   56   57   58   59   60
                                       I    I    K    I    H    W    Q    E    K    K    S    N    T    I    L    G    S    Q    E    G
M15002   ,TRGC2(2x)*01,lambdaD7  (EX1) ATT  ATT  AAG  ATA  CAT  TGG  CAA  GAA  AAG  AAG  AGC  AAC  ACG  ATT  CTG  GGA  TCC  CAG  GAG  GGG

M13231   ,TRGC2(2x)*01,HPB-MLT  (cDNA) ---  ---  ---  ---  ---  ---  ---  ---  ---  ---  ---  ---  ---  ---  ---  ---  ---  ---  ---  ---

M15001   ,TRGC2(2x)*02,lambdaD11 (EX1) ---  ---  ---  ---  ---  ---  ---  ---  ---  ---  ---  ---  ---  ---  ---  ---  ---  ---  ---  ---

M17324   ,TRGC2(2x)*03,Fgamma7  (cDNA) ---  ---  ---  ---  ---  ---  ---  ---  ---  ---  ---  ---  ---  ---  ---  ---  ---  ---  ---  ---

AF159056,TRGC2(2x)*04                  ---  ---  ---  ---  ---  ---  ---  ---  ---  ---  ---  ---  ---  ---  ---  ---  ---  ---  ---  ---

                                      61   62   63   64   65   66   67   68   69   70   71   72   73   74   75   76   77   78   79   80
                                       N    T    M    K    T    N    D    T    Y    M    K    F    S    W    L    T    V    P    E    E
M15002   ,TRGC2(2x)*01,lambdaD7  (EX1) AAC  ACC  ATG  AAG  ACT  AAC  GAC  ACA  TAC  ATG  AAA  TTT  AGC  TGG  TTA  ACG  GTG  CCA  GAA  GAG

M13231   ,TRGC2(2x)*01,HPB-MLT  (cDNA) ---  ---  ---  ---  ---  ---  ---  ---  ---  ---  ---  ---  ---  ---  ---  ---  ---  ---  ---  ---

M15001   ,TRGC2(2x)*02,lambdaD11       ---  ---  ---  ---  ---  ---  ---  ---  ---  ---  ---  ---  ---  ---  ---  ---  ---  ---  ---  ---

M17324   ,TRGC2(2x)*03,Fgamma7  (cDNA) ---  ---  ---  ---  ---  ---  ---  ---  ---  ---  ---  ---  ---  ---  ---  ---  ---  ---  ---  ---

AF159056,TRGC2(2x)*04                  ---  ---  ---  ---  ---  ---  ---  ---  ---  ---  ---  ---  ---  ---  ---  ---  ---  ---  ---  ---
```

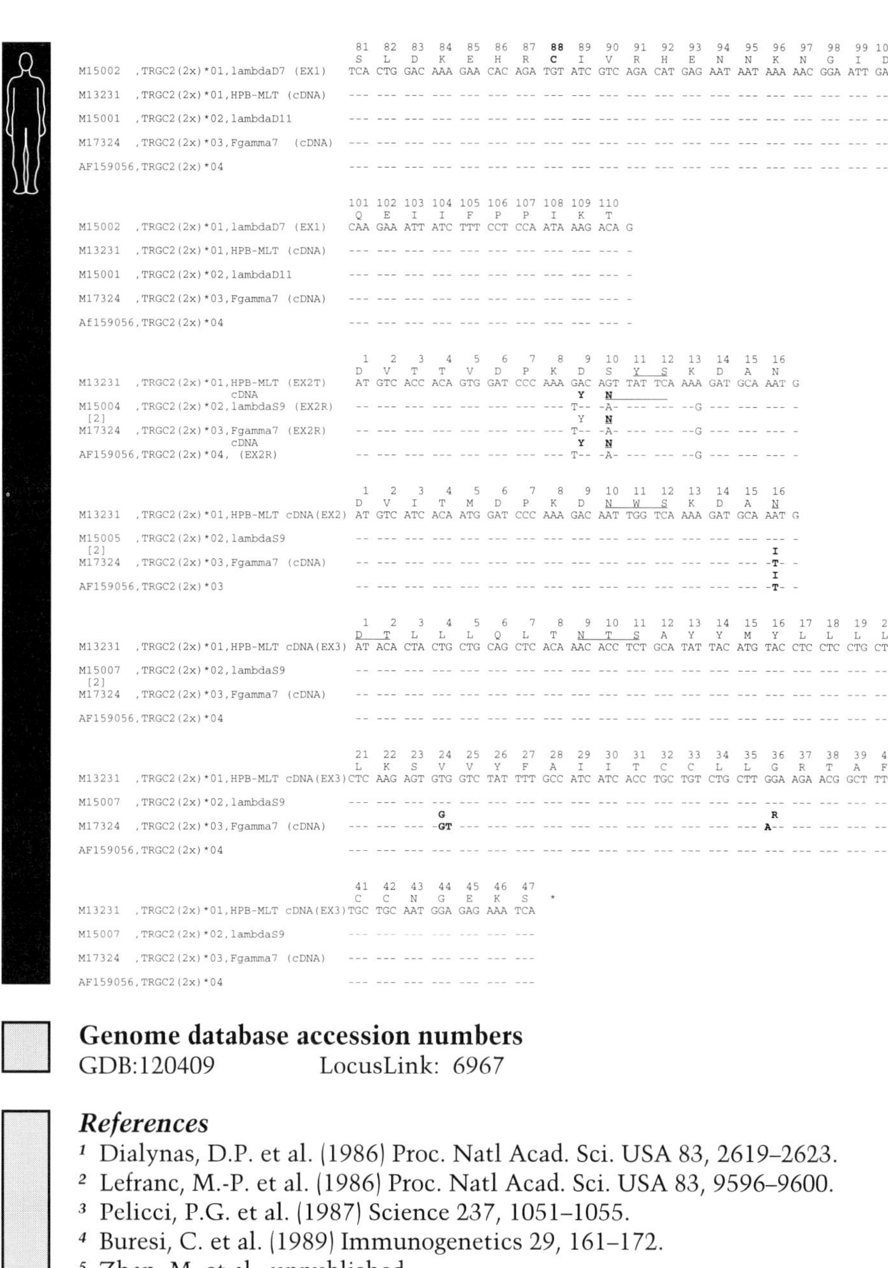

```
                                    81  82  83  84  85  86  87  88  89  90  91  92  93  94  95  96  97  98  99 100
                                     S   L   D   K   E   H   R   C   I   V   R   H   E   N   N   K   N   G   I   D
M15002  ,TRGC2(2x)*01,lambdaD7 (EX1) TCA CTG GAC AAA GAA CAC AGA TGT ATC GTC AGA CAT GAG AAT AAT AAA AAC GGA ATT GAT
M13231  ,TRGC2(2x)*01,HPB-MLT (cDNA) --- --- --- --- --- --- --- --- --- --- --- --- --- --- --- --- --- --- --- ---
M15001  ,TRGC2(2x)*02,lambdaD11       --- --- --- --- --- --- --- --- --- --- --- --- --- --- --- --- --- --- --- ---
M17324  ,TRGC2(2x)*03,Fgamma7  (cDNA) --- --- --- --- --- --- --- --- --- --- --- --- --- --- --- --- --- --- --- ---
AF159056,TRGC2(2x)*04                 --- --- --- --- --- --- --- --- --- --- --- --- --- --- --- --- --- --- --- ---

                                    101 102 103 104 105 106 107 108 109 110
                                     Q   E   I   I   F   P   P   I   K   T
M15002  ,TRGC2(2x)*01,lambdaD7 (EX1) CAA GAA ATT ATC TTT CCT CCA ATA AAG ACA G
M13231  ,TRGC2(2x)*01,HPB-MLT (cDNA) --- --- --- --- --- --- --- --- --- --- -
M15001  ,TRGC2(2x)*02,lambdaD11       --- --- --- --- --- --- --- --- --- --- -
M17324  ,TRGC2(2x)*03,Fgamma7 (cDNA) --- --- --- --- --- --- --- --- --- --- -
Af159056,TRGC2(2x)*04                 --- --- --- --- --- --- --- --- --- --- -

                                     1   2   3   4   5   6   7   8   9  10  11  12  13  14  15  16
                                     D   V   T   T   V   D   P   K   D   S   Y   S   K   D   A   N
M13231  ,TRGC2(2x)*01,HPB-MLT (EX2T) AT GTC ACC ACA GTG GAT CCC AAA GAC AGT TAT TCA AAA GAT GCA AAT G
                 cDNA                                                 Y   N
M15004  ,TRGC2(2x)*02,lambdaS9 (EX2R) -- --- --- --- --- --- --- --- T-- -A- --- --- --G --- --- --- -
  [2]                                                                 Y   N
M17324  ,TRGC2(2x)*03,Fgamma7 (EX2R)  -- --- --- --- --- --- --- --- T-- -A- --- --- --G --- --- --- -
                 cDNA                                                 Y   N
AF159056,TRGC2(2x)*04,  (EX2R)        -- --- --- --- --- --- --- --- T-- -A- --- --- --G --- --- --- -

                                     1   2   3   4   5   6   7   8   9  10  11  12  13  14  15  16
                                     D   V   I   T   M   D   P   K   D   N   W   S   K   D   A   N
M13231  ,TRGC2(2x)*01,HPB-MLT cDNA(EX2) AT GTC ATC ACA ATG GAT CCC AAA GAC AAT TGG TCA AAA GAT GCA AAT G
M15005  ,TRGC2(2x)*02,lambdaS9        -- --- --- --- --- --- --- --- --- --- --- --- --- --- --- --- -
  [2]                                                                                             I
M17324  ,TRGC2(2x)*03,Fgamma7 (cDNA)  -- --- --- --- --- --- --- --- --- --- --- --- --- --- --- -T- -
                                                                                                  I
AF159056,TRGC2(2x)*03                 -- --- --- --- --- --- --- --- --- --- --- --- --- --- --- -T- -

                                     1   2   3   4   5   6   7   8   9  10  11  12  13  14  15  16  17  18  19  20
                                     D   T   L   L   L   Q   L   T   N   T   S   A   Y   Y   M   Y   L   L   L   L
M13231  ,TRGC2(2x)*01,HPB-MLT cDNA(EX3) AT ACA CTA CTG CTG CAG CTC ACA AAC ACC TCT GCA TAT TAC ATG TAC CTC CTC CTG CTC
M15007  ,TRGC2(2x)*02,lambdaS9        -- --- --- --- --- --- --- --- --- --- --- --- --- --- --- --- --- --- --- ---
  [2]
M17324  ,TRGC2(2x)*03,Fgamma7 (cDNA)  -- --- --- --- --- --- --- --- --- --- --- --- --- --- --- --- --- --- --- ---
AF159056,TRGC2(2x)*04                 -- --- --- --- --- --- --- --- --- --- --- --- --- --- --- --- --- --- --- ---

                                    21  22  23  24  25  26  27  28  29  30  31  32  33  34  35  36  37  38  39  40
                                     L   K   S   V   V   Y   F   A   I   I   T   C   C   L   L   G   R   T   A   F
M13231  ,TRGC2(2x)*01,HPB-MLT cDNA(EX3) CTC AAG AGT GTG GTC TAT TTT GCC ATC ATC ACC TGC TGT CTG CTT GGA AGA ACG GCT TTC
M15007  ,TRGC2(2x)*02,lambdaS9        --- --- --- --- --- --- --- --- --- --- --- --- --- --- --- --- --- --- --- ---
  [2]                                             G                                           R
M17324  ,TRGC2(2x)*03,Fgamma7 (cDNA)  --- --- --- -GT --- --- --- --- --- --- --- --- --- --- --- A-- --- --- --- ---
AF159056,TRGC2(2x)*04                 --- --- --- --- --- --- --- --- --- --- --- --- --- --- --- --- --- --- --- ---

                                    41  42  43  44  45  46  47
                                     C   C   N   G   E   K   S   *
M13231  ,TRGC2(2x)*01,HPB-MLT cDNA(EX3) TGC TGC AAT GGA GAG AAA TCA
M15007  ,TRGC2(2x)*02,lambdaS9        --- --- --- --- --- --- ---
M17324  ,TRGC2(2x)*03,Fgamma7 (cDNA)  --- --- --- --- --- --- ---
AF159056,TRGC2(2x)*04                 --- --- --- --- --- --- ---
```

Genome database accession numbers

GDB:120409   LocusLink: 6967

References

1 Dialynas, D.P. et al. (1986) Proc. Natl Acad. Sci. USA 83, 2619–2623.
2 Lefranc, M.-P. et al. (1986) Proc. Natl Acad. Sci. USA 83, 9596–9600.
3 Pelicci, P.G. et al. (1987) Science 237, 1051–1055.
4 Buresi, C. et al. (1989) Immunogenetics 29, 161–172.
5 Zhan, M. et al., unpublished.

Protein Display

Protein display of the TRGC2(2x) gene is shown on page 372.

Nomenclature

TRGC2(3x) : T cell receptor gamma constant 2 (3x).

Definition and functionality

TRGC2 is one of the two functional genes of the TRGC group which comprises two mapped genes, TRGC1 and TRGC2. TRGC1 and TRGC2 result from a recent duplication. The TRGC2 gene has four or five exons due to the duplication or triplication of exon 2. TRGC2(3x) designates the polymorphic TRGC2 gene with triplication of exon 2 (from 5' to 3': EX2T, EX2R, EX2)[2].

Gene location

TRGC2 is in the TRG locus on chromosome 7 at 7p14. TRGC2 is preceded by two functional joining genes TRGJP2 and TRGJ2.

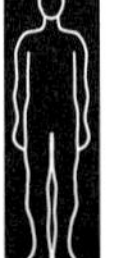

Nucleotide and amino acid sequences for human TRGC2(3x)

The nucleotide between parentheses at the beginning of exons comes from a DONOR–SPLICE (n from ngt).
The Cysteines involved in the intrachain disulfide bridges are shown with their number and letter **C** in bold.
N-glycosylation sites (NXS/T, where X is different from P) are underlined.

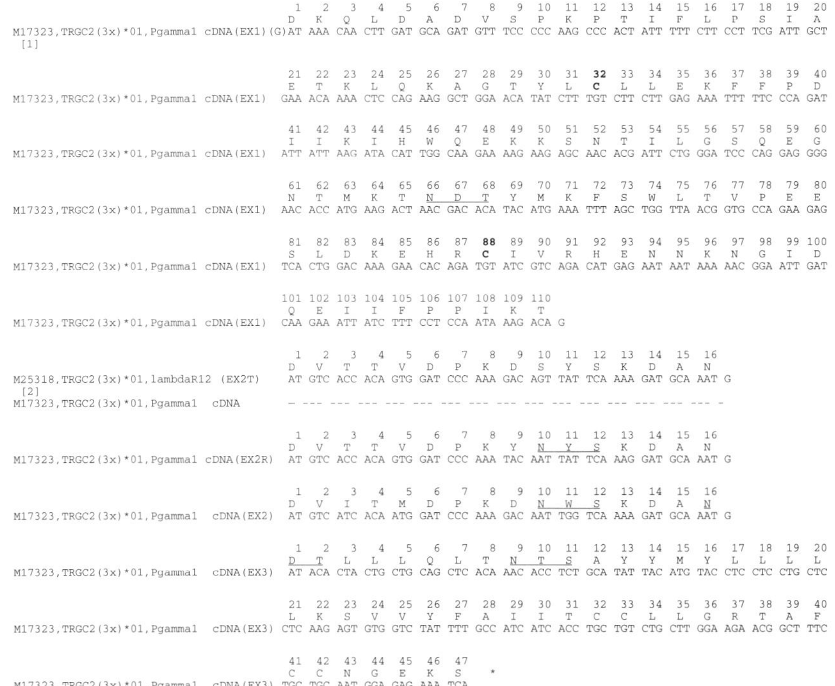

```
                                              1   2   3   4   5   6   7   8   9  10  11  12  13  14  15  16  17  18  19  20
                                              D   K   Q   L   D   A   D   V   S   P   K   P   T   I   F   L   P   S   I   A
M17323,TRGC2(3x)*01,Pgamma1 cDNA(EX1)(G)AT AAA CAA CTT GAT GCA GAT GTT TCC CCC AAG CCC ACT ATT TTT CTT CCT TCG ATT GCT
    [1]

                                             21  22  23  24  25  26  27  28  29  30  31  32  33  34  35  36  37  38  39  40
                                              E   T   K   L   Q   K   A   G   T   Y   L   C   L   L   E   K   F   F   P   D
M17323,TRGC2(3x)*01,Pgamma1 cDNA(EX1)   GAA ACA AAA CTC CAG AAG GCT GGA ACA TAT CTT TGT CTT CTT GAG AAA TTT TTC CCA GAT

                                             41  42  43  44  45  46  47  48  49  50  51  52  53  54  55  56  57  58  59  60
                                              I   I   K   I   H   W   Q   E   K   K   S   N   T   I   L   G   S   Q   E   G
M17323,TRGC2(3x)*01,Pgamma1 cDNA(EX1)   ATT ATT AAG ATA CAT TGG CAA GAA AAG AAG AGC AAC ACG ATT CTG GGA TCC CAG GAG GGG

                                             61  62  63  64  65  66  67  68  69  70  71  72  73  74  75  76  77  78  79  80
                                              N   T   M   K   T   N   D   T   Y   M   K   F   S   W   L   T   V   P   E   E
M17323,TRGC2(3x)*01,Pgamma1 cDNA(EX1)   AAC ACC ATG AAG ACT AAC GAC ACA TAC ATG AAA TTT AGC TGG TTA ACG GTG CCA GAA GAG

                                             81  82  83  84  85  86  87  88  89  90  91  92  93  94  95  96  97  98  99 100
                                              S   L   D   K   E   H   R   C   I   V   R   H   E   N   N   K   N   G   I   D
M17323,TRGC2(3x)*01,Pgamma1 cDNA(EX1)   TCA CTG GAC AAA GAA CAC AGA TGT ATC GTC AGA CAT GAG AAT AAT AAA AAC GGA ATT GAT

                                            101 102 103 104 105 106 107 108 109 110
                                              Q   E   I   I   F   P   P   I   K   T
M17323,TRGC2(3x)*01,Pgamma1 cDNA(EX1)   CAA GAA ATT ATC TTT CCT CCA ATA AAG ACA G

                                              1   2   3   4   5   6   7   8   9  10  11  12  13  14  15  16
                                              D   V   T   T   V   D   P   K   D   S   Y   S   K   D   A   N
M25318,TRGC2(3x)*01,lambdaR12  (EX2T)   AT GTC ACC ACA GTG GAT CCC AAA GAC AGT TAT TCA AAA GAT GCA AAT G
    [2]
M17323,TRGC2(3x)*01,Pgamma1    cDNA     - --- --- --- --- --- --- --- --- --- --- --- --- --- --- --- -

                                              1   2   3   4   5   6   7   8   9  10  11  12  13  14  15  16
                                              D   V   T   T   V   D   P   K   Y   N   Y   S   K   D   A   N
M17323,TRGC2(3x)*01,Pgamma1 cDNA(EX2R)  AT GTC ACC ACA GTG GAT CCC AAA TAC AAT TAT TCA AAG GAT GCA AAT G

                                              1   2   3   4   5   6   7   8   9  10  11  12  13  14  15  16
                                              D   V   I   T   M   D   P   K   D   N   W   S   K   D   A   N
M17323,TRGC2(3x)*01,Pgamma1  cDNA(EX2)  AT GTC ATC ACA ATG GAT CCC AAA GAC AAT TGG TCA AAA GAT GCA AAT G

                                              1   2   3   4   5   6   7   8   9  10  11  12  13  14  15  16  17  18  19  20
                                              D   T   L   L   L   Q   L   T   N   T   S   A   Y   Y   M   Y   L   L   L   L
M17323,TRGC2(3x)*01,Pgamma1  cDNA(EX3)  AT ACA CTA CTG CTG CAG CTC ACA AAC ACC TCT GCA TAT TAC ATG TAC CTC CTC CTG CTC

                                             21  22  23  24  25  26  27  28  29  30  31  32  33  34  35  36  37  38  39  40
                                              L   K   S   V   V   Y   F   A   I   I   T   C   C   L   L   G   R   T   A   F
M17323,TRGC2(3x)*01,Pgamma1  cDNA(EX3)  CTC AAG AGT GTG GTC TAT TTT GCC ATC ATC ACC TGC TGT CTG CTT GGA AGA ACG GCT TTC

                                             41  42  43  44  45  46  47
                                              C   C   N   G   E   K   S   *
M17323,TRGC2(3x)*01,Pgamma1  cDNA(EX3)  TGC TGC AAT GGA GAG AAA TCA
```

Genome database accession numbers
GDB:120409   LocusLink: 6967

References
[1] Pelicci, P.G. et al. (1987) Science 237, 1051–1055.
[2] Buresi, C. et al. (1989) Immunogenetics 29, 161–172.

Protein display
Protein display of the TRGC2(3x) gene is shown on page 372.

Part 2

TRGJ

TRGJ group

Nomenclature

T cell receptor gamma joining group.

Definition and functionality

The human TRGJ group comprises five functional mapped genes: TRGJ1, TRGJ2, TRGJP, TRGJP1, and TRGJP2[1].

Gene location

The human TRGJ genes are located in the TRG locus on chromosome 7 at 7p14. TRGJP1, TRGJP, and TRGJ1 are located upstream from TRGC1. TRGJ2 and TRGJP2 are located upstream from TRGC2. That genomic organization results from a recent duplication. However, there is no equivalent of TRGJP (by far, the most frequently used J gene in the human peripheral γδ T cells) in the TRGJP2, TRGJ2, TRGC2 cluster.

Nucleotide and amino acid sequences for the human functional TRGJ genes with nomenclature

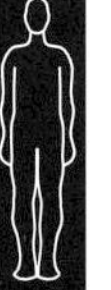

The conserved **FGXG** motif, characteristic of the TRG J-REGION is underlined.

```
TRGJ1
T cell receptor gamma joining 1

                                   N   Y   Y   K   K   L   F   G   S   G   T   T   L   V   V   T
   M12960  ,TRGJ1*01     [2]     G AAT TAT TAT AAG AAA CTC TTT GGC AGT GGA ACA ACA CTG GTT GTC ACA G

   [3][4]  ,TRGJ1*02             - --- --- --- --- --- --- --- --- --- --- --- --- --T --- --- --- -


TRGJ2
T cell receptor gamma joining 2

                                   N   Y   Y   K   K   L   F   G   S   G   T   T   L   V   V   T
   M12961  ,TRGJ2*01     [2]     G AAT TAT TAT AAG AAA CTC TTT GGC AGT GGA ACA ACT CTT GTT GTC ACA G


TRGJP
T cell receptor gamma joining P

                               G   Q   E   L   G   K   K   I   K   V   F   G   P   G   T   K   L   I   I   T
   M12950  ,TRGJP*01     [3]  GGG CAA GAG TTG GGC AAA AAA ATC AAG GTA TTT GGT CCC GGA ACA AAG CTT ATC ATT ACA G


TRGJP1
T cell receptor gamma joining P1

                                    T   T   G   W   F   K   I   F   A   E   G   T   K   L   I   V   T   S   P
   X08084  ,TRGJP1*01    [4]     AT ACC ACT GGT TGG TTC AAG ATA TTT GCT GAA GGG ACT AAG CTC ATA GTA ACT TCA CCT G


TRGJP2
T cell receptor gamma joining P2

                                    S   S   D   W   I   K   T   F   A   K   G   T   R   L   I   V   T   S   P
   M16016  ,TRGJP2*01    [5]     AT AGT AGT GAT TGG ATC AAG ACG TTT GCA AAA GGG ACT AGG CTC ATA GTA ACT TCG CCT G
```

Recombination signals

J Recombination Signal (J-RS)			TRGJ gene and allele name
J-NONAMER	(bp)	J-HEPTAMER	
AGTTTTTGA	12	CACTGTG	TRGJ1*01
AGTTTTTGA	12	CACTGTG	TRGJ1*02
AGTTTTTGA	12	CACTGTG	TRGJ2*01
GAGATTCTT	12	CAGGTGG	TRGJP*01
GATTTTTCT	12	CGGTGTG	TRGJP1*01
GATTTTTGT	12	CAGTGTG	TRGJP2*01

References:
[1] Lefranc, M.-P. and Rabbitts, T.H. (1986) Nature 316, 464–466.
[2] Lefranc, M.-P. et al. (1986) Nature 319, 420–422.
[3] Lefranc, M.-P. et al. (1986) Cell 45, 237–246.
[4] Huck, S. and Lefranc, M.-P. (1987) FEBS Lett. 224, 291–296.
[5] Quertermous, T. et al. (1987) J. Immunol. 138, 2687–2690.

Part 3

TRGV

TRGV1

Nomenclature

TRGV1: T cell receptor gamma variable 1.

Definition and functionality

TRGV1 is the unique ORF of the TRGV1 subgroup which comprises 7–9 mapped genes (of which 3–5 are functional) in the TRG locus, depending on the haplotypes[4,5].TRGV1 is an ORF due to an unusual V-SPACER length: DELETION of 14 nucleotides.

Gene location

TRGV1 is in the TRG locus on chromosome 7 at 7p14.

Nucleotide and amino acid sequences for human TRGV1

```
                                 1   2   3   4   5   6   7   8   9  10  11  12  13  14  15  16  17  18  19  20
                                 S   S   N   L   E   G   R   T   K   S   V   T   R   L   T   G   S   S   A   E
       M12949   ,TRGV1*01   [8]  TCT TCC AAC TTG GAA GGG AGA ACG AAG TCA GTC ACC AGG CTG ACT GGG TCA TCT GCT GAA

       AF159056,TRGV1*01 (1) [12] --- --- --- --- --- --- --- --- --- --- --- --- --- --- --- --- --- --- --- ---


                                                                  ____________________CDR1-IMGT______________
                                21  22  23  24  25  26  27  28  29  30  31  32  33  34  35  36  37  38  39  40
                                 I   T   C   D   L   P   G   A   S   T   L   Y                           I   H
       M12949   ,TRGV1*01       ATC ACC TGT GAT CTT CCT GGA GCA AGT ACC TTA TAC ... ... ... ... ... ... ATC CAC

       AF159056,TRGV1*01        --- --- --- --- --- --- --- --- --- --- --- --- ... ... ... ... ... ... --- ---


                                                                                      ________________CDR2-
                                41  42  43  44  45  46  47  48  49  50  51  52  53  54  55  56  57  58  59  60
                                 W   Y   L   H   Q   E   G   K   A   P   Q   C   L   L   Y   Y   E   P   Y   Y
       M12949   ,TRGV1*01       TGG TAC CTG CAC CAG GAG GGG AAG GCC CCA CAG TGT CTT CTG TAC TAT GAA CCC TAC TAC

       AF159056,TRGV1*01        --- --- --- --- --- --- --- --- --- --- --- --- --- --- --- --- --- --- --- ---


                                IMGT____
                                61  62  63  64  65  66  67  68  69  70  71  72  73  74  75  76  77  78  79  80
                                 S   R   V           V   L   E   S   G   I   T   P   G   K   Y   D   T       G
       M12949   ,TRGV1*01       TCC AGG GTT ... ... GTG CTG GAA TCA GGA ATC ACT CCA GGA AAG TAT GAC ACT ... GGA

       AF159056,TRGV1*01        --- --- --- ... ... --- --- --- --- --- --- --- --- --- --- --- --- --- ... ---


                                81  82  83  84  85  86  87  88  89  90  91  92  93  94  95  96  97  98  99 100
                                 S       T   R   S   N   W   N   L   R   L   Q   N   L   I   K   N   D   S   G
       M12949   ,TRGV1*01       AGC ... ACA AGG AGC AAT TGG AAT TTG AGA CTG CAA AAT CTA ATT AAA AAT GAT TCT GGG

       AF159056,TRGV1*01        --- ... --- --- --- --- --- --- --- --- --- --- --- --- --- --- --- --- --- ---


                                            ______CDR3-IMGT______
                               101 102 103 104 105 106 107 108 109
                                 F   Y   Y   C   A   T   W   D   R
       M12949   ,TRGV1*01       TTC TAT TAC TGT GCC ACC TGG GAC AGG

       AF159056,TRGV1*01        --- --- --- --- --- --- --- --- ---
```

Note:

(1) The allele TRGV1*01 from AF057177 is not reported in this alignment to avoid redundancy, AF057177 being included in AF159056.

Framework and complementarity determining regions

FR1-IMGT: 26

FR2-IMGT: 17

FR3-IMGT: 37 (-2 aa: 79,82)

CDR1-IMGT: 6

CDR2-IMGT: 8

CDR3-IMGT: 5

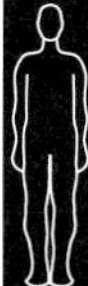

Collier de Perles for human TRGV1*01

Accession number: IMGT M12949   EMBL/GenBank/DDBJ: M12949

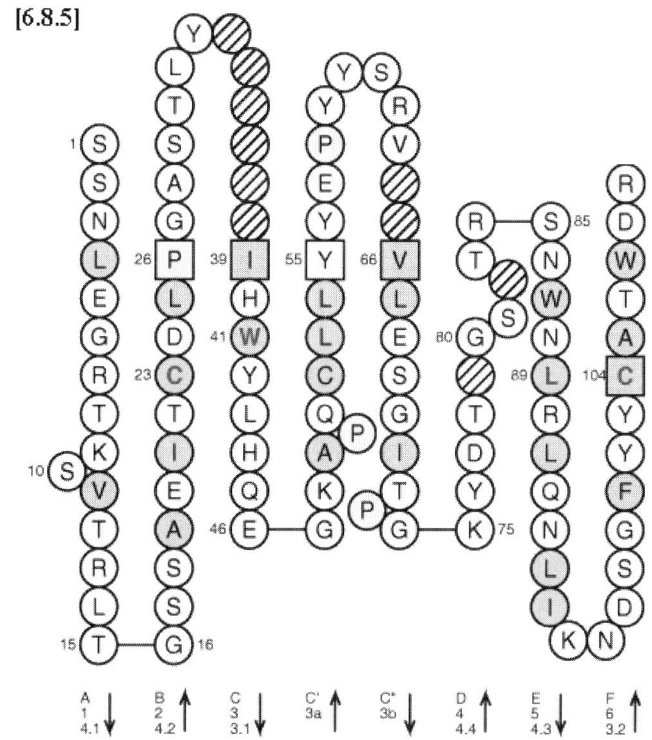

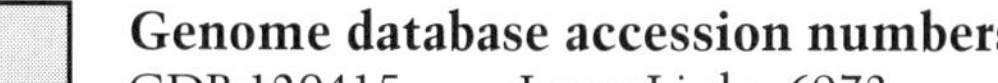

Genome database accession numbers
GDB:120415   LocusLink: 6973

TRGV2

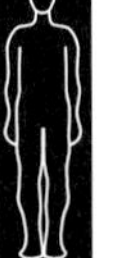

Nomenclature

TRGV2: T cell receptor gamma variable 2.

Definition and functionality

TRGV2 is one of the 3–5 mapped functional genes of the TRGV1 subgroup which comprises 7–9 mapped genes, depending on the haplotypes[4,5].

Gene location

TRGV2 is in the TRG locus on chromosome 7 at 7p14.

Nucleotide and amino acid sequences for human TRGV2

```
                    1   2   3   4   5   6   7   8   9  10  11  12  13  14  15  16  17  18  19  20
                    S   S   N   L   E   G   R   T   K   S   V   I   R   Q   T   G   S   S   A   E
M13429   ,TRGV2*01      [8]  TCT TCC AAC TTG GAA GGG AGA ACG AAG TCA GTC ATC AGG CAG ACT GGG TCA TCT GCT GAA

AF159056,TRGV2*01 (1) [12]  --- --- --- --- --- --- --- --- --- --- --- --- --- --- --- --- --- --- --- ---

M27337   ,TRGV2*02     [11]  --- --- --- --- --- --- --- --- --- --- --- --- --- --- --- --- --- --- --- ---


                                                                        ____________CDR1-IMGT____________
                   21  22  23  24  25  26  27  28  29  30  31  32  33  34  35  36  37  38  39  40
                    I   T   C   D   L   A   E   G   S   N   G   Y                           I   H
M13429   ,TRGV2*01  ATC ACT TGT GAT CTT GCT GAA GGA AGT AAC GGC TAC ... ... ... ... ... ... ATC CAC

AF159056,TRGV2*01   --- --- --- --- --- --- --- --- --- --- --- --- ... ... ... ... ... ... --- ---

M27337   ,TRGV2*02  --- --- --- --- --- --- --- --- --- --- --- --- ... ... ... ... ... ... --- ---


                                                                                        ____CDR2-
                   41  42  43  44  45  46  47  48  49  50  51  52  53  54  55  56  57  58  59  60
                    W   Y   L   H   Q   E   G   K   A   P   Q   R   L   Q   Y   Y   D   S   Y   N
M13429   ,TRGV2*01  TGG TAC CTA CAC CAG GAG GGG AAG GCC CCA CAG CGT CTT CAG TAC TAT GAC TCC TAC AAC

AF159056,TRGV2*01   --- --- --- --- --- --- --- --- --- --- --- --- --- --- --- --- --- --- --- ---

M27337   ,TRGV2*02  --- --- --- --- --- --- --- --- --- --- --- --- --- --- --- --- --- --- --- ---


                   IMGT__________________
                   61  62  63  64  65  66  67  68  69  70  71  72  73  74  75  76  77  78  79  80
                    S   K   V           V   L   E   S   G   V   S   P   G   K   Y   Y   T   Y   A
M13429   ,TRGV2*01  TCC AAG GTT ... ... GTG TTG GAA TCA GGA GTC AGT CCA GGG AAG TAT TAT ACT TAC GCA

AF159056,TRGV2*01   --- --- --- ... ... --- --- --- --- --- --- --- --- --- --- --- --- --- --- ---

M27337   ,TRGV2*02  --- --- --- ... ... --- --- --- --- --- --- --- --- --- --- --- --- --- --- ---


                   81  82  83  84  85  86  87  88  89  90  91  92  93  94  95  96  97  98  99 100
                    S       T   R   N   N   L   R   L   I   L   R   N   L   I   E   N   D   S   G
M13429   ,TRGV2*01  AGC ... ACA AGG AAC AAC TTG AGA TTG ATA CTG CGA AAT CTA ATT GAA AAT GAC TCT GGG

AF159056,TRGV2*01   --- ... --- --- --- --- --- --- --- --- --- --- --- --- --- --- --- --- --- ---

                                                                Q
M27337   ,TRGV2*02  --- ... --- --- --- --- --- --- --- --- --- -A- --- --- --- --- --- --- --- ---


                           ______CDR3-IMGT______
                  101 102 103 104 105 106 107 108 109
                    V   Y   Y   C   A   T   W   D   G
M13429   ,TRGV2*01  GTC TAT TAC TGT GCC ACC TGG GAC GGG

AF159056,TRGV2*01   --- --- --- --- --- --- --- --- ---

M27337   ,TRGV2*02  --- --- --- --- --- --- --- ---        #c

#c: Rearranged cDNA.
```

Note:

(1) The allele TRGV2*01 from AF057177 is not reported in this alignment to avoid redundancy, AF057177 being included in AF159056.

Framework and complementarity determining regions

FR1-IMGT: 26   CDR1-IMGT: 6
FR2-IMGT: 17   CDR2-IMGT: 8
FR3-IMGT: 38 (-1 aa: 82)   CDR3-IMGT: 5

Collier de Perles for human TRGV2*01

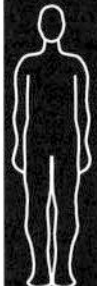

Accession number: IMGT M13429   EMBL/GenBank/DDBJ: M13429

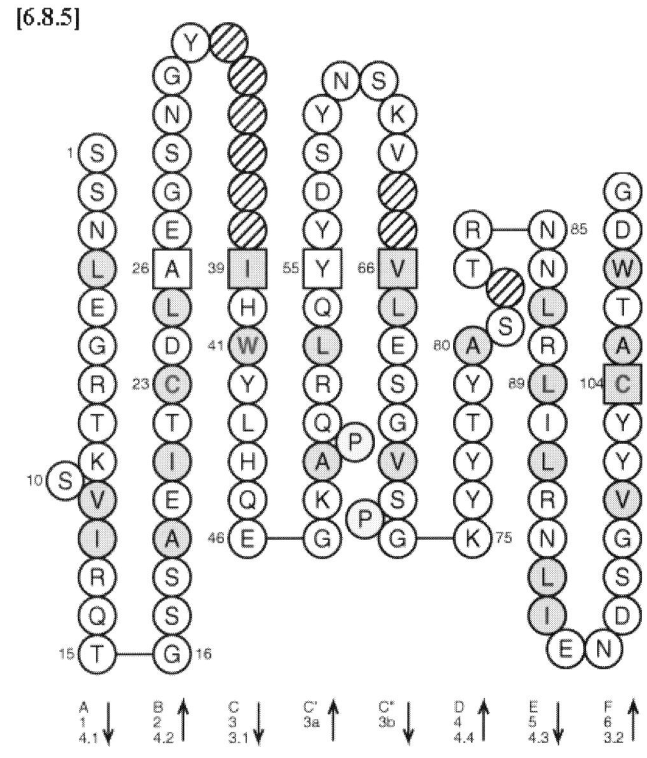

Genome database accession numbers
GDB:120418   LocusLink: 6974

Nomenclature

TRGV3: T cell receptor gamma variable 3.

Definition and functionality

TRGV3 is one of the 3–5 mapped functional genes of the TRGV1 subgroup which comprises 7–9 mapped genes, depending on the haplotypes[4,5].

Gene location

TRGV3 is in the TRG locus on chromosome 7 at 7p14.

Nucleotide and amino acid sequences for human TRGV3

```
                        1   2   3   4   5   6   7   8   9  10  11  12  13  14  15  16  17  18  19  20
                        S   S   N   L   E   G   R   T   K   S   V   T   R   Q   T   G   S   S   A   E
M13430  ,TRGV3*01    [8] TCT TCC AAC TTG GAA GGG AGA ACG AAG TCA GTC ACC AGG CAG ACT GGG TCA TCT GCT GAA

AF159056,TRGV3*01(1) [12] --- --- --- --- --- --- --- --- --- --- --- --- --- --- --- --- --- --- --- ---

X04038  ,TRGV3*02    [10] --- --- --- --- --- --- --- --- --- --- --- --- --- --- --- --- --- --- --- ---

                                                             ______________CDR1-IMGT______
                        21  22  23  24  25  26  27  28  29  30  31  32  33  34  35  36  37  38  39  40
                        I   T   C   D   L   T   V   T   N   T   F   Y                           I   H
M13430  ,TRGV3*01        ATC ACT TGC GAT CTT ACT GTA ACA AAT ACC TTC TAC ... ... ... ... ... ... ATC CAC

AF159056,TRGV3*01        --- --- --- --- --- --- --- --- --- --- --- --- ... ... ... ... ... ... --- ---

X04038  ,TRGV3*02        --- --- --- --- --- --- --- --- --- --- --- --- ... ... ... ... ... ... --- ---

                                                                             ________________CDR2-
                        41  42  43  44  45  46  47  48  49  50  51  52  53  54  55  56  57  58  59  60
                        W   Y   L   H   Q   E   G   K   A   P   Q   R   L   L   Y   Y   D   V   S   T
M13430  ,TRGV3*01        TGG TAC CTA CAC CAG GAG GGG AAG GCC CCA CAG CGT CTT CTG TAC TAT GAC GTC TCC ACC

AF159056,TRGV3*01        --- --- --- --- --- --- --- --- --- --- --- --- --- --- --- --- --- --- --- ---

X04038  ,TRGV3*02        --- --- --- --- --- --- --- --- --- --- --- --- --- --- --- --- --- --- --- --T

                        IMGT_____________________
                        61  62  63  64  65  66  67  68  69  70  71  72  73  74  75  76  77  78  79  80
                        A   R   D           V   L   E   S   G   L   S   P   G   K   Y   Y   T   H   T
M13430  ,TRGV3*01        GCA AGG GAT ... ... GTG TTG GAA TCA GGA CTC AGT CCA GGA AAG TAT TAT ACT CAT ACA

AF159056,TRGV3*01        --- --- --- ... ... --- --- --- --- --- --- --- --- --- --- --- --- --- --- ---

X04038  ,TRGV3*02        --- --- --- ... ... --- --- --- --- --- --- --- --- --- --- --- --- --- --- ---

                        81  82  83  84  85  86  87  88  89  90  91  92  93  94  95  96  97  98  99 100
                        P       R   R   W   S   W   I   L   R   L   Q   N   L   I   E   N   D   S   G
M13430  ,TRGV3*01        CCC ... AGG AGG TGG AGC TGG ATA TTG AGA CTG CAA AAT CTA ATT GAA AAT GAT TCT GGG

AF159056,TRGV3*01        --- ... --- --- --- --- --- --- --- --- --- --- --- --- --- --- --- --- --- ---

X04038  ,TRGV3*02        --- ... --- --- --- --- --- --- --- --- --- --- --- --- --- --- --- --- --- ---

                            ______CDR3-IMGT______
                        101 102 103 104 105 106 107 108 109
                        V   Y   Y   C   A   T   W   D   R
M13430  ,TRGV3*01        GTC TAT TAC TGT GCC ACC TGG GAC AGG

AF159056,TRGV3*01        --- --- --- --- --- --- --- --- ---

X04038  ,TRGV3*02        --- --- --- --- --- --- --- --- ---
```

Note:

(1) The allele TRGV3*01 from AF057177 is not reported in this alignment to avoid redundancy, AF057177 being included in AF159056. Note that g181 (codon 61) in AF159056 was undefined (r181, r being a or g) in AF057177.

Framework and complementarity determining regions

FR1-IMGT: 26	CDR1-IMGT: 6
FR2-IMGT: 17	CDR2-IMGT: 8
FR3-IMGT: 38 (-1 aa: 82)	CDR3-IMGT: 5

Collier de Perles for human TRGV3*01

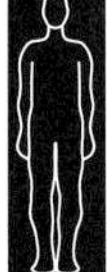

Accession number: IMGT M13430   EMBL/GenBank/DDBJ: M13430

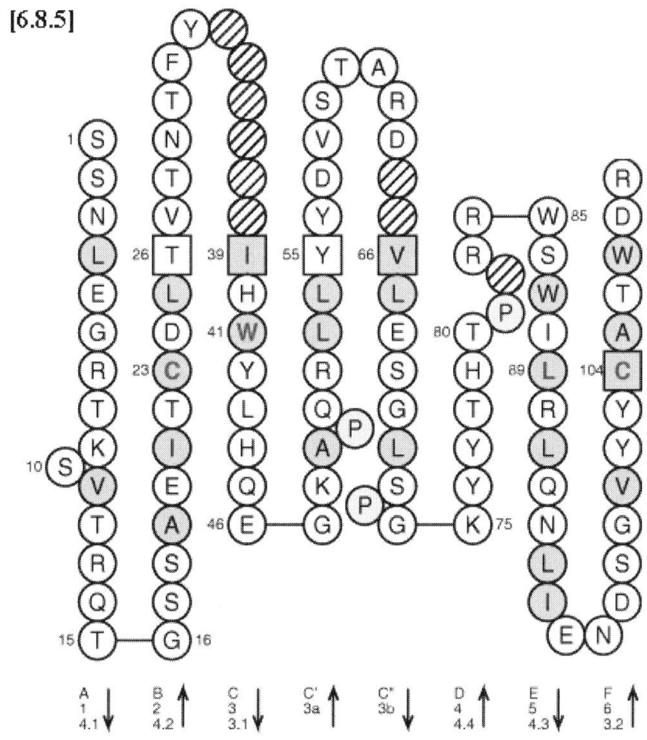

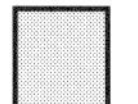

Genome database accession numbers
GDB:120419   LocusLink: 6976

Nomenclature

TRGV4: T cell receptor gamma variable 4.

Definition and functionality

TRGV4 is a mapped functional gene, which may, or may not, be present due to a polymorphism by insertion/deletion[4,5]. TRGV4 belongs to the TRGV1 subgroup which comprises 7–9 mapped genes (of which 3–5 are functional), depending on the haplotypes[4,5].

Gene location

TRGV4 is in the TRG locus on chromosome 7 at 7p14.

Nucleotide and amino acid sequences for human TRGV4

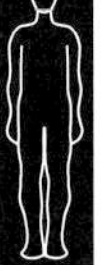

```
                                1   2   3   4   5   6   7   8   9  10  11  12  13  14  15  16  17  18  19  20
                                S   S   N   L   E   G   R   T   K   S   V   I   R   Q   T   G   S   S   A   E
X15272   ,TRGV4*01    [2] [8]  TCT TCC AAC TTG GAA GGG AGA ACG AAG TCA GTC ATC AGG CAG ACT GGG TCA TCT GCT GAA

AF159056,TRGV4*01    (1)[12]  --- --- --- --- --- --- --- --- --- --- --- --- --- --- --- --- --- --- --- ---

X13354/M36285,TRGV4*02  [3]   --- --- --- --- --- --- --- --- --- --- --- --- --- --- --- --- --- --- --- ---


                                                                   __________________CDR1-IMGT___________________
                               21  22  23  24  25  26  27  28  29  30  31  32  33  34  35  36  37  38  39  40
                                I   T   C   D   L   A   E   G   S   T   G   Y                           I   H
X15272   ,TRGV4*01            ATC ACT TGT GAT CTT GCT GAA GGA AGT ACC GGC TAC ... ... ... ... ... ... ATC CAC

AF159056,TRGV4*01             --- --- --- --- --- --- --- --- --- --- --- ---             ... ... --- ---

X13354/M36285,TRGV4*02        --- --- --- --- --- --- --- --- --- --- --- ---         ... ... ... ... --- ---


                                                                                       ________________CDR2-
                               41  42  43  44  45  46  47  48  49  50  51  52  53  54  55  56  57  58  59  60
                                W   Y   L   H   Q   E   G   K   A   P   Q   R   L   L   Y   Y   D   S   Y   T
X15272   ,TRGV4*01            TGG TAC CTA CAC CAG GAG GGG AAG GCC CCA CAG CGT CTT CTG TAC TAT GAC TCC TAC ACC

AF159056,TRGV4*01             --- --- --- --- --- --- --- --- --- --- --- --- --- --- --- --- --- --- --- ---

X13354/M36285,TRGV4*02        --- --- --- --- --- --- --- --- --- --- --- --- --- --- --- --- --- --- --- ---


                               IMGT__________________
                               61  62  63  64  65  66  67  68  69  70  71  72  73  74  75  76  77  78  79  80
                                S   S   V           V   L   E   S   G   I   S   P   G   K   Y   D   T   Y   G
X15272   ,TRGV4*01            TCC AGC GTT ... ... GTG TTG GAA TCA GGA ATC AGC CCA GGG AAG TAT GAT ACT TAT GGA

AF159056,TRGV4*01             --- --- --- ... ... --- --- --- --- --- --- --- --- --- --- --- --- --- --- ---

X13354/M36285,TRGV4*02        --- --- --- ... ... --- --- --- --- --- --- --- --- --- --- --- --- --- --C ---


                               81  82  83  84  85  86  87  88  89  90  91  92  93  94  95  96  97  98  99 100
                                S       T   R   K   N   L   R   M   I   L   R   N   L   I   E   N   D   S   G
X15272   ,TRGV4*01            AGC ... ACA AGG AAG AAC TTG AGA ATG ATA CTG CGA AAT CTT ATT GAA AAT GAC TCT GGA

AF159056,TRGV4*01             --- ... --- --- --- --- --- --- --- --- --- --- --- --- --- --- --- --- --- ---

X13354/M36285,TRGV4*02        --- ... --- --- --- --- --- --- --- --- --- --- --- --- --- --- --- --- --- ---


                                            ______CDR3-IMGT______
                              101 102 103 104 105 106 107 108 109
                                V   Y   Y   C   A   T   W   D   G
X15272   ,TRGV4*01            GTC TAT TAC TGT GCC ACC TGG GAT GGG

AF159056,TRGV4*01             --- --- --- --- --- --- --- --- ---

X13354/M36285,TRGV4*02        --- --- --- --- --- --- --- --- ---
```

Note:

(1) The allele TRGV4*01 from AF057177 is not reported in this alignment to avoid redundancy, AF057177 being included in AF159056.

g18>c (codon 6) and t237>c (codon 79) mutations originally in AF057177 are not found in AF159056 and therefore probably resulted from sequencing or typing errors.

Framework and Complementarity Determining Regions

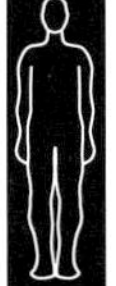

FR1-IMGT: 26
FR2-IMGT: 17
FR3-IMGT: 38 (-1 aa: 82)

CDR1-IMGT: 6
CDR2-IMGT: 8
CDR3-IMGT: 5

Collier de Perles for human TRGV4*01

Accession number: IMGT X15272

EMBL/GenBank/DDBJ: X15272

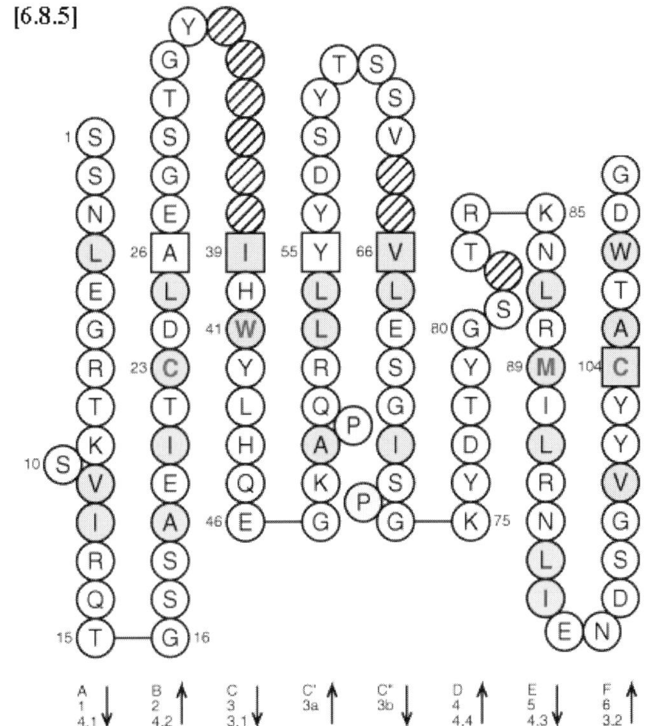

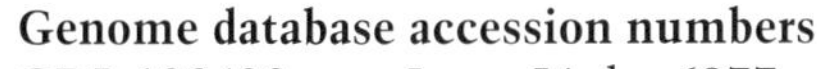

Genome database accession numbers
GDB:120420   LocusLink: 6977

TRGV5

Nomenclature

TRGV5: T cell receptor gamma variable 5.

Definition and functionality

TRGV5 is a mapped functional gene, which may, or may not, be present due to a polymorphism by insertion/deletion[4,5]. TRGV5 belongs to the TRGV1 subgroup which comprises 7–9 mapped genes (of which 3–5 are functional), depending on the haplotypes[4,5].

Gene location

TRGV5 is in the TRG locus on chromosome 7 at 7p14.

Nucleotide and amino acid sequences for human TRGV5

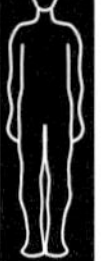

```
                          1   2   3   4   5   6   7   8   9   10  11  12  13  14  15  16  17  18  19  20
                          S   S   N   L   E   G   G   T   K   S   V   T   R   P   T   R   S   S   A   E
X13355/M36286,TRGV5*01 [3] TCT TCC AAC TTG GAA GGG GGA ACG AAG TCA GTC ACG AGG CCG ACT AGG TCA TCT GCT GAA

AF159056,TRGV5*01(1)  [12] --- --- --- --- --- --- --- --- --- --- --- --- --- --- --- --- --- --- --- ---


                                                                   ________CDR1-IMGT________________
                          21  22  23  24  25  26  27  28  29  30  31  32  33  34  35  36  37  38  39  40
                          I   T   C   D   L   T   V   I   N   A   F   Y                           I   H
X13355/M36286,TRGV5*01    ATC ACT TGT GAC CTT ACT GTA ATA AAT GCC TTC TAC ... ... ... ... ... ... ATC CAC

AF159056,TRGV5*01         --- --- --- --- --- --- --- --- --- --- --- ---         ... ... ... ... --- ---


                                                                                      ____________CDR2-
                          41  42  43  44  45  46  47  48  49  50  51  52  53  54  55  56  57  58  59  60
                          W   Y   L   H   Q   E   G   K   A   P   Q   R   L   L   Y   Y   D   V   S   N
X13355/M36286,TRGV5*01    TGG TAC CTA CAC CAG GAG GGG AAG GCC CCA CAG CGT CTT CTG TAC TAT GAC GTC TCC AAC

AF159056,TRGV5*01         --- --- --- --- --- --- --- --- --- --- --- --- --- --- --- --- --- --- --- ---


                          IMGT____________
                          61  62  63  64  65  66  67  68  69  70  71  72  73  74  75  76  77  78  79  80
                          S   K   D           V   L   E   S   G   L   S   P   G   K   Y   Y   T   H   T
X13355/M36286,TRGV5*01    TCA AAG GAT ... ... GTG TTG GAA TCA GGA CTC AGT CCA GGA AAG TAT TAT ACT CAT ACA

AF159056,TRGV5*01         --- --- --- --- --- --- --- --- --- --- --- --- --- --- --- --- --- --- --- ---


                          81  82  83  84  85  86  87  88  89  90  91  92  93  94  95  96  97  98  99  100
                          P   R   R   W   S   W   I   L   I   L   R   N   L   I   E   N   D   S   G
X13355/M36286,TRGV5*01    CCC ... AGG AGG TGG AGC TGG ATA TTG ATA CTA CGA AAT CTA ATT GAA AAT GAT TCT GGG

AF159056,TRGV5*01         --- ... --- --- --- --- --- --- --- --- --- --- --- --- --- --- --- --- --- ---


                                           ____CDR3-IMGT_____
                          101 102 103 104 105 106 107 108 109
                          V   Y   Y   C   A   T   W   D   R
X13355/M36286,TRGV5*01    GTC TAT TAC TGT GCC ACC TGG GAC AGG

AF159056,TRGV5*01         --- --- --- --- --- --- --- --- ---
```

Note:

(1) The allele TRGV5*01 from AF057177 is not reported in this alignment to avoid redundancy, AF057177 being included in AF159056.

Framework and complementarity determining regions

FR1-IMGT: 26
FR2-IMGT: 17
FR3-IMGT: 38 (-1 aa: 82)

CDR1-IMGT: 6
CDR2-IMGT: 8
CDR3-IMGT: 5

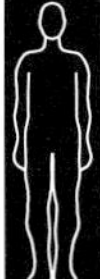

Collier de Perles for human TRGV5*01

Accession number: IMGT X13355   EMBL/GenBank/DDBJ: X13355

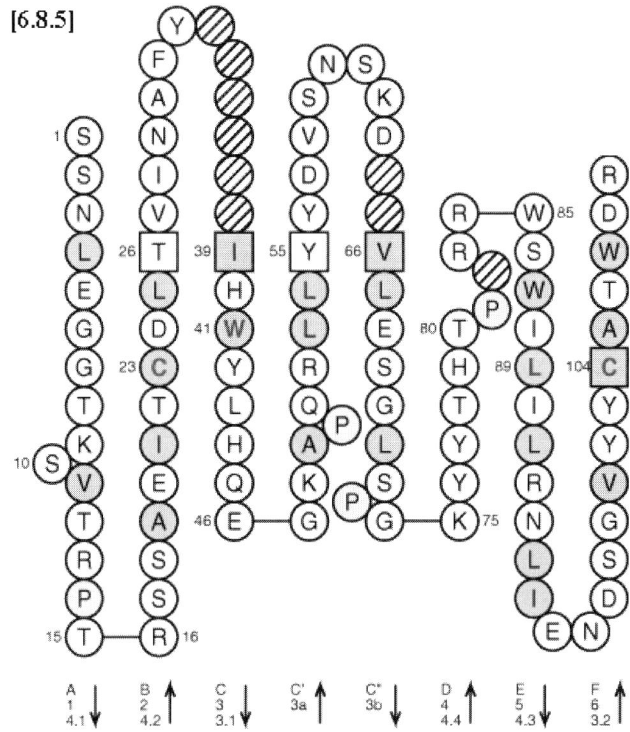

Genome database accession numbers

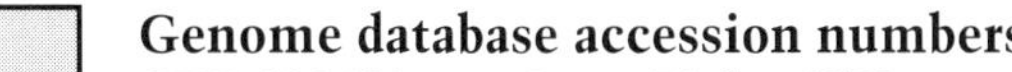

GDB:120421   LocusLink: 6978

Nomenclature

TRGV8: T cell receptor gamma variable 8.

Definition and functionality

TRGV8 is one of the 3–5 mapped functional genes of the TRGV1 subgroup which comprises 7–9 mapped genes in the TRG locus, depending on the haplotypes[4,5].

Gene location

TRGV8 is in the TRG locus on chromosome 7 at 7p14.

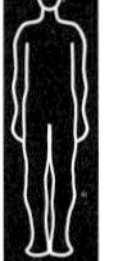

Nucleotide and amino acid sequences for human TRGV8

```
                            1   2   3   4   5   6   7   8   9  10  11  12  13  14  15  16  17  18  19  20
                            S   S   N   L   E   G   R   T   K   S   V   T   R   P   T   G   S   S   A   V
M13434   ,TRGV8*01     [8]  TCT TCC AAC TTG GAA GGG AGA ACA AAG TCA GTC ACC AGG CCA ACT GGG TCA TCA GCT GTA

AF159056,TRGV8*01 (1) [12]  --- --- --- --- --- --- --- --- --- --- --- --- --- --- --- --- --- --- --- ---

                                                                           ________________CDR1-IMGT____________________
                            21  22  23  24  25  26  27  28  29  30  31  32  33  34  35  36  37  38  39  40
                            I   T   C   D   L   P   V   E   N   A   V   Y                           T   H
M13434   ,TRGV8*01          ATC ACT TGT GAT CTT CCT GTA GAA AAT GCC GTC TAC ... ... ... ... ... ... ACC CAC

AF159056,TRGV8*01          --- --- --- --- --- --- --- --- --- --- --- --- ... ... ... ... ... ... --- ---

                                                                                       ___________________CDR2-
                            41  42  43  44  45  46  47  48  49  50  51  52  53  54  55  56  57  58  59  60
                            W   Y   L   H   Q   E   G   K   A   P   Q   R   L   L   Y   Y   D   S   Y   N
M13434   ,TRGV8*01          TGG TAC CTA CAC CAG GAG GGG AAG GCC CCA CAG CGT CTT CTG TAC TAT GAC TCC TAC AAC

AF159056,TRGV8*01          --- --- --- --- --- --- --- --- --- --- --- --- --- --- --- --- --- --- --- ---

                            IMGT_____________________
                            61  62  63  64  65  66  67  68  69  70  71  72  73  74  75  76  77  78  79  80
                            S   R   V           V   L   E   S   G   I   S   R   E   K   Y   H   T   Y   A
M13434   ,TRGV8*01          TCC AGG GTT ... ... GTG TTG GAA TCA GGA ATC AGT CGA GAA AAG TAT CAT ACT TAT GCA

AF159056,TRGV8*01          --- --- --- ... ... --- --- --- --- --- --- --- --- --- --- --- --- --- --- ---

                            81  82  83  84  85  86  87  88  89  90  91  92  93  94  95  96  97  98  99 100
                            S       T   G   K   S   L   K   F   I   L   E   N   L   I   E   R   D   S   G
M13434   ,TRGV8*01          AGC ... ACA GGG AAG AGC CTT AAA TTT ATA CTG GAA AAT CTA ATT GAA CGT GAC TCT GGG

AF159056,TRGV8*01          --- ... --- --- --- --- --- --- --- --- --- --- --- --- --- --- --- --- --- ---

                                            ______CDR3-IMGT______
                           101 102 103 104 105 106 107 108 109
                            V   Y   Y   C   A   T   W   D   R
M13434   ,TRGV8*01          GTC TAT TAC TGT GCC ACC TGG GAT AGG

AF159056,TRGV8*01          --- --- --- --- --- --- --- --- ---
```

Note:
(1) The allele TRGV8*01 from AF057177 is not reported in this alignment to avoid redundancy, AF057177 being included in AF159056.

Framework and complementarity determining regions

FR1-IMGT: 26   CDR1-IMGT: 6
FR2-IMGT: 17   CDR2-IMGT: 8
FR3-IMGT: 38 (-1 aa: 82)   CDR3-IMGT: 5

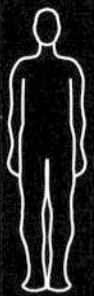

Collier de Perles for human TRGV8*01

Accession number: IMGT M13434   EMBL/GenBank/DDBJ: M13434

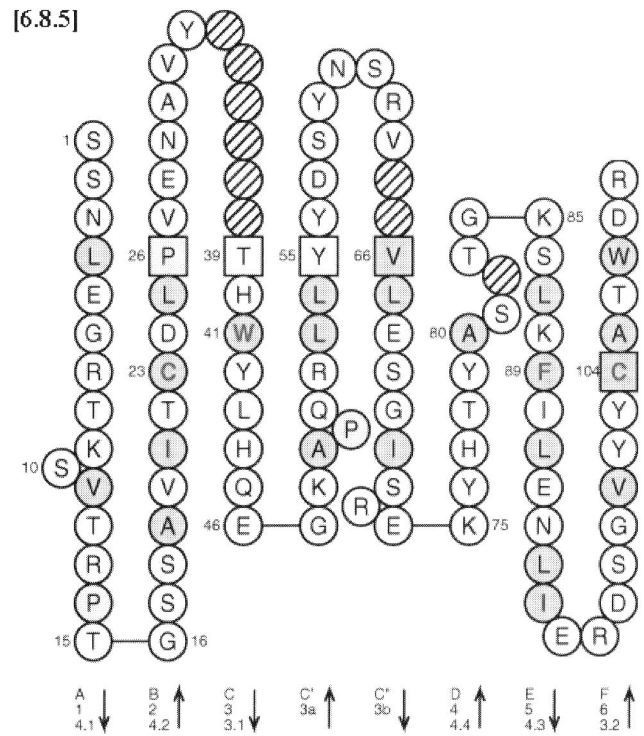

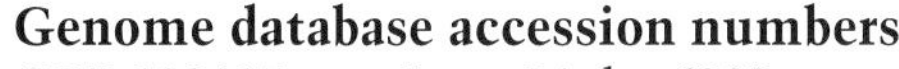

Genome database accession numbers
GDB:120425   LocusLink: 6982

Nomenclature

TRGV9: T cell receptor gamma variable 9.

Definition and functionality

TRGV9 is the unique mapped functional gene of the TRGV2 subgroup which only comprises that gene[7-9].

Gene location

TRGV9 is in the TRG locus on chromosome 7 at 7p14.

Nucleotide and amino acid sequences for human TRGV9

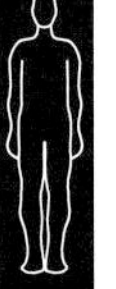

```
                         1    2    3    4    5    6    7    8    9   10   11   12   13   14   15   16   17   18   19   20
                         A    G    H    L    E    Q    P    Q    I    S    S    T    K    T    L    S    K    T    A    R
X07205   ,TRGV9*01  [4]  GCA  GGT  CAC  CTA  GAG  CAA  CCT  CAA  ATT  TCC  AGT  ACT  AAA  ACG  CTG  TCA  AAA  ACA  GCC  CGC

AF159056,TRGV9*01   [8]  ---  ---  ---  ---  ---  ---  ---  ---  ---  ---  ---  ---  ---  ---  ---  ---  ---  ---  ---  ---

X15274   ,TRGV9*02  [2]  ---  ---  ---  ---  ---  ---  ---  ---  ---  ---  ---  ---  ---  ---  ---  ---  ---  ---  ---  ---


                                                        _______________________CDR1-IMGT_______________________
                        21   22   23   24   25   26   27   28   29   30   31   32   33   34   35   36   37   38   39   40
                         L    E    C    V    V    S    G    I    T    I    S    A    T    S                        V    Y
X07205   ,TRGV9*01      CTG  GAA  TGT  GTG  GTG  TCT  GGA  ATA  ACA  ATT  TCT  GCA  ACA  TCT  ...  ...  ...  ...  GTA  TAT

AF159056,TRGV9*01       ---  ---  ---  ---  ---  ---  ---  ---  ---  ---  ---  ---  ---  ---  ...  ...  ...  ...  ---  ---
                                                           K
X15274   ,TRGV9*02      ---  ---  ---  ---  ---  ---  ---  ---  -A-  ---  ---  ---  ---  ---  ...  ...  ...  ...  ---  ---


                                                                                            _______________________CDR2-
                        41   42   43   44   45   46   47   48   49   50   51   52   53   54   55   56   57   58   59   60
                         W    Y    R    E    R    P    G    E    V    I    Q    F    L    V    S    I    S    Y    D    G
X07205   ,TRGV9*01      TGG  TAT  CGA  GAG  AGA  CCT  GGT  GAA  GTC  ATA  CAG  TTC  CTG  GTG  TCC  ATT  TCA  TAT  GAC  GGC

AF159056,TRGV9*01       ---  ---  ---  ---  ---  ---  ---  ---  ---  ---  ---  ---  ---  ---  ---  ---  ---  ---  ---  ---

X15274   ,TRGV9*02      ---  ---  ---  ---  ---  ---  ---  ---  ---  ---  ---  ---  ---  ---  ---  ---  ---  ---  ---  ---


                        IMGT________________________
                        61   62   63   64   65   66   67   68   69   70   71   72   73   74   75   76   77   78   79   80
                         T    V                        R    K    E    S    G    I    P    S    G    K    F    E    V    D    R
X07205   ,TRGV9*01      ACT  GTC  ...  ...  ...  AGA  AAG  GAA  TCC  GGC  ATT  CCG  TCA  GGC  AAA  TTT  GAG  GTG  GAT  AGG

AF159056,TRGV9*01       ---  ---  ...  ...  ...  ---  ---  ---  ---  ---  ---  ---  ---  ---  ---  ---  ---  ---  ---  ---

X15274   ,TRGV9*02      ---  ---  ...  ...  ...  ---  ---  ---  --T  ---  ---  ---  ---  ---  ---  ---  ---  ---  ---  ---


                        81   82   83   84   85   86   87   88   89   90   91   92   93   94   95   96   97   98   99  100
                         I    P    E    T    S    T    S    T    L    T    I    H    N    V    E    K    Q    D    I    A
X07205   ,TRGV9*01      ATA  CCT  GAA  ACG  TCT  ACA  TCC  ACT  CTC  ACC  ATT  CAC  AAT  GTA  GAG  AAA  CAG  GAC  ATA  GCT

AF159056,TRGV9*01       ---  ---  ---  ---  ---  ---  ---  ---  ---  ---  ---  ---  ---  ---  ---  ---  ---  ---  ---  ---

X15274   ,TRGV9*02      ---  ---  ---  ---  ---  ---  ---  ---  ---  ---  ---  ---  ---  ---  ---  ---  ---  ---  ---  ---


                                          ________CDR3-IMGT________
                       101  102  103  104  105  106  107  108  109
                         T    Y    Y    C    A    L    W    E    V
X07205   ,TRGV9*01      ACC  TAC  TAC  TGT  GCC  TTG  TGG  GAG  GTG

AF159056,TRGV9*01       ---  ---  ---  ---  ---  ---  ---  ---  ---

X15274   ,TRGV9*02      ---  ---  ---  ---  ---  ---  ---  ---  ---
```

Framework and complementarity determining regions

FR1-IMGT: 26	CDR1-IMGT: 8
FR2-IMGT: 17	CDR2-IMGT: 7
FR3-IMGT: 39	CDR3-IMGT: 5

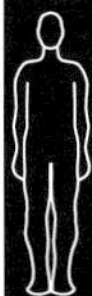

Collier de Perles for human TRGV9*01

Accession number: IMGT X07205   EMBL/GenBank/DDBJ: X70205

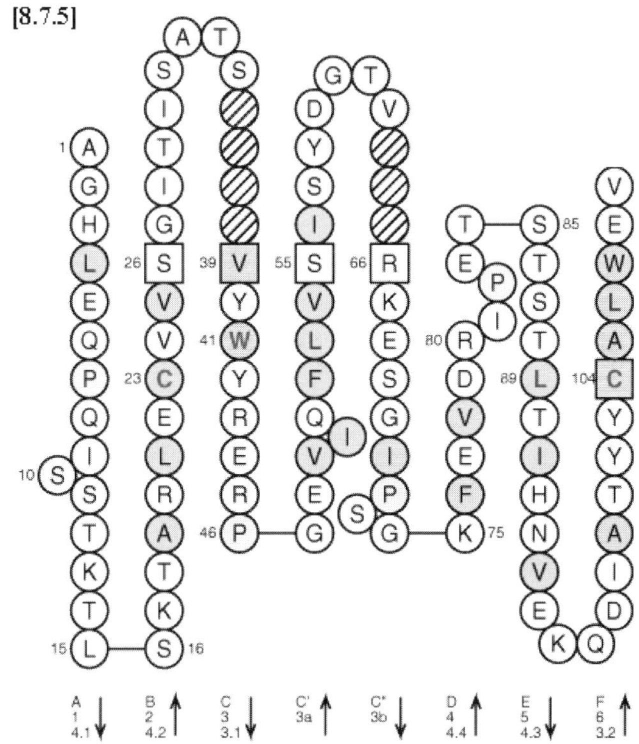

Genome database accession numbers
GDB:120426   LocusLink: 6983

Nomenclature

TRGV10: T cell receptor gamma variable 10.

Definition and functionality

TRGV10 is the unique mapped ORF of the TRGV3 subgroup which only comprises that gene[6].

TRGV10 is an ORF due to a defective DONOR–SPLICE: nct instead of ngt, and to the absence of splicing of the V10 leader intron[13,14].

Gene location

TRGV10 is in the TRG locus on chromosome 7 at 7p14.

Nucleotide and amino acid sequences for human TRGV10

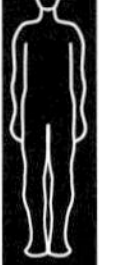

```
                        1   2   3   4   5   6   7   8   9  10  11  12  13  14  15  16  17  18  19  20
                        L   S   K   V   E   Q   F   Q   L   S   I   S   T   E   V   K   K   S   I   D
X07206   ,TRGV10*01 [4] TTA TCA AAA GTG GAG CAG TTC CAG CTA TCC ATT TCC ACG GAA GTC AAG AAA AGT ATT GAC
X74798   ,TRGV10*02 [9] --- --- --- --- --- --- --- --- --- --- --- --- --- --- --- --- --- --- --- ---
AF159056,TRGV10*02 [8] --- --- --- --- --- --- --- --- --- --- --- --- --- --- --- --- --- --- --- ---


                                                            __________________CDR1-IMGT________________
                       21  22  23  24  25  26  27  28  29  30  31  32  33  34  35  36  37  38  39  40
                        I   P   C   K   I   S   S   T   R   F   E   T   D   V                   I   H
X07206   ,TRGV10*01    ATA CCT TGC AAG ATA TCG AGC ACA AGG TTT GAA ACA GAT GTC ... ... ... ... ATT CAC
X74798   ,TRGV10*02    --- --- --- --- --- --- --- --- --- --- --- --- --- --- ... ... ... ... --- ---
AF159056,TRGV10*02    --- --- --- --- --- --- --- --- --- --- --- --- --- --- ... ... ... ... --- ---


                                                                                 _________________CDR2-
                       41  42  43  44  45  46  47  48  49  50  51  52  53  54  55  56  57  58  59  60
                        W   Y   R   Q   K   P   N   Q   A   L   E   H   L   I   Y   I   V   S   T   K
X07206   ,TRGV10*01    TGG TAC CGG CAG AAA CCA AAT CAG GCT TTG GAG CAC CTG ATC TAT ATT GTC TCA ACA AAA
X74798   ,TRGV10*02    --- --- --- --- --- --- --- --- --- --- --- --- --- --- --- --- --- --- --- ---
AF159056,TRGV10*02    --- --- --- --- --- --- --- --- --- --- --- --- --- --- --- --- --- --- --- ---


                       IMGT_________________
                       61  62  63  64  65  66  67  68  69  70  71  72  73  74  75  76  77  78  79  80
                        S   A   A               R   R   S   M   G   K   T   S   N   K   V   E   A   R   K
X07206   ,TRGV10*01    TCC GCA GCT ... ... CGA CGC AGC ATG GGT AAG ACA AGC AAC AAA GTG GAG GCA AGA AAG
X74798   ,TRGV10*02    --- --- --- ... ... --- --- --- --- --- --- --- --- --- --- --- --- --- --- ---
AF159056,TRGV10*02    --- --- --- ... ... --- --- --- --- --- --- --- --- --- --- --- --- --- --- ---


                       81  82  83  84  85  86  87  88  89  90  91  92  93  94  95  96  97  98  99 100
                        N   S   Q   T   L   T   S   I   L   T   I   K   S   V   E   K   E   D   M   A
X07206   ,TRGV10*01    AAT TCT CAA ACT CTC ACT TCA ATC CTT ACC ATC AAG TCC GTA GAG AAA GAA GAC ATG GCC
X74798   ,TRGV10*02    --- --- --- --- --- --- --- --- --- --- --- --- --- --- --- --- --- --- --- ---
AF159056,TRGV10*02    --- --- --- --- --- --- --- --- --- --- --- --- --- --- --- --- --- --- --- ---


                                       ________CDR3-IMGT________
                      101 102 103 104 105 106 107 108 109
                        V   Y   Y   C   A   A   W   W   V
X07206   ,TRGV10*01    GTT TAC TAC TGT GCT GCG TGG TGG GTG GC
                                                                D
X74798   ,TRGV10*02    --- --- --- --- --- --- --- ... -AT TA
                                                                D
AF159056,TRGV10*02    --- --- --- --- --- --- --- ... -AT TA
```

Framework and complementarity determining regions

FR1-IMGT: 26	CDR1-IMGT: 8
FR2-IMGT: 17	CDR2-IMGT: 8
FR3-IMGT: 39	CDR3-IMGT: 5

Collier de Perles for human TRGV10*01

Accession number: IMGT X07206   EMBL/GenBank/DDBJ: X07206

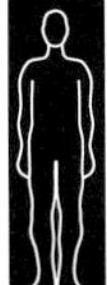

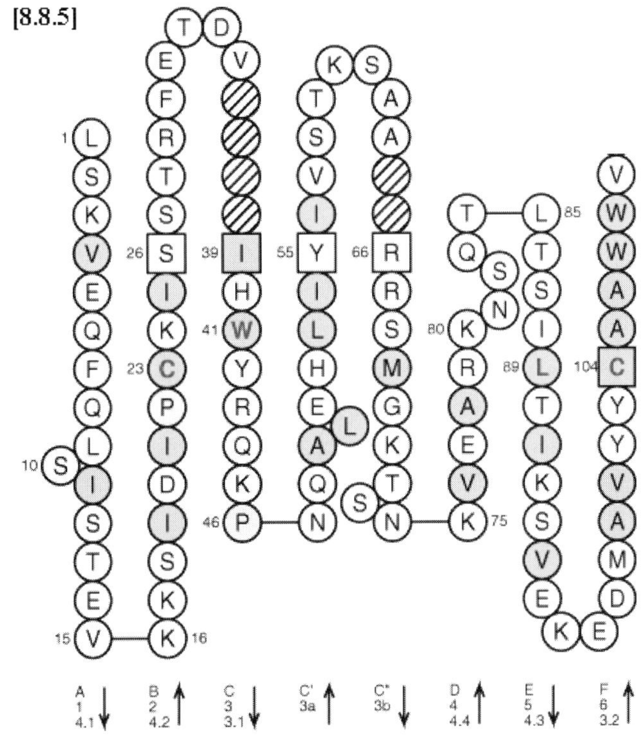

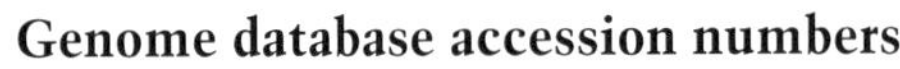

Genome database accession numbers
GDB:120416   LocusLink: 6984

Nomenclature

TRGV11: T cell receptor gamma variable 11

Definition and functionality

TRGV11 is the unique mapped ORF of the TRGV4 subgroup which only comprises that gene[1,6].

TRGV11 is an ORF due to a defective DONOR–SPLICE: nct instead of ngt, and to the absence of splicing of the V11 leader intron, and 1st–CYS replaced by Tryptophan (tgg) in FR1-IMGT[13,14].

Gene location

TRGV11 is in the TRG locus on chromosome 7 at 7p14.

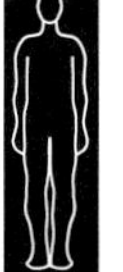

Nucleotide and amino acid sequences for human TRGV11

```
                    1   2   3   4   5   6   7   8   9   10  11  12  13  14  15  16  17  18  19  20
                    L   G   Q   L   E   Q   P   E   I   S   I   S   R   P   A   N   K   S   A   H
Y11227  ,TRGV11*01  [1] CTT GGG CAG TTG GAA CAA CCT GAA ATA TCT ATT TCC AGA CCA GCA AAT AAG AGT GCC CAC

AF159056,TRGV11*02  [8] --- --- --- --- --- --- --- --- --- --- --- --- --- --- --- --- --- --- --- ---


                                                            ____________________CDR1-IMGT____________________
                    21  22  23  24  25  26  27  28  29  30  31  32  33  34  35  36  37  38  39  40
                    I   S   W   K   A   S   I   Q   G   F   S   S   K   I                   I   H
Y11227  ,TRGV11*01  ATA TCT TGG AAG GCA TCC ATC CAA GGC TTT AGC AGT AAA ATC ... ... ... ... ATA CAC

AF159056,TRGV11*02  --- --- --- --- --- --- --- --- --- --- --- --- --- --- ... ... ... ... --- ---


                                                                            ________________________CDR2-
                    41  42  43  44  45  46  47  48  49  50  51  52  53  54  55  56  57  58  59  60
                    W   Y   W   Q   K   P   N   K   G   L   E   Y   L   L   H   V   F   L   T   I
Y11227  ,TRGV11*01  TGG TAC TGG CAG AAA CCA AAC AAA GGC TTA GAA TAT TTA TTA CAT GTC TTC TTG ACA ATC

AF159056,TRGV11*02  --- --- --- --- --- --- --- --- --- --- --- --- --- --- --- --- --- --- --- ---


                    IMGT________________
                    61  62  63  64  65  66  67  68  69  70  71  72  73  74  75  76  77  78  79  80
                    S   A                   Q   D   C   S   G   G   K   T   K   K   L   E   V   S   K
Y11227  ,TRGV11*01  TCT GCT ... ... ... CAA GAT TGC TCA GGT GGG AAG ACT AAG AAA CTT GAG GTA AGT AAA

AF159056,TRGV11*02  --- --- ... ... ... --- --- --- --- --- --- --- --- --- --- --- --- A-- --- ---


                    81  82  83  84  85  86  87  88  89  90  91  92  93  94  95  96  97  98  99  100
                    N   A   H   T   S   T   S   T   L   K   I   K   F   L   E   K   E   D   E   V
Y11227  ,TRGV11*01  AAT GCT CAC ACT TCC ACT TCC ACT TTG AAA ATA AAG TTC TTA GAG AAA GAA GAT GAG GTG

AF159056,TRGV11*02  --- --- --- --- --- --- --- --- --- --- --- --- --- --- --- --- --- --- --- ---


                                        ________CDR3-IMGT________
                    101 102 103 104 105 106 107 108 109 110
                    V   Y   H   C   A   C   W   I   R   H
Y11227  ,TRGV11*01  GTG TAC CAC TGT GCC TGC TGG ATT AGG CAC

AF159056,TRGV11*02  --- --- --- --- --- --- --- --- --- ---
```

Framework and complementarity determining regions

FR1-IMGT: 26   CDR1-IMGT: 8
FR2-IMGT: 17   CDR2-IMGT: 7
FR3-IMGT: 39   CDR3-IMGT: 6

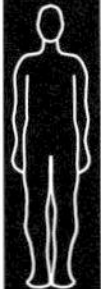

Collier de Perles for human TRGV11*01

Accession number: IMGT Y11227   EMBL/GenBank/DDBJ: Y11227

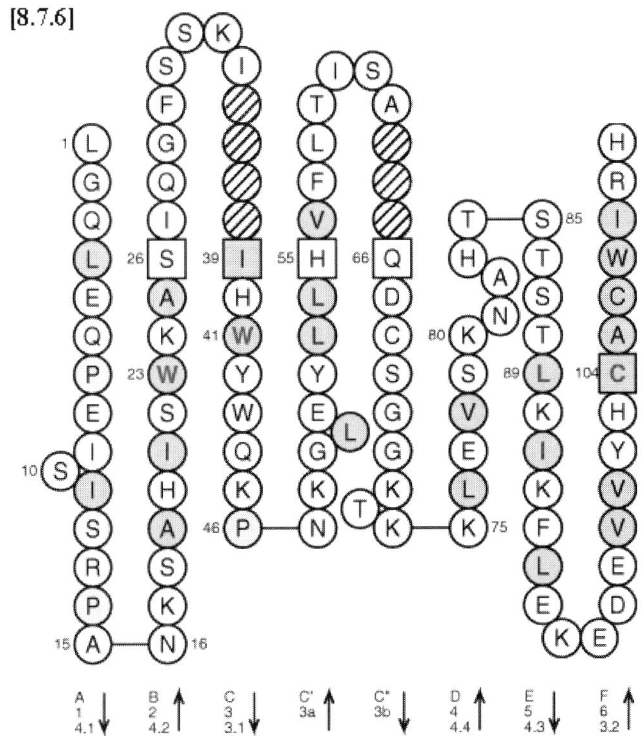

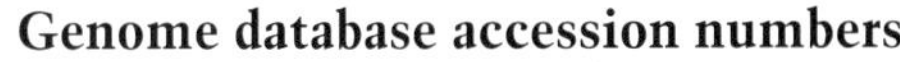

Genome database accession numbers
GDB:120417   LocusLink: 6985

TRGV protein display

Protein display of the human TRG V-REGIONs.

*Only the *01 allele of each functional or ORF V-REGION is shown. TRGV genes are listed, for each subgroup, according to their position from 5' to 3' in the locus. N-glycosylation sites (NXS/T, where X is different from P) are underlined.*

```
TRGV                      FR1-IMGT            CDR1-IMGT     FR2-IMGT          CDR2-IMGT       FR3-IMGT                              CDR3-IMGT
gene                      (1-26)              (27-38)       (39-55)           (56-65)         (66-104)                              (105-115)

                    1        10        20        30        40        50        60        70        80        90       100        110
                    .........|.........|.... ...|........ .|.........|.... ....|.... ....|.........|.........|.........|.... ....|....
M12949    ,TRGV1    SSNLEGRTKSVTRLTGSSAEITCDLP GASTLY...... IHWYLHQEGKAPQCLLY YEPYYSRV.. VLESGITPGKYDT.GS.TRSNWNLRLQNLIKNDSGFYYC ATWDR.....
M13429    ,TRGV2    SSNLEGRTKSVIRQTGSSAEITCDLA EGSNGY...... IHWYLHQEGKAPQRLQY YDSYNSKV.. VLESGVSPGKYYTYAS.TRNNLRLILRNLIENDSGVYYC ATWDG.....
M13430    ,TRGV3    SSNLEGRTKSVTRQTGSSAEITCDLT VTNTFY...... IHWYLHQEGKAPQRLLY YDVSTARD.. VLESGLSPGKYYTHTP.RRWSWILRLQNLIENDSGVYYC ATWDR.....
X15272    ,TRGV4    SSNLEGRTKSVIRQTGSSAEITCDLA EGSTGY...... IHWYLHQEGKAPQRLLY YDSYTSSV.. VLESGISPGKYDTYGS.TRKNLRMILRNLIENDSGVYYC ATWDG.....
X13355/M36286,TRGV5 SSNLEGGTKSVTRPTRSSAEITCDLT VINAFY...... IHWYLHQEGKAPQRLLY YDVSNSKD.. VLESGLSPGKYYTHTP.RRWSWILILRNLIENDSGVYYC ATWDR.....
M13434    ,TRGV8    SSNLEGRTKSVTRPTGSSAVITCDLP VENAVY...... THWYLHQEGKAPQRLLY YDSYNSRV.. VLESGISREKYHTYAS.TGKSLKFILENLIERDSGVYYC ATWDR.....

X07205    ,TRGV9    AGHLEQPQISSTKTLSKTARLECVVS GITISATS.... VYWYRERPGEVIQFLVS ISYDGTV... RKESGIPSGKFEVDRIPETSTSTLTIHNVEKQDIATYYC ALWEV.....

X07206    ,TRGV10   LSKVEQFQLSISTEVKKSIDIPCKIS STRFETDV.... IHWYRQKPNQALEHLIY IVSTKSAA.. RRSMGKTSNKVEARKNSQTLTSILTIKSVEKEDMAVYYC AAWWV.....

Y11227    ,TRGV11   LGQLEQPEISISRPANKSAHISWKAS IQGFSSKI.... IHWYWQKPNKGLEYLLH VFLTISA... QDCSGGKTKKLEVSKNAHTSTSTLKIKFLEKEDEVVYHC ACWIRH.....
```

TRGV recombination signals and references

Recombination signals

Only the recombination signals of the allele *01 of each functional or ORF V-REGION are shown.

| TRGV | V Recombination Signal (V-RS) | | |
gene name	V-HEPTAMER	(bp)	V-NONAMER
TRGV1*01 (ORF)	CACAGTG	9	CTGAAAATC
TRGV2*01	CACAGTG	23	CTGAAAATC
TRGV3*01	CACAGTG	23	CTGAAAATC
TRGV4*01	CACAGTG	23	CTGAAAATC
TRGV5*01	CACAGTG	23	CTGAAAATC
TRGV8*01	CACAGTG	23	CTGAAAATC
TRGV9*01	CACAGCA	23	TCAATAAAT
TRGV10*01 (ORF)	CACATAC	23	CAAAATCCC
TRGV11*01 (ORF)	CACAGTG	23	ACAGAAACT

References

[1] Chen, Z. et al. (1988) Blood 72, 776–783.

[2] Dariavach, P. and Lefranc, M.-P. (1989) FEBS Lett. 256, 185–191.

[3] Font, M.P. et al. (1988) J. Exp. Med. 168, 1383–1394.

[4] Ghanem, N. et al. (1991) Hum. Genet. 86, 450–456.

[5] Ghanem, N. et al. (1989) Immunogenetics 30, 350–360.

[6] Huck, S. et al. (1988) EMBO J. 7, 719–726.

[7] Lefranc, M.-P. et al. (1985) Nature 316, 464–466.

[8] Lefranc, M.-P. et al. (1986) Cell 45, 237–246.

[9] Lefranc, M.-P. et al. (1989) Eur. J. Immunol. 19, 989–994.

[10] Quertermous, T. et al. (1986) Nature 322, 184–187.

[11] Yoshikai, Y. et al. (1987) Eur. J .Immunol. 17, 119–126.

[12] Zhan, M. et al., unpublished.

[13] Zhang, X.M. et al. (1994) Eur. J. Immunol. 24, 571–578.

[14] Zhang, X.M. et al. (1996) Immunogenetics 43, 196–203.

THE HUMAN
T CELL RECEPTOR
TRD GENES

Part 1

TRDC

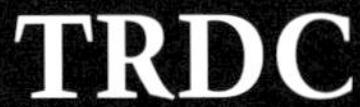

Nomenclature

TRDC: T cell receptor delta constant.

Definition and functionality

TRDC is the functional and unique constant gene in the TRD locus.

Gene location

TRDC is in the TRD locus on chromosome 14 at 14q11.2.
The TRD locus is embedded in the TRA locus, between the TRAV and TRAJ genes.

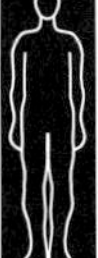

Nucleotide and amino acid sequences for human TRDC

The nucleotide between parentheses at the beginning of exons comes from a DONOR–SPLICE (n from ngt).

The Cysteines involved in the intrachain disulfide bridges are shown with their number and letter **C** in bold.

N-Glycosylation sites (NXS/T, where X is different from P) are underlined.

Poly(A) signals are shown in bold and underlined.

A DONOR–SPLICE, located just after the termination codon, uses a downstream ACCEPTOR–SPLICE, placing part of the 3' non-coding sequence on a separate untranslated exon, designated as EX4. Since EX4 is untranslated, nucleotide differences observed in EX4 are not taken into account for the description of alleles, according to IMGT allele nomenclature and sequence polymorphisms.

Note that AE000661 encompasses M94081.

```
                               1   2   3   4   5   6   7   8   9  10  11  12  13  14  15  16  17  18  19  20
                               R   S   Q   P   H   T   K   P   S   V   F   V   M   K   N   G   T   N   V   A
M22148   ,TRDC*01 (EX1)    [1] (C)GA AGT CAG CCT CAT ACC AAA CCA TCC GTT TTT GTC ATG AAA AAT GGA ACA AAT GTC GCT

X07019   ,TRDC*01         [2] (-)-- --- --- --- --- --- --- --- --- --- --- --- --- --- --- --- --- --- --- ---

M94081   ,TRDC*01         [4] (-)-- --- --- --- --- --- --- --- --- --- --- --- --- --- --- --- --- --- --- ---

AE000661,TRDC*01          [5] (-)-- --- --- --- --- --- --- --- --- --- --- --- --- --- --- --- --- --- --- ---

M20288   ,TRDC*01         [3] (-)-- --- --- --- --- --- --- --- --- --- --- --- --- --- --- --- --- --- --- ---


                               21  22  23  24  25  26  27  28  29  30  31  32  33  34  35  36  37  38  39  40
                               C   L   V   K   E   F   Y   P   K   D   I   R   I   N   L   V   S   S   K   K
M22148   ,TRDC*01 (EX1)        TGT CTG GTG AAG GAA TTC TAC CCC AAG GAT ATA AGA ATA AAT CTC GTG TCA TCC AAG AAG

X07019   ,TRDC*01              --- --- --- --- --- --- --- --- --- --- --- --- --- --- --- --- --- --- --- ---

M94081   ,TRDC*01              --- --- --- --- --- --- --- --- --- --- --- --- --- --- --- --- --- --- --- ---

AE000661,TRDC*01               --- --- --- --- --- --- --- --- --- --- --- --- --- --- --- --- --- --- --- ---

M20288   ,TRDC*01              --- --- --- --- --- ---


                               41  42  43  44  45  46  47  48  49  50  51  52  53  54  55  56  57  58  59  60
                               I   T   E   F   D   P   A   I   V   I   S   P   S   G   K   Y   N   A   V   K
M22148   ,TRDC*01 (EX1)        ATA ACA GAG TTT GAT CCT GCT ATT GTC ATC TCT CCC AGT GGG AAG TAC AAT GCT GTC AAG

X07019   ,TRDC*01              --- --- --- --- --- --- --- --- --- --- --- --- --- --- --- --- --- --- --- ---

M94081   ,TRDC*01              --- --- --- --- --- --- --- --- --- --- --- --- --- --- --- --- --- --- --- ---

AE000661,TRDC*01               --- --- --- --- --- --- --- --- --- --- --- --- --- --- --- --- --- --- --- ---

M20288   ,TRDC*01
```

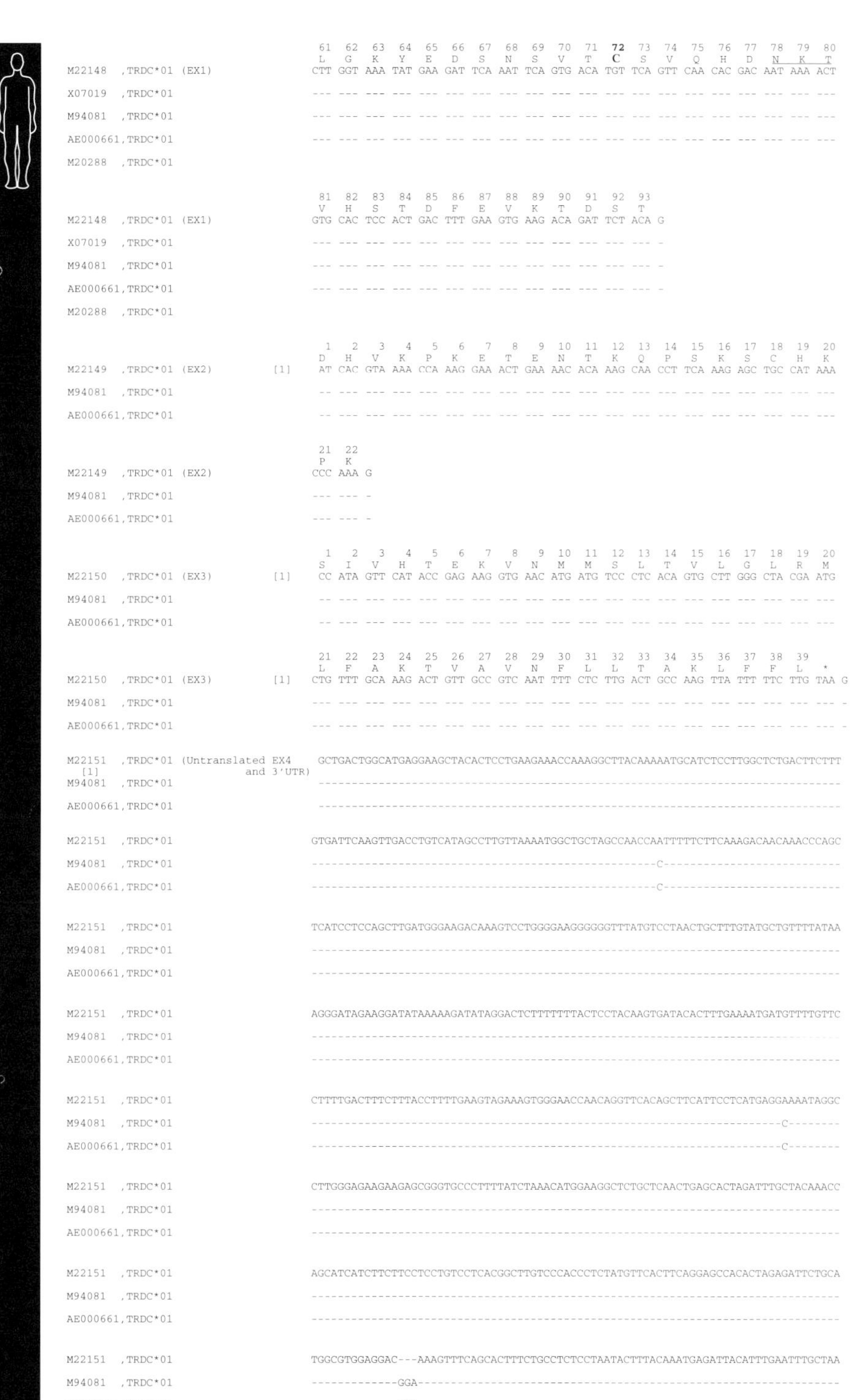

```
                         61  62  63  64  65  66  67  68  69  70  71  72  73  74  75  76  77  78  79  80
                          L   G   K   Y   E   D   S   N   S   V   T   C   S   V   Q   H   D   N   K   T
M22148   ,TRDC*01 (EX1)  CTT GGT AAA TAT GAA GAT TCA AAT TCA GTG ACA TGT TCA GTT CAA CAC GAC AAT AAA ACT
X07019   ,TRDC*01       --- --- --- --- --- --- --- --- --- --- --- --- --- --- --- --- --- --- --- ---
M94081   ,TRDC*01       --- --- --- --- --- --- --- --- --- --- --- --- --- --- --- --- --- --- --- ---
AE000661 ,TRDC*01       --- --- --- --- --- --- --- --- --- --- --- --- --- --- --- --- --- --- --- ---
M20288   ,TRDC*01

                         81  82  83  84  85  86  87  88  89  90  91  92  93
                          V   H   S   T   D   F   E   V   K   T   D   S   T
M22148   ,TRDC*01 (EX1)  GTG CAC TCC ACT GAC TTT GAA GTG AAG ACA GAT TCT ACA G
X07019   ,TRDC*01       --- --- --- --- --- --- --- --- --- --- --- --- --- -
M94081   ,TRDC*01       --- --- --- --- --- --- --- --- --- --- --- --- --- -
AE000661 ,TRDC*01       --- --- --- --- --- --- --- --- --- --- --- --- --- -
M20288   ,TRDC*01

                              1   2   3   4   5   6   7   8   9  10  11  12  13  14  15  16  17  18  19  20
                              D   H   V   K   P   K   E   T   E   N   T   K   Q   P   S   K   S   C   H   K
M22149   ,TRDC*01 (EX2)  [1]  AT CAC GTA AAA CCA AAG GAA ACT GAA AAC ACA AAG CAA CCT TCA AAG AGC TGC CAT AAA
M94081   ,TRDC*01            -- --- --- --- --- --- --- --- --- --- --- --- --- --- --- --- --- --- --- ---
AE000661 ,TRDC*01            -- --- --- --- --- --- --- --- --- --- --- --- --- --- --- --- --- --- --- ---

                             21  22
                              P   K
M22149   ,TRDC*01 (EX2)  CCC AAA G
M94081   ,TRDC*01       --- --- -
AE000661 ,TRDC*01       --- --- -

                              1   2   3   4   5   6   7   8   9  10  11  12  13  14  15  16  17  18  19  20
                              S   I   V   H   T   E   K   V   N   M   M   S   L   T   V   L   G   L   R   M
M22150   ,TRDC*01 (EX3)  [1]  CC ATA GTT CAT ACC GAG AAG GTG AAC ATG ATG TCC CTC ACA GTG CTT GGG CTA CGA ATG
M94081   ,TRDC*01            -- --- --- --- --- --- --- --- --- --- --- --- --- --- --- --- --- --- --- ---
AE000661 ,TRDC*01            -- --- --- --- --- --- --- --- --- --- --- --- --- --- --- --- --- --- --- ---

                             21  22  23  24  25  26  27  28  29  30  31  32  33  34  35  36  37  38  39
                              L   F   A   K   T   V   A   V   N   F   L   L   T   A   K   L   F   F   L   *
M22150   ,TRDC*01 (EX3)  [1]  CTG TTT GCA AAG ACT GTT GCC GTC AAT TTT CTC TTG ACT GCC AAG TTA TTT TTC TTG TAA G
M94081   ,TRDC*01            --- --- --- --- --- --- --- --- --- --- --- --- --- --- --- --- --- --- --- -
AE000661 ,TRDC*01            --- --- --- --- --- --- --- --- --- --- --- --- --- --- --- --- --- --- --- -
```

```
M22151   ,TRDC*01 (Untranslated EX4    GCTGACTGGCATGAGGAAGCTACACTCCTGAAGAAACCAAAGGCTTACAAAAATGCATCTCCTTGGCTCTGACTTCTTT
     [1]                 and 3'UTR)
M94081   ,TRDC*01       ------------------------------------------------------------------------------
AE000661 ,TRDC*01       ------------------------------------------------------------------------------

M22151   ,TRDC*01       GTGATTCAAGTTGACCTGTCATAGCCTTGTTAAAATGGCTGCTAGCCAACCAATTTTTCTTCAAAGACAACAAACCCAGC
M94081   ,TRDC*01       ----------------------------------------------------C-------------------------
AE000661 ,TRDC*01       ----------------------------------------------------C-------------------------

M22151   ,TRDC*01       TCATCCTCCAGCTTGATGGGAAGACAAAGTCCTGGGGAAGGGGGGGTTTATGTCCTAACTGCTTTGTATGCTGTTTTATAA
M94081   ,TRDC*01       ------------------------------------------------------------------------------
AE000661 ,TRDC*01       ------------------------------------------------------------------------------

M22151   ,TRDC*01       AGGGATAGAAGGATATAAAAAGATATAGGACTCTTTTTTTACTCCTACAAGTGATACACTTTGAAAATGATGTTTTGTTC
M94081   ,TRDC*01       ------------------------------------------------------------------------------
AE000661 ,TRDC*01       ------------------------------------------------------------------------------

M22151   ,TRDC*01       CTTTTGACTTTCTTTACCTTTTGAAGTAGAAAGTGGGAACCAACAGGTTCACAGCTTCATTCCTCATGAGGAAAATAGGC
M94081   ,TRDC*01       ---------------------------------------------------------------------C--------
AE000661 ,TRDC*01       ---------------------------------------------------------------------C--------

M22151   ,TRDC*01       CTTGGGAGAAGAAGAGCGGGTGCCCTTTTATCTAAACATGGAAGGCTCTGCTCAACTGAGCACTAGATTTGCTACAAACC
M94081   ,TRDC*01       ------------------------------------------------------------------------------
AE000661 ,TRDC*01       ------------------------------------------------------------------------------

M22151   ,TRDC*01       AGCATCATCTTCTTCCTCCTGTCCTCACGGCTTGTCCCACCCTCTATGTTCACTTCAGGAGCCACACTAGAGATTCTGCA
M94081   ,TRDC*01       ------------------------------------------------------------------------------
AE000661 ,TRDC*01       ------------------------------------------------------------------------------

M22151   ,TRDC*01       TGGCGTGGAGGAC---AAAGTTTCAGCACTTTCTGCCTCTCCTAATACTTTACAAATGAGATTACATTTGAATTTGCTAA
M94081   ,TRDC*01       -------------GGA--------------------------------------------------------------
AE000661 ,TRDC*01       -------------GGA--------------------------------------------------------------
```

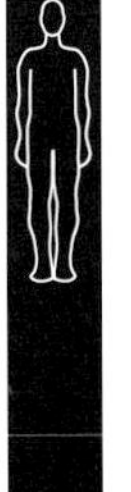

```
M22151   ,TRDC*01    TACTTTATGAGCAGGCAATGAGGTTTCCAAAATCTCATCTAAATACTCTCCAATCTATTAGCAAAAATCAGAGTAAAATA
M94081   ,TRDC*01    --------------------------------------------------------------------------------
AE000661 ,TRDC*01    --------------------------------------------------------------------------------

M22151   ,TRDC*01    CAGAGGAAAGGCACTGCTTTCTGTTAATTGATTTAACATGCATGAATTAGCTCCCTCTGAGTTCCAGGCACTATGCTGAG
M94081   ,TRDC*01    --------------------------------------------------------------------------------
AE000661 ,TRDC*01    --------------------------------------------------------------------------------

M22151   ,TRDC*01    AGTACAAAGAAGACACAAGTCTGCTTTCAAGCAACTCACTGTGAAAGTGTTTTTGAAGGGAGGAACAGAAATGAGACCCC
M94081   ,TRDC*01    --------------------------------------------------------------------------------
AE000661 ,TRDC*01    --------------------------------------------------------------------------------

M22151   ,TRDC*01    TATCTTTCCCTATAAAAACAACATTTTTACTGTGTTTTGCCTGCCAATCTGTATTTGAAACCATTGGACACTGATTCTCT
M94081   ,TRDC*01    ---------------------------------C----------------------------------------------
AE000661 ,TRDC*01    ---------------------------------C----------------------------------------------

M22151   ,TRDC*01    GGCCTGGGACTTTGGCATTGATGGTTTTCTGCCTTTCTTCTCAGCCTCTGCCTCTATTGCATTTATTAAACTGCATTGTG
M94081   ,TRDC*01    --------------------------------------------------------------------------------
AE000661 ,TRDC*01    --------------------------------------------------------------------------------

M22151   ,TRDC*01    TGC
M94081   ,TRDC*01    ---
AE000661 ,TRDC*01    ---
```

Genome database accession numbers

GDB:9954211   LocusLink: 28526

References

[1] Takihara, Y. et al. (1988) Proc. Natl Acad. Sci. USA 85, 6097–6101.
[2] Boehm, T. et al. (1988) EMBO J. 7, 385–394.
[3] Isobe, M. et al. (1988) Proc. Natl Acad. Sci. USA 85, 3933–3937.
[4] Koop, B.F. et al. (1994) Genomics 19, 478–493.
[5] Boysen, C. et al., unpublished.

Protein display

Protein display of the TRDC gene is shown on page 372.

Part 2

TRDD

TRDD group

Nomenclature

T cell receptor delta diversity group.

Definition and functionality

The human TRDD group comprises three functional mapped genes, TRDD1, TRDD2, and TRDD3. The TRDD genes have two or three open reading frames in both the direct and inverted orientations.

Gene location

The human TRDD genes are located in the TRA/TRD locus on chromosome 14 at 14q11.2, upstream from the TRDJ genes.

Nucleotide and amino acid sequences for the human TRDD genes with nomenclature

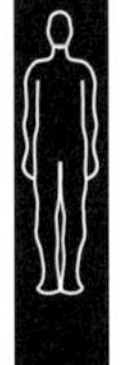

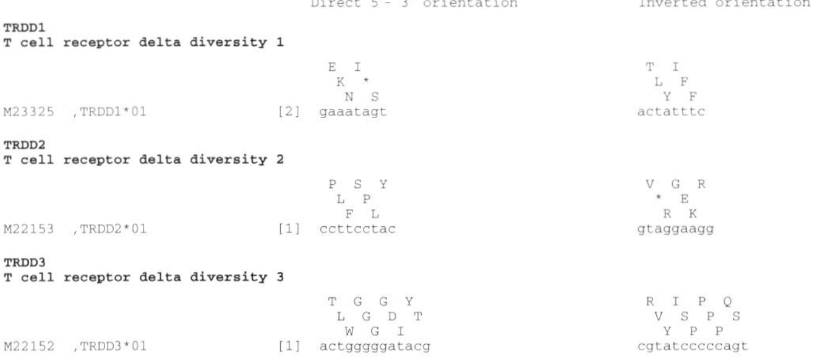

```
                                  Direct 5'- 3' orientation          Inverted orientation
TRDD1
T cell receptor delta diversity 1
                                        E  I                           T  I
                                        K  *                           L  F
                                        N  S                           Y  F
      M23325   ,TRDD1*01          [2]  gaaatagt                        actatttc

TRDD2
T cell receptor delta diversity 2
                                        P  S  Y                        V  G  R
                                        L  P                           *  E
                                        F  L                           R  K
      M22153   ,TRDD2*01          [1]  ccttcctac                      gtaggaagg

TRDD3
T cell receptor delta diversity 3
                                        T  G  G  Y                     R  I  P  Q
                                        L  G  D  T                     V  S  P  S
                                        W  G  I                        Y  P  P
      M22152   ,TRDD3*01          [1]  actgggggatacg                  cgtatcccccagt
```

Recombination signals

5'D Recombination Signal (5'D-RS)			TRDD gene and allele name	3'D Recombination Signal (3'D-RS)		
5'D-NONAMER	(bp)	5'D-HEPTAMER		3'D-HEPTAMER	(bp)	3'D-NONAMER
ATTTTTTCA	12	CAAAGTG	TRDD1*01	CACTCAA	23	ATTAACCAA
GGTTTTTAT	12	CATTGTG	TRDD2*01	CACACAG	23	CCAAAAACA
AGTTTTTGT	12	CACTGTG	TRDD3*01	CACAGTG	23	ACAAAAACT

References

[1] Takihara, Y. et al. (1988) Proc. Natl Acad. Sci. USA 85, 6097–6101.
[2] Loh, M. et al. (1988) Proc. Natl Acad. Sci. USA 85, 9714–9718.

Part 3

TRDJ

TRDJ group

Nomenclature

T cell receptor delta joining group.

Definition and functionality

The human TRDJ group comprises four functional mapped genes: TRDJ1, TRDJ2, TRDJ3, and TRDJ4.

Gene location

The human TRDJ genes are located in the TRA/TRD locus on chromosome 14 at 14q11.2, upstream from the TRDC gene.

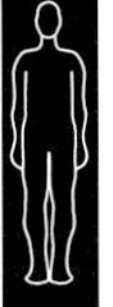

Nucleotide and amino acid sequences for the human functional TRDJ genes with nomenclature

The conserved **FGXG** motif, characteristic of the TRD J-REGION is underlined.

```
TRDJ1
T cell receptor delta joining 1
                                       T   D   K   L   I   F   G   K   G   T   R   V   T   V   E   P
   M20289  ,TRDJ1*01      [2]         AC ACC GAT AAA CTC ATC TTT GGA AAA GGA ACC CGT GTG ACT GTG GAA CCA A

TRDJ2
T cell receptor delta joining 2
                                     L   T   A   Q   L   F   F   G   K   G   T   Q   L   I   V   E   P
   L36386  ,TRDJ2*01      [3]      CT TTG ACA GCA CAA CTC TTC TTT GGA AAG GGA ACA CAA CTC ATC GTG GAA CCA G

TRDJ3
T cell receptor delta joining 3
                                 S   W   D   T   R   Q   M   F   F   G   T   G   I   K   L   F   V   E   P
   M21508  ,TRDJ3*01      [4]   C TCC TGG GAC ACC CGA CAG ATG TTT TTC GGA ACT GGC ATC AAA CTC TTC GTG GAG CCC C

TRDJ4
T cell receptor delta joining 4
                                     R   P   L   I   F   G   K   G   T   Y   L   E   V   Q   Q
   AJ249814,TRDJ4*01      [1]      CC AGA CCC CTG ATC TTT GGC AAA GGA ACC TAT CTG GAG GTA CAA CAA C
```

Recombination signals

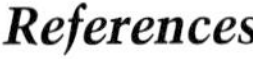

J Recombination Signal (J-RS)			TRDJ gene and allele name
J-NONAMER	(bp)	J-HEPTAMER	
GGTTTTTGG	12	TGCTGTG	TRDJ1*01
GGTTTTTCG	13	GGTAGTG	TRDJ2*01
GTTACCTGT	12	TAATGTG	TRDJ3*01
GGTTTTTCG	13	GGTAGTG	TRDJ4*01

References

[1] Davodeau, F. et al. (1994) J. Immunol. 153, 137–142.

[2] Isobe, M. et al. (1988) Proc. Natl Acad. Sci. USA 85, 3933–3937.

[3] Loh, E.Y. et al. (1988) Proc. Natl Acad. Sci. USA 85, 9714–9718.

[4] Satyanarayana, K. et al. (1988) Proc. Natl Acad. Sci. USA 85, 8166–8170.

Part 4

TRDV

TRDV1

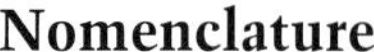

Nomenclature

TRDV1: T cell receptor delta variable 1.

Definition and functionality

TRDV1 is the unique mapped functional gene of the TRDV1 subgroup which only comprises that gene.

Gene location

TRDV1 is in the TRA/TRD locus on chromosome 14 at 14q11.2. TRDV1 is localized at 360 kb upstream of the TRDC gene, among the TRAV genes[2].

Nucleotide and amino acid sequences for human TRDV1

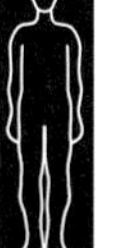

```
                 1    2    3    4    5    6    7    8    9   10   11   12   13   14   15   16   17   18   19   20
                 A    Q    K    V    T    Q    A    Q    S    S    V    S    M    P    V    R    K    A    V    T
M22198   ,TRDV1*01  [7]  GCC  CAG  AAG  GTT  ACT  CAA  GCC  CAG  TCA  TCA  GTA  TCC  ATG  CCA  GTG  AGG  AAA  GCA  GTC  ACC
U32547   ,TRDV1*01  [1]  ---  ---  ---  ---  ---  ---  ---  ---  ---  ---  ---  ---  ---  ---  ---  ---  ---  ---  ---  ---
AE000660,TRDV1*01  [2]  ---  ---  ---  ---  ---  ---  ---  ---  ---  ---  ---  ---  ---  ---  ---  ---  ---  ---  ---  ---


                                                             ________________________CDR1-IMGT________________________
                21   22   23   24   25   26   27   28   29   30   31   32   33   34   35   36   37   38   39   40
                 L    N    C    L    Y    E    T    S    W    W    S    Y    Y                        I    F
M22198   ,TRDV1*01  CTG  AAC  TGC  CTG  TAT  GAA  ACA  AGT  TGG  TGG  TCA  TAT  TAT  ...  ...  ...  ...  ...  ATT  TTT
U32547   ,TRDV1*01  ---  ---  ---  ---  ---  ---  ---  ---  ---  ---  ---  ---  ---  ...  ...  ...  ...  ...  ---  ---
AE000660,TRDV1*01  ---  ---  ---  ---  ---  ---  ---  ---  ---  ---  ---  ---  ---  ...  ...  ...  ...  ...  ---  ---


                                                                                         ______________________CDR2-
                41   42   43   44   45   46   47   48   49   50   51   52   53   54   55   56   57   58   59   60
                 W    Y    K    Q    L    P    S    K    E    M    I    F    L    I    R    Q    G    S
M22198   ,TRDV1*01  TGG  TAC  AAG  CAA  CTT  CCC  AGC  AAA  GAG  ATG  ATT  TTC  CTT  ATT  CGC  CAG  GGT  TCT  ...  ...
U32547   ,TRDV1*01  ---  ---  ---  ---  ---  ---  ---  ---  ---  ---  ---  ---  ---  ---  ---  ---  ---  ---  ...  ...
AE000660,TRDV1*01  ---  ---  ---  ---  ---  ---  ---  ---  ---  ---  ---  ---  ---  ---  ---  ---  ---  ---  ---  ...  ...


                IMGT________________
                61   62   63   64   65   66   67   68   69   70   71   72   73   74   75   76   77   78   79   80
                                      D    E    Q    N    A    K    S         G    R    Y    S    V    N    F
M22198   ,TRDV1*01  ...  ...  ...  ...  ...  GAT  GAA  CAG  AAT  GCA  AAA  AGT  ...  GGT  CGC  TAT  TCT  GTC  AAC  TTC
U32547   ,TRDV1*01  ...  ...  ...  ...  ...  ---  ---  ---  ---  ---  ---  ---  ...  ---  ---  ---  ---  ---  ---  ---
AE000660,TRDV1*01  ...  ...  ...  ...  ...  ---  ---  ---  ---  ---  ---  ---  ...  ---  ---  ---  ---  ---  ---  ---


                81   82   83   84   85   86   87   88   89   90   91   92   93   94   95   96   97   98   99  100
                 K    K    A    A    K    S    V    A    L    T    I    S    A    L    Q    L    E    D    S    A
M22198   ,TRDV1*01  AAG  AAA  GCA  GCG  AAA  TCC  GTC  GCC  TTA  ACC  ATT  TCA  GCC  TTA  CAG  CTA  GAA  GAT  TCA  GCA
U32547   ,TRDV1*01  ---
AE000660,TRDV1*01  ---  ---  ---  ---  ---  ---  ---  ---  ---  ---  ---  ---  ---  ---  ---  ---  ---  ---  ---  ---


                              ______CDR3-IMGT______
                101  102  103  104  105  106  107  108
                 K    Y    F    C    A    L    G    E
M22198   ,TRDV1*01  AAG  TAC  TTT  TGT  GCT  CTT  GGG  GAA  CT
U32547   ,TRDV1*01
AE000660,TRDV1*01  ---  ---  ---  ---  ---  ---  ---  ---  -
```

Framework and complementarity determining regions

FR1-IMGT: 26	CDR1-IMGT: 7
FR2-IMGT: 17	CDR2-IMGT: 3
FR3-IMGT: 38 (-1 aa: 73)	CDR3-IMGT: 4

Collier de Perles for human TRDV1*01

Accession number: IMGT M22198   EMBL/GenBank/DDBJ: M22198

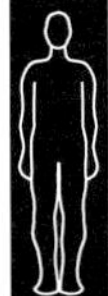

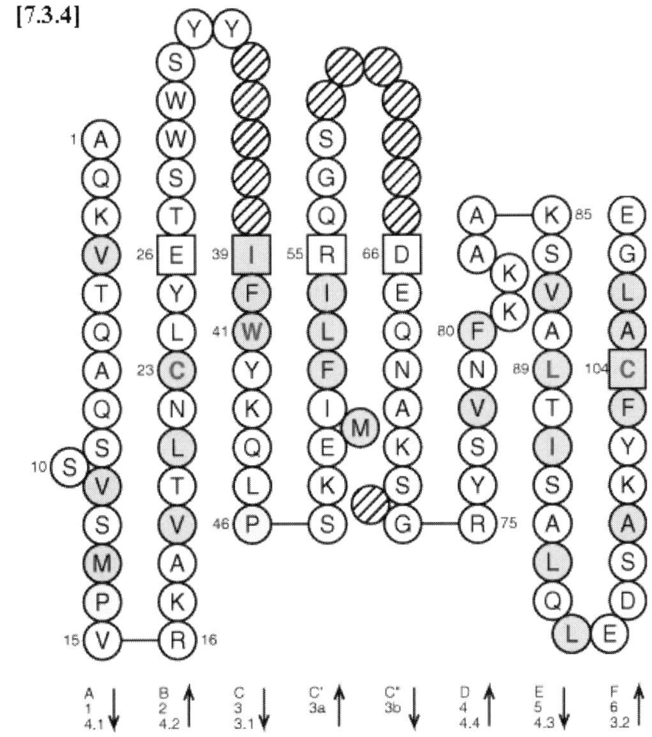

Genome database accession numbers
GDB:9953671   LocusLink: 28518

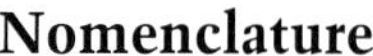

Nomenclature

TRDV2: T cell receptor delta variable 2.

Definition and functionality

TRDV2 is the unique mapped functional gene of the TRDV2 subgroup which only comprises that gene.

Gene location

TRDV2 is in the TRA/TRD locus on chromosome 14 at 14q11.2. TRDV2 is localized upstream of the TRD D-J-C-CLUSTER [3].

Nucleotide and amino acid sequences for human TRDV2

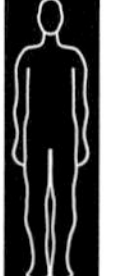

```
                       1    2    3    4    5    6    7    8    9   10   11   12   13   14   15   16   17   18   19   20
                       A    I    E    L    V    P    E    H    Q    T    V    P    V    S    I    G    V    P    A    T
X15207   ,TRDV2*01 [3] GCC  ATT  GAG  TTG  GTG  CCT  GAA  CAC  CAA  ACA  GTG  CCT  GTG  TCA  ATA  GGG  GTC  CCT  GCC  ACC
U32548   ,TRDV2*01 [1]                          ---  ---  ---  ---  ---  ---  ---  ---  ---  ---  ---  ---  ---  ---  ---
                                                                                                  I
Y13426   ,TRDV2*02 [10]     ---  ---  ---  ---  ---  ---  ---  ---  ---  ---  ---  ---  ---  ---  ---  A--  ---  ---  ---
AE000661 ,TRDV2*03 [2] ---  ---  ---  ---  ---  ---  ---  ---  ---  ---  ---  ---  ---  ---  ---  ---  ---  ---  ---  ---
X53849   ,TRDV2*03 [9] ---  ---  ---  ---  ---  ---  ---  ---  ---  ---  ---  ---  ---  ---  ---  ---  ---  ---  ---  ---


                                                 ___________________________CDR1-IMGT___________________________
                      21   22   23   24   25   26   27   28   29   30   31   32   33   34   35   36   37   38   39   40
                       L    R    C    S    M    K    G    E    A    I    G    N    Y    Y                        I    N
X15207   ,TRDV2*01   CTC  AGG  TGC  TCC  ATG  AAA  GGA  GAA  GCG  ATC  GGT  AAC  TAC  TAT  ...  ...  ...  ...  ATC  AAC
U32548   ,TRDV2*01   ---  ---  ---  ---  ---  ---  ---  ---  ---  ---  ---  ---  ---  ---  ...  ...  ...  ...  ---  ---
Y13426   ,TRDV2*02   ---  ---  ---  ---  ---  ---  ---  ---  ---  ---  ---  ---  ---  ---  ...  ...  ...  ...  ---  ---
AE000661 ,TRDV2*03   ---  ---  ---  ---  ---  ---  ---  ---  ---  ---  ---  ---  ---  ---  ...  ...  ...  ...  ---  ---
X53849   ,TRDV2*03   ---  ---  ---  ---  ---  ---  ---  ---  ---  ---  ---  ---  ---  ---  ...  ...  ...  ...  ---  ---


                                                                           ________________CDR2-
                      41   42   43   44   45   46   47   48   49   50   51   52   53   54   55   56   57   58   59   60
                       W    Y    R    K    T    Q    G    N    T    I    T    F    I    Y    R    E    K    D
X15207   ,TRDV2*01   TGG  TAC  AGG  AAG  ACC  CAA  GGT  AAC  ACA  ATC  ACT  TTC  ATA  TAC  CGA  GAA  AAG  GAC  ...  ...
U32548   ,TRDV2*01   ---  ---  ---  ---  ---  ---  ---  ---  ---  ---  ---  ---  ---  ---  ---  ---  ---  ---  ...  ...
Y13426   ,TRDV2*02   ---  ---  ---  ---  ---  ---  ---  ---  ---  ---  ---  ---  ---  ---  ---  ---  ---  ---  ...  ...
                                                                      M
AE000661 ,TRDV2*03   ---  ---  ---  ---  ---  ---  ---  ---  ---  --G  ---  ---  ---  ---  ---  ---  ---  ---  ...  ...
                                                                      M
X53849   ,TRDV2*03   ---  ---  ---  ---  ---  ---  ---  ---  ---  --G  ---  ---  ---  ---  ---  ---  ---  ---  ...  ...


IMGT________________
                      61   62   63   64   65   66   67   68   69   70   71   72   73   74   75   76   77   78   79   80
                                                  I    Y    G    P    G    F    K         D    N    F    Q    G    D    I
X15207   ,TRDV2*01   ...  ...  ...  ...  ...  ATC  TAT  GGC  CCT  GGT  TTC  AAA  ...  GAC  AAT  TTC  CAA  GGT  GAC  ATT
U32548   ,TRDV2*01   ...  ...  ...  ...  ...  ---  ---  ---  ---  ---  ---  ---  ...  ---  ---  ---  ---  ---  ---  ---
Y13426   ,TRDV2*02   ...  ...  ...  ...  ...  ---  ---  ---  ---  ---  ---  ---  ...  ---  ---  ---  ---  ---  ---  ---
AE000661 ,TRDV2*03   ...  ...  ...  ...  ...  ---  ---  ---  ---  ---  ---  ---  ...  ---  ---  ---  ---  ---  ---  ---
X53849   ,TRDV2*03   ...  ...  ...  ...  ...  ---  ---  ---  ---  ---  ---  ---  ...  ---  ---  ---  ---  ---  ---  ---


                      81   82   83   84   85   86   87   88   89   90   91   92   93   94   95   96   97   98   99  100
                       D    I    A    K    N    L    A    V    L    K    I    L    A    P    S    E    R    D    E    G
X15207   ,TRDV2*01   GAT  ATT  GCA  AAG  AAC  CTG  GCT  GTA  CTT  AAG  ATA  CTT  GCA  CCA  TCA  GAG  AGA  GAT  GAA  GGG
U32548   ,TRDV2*01   ---  ---  ---  ---  ---  ---  ---  ---  ---  ---  ---
Y13426   ,TRDV2*02   ---  ---  ---  ---  ---  ---  ---  ---  ---  ---  ---  ---  ---  ---  ---  ---  ---  ---  ---  ---
AE000661 ,TRDV2*03   ---  ---  ---  ---  ---  ---  ---  ---  ---  ---  ---  ---  ---  ---  ---  ---  ---  ---  ---  ---
X53849   ,TRDV2*03   ---  ---  ---  ---  ---  ---  ---  ---  ---  ---  ---  ---  ---  ---  ---  ---  ---  ---  ---  ---


                                        ____CDR3-IMGT____
                     101  102  103  104  105  106  107  108
                       S    Y    Y    C    A    C    D    T
X15207   ,TRDV2*01   TCT  TAC  TAC  TGT  GCC  TGT  GAC  ACC
U32548   ,TRDV2*01
Y13426   ,TRDV2*02   ---  ---  ---  ---  ---  ---  ---  -
AE000661 ,TRDV2*03   ---  ---  ---  ---  ---  ---  ---  --
X53849   ,TRDV2*03   ---  ---  ---  ---  ---  ---  ---  --       #c
```

#c: Rearranged cDNA

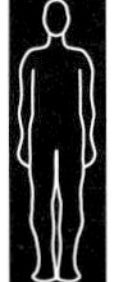

Framework and complementarity determining regions

FR1-IMGT: 26

FR2-IMGT: 17

FR3-IMGT: 38 (-1 aa: 73)

CDR1-IMGT: 8

CDR2-IMGT: 3

CDR3-IMGT: 4

Collier de Perles for human TRDV2*01

Accession number: IMGT X15207

EMBL/GenBank/DDBJ: X15207

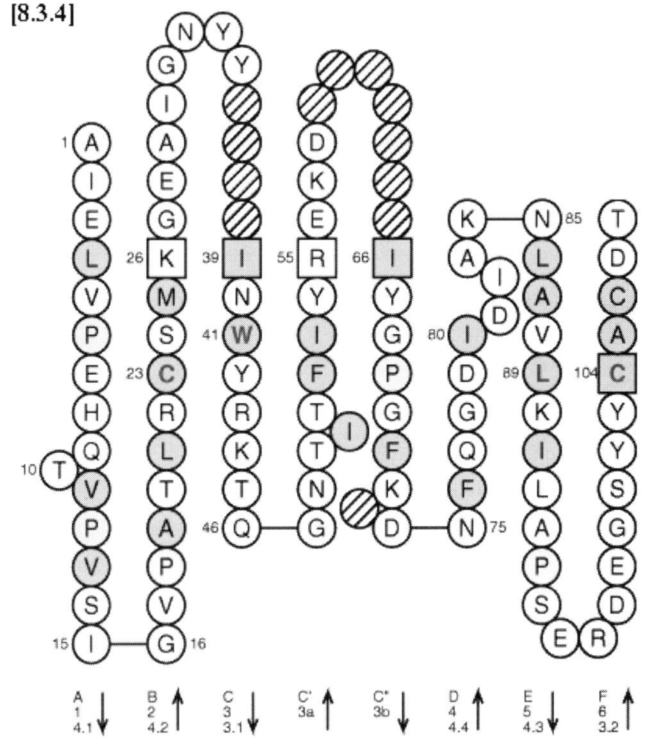

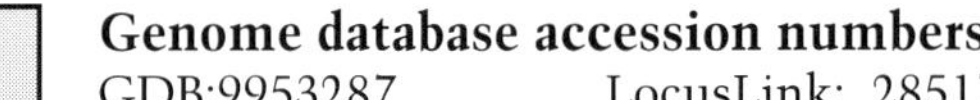

Genome database accession numbers

GDB:9953287   LocusLink: 28517

Nomenclature

TRDV3: T cell receptor delta variable 3.

Definition and functionality

TRDV3 is the unique mapped functional gene of the TRDV3 subgroup which only comprises that gene.

Gene location

TRDV3 is in the TRA/TRD locus on chromosome 14 at 14q11.2. TRDV3 is localized downstream of the TRDC gene, in inverted orientation of trancription, and rearranges by an inversion mechanism[4,6,8].

Nucleotide and amino acid sequences for human TRDV3

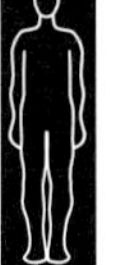

```
                        1   2   3   4   5   6   7   8   9   10  11  12  13  14  15  16  17  18  19  20
                        C   D   K   V   T   Q   S   S   P   D   Q   T   V   A   S   G   S   E   V   V
M23326    ,TRDV3*01 [6] TGT GAC AAA GTA ACC CAG AGT TCC CCG GAC CAG ACG GTG GCG AGT GGC AGT GAG GTG GTA
X13954    ,TRDV3*01 [4] --- --- --- --- --- --- --- --- --- --- --- --- --- --- --- --- --- --- --- ---
U32549    ,TRDV3*01 [1] --- --- --- --- --- --- --- --- --- --- --- --- --- --- --- --- --- --- --- ---
M94081    ,TRDV3*01 [5] --- --- --- --- --- --- --- --- --- --- --- --- --- --- --- --- --- --- --- ---
AE000661  ,TRDV3*01 [2] --- --- --- --- --- --- --- --- --- --- --- --- --- --- --- --- --- --- --- ---
X15261    ,TRDV3*02 [8] --- --- --- --- --- --- --- --- --- --- --- --- --- --- --- --- --- --- --- ---

                                                              ________________CDR1-IMGT________________
                        21  22  23  24  25  26  27  28  29  30  31  32  33  34  35  36  37  38  39  40
                        L   L   C   T   Y   D   T   V   Y   S   N   P   D                       L   F
M23326    ,TRDV3*01     CTG CTC TGC ACT TAC GAC ACT GTA TAT TCA AAT CCA GAT ... ... ... ... ... TTA TTC
X13954    ,TRDV3*01     --- --- --- --- --- --- --- --- --- --- --- --- --- ... ... ... ... ... --- ---
U32549    ,TRDV3*01     --- --- --- --- --- --- --- --- --- --- --- --- --- ... ... ... ... ... --- ---
M94081    ,TRDV3*01     --- --- --- --- --- --- --- --- --- --- --- --- --- ... ... ... ... ... --- ---
AE000661  ,TRDV3*01     --- --- --- --- --- --- --- --- --- --- --- --- --- ... ... ... ... ... --- ---
X15261    ,TRDV3*02     --- --- --- --- --- --- --- --- --- --- --- --- --- ... ... ... ... ... --- ---

                                                                                            ________CDR2-
                        41  42  43  44  45  46  47  48  49  50  51  52  53  54  55  56  57  58  59  60
                        W   Y   R   I   R   P   D   Y   S   F   Q   F   V   F   Y   G   D   N   S   R
M23326    ,TRDV3*01     TGG TAC CGG ATA AGG CCA GAT TAT TCC TTT CAG TTT GTC TTT TAT GGG GAT AAC AGC AGA
X13954    ,TRDV3*01     --- --- --- --- --- --- --- --- --- --- --- --- --- --- --- --- --- --- --- ---
U32549    ,TRDV3*01     --- --- --- --- --- --- --- --- --- --- --- --- --- --- --- --- --- --- --- ---
M94081    ,TRDV3*01     --- --- --- --- --- --- --- --- --- --- --- --- --- --- --- --- --- --- --- ---
AE000661  ,TRDV3*01     --- --- --- --- --- --- --- --- --- --- --- --- --- --- --- --- --- --- --- ---
                                    W
X15261    ,TRDV3*02     --- --- T-- --- --- --- --- --- --- --- --- --- --- --- --- --- --- --- --- ---

                        IMGT________________
                        61  62  63  64  65  66  67  68  69  70  71  72  73  74  75  76  77  78  79  80
                                                S   E   G   A   D   F   T   Q   G   R   F   S   V   K   H
M23326    ,TRDV3*01     ... ... ... ... ... TCA GAA GGT GCA GAT TTT ACT CAA GGA CGG TTT TCT GTG AAA CAC
X13954    ,TRDV3*01     ... ... ... ... ... --- --- --- --- --- --- --- --- --- --- --- --- --- --- ---
U32549    ,TRDV3*01     ... ... ... ... ... --- --- --- --- --- --- --- --- --- --- --- --- --- --- ---
M94081    ,TRDV3*01     ... ... ... ... ... --- --- --- --- --- --- --- --- --- --- --- --- --- --- ---
AE000661  ,TRDV3*01     ... ... ... ... ... --- --- --- --- --- --- --- --- --- --- --- --- --- --- ---
X15261    ,TRDV3*02     ... ... ... ... ... --- --- --- --- --- --- --- --- --- --- --- --- --- --- ---

                        81  82  83  84  85  86  87  88  89  90  91  92  93  94  95  96  97  98  99  100
                        I   L   T   Q   K   A   F   H   L   V   I   S   P   V   R   T   E   D   S   A
M23326    ,TRDV3*01     ATT CTG ACC CAG AAA GCC TTT CAC TTG GTG ATC TCT CCA GTA AGG ACT GAA GAC AGT GCC
X13954    ,TRDV3*01     --- --- --- --- --- --- --- --- --- --- --- --- --- --- --- --- --- --- --- ---
U32549    ,TRDV3*01     --- --- --- --- --- --- --- --- --- --- --- --- --- --- --- --- --- --- --- ---
M94081    ,TRDV3*01     --- --- --- --- --- --- --- --- --- --- --- --- --- --- --- --- --- --- --- ---
AE000661  ,TRDV3*01     --- --- --- --- --- --- --- --- --- --- --- --- --- --- --- --- --- --- --- ---
X15261    ,TRDV3*02     --- --- --- --- --- --- --- --- --- --- --- --- --- --- --- --- --- --- --- ---
```

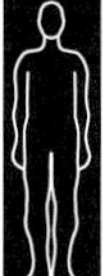

```
                                    _CDR3-IMGT_
                        101 102 103 104 105 106 107
                         T   Y   Y   C   A   F
M23326   ,TRDV3*01      ACT TAC TAC TGT GCC TTT AG
X13954   ,TRDV3*01      --- --- --- --- --- --- -
U32549   ,TRDV3*01      --- --- --- --- --- --- -
M94081   ,TRDV3*01      --- --- --- --- --- --- -
AE000661,TRDV3*01       --- --- --- --- --- --- -
X15261   ,TRDV3*02      --- --- --- --- --- --- -
```

Framework and complementarity determining regions

FR1-IMGT: 26　　　　　　　　　　CDR1-IMGT: 7
FR2-IMGT: 17　　　　　　　　　　CDR2-IMGT: 5
FR3-IMGT: 39　　　　　　　　　　CDR3-IMGT: 2

Collier de Perles for human TRDV3*01

Accession number: IMGT M23326　　EMBL/GenBank/DDBJ: M23326

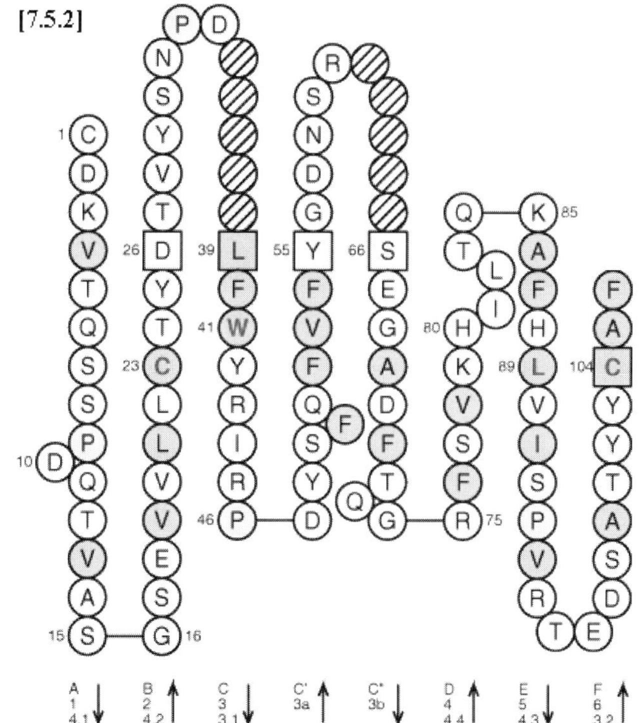

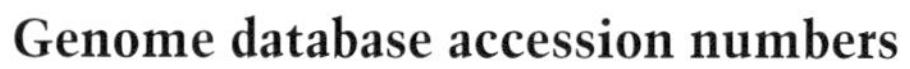

TRDV protein display

Protein display of the human TRD V-REGIONs.

*Only the *01 allele of each functional V-REGION is shown. TRDV genes are listed, for each subgroup, according to their position from 5′ to 3′ in the locus.*

```
TRDV            FR1-IMGT                 CDR1-IMGT    FR2-IMGT          CDR2-IMGT    FR3-IMGT                                CDR3-IMGT
gene            (1-26)                   (27-38)      (39-55)           (56-65)      (66-104)                                (105-115)

                1        10        20     30          40        50      60          70        80        90        100       110
                .........|.........|.....  ...|....   .|.........|....  ....|....   ....|.........|.........|.........|....  .....|....
M22198  ,TRDV1  AQKVTQAQSSVSMPVRKAVTLNCLYE TSWWSYY..... IFWYKQLPSKEMIFLIR QGS.......  DEQNAKS.GRYSVNFKKAAKSVALTISALQLEDSAKYFC ALGE.......

X15207  ,TRDV2  AIELVPEHQTVPVSIGVPATLRCSMK GEAIGNYY.... INWYRKTQGNTITFIYR EKD.......  IYGPGFK.DNFQGDIDIAKNLAVLKILAPSERDEGSYYC ACDT.......

M23326  ,TRDV3  CDKVTQSSPDQTVASGSEVVLLCTYD TVYSNPD..... LFWYRIRPDYSFQFVFY GDNSR.....  SEGADFTQGRFSVKHILTQKAFHLVISPVRTEDSATYYC AF.........
```

TRDV recombination signals and references

Recombination signals

Only the recombination signals of the allele *01 of each functional V-REGION are shown.

TRDV	V Recombination Signal (V-RS)		
gene name	V-HEPTAMER	(bp)	V-NONAMER
TRDV1*01	CACAGTG	23	ACAAAAACC
TRDV2*01	CACCCTG	23	TCAAAAACC
TRDV3*01	CACTATG	22	AACACAAAC

References
[1] Boysen, C. et al. (1996) Immunogenetics 44, 121–127.
[2] Boysen, C. et al., unpublished.
[3] Dariavach, P. and Lefranc, M.-P. (1989) Nucleic Acids Res. 17, 4880.
[4] Hata, S. et al. (1989) J. Exp. Med. 169, 41–57.
[5] Koop, B.F. et al., unpublished.
[6] Loh, E.Y. et al. (1988) Proc. Natl Acad. Sci. USA 85, 9714–9718.
[7] Satyanarayana, K. et al. (1988) Proc. Natl Acad. Sci. USA 85, 8166–8170.
[8] Takihara, Y. et al. (1989) Eur. J. Immunol. 19, 571–574.
[9] Triebel, F. et al. (1988) Eur. J. Immunol. 18, 2021–2027.
[10] Zhang, X.M. and Lefranc, M.-P. (1993) Hum. Genet. 92, 100.

TRAC, TRBC, TRGC, and TRDC protein displays

```
EX1
TRAC        (N)IQNPDPAVYQLRDSK....SSDKSVCLFTDFD.SQTNVSQSKDDVYIT.DKTVLDMRSMDF.....KSNSAVAWSNKS.........DFACANAFNN...SIIPEDTFFPSP
TRBC1       (E)DLNKVFPPEVAVFEPSEAEISHTQKATLVCLATGFFPDHVELSWWVNGKEVHSGVSTDPQPLKEQPALNDSRYCLSSRLRVSATFWQNPRNHFRCQVQFYG..LSENDEWTQDRAKPVTQIVSAEAWGRA
TRBC2       (E)DLKNVFPPEVAVFEPSEAEISHTQKATLVCLATGFYPDHVELSWWVNGKEVHSGVSTDPQPLKEQPALNDSRYCLSSRLRVSATFWQNPRNHFRCQVQFYG..LSENDEWTQDRAKPVTQIVSAEAWGRA
TRDC        (R)SQPHTKPSVFVM.....KNGTNVACLVKEFYPKDIRINLVSSKKITEFDPAIVISPS........GKYNAVKLGKYED......SNSVTCSVQHDN..KTVHSTDFEVKTDST
TRGC1       (D)KQLDADVSPKPTIFLPSIAETKLQKAGTYLCLLEKFFPDVIKIHWQEKKSNTILGSQEGNTMKTN......DTYMKFSWLTVPESL....DKEHRCIVRHEN.NKNGVQEIIFPPIKT
TRGC2(2x)   (D)KQLDADVSPKPTIFLPSIAETKLQKAGTYLCLLEKFFPDIIKIHWQEKKSNTILGSQEGNTMKTN......DTYMKFSWLTVPEESL...DKEHRCIVRHEN.NKNGIQEIIFPPIKT
TRGC2(3x)   (D)KQLDADVSPKPTIFLPSIAETKLQKAGTYLCLLEKFFPDIIKIHWQEKKSNTILGSQEGNTMKTN......DTYMKFSWLTVPEESL...DKEHRCIVRHEN.NKNGIDQEIIFPPIKT


TRAC                                                       EX2                     (E)SSCDVKLVEKSFET
TRBC1                                                      EX2                        (D)CGFTS
TRBC2                                                      EX2                        (D)CGFTS
TRDC                                                       EX2   (D)HVKPKETENTKQPSKSCHKPK
TRGC1                                                      EX2                   (D)VITMDPKDNCSKDAN
TRGC2(2x)*01  EX2T   DVTTVDPKDSYSKDAN                      EX2                   (D)VITMDPKDNWSKDAN
TRGC2(2x)*02                     EX2R   DVTTVDPKYNYSKDAN   EX2                   (D)VITMDPKDNWSKDAN
TRGC2(3x)     EX2T   DVTTVDPKDSYSKDAN   EX2R   DVTTVDPKYNYSKDAN   EX2             (D)VITMDPKDNWSKDAN


EX3
TRAC        (D)TNLNFQNLSVIGFRILLLKVAGFNLLMTLRL.........WSS
TRBC1       (V)SYQQGVLSATILYEILLGKATLYAVLVSALVLMAM     VKRKDF      EX4
TRBC2       (E)SYQQGVLSATILYEILLGKATLYAVLVSALVLMAM     VKRKDSRG   EX4
TRDC        (S)IVHTEKVNMMSLTVLGLRMLFAKTVAVNFLLTAKLFFL
TRGC1       (D)TLLLQLTNMYLLLLTSAYYLKSVVYFAIITCCLLRRTAFCCNGEKS
TRGC2(2x)   (D)TLLLQLTNTSAYYMYLLLLLKSVVYFAIITCCLLGRTAFCCNGEKS
TRGC2(3x)   (D)TLLLQLTNTSAYYMYLLLLLKSVVYFAIITCCLLGRTAFCCNGEKS
            Extracellular region | Transmembrane region |Intracytoplasmic region
```

Amino acids resulting from the splicing are shown in parentheses.
N-glycosylation sites (NXS/T, where X is different from P) are boxed.
Amino acid sequences are deduced from the alleles *01.